Healthcare Interoperability Standards Compliance Handbook

Frank Oemig · Robert Snelick

Healthcare Interoperability Standards Compliance Handbook

Conformance and Testing of Healthcare Data Exchange Standards

Springer

Frank Oemig
Deutsche Telekom Healthcare
and Security Solutions GmbH
Mülheim
Germany

Robert Snelick
National Institute of Standards
and Technology (NIST)
Gaithersburg, MD
USA

ISBN 978-3-319-44837-4 ISBN 978-3-319-44839-8 (eBook)
DOI 10.1007/978-3-319-44839-8

Library of Congress Control Number: 2016949613

Printed on acid-free paper

This Springer imprint is published by Springer Nature
The registered company is Springer International Publishing AG
The registered company address is: Gewerbestrasse 11, 6330 Cham, Switzerland

Foreword

Interoperability is essential for information to flow freely, accurately, efficiently, and securely between health information technology (HIT) systems and across healthcare networks—systems and networks that support hospitals and clinicians in the delivery of patient care. This information flow can enable the healthcare industry to achieve its goals related to preventive care, population health management, cost-effectiveness, and, that particularly elusive factor, patient safety.

Actually achieving interoperability through use of HIT has been compared, as far as the difficulty involved and the likelihood of it happening, to traveling to another planet; however, the initial building blocks needed for successfully realizing the information flow envisioned with true interoperability are identifiable today, including well-designed and clearly articulated data exchange standards and the test tools that evaluate conformance of HIT systems to those standards.

In *Healthcare Interoperability Standards Compliance Handbook: Conformance and Testing of Healthcare Data Exchange Standards*, Mr. Oemig and Mr. Snelick explain the challenges, methodologies, and mechanisms related to developing the standards and measuring the conformance of HIT systems. Having been co-chairs of the *HL7 Conformance and Guidance for Implementation/Testing Working Group* for numerous years, these authors are able to impart knowledge gleaned from real-world experience in development of conformance tools as well as from detailed discussions with clinical informatics experts in development of official standards that are in use today. With their in-depth understanding and their international perspective about the subject matter, the authors convey valuable information about the different families of data exchange standards—HL7 version 2.x, HL7 V3, and others—and about the need for an underlying system architecture and standards that provide the foundation for electronic communication of healthcare data at the national level in various countries and that also are flexible enough to allow for local adaptations and enhancements.

The format of interoperability standards documents themselves does not provide the means to disclose the details of the discussions that occur among the standards developers. In this book, however, the authors are able to give the readers insight into the topics that are discussed as well as how the conclusions included in the standards were reached.

Using the basic interoperability guidelines, the foundation for which is provided in this book, the readers should be able to participate actively in efforts toward achieving the goals of compatible and interoperable implementations when applying the standards that are discussed herein. Furthermore, as the various concepts described are independent of these standards, the interoperability guidelines can be utilized with standards other than the ones highlighted in this text.

By providing this book as a source of up-to-date information about conformance testing and the development of testable data exchange standards, the authors are facilitating the healthcare industry's progress toward achieving HIT interoperability and reaching the goal of safer and more cost-effective patient care.

Gaithersburg, Maryland, USA

Sheryl L. Taylor, BSN, RN
IT Specialist, NIST

Preface

This book is organized into three parts. Part I, *Healthcare Information Technology*, outlines the motivation for writing the book, the background for the discussions, and the foundation upon which the subsequent parts of the book are based, and establishes the context for descriptions of the included conformance, interoperability, and testing concepts. Chapter 1, *Introduction*, gives an overview of the concepts, the targeted issues, and how the concepts are interrelated. This chapter describes a complete conformance testing process lifecycle from the development of standards to the certification of products. Chapter 2, *Architecture*, describes common architectures for distributed healthcare systems. The remaining concepts of the book are discussed against the backdrop of this context. Chapter 3, *Healthcare Data Exchange Landscape,* provides an overview of the Standards Development Organizations (SDO) and Standards Profiling Enforcement Organizations (PEO). In general, SDOs create the standards and PEOs apply the standards to address various workflows. Chapter 4, *Healthcare Data Exchange Standards*, provides a survey of the most relevant standards in use for healthcare data exchange today, while giving the reader a perspective on the standards-related technologies that are available along with the means to compare and contrast them at a high level. To explain the various data exchange concepts, case studies using specific standards are presented extensively throughout this book. Although any standard could have been used in the case studies, the HL7 v2.x standard is used for the most part since it is the most widely deployed standard, and the authors have extensive experience with it.

Part II, *Conformance,* focuses on the definition and explanation of conformance concepts and techniques for unambiguously specifying requirements, including applying the concepts of profiling. In the opinion of the authors, the lack of quality standard specifications is the biggest impediment to achieving interoperability among healthcare information systems. We encourage all standards developers to employ the concepts presented in Part II. Chapter 5, *Conformance Constructs*, provides a detailed explanation of conformance concepts that are applicable in a standard-agnostic manner to most standard specifications. This explanation sets the foundation for much of the discussion in later chapters, and the reader's understanding of the information provided in this chapter is essential. Chapter 6, *Principles of Specifying Conformance*, describes how specifications should state requirements (conformance) in a general sense. This discussion includes the necessary conformance components and what they mean. A list of principles is given with explicit examples. Chapter 7, *Principles of Effective Profiling*, introduces the concept of profiling and how to use profiles effectively for managing standard specifications and for developing implementations. Chapter 8, *Profile Relationships*, gives an in-depth analysis of how profiles relate to each other in multiple dimensions (e.g., profile hierarchy and sender/receiver perspectives). A set of rules for creating and determining profile compliance and compatibility is given. Chapter 9, *Tools for Conformance Profiling*, provides a survey of the tools that help in effective application of the profiling mechanisms.

Part III, *Testing and Tools*, focuses on the concepts and techniques of conformance and interoperability testing. Principles of testing are discussed along with application of those principles via testing models, frameworks, architecture, tools, and testing programs. Parts I and II laid the foundation for a clear understanding of what conformance means, why it is necessary, and its benefits. Given that information as the background, how does anyone verify that implementers and users are applying the concepts appropriately in practice? *Testing and Tools* examines this topic by exploring the process, strategy, assessment, and instantiation of conformance and interoperability testing. A foundational chapter, Chap. 10, *Testing Models*, begins this part of the book by defining, in an abstract manner, the various testing models and describing the types of testing that can be performed within the models. Chapter 11, *Principles of Conformance Testing*, explains how to conduct conformance testing, including the creation and execution of test plans. Various types of conformance testing are examined. Chapter 12, *Conformity Assessment*, presents the assessment tables and interpretation of conformance for the conformance constructs presented in Chap. 5. The assessments provide the requirements for building validation tools to evaluate conformance. Through use of concrete examples, Chap. 13, *Testing Architectures*, provides a realization of the concepts and methodologies described in Chaps. 10 and 11. This realization includes a description of a testing infrastructure, testing framework, and an interoperability test bed. Case studies are provided to emphasize the utility of the modular approach. Chapter 14 builds upon this theme by providing a sampling of test tools created from the ideas (framework) explained in Chap. 13. Finally, Chap. 15 describes how testing programs operate and how they utilize the testing tools. An overview is given of the most prevalent testing and certification programs, such as the IHE Connect-a-thon and the ONC Health IT Certification Program that supports the CMS EHR Meaningful Use Programs.

Finally, Appendix, *Additional Healthcare Data Exchange Standards*, provides additional background information about some of the data exchange standards that are in use worldwide.

Trademarks and Disclaimer

Use of trademarks and referenced materials does not represent endorsement by these organizations for the text provided with this book. Trademark information can be found on page iii.

The information in this book was compiled with great care. However, mistakes cannot be completely ruled out. Authors assume no legal responsibility or liability of possible errors, incorrect data or the resulting consequences thereof.

All product names are used without guarantee of their unrestricted applicability and are possibly registered trademarks.

Certain commercial products or materials are identified in this book in order to explain a concept or to provide realistic examples adequately. Such identification is not intended to imply recommendation or endorsement by the National Institute of Standards and Technology, nor is it intended to imply that the products or materials identified are necessarily the best available for the purpose.

Copy-Editor

We can't thank Sheryl Taylor (NIST) enough for the detailed edits she made in multiple drafts of the book, improving the readability and content immensely.

Contributors

The section "EHR Certification and Meaningful Use Programs" in Chap. 15 was contributed by Sheryl Taylor of NIST. We are delighted that Sheryl shared her knowledge about the CMS Meaningful Use and ONC Health IT Certification Programs and the associated testing efforts. Another special thank you goes to those persons and institutions/organizations that have provided us with supportive material which we are allowed to use to underline our statements and explanations: Bernd Blobel, Kai Heitmann, Ioana Singureanu, Pete Rontey, Sheryl Taylor, Ted Klein, Friedemann Schulz von Thun, HL7 International, National Electrical Manufacturers Association (NEMA), IHE-Integrating the Healthcare Enterprise, International Standardization Organization (ISO), Deutsches Institut für Normung (DIN), ASTM, OASIS, IETF, United Nations, DVTk, Hprim Santé, Phast, ART-DECOR Experts Group, Lantana Consulting Group, Furore, Qualitätsring Medizinische Software, and finally Australian Healthcare Messaging Laboratory (AHML).

Reviewers

We would like to thank Craig Newman, who was the technical reviewer for the book. Craig provided thoughtful and detailed comments that led to many clarifications, improvements, and additional content.

We would like to thank other reviewers who also provided comments that led to many quality improvements in one or more chapters: Bernd Blobel, Peter Geibel, Ted Klein (contributed to, and reviewed various sections in vocabulary), Riki Merrick, Nathan Bunker, John Garguilo and Marek Vaçlavik.

Finally, we would like to thank those who partially reviewed specific sections for their correctness: Francois Macary/Franck Gener/Olivier Boux (InteropSante, ASIP.SANTE, Hprim Santé, PN13), Michel Rutten (Forge profile editing tool), Kai Heitmann (ART-DECOR), Reinhold Mainz (xDT standards family), Nicolas Canu (PN13), Ewout Kramer (FHIR), Liora Alschuler/Rick Geimer/Sean P. McIlvenna (Trifolia), and Andreas Schultz (EDIFACT).

HL7 Conformance Working Group

We would like to thank the members of the HL7 Conformance, Vocabulary, and Order and Observations Working Groups for the many fruitful and insightful conversations through the years that helped formulate many of the concepts and principles documented in this book.

Robert Snelick Acknowledgments

I would like to thank the numerous colleagues with whom I have worked at NIST. Many of the concepts explained in this book were generated from our projects. Caroline Rosin is the senior developer for the suite of laboratory conformance HL7 v2 testing tools. Harold Affo is the architect and senior developer of the NIST HL7 v2 testing framework. He is also the project lead and architect of the NIST Implementation Guide Authoring and Management Tool (IGAMT). Woo Jungyub is the architect and senior developer of the NIST Test Case Authoring and Management Tool (TCAMT). Sydney Henrard, Salifou Malick, and Hossam Tamri have developed and refined the validation engine over many years. Sandra Martinez is the tool analyst for the Immunization and Vital Records domains. I would like to thank Sheryl Taylor for her unyielding work ethic and for sharing her knowledge of clinical informatics as we developed the three iterations of ONC certification test procedures and test tools. Others who also contributed as tool analysts or developers include Len Gebase, Sheryl Taylor, Roch Bertucat, Nico Couzier, and Mike Indovina. NIST management, past and present, must be thanked for their forward-thinking vision in establishing the conformance testing project and for providing a first-class working environment.

I would also like to thank the NIST contractors, associates, and collaborators, of whom there are too many to name. I would especially like to thank the subject matter experts who provided domain expertise, test data, and feedback during the process of the tool development: Rob Savage, Craig Newman, Nathan Bunker, and Eric Larson (Immunization); Riki Merrick, Eric Haas, and Bob Dieterle (Laboratory); and others in the various domains. I am appreciative of the efforts of the S&I Framework Laboratory Work Group, through which many of the profiling ideas and concepts were proposed, applied, vetted, and refined. I would also like to thank my colleagues at the CDC, HL7, and IHE.

And, finally, I would like to thank my wife Donna for always being there for me and to thank my children Victoria, Austin, and Connor for their support and patience; it is finally finished!

Frank Oemig Acknowledgments

I would like to thank my mentor and long-time friend Bernd Blobel for an uncountable number of discussions in this domain. Without his outstanding support I wouldn't be in the position I am in today.

A lot of my work is supported not only by my employer, but also HL7 Germany. Here I would like to say thank you to my friends and colleagues Kai, Christof, Sylvia, Bernd (2x), Alex, Markus, Mathias, Daniel, Peter (2x), Marek, Simone, Ralf and Tarik. I am sorry if I missed anyone here.

Furthermore, I appreciate the discussions with my friends from the international and national community and would like to thank them for their patience with me. I know it is not that easy.

Another special thank you goes to Sheryl, who has done an incredible job in taking care of my English. As a non-native speaker it was a great exercise for me, and I have learned a lot.

Finally, I would like to thank my wife Anja and our children Alina and Fabian for their continuous support and encouragement, especially when I have to start a new trip to USA.

After several years of work and huge amount of intermediate versions of the individual chapters the first release of our book is ready.

Dedication

The authors would like to dedicate this book to friend and colleague Pete Rontey. Pete was a leader in establishing conformance principles and implemented those principles in his development of the highly successful messaging workbench (MWB). We recall fond memories of Pete at the HL7 working group meetings discussing conformance issues over a cold beer (or two…). This one is for you Pete!

Mülheim, Germany Frank Oemig
Gaithersburg, USA Robert Snelick

Contents

About the Authors

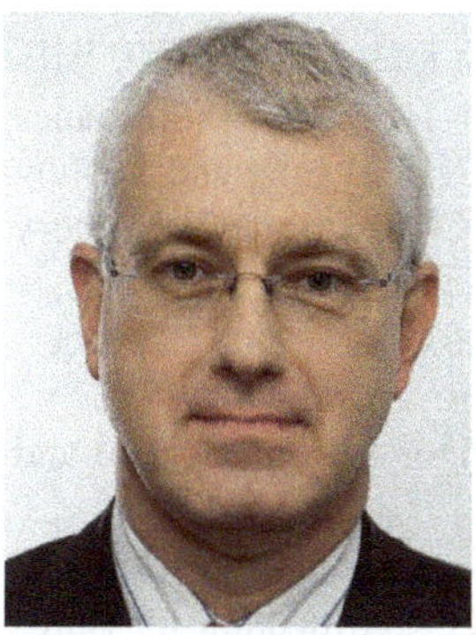

Frank Oemig, Ph.D., FHL7 has studied computer science and theoretical medicine at the Universities in Dortmund and Bochum (both located in Germany) in the mid-eighties. Although he concentrated on artificial intelligence (AI) he also worked for a software company developing programs for radiology departments, diagnosis coding and other healthcare related problems. Having said that, Mr. Oemig has been active in the healthcare domain for more than 30 years.

Immediately after finalizing his diploma thesis and leaving his first employment in a research department he started concentrating on ICT—information communication technology—in healthcare. One of his first topics was enabling a subsystem to receive patient related data. During that time (1993) he started a more intensive work with HL7 v2.1 in Germany. When joining the internal HL7 community in 1998 he became one of the first international co-chairs for the Personnel Management Work Group which he led together with Bernd Blobel till 2003. Since 2005 Frank is one of the co-chairs to the Conformance and Guidance for Implementation and Testing Work Group (CGIT, formerly known as Conformance WG).

Frank is also co-founder of IHE in Germany, initiator of HL7 Switzerland, HL7 Austria, HL7 Luxembourg and HL7 Bosnia & Herzegovina.

For more than 9 years Frank has worked for Agfa Healthcare GmbH, Bonn, Germany, a vendor company being the HIS leader in Germany. Now he is employed by Deutsche Telekom Healthcare and Security Solutions GmbH, a subsidiary of T-System International.

Using all that knowledge, Frank could intensify his engagement with HL7 by writing a Ph.D. thesis about knowledge representation in healthcare using formal ontologies. The most important result was the development of a communication standards ontology (CSO) formally allowing to bridge different communication standards like HL7 v2.x and Version 3.

Mr. Oemig has published approximately 180 of his works, including articles in journals, papers for conferences, and chapters for technical books.

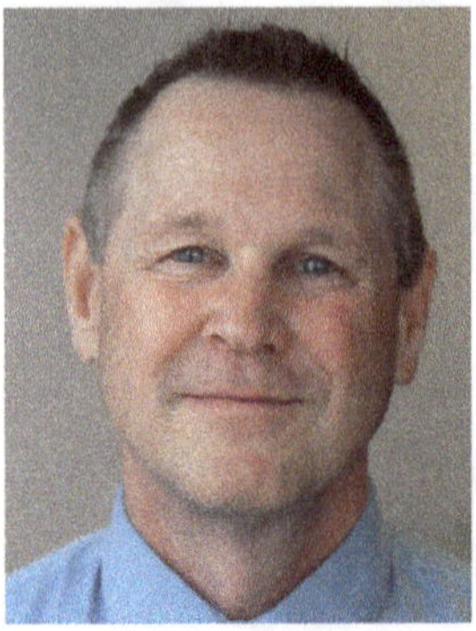

Robert Snelick, M.Sc. has a B.S. (Computer Science) from Clarion University of Pennsylvania (1986) and a M.S. (Computer Science) from the Johns Hopkins University (1991). Mr. Snelick has been employed at the National Institute of Standards and Technology (NIST) since 1986. He began working in the healthcare technology domain in 2004. Mr. Snelick is currently the project lead and chief architect for the NIST HL7 v2 Testing Framework and Tools, the Implementation Guide Authoring and Management Tool (IGAMT), and the Test Case Authoring and Management Tool (TCAMT).

Mr. Snelick is active in standards development organizations such as HL7, IHE, and ONC S&I Framework. He has served as a co-chair for HL7 Conformance working group for the past eight years, is a member of the IHE Testing and Tooling Committee, and is the S&I Framework Validation Suite Chair for the Laboratory domain. His technical focus is on improving the specification of conformance requirements and the testing of implementations for conformance and interoperability. Mr. Snelick's proposals have led to numerous improvements to the HL7 v2 conformance model and to the increased efficiency and rigor in conformance and interoperability testing.

Mr. Snelick has lead the development of the test procedures and test tools to support the ONC 2012, 2014, and 2015 Edition Health IT Certification measures that included HL7 v2 standards. He has also led tool development efforts to support testing activities at the CDC, IHE, AIRA, HL7, HITSP, and CCHIT.

Prior to working in the healthcare information technology domain, Mr. Snelick conducted research and development in performance evaluation of parallel and supercomputing, cluster computing, interactive digital television, biometrics, and multi-model biometrics methods and testing.

Mr. Snelick has published over 30 of his works, including articles in journals, papers for conferences, and chapters for technical books.

Acronyms

ACB	Authorized Certification Body
ACK	Acknowledgement
ACR	American College of Radiology
ACRNEMA	American College of Radiology—National Electrical Manufacturers Association predecessor of the DICOM standard defined by ACR and NEMA
ADT	Abrechnungsdatentransfer (xDT)—aka financial transaction ⇒ QMS
ADT	Admission, Discharge and Transfer ⇒ HL7
AHIC	American Health Information Community
AHML	Australian Healthcare Messaging Laboratory, University of Ballarat, Australia, www.ahml.com.au
AMS	Abstract Message Syntax ⇒ HL7 v2.x
ANSI	American National Standards Institute
API	Application Programming Interface
ART	Advanced Requirement tooling ⇒ ART-DECOR
ASC	Accredited Standards Committee
ASCII	American Standard Code for Information Interchange
ASIP	Agence des systèmes d'information partagés de santé ⇒ ASIP Santé
ASTM	American Society for Testing and Materials
ATL	Accredited Testing Laboratory
ATL	Archetype Type Library
B2B	Business to Business
BDT	Behandlungsdatentransfer (xDT)—aka administrative data transfer ⇒ QMS
BNF	Backus Naur Form
BOM	Byte Order Mark
BPEL	Business Process Execution Language

CCOW	Clinical Context Object Working Group ⇒ HL7
CDA	Clinical Document Architecture ⇒ HL7
CDC	Center for Disease Control and Prevention
CEHRT	Certified EHR Technology
CEN	Comité Européen de Normalisation, http://www.cen.org
CGIT	Conformance and Guidance for Implementation/Testing, an HL7 Work group, www.hl7.org
CHI	Canada Health Infoway
ClaML	Classification Markup Language ⇒ ISO
CLIA	Clinical Laboratory Improvement Amendments
CMET	Common Message Element Types ⇒ HL7 V3
CMS	Centers for Medicare and Medicaid Services
CORBA	Common Object Request Broker Architecture
CT	Computer Tomography
CTS	Common Terminology Services ⇒ HL7, OMG
CTS2	Common Terminology Services, Release 2 ⇒ HL7, OMG
D2D	Doctor-to-Doctor Communication
DECOR	Data Elements, Codes, OIDs and Rules ⇒ ART-DECOR
DICOM	Digital Imaging and COmmunication in Medicine, www.rsna.org
DIMSE	DICOM Message Service Element
DIN	Deutsches Institut für Normung, German branch of CEN
DITA	Darwin Information Typing Architecture ⇒ OASIS
D-MIM	Domain Message Information Model ⇒ HL7 V3
DMP	Dossier Médical Personnel ⇒ ASIP Santé
DQA	Data Quality Assurance
DRG	Diagnosis Related Group
DSTU	Draft Standard for Trial Use ⇒ HL7, IHE, now replaced by STU
EBCDIC	Extended Binary Coded Decimal Interchange Code
ebRIM	Electronic business Registry Information Model ⇒ OASIS
ebXML	Electronic business XML ⇒ OASIS
ECCF	Enterprise Compliance and Conformance Framework ⇒ HL7, SAIF
EDI	Electronic Data Interchange
EDIFACT	Electronic Data Interchange For Administration, Commerce and Transport
EHR	Electronic Health Record
EHR-S	Electronic Health Record System
ELR	Electronic Laboratory Reports
ER7	Encoding Rules 7, the standard encoding format for HL7 v2 messaging ⇒ HL7
ESB	Enterprise Service Bus
EU	European Union
EUP	EHR Usability Protocol, www.nist.gov

FHIR	Fast Healthcare Interoperability Resources ⇒ HL7
GCM	Generic Component Model
GDT	Gerätedatentransfer (xDT), aka of device data transfer ⇒ KBV
GELLO	An OCL-Like Common Expression Language ⇒ HL7
Gematik	"Gesellschaft für Telematik im Gesundheitswesen", http://www.gematik.de
GLIF	Guideline Interchange Format ⇒ HL7
GMSIH	Groupement pour la Modernisation du Système s'Information Hospitalier
GP	General Practitioner
H.PR.I.M.	Harmonie et Promotion de l'Information Médicale
HAPI	HL7 API, a Java-based toolkit
HDF	HL7 Development Framework ⇒ HL7
HIMSS	Healthcare Information and Management Systems Society
HIS	Hospital Information System
HISSP	Health Information System Strategic Plan
HIT	Health(care) Information Technology
HITSP	Health(care) Information Technology Standards Panel
HL7	Health Level Seven, Inc., www.hl7.org
HL7v2.6	HL7 Version 2.6 ⇒ HL7
HL7v2.7	HL7 Version 2.7 ⇒ HL7
HL7V3NE2008	HL7 Version 3 Normative Edition 2008 ⇒ HL7
HLLP	Hybrid Lower Layer Protocol
HPC	Health Professional Card
HTML	Hyper Text Markup Language
IATM	International Association for Testing and Materials
ICT	Information and Communication Technology
IE	Information Entity ⇒ DICOM
IEEE	Institute of Electrical and Electronics Engineers
IG	Implementation Guide
IHE	Integrating the Healthcare Enterprise, www.ihe.net
IHTSDO	International Health Terminology Standards Development Organization, www.ihtsdo.org
IOM	Institute of Medicine's
IP	Internet Protocol
ISO	International Standardisation Organisation, http://www.iso.org
IT	Information Technology
ITB	Interoperability Test Bed
ITI	IT-Infrastructure: IHE Domain, ⇒ IHE, www.ihe.net
ITS	Implementation Technology Specification ⇒ HL7 V3
JSON	Java Script Object Notation
KADT	Kurärztliche Abrechnungsdaten (xDT)
KBV	"Kassenärztliche Bundesvereinigung", a German institution being responsible for handling the reimbursement of general practitioners, www.kbv.de

KdÖR	www.kbv.de/html/ita.php
KH-IT	Bundesverband der Krankenhaus-IT-Leiterinnen/Leiter e.V., professional association of head of IT departments in hospitals, www.kh-it.de
KV	"Kassenärztliche Vereinigung", diverse branches of the KBV in the different German federal states
LDT	Labordatentransfer (xDT)—aka laboratory data transfer ⇒ KBV
LIS	Laboratory Information System
LOI	Laboratory Order Interface, www.healthit.gov
LOINC	Logical Observation Identifier Names and Codes, www.loinc.org, www.regenstrief.org
LRI	Laboratory Results Interface, www.healthit.gov
LTPAC	Long Term and Past Acute Care
MDF	Message Development Framework, 1999 ⇒ HL7
MDHT	Model Driven Health Tool ⇒ HL7 V3
MIF	Model Interchange Format ⇒ HL7 V3
MLLP	Minimal Lower Layer Protocol ⇒ HL7 v2
MR	Magnetic Resonance
MSH	Message Header ⇒ HL7 v2
MU	Meaningful Use ⇒ CMS
NATA	National Association of Testing Authorities
NCPDP	National Council for Prescription Drug Programs
NEMA	National Electrical Manufacturing Association, a US trade organization
NHS	National Health Service (UK)
NICTIZ	Nationaal ICT Instituut in der Zorg, www.nictiz.nl
NIST	National Institute of Standards and Technology, www.nist.gov
OASIS	Organization for the Advancement of Structured Information Standards, www.oasis-open.org
OCL	Object Constraint Language
OHT	Open Health Tools
OMG	Object Management Group, www.omg.org
ONC	Office of the National Coordinator
OSI	Open Systems Interconnection
PACS	Picture Archiving and Communication System
PAM	Patient Administration Management ⇒ IHE IT-Infrastructure
PCC	Patient Care Coordination: Domain ⇒ IHE
PCD	Patient Care Devices: Domain ⇒ IHE
PDF	Portable Document Format, http://www.pdfassociation.org
PDF/A	PDF Archive
PDO	Profile Development Organization
PDQ	Patient Demographics Query ⇒ IHE IT-Infrastructure
PET	Positron Emission Tomography

PHAST	Association Réseau Phast, L'Information de santé Standardisée, http://www.phast.fr
PIF	Patient Identity Feed ⇒ IHE ITI XDS
PIX	Patient Information Cross Referencing ⇒ IHE IT-Infrastructure
QMS	Qualitätsring Medizinische Software, www.qms-standards.de
QRPH	Quality, Research and Public Health ⇒ IHE
REST	Representational State Transfer
RIM	Reference Information Model
RM-ODP	Reference Model for Open Distributed Processing
RSNA	Radiological Society of North America, www.rsna.org
RTF	Rich Text Format
RTM	Rosetta Terminology Mapping ⇒ IHE PCD
SAEAF	Services Aware Enterprise Architecture Framework (old term ⇒ SAIF)
SAIF	Services Aware Interoperability Framework (new term ⇐ SAEAF)
SAML	Security Assertion Markup Language ⇒ OASIS
SCIPHOX	Standardized Communication in Physician Offices and Hospitals using XML, www.sciphox.de, relinked to www.hl7.de
SCP	Service Class Provider ⇒ DICOM
SCU	Service Class User ⇒ DICOM
SDA	Structured Document Architecture ⇒ HL7
SDO	Standards Developing Organisation
SFM	Service functional model
SGML	Standard Generalized Markup Language ⇒ OASIS
Snomed CT	Snomed Clinical Terms ⇒ IHTSDO
SNOMED	Systemized NOmenclature in MEDicine ⇒ IHTSDO
SOAP	Service oriented access protocol
SOP	Service Object Pair ⇒ DICOM
SPL	Structured Product Labeling
STU	Standard for Trial Use ⇒ HL7
SUT	System under test
SWF	Scheduled Workflow ⇒ IHE Radiology
TCP/IP	Transmission Control Program/Internet Protocol
TeveGe	"Telematikgesellschaft für ein vernetztes Gesundheitswesen", www.tevege.de
UCS	Universal Multiple-Octet Coded Character Set
UCUM	Unified Code for Units of Measure
UDDI	Universal Description, Discovery and Integration ⇒ OASIS
UDP/IP	User Datagram Protocol/Internet Protocol
UID	Unique Identifier
UML	Unified Modeling Language, www.omg.org
UN/EDIFACT	United Nations Electronic Data Interchange for Administration, Commerce and Transport

UNECE	United Nations Economic Commission for Europe
UNICODE	www.unicode.org
UNSM	United Nations Standards Message ⇒ UN/EDIFACT
URL	Uniform Resource Locator
UTF	Universal Multiple-Octet Coded Character Set (UCS) Transformation Format
VCS	VdAP Communication Standard—aka secure transmission protocol for GPs in Germany
VM	Value Multiplicity ⇒ DICOM
VR	Value Representation ⇒ DICOM
WHO	World Health Organisation
WoHIT	World of Health IT
XACML	eXtensible Access Control Markup Language
XDS	Cross-Enterprise Document Sharing ⇒ IHE IT-Infrastructure
xDT	“Datenträgeraustausch” of the KBV (“Kassenärztliche Bundesvereinigung”), an encoding format and a family of content standards, www.kbv.de ⇒ KBV
XML	eXtensible Markup Language, www.w3.org ⇒ W3C
XSL	XML Stylesheet Language, www.w3.org ⇒ XML
XSLT	XSL Translation, www.w3.org ⇒ XML
ZI	Zentralinstitut für die kassenärztliche Versorgung in der Bundesrepublik Deutschland (central institute for public insurances), http://www.zi.de

List of Figures

List of Tables

Part I
Healthcare Information Technology

Chapter 1
Introduction

Perhaps the biggest impediment to achieving reliable and interoperable healthcare information systems is the absence of widespread standards adoption; and not just standards, but standards that are clear and unambiguous. These standards must provide precise specifications in a language that can be universally understood and interpreted—the *language* of conformance. This *conformance language* provides the means and constructs for defining requirements and solutions exactly and consistently so that systems, products, etc. can achieve conformance that ultimately leads to interoperability. These means and constructs are embodied in the principles of conformance, the subject and focus of this book.

The importance of clear and unambiguous specifications in standards cannot be overstated. Well-defined standards, and conformance to those standards, provide the foundation for reliable, functioning, usable, and interoperable healthcare information systems. Recent federal programs (in the US) have included incentive payments for healthcare providers who adopt and "meaningfully use" certified electronic health record (EHR) technologies; however, unless these products are developed using clearly-defined standards, the adoption rate will increase, but the promise of improved quality of healthcare will not be realized. The proliferation of healthcare information systems not designed according to standards will likely exacerbate, not lessen, current patient care challenges by creating a landscape saturated with systems that are deficient in usefulness, usability, and interoperability, consequently lacking acceptance by the end-user community. Additionally, standards need to be written to meet a desired state, and not merely document the current state; however, all too often the latter has too much influence in the standard development process.

The most effective solutions include standards[1] that encompass the transport, functional requirements and interoperability aspects. If the *right* standards are prescribed and those standards are well-defined, then creation of highly useful healthcare information systems is possible without having a negative impact on

[1]Specified separately and independently.

F. Oemig and R. Snelick, *Healthcare Interoperability Standards Compliance Handbook*, DOI 10.1007/978-3-319-44839-8_1

innovation. So, with the urgent push for better systems bearing down on the community, how can we produce better quality standards? How can we enable a common understanding of a standard by all stakeholders involved? Knowing that a sound foundation saves *x-fold*[2] in effort and cost related to system development, integration, and maintenance, what will it take to put this foundation in place? Directed investment combined with knowledge and skills to develop quality standards are crucial aspects of the solution. Development of the standard and conformance to that standard are essential for success. The standard development life-cycle is an incremental process involving three key phases: (1) standard development, (2) implementation, and (3) testing. Each of these phases is necessary and each one influences the outcome of the others. It is a mistake not to invest the necessary time and resources to the entire standards development life-cycle. Taking shortcuts and rushing to meet unrealistic deadlines usually leads to the creation and implementation of poor standards. When market or regulatory forces compress timelines, appropriate resources need to be provided to meet such timelines. Skipping a phase in the life-cycle is not advisable.

Following the principles for specifying and testing standards presented in this book is one (essential) piece of the puzzle. Standards Development Organizations (SDOs), authors of standards, and (tool) developers should understand and apply these principles.

Most SDOs have long known the importance of standards specification, piloting, and testing, but many have not fully embraced the inclusion of these components into their processes. Following the guidance of the Object Management Group (OMG) [1], SDOs should publish a standard[3] only after including formal pilot testing, a reference implementation, and a conformance test tool in the standards development process. Would all stakeholders not be better off in the long run if these components were completed successfully prior to the release of a standard? The goal of this approach is not to slow progress toward the adoption of standards; on the contrary, we believe more effort, resources, and money should be placed on the development of standards. An argument can be made for shifting resources to the foundational layers, emphasizing the necessity for clarity in requirement specification, and ensuring that each standard has a precise definition of conformance constructs that are used consistently and correctly throughout the standard definitions. The specification and use of quality standards and the testing of implementations that use those standards are imperative for making progress towards out-of-the-box interoperability (or at least for reducing the amount of translation needed for integration).

---

[2]It is hard to assign a definitive value to the savings, but typical estimates found in the literature conservatively place the amount spent when issues are discovered during the operations phase at 100 times the amount spent for discovering and resolving the issues during the requirements definition phase. See the [2] study for details on the subject.

[3]Meaning the normative standard; intermediate standards for trial use (STU) are integral parts of the standard's development life-cycle.

In the absent of not adhering to the complete standards development process, what remedies can mitigate the pitfalls of subpar standards? Understanding the concepts of conformance and how to apply them is critical—education is the key. Our goal is to convey these concepts to the reader, with the intent that the principles will be used in developing standards. This knowledge will equip standards developers with the skills necessary to develop better standards in compressed timelines.

1.1 The Case for Common Understanding

A terminology is a mechanism that provides definitions of the terms used by a particular discipline or domain. In healthcare, "terminology" is commonly associated with the set of terms used by the medical domain. It is clear that a medical term like "COLD" requires a standard definition so that its meaning, whether it is a "simple cough" or "chronic obstructive lung disease", is unambiguously communicated and understood.

Analogous to the medical domain, a common definition (and understanding) of terms must be established in order to develop and interpret specifications in the technical domain. Unfortunately, in current practice having a common definition for a given term is often not the case. One prevalent example is the term "required",[4] which has a subtle difference in meaning among the various technical communication standards. As a consequence, the definition of "required" in one standard cannot be assumed to be the same in another standard. Even more troublesome is when the definition of a concept within a standard is not interpreted uniformly, as is the case with the usage indicator "RE—Required, but may be Empty"[5] usage indicator in HL7 v2.x. This misinterpretation leads directly to incorrect implementations, which contributes to data exchange problems. Preventing these types of difficulties is one of the incentives for writing this book.

One key goal of this work is to explain the terms, and more importantly the concepts they represent, that are used to write specifications (e.g., technical frameworks in IHE—Integrating the Healthcare Enterprise).

In this book, we formulate and explain concepts in an abstract manner and employ specific standard instances such as HL7 version 2.x as case studies. This book demonstrates that all of the concepts used in data exchange standards are more or less applicable to other standards; but these concepts are not used in the same way across the various standards. We will point out where and why variations exist, but will not address every instance. As an example, DICOM provides the concept

[4]Although the term "required" is quite common in various data exchange standards, the detailed semantics varies. Sometimes it includes null values, sometimes not. Sometimes it refers to the presence of real data, sometimes the presence of the element (without) data is sufficient.

[5]In general, the concept of "RE" means that an implementation must support the capability but operationally data may or may not be present. The subtleties of this concept will be explained in-depth over the course of this book.

of "optional" as a possible usage for data elements (see part 5, Sect. 7.4.5 in the DICOM standard [3]), but does not provide a robust profiling mechanism[6] as in HL7 v2.x. Instead, DICOM requires high-level conformance statements. Therefore, statements about the consideration (implementation choices) of those optional elements in implementations can also be named *implementable profiles* (i.e., *defined precisely enough to be implemented*), a term originated in HL7 v2 and not used in the DICOM world. In essence both approaches accomplish the same thing using different tactics, and it is open to debate which approach is superior.

1.1.1 The Need for Consistency

IHE[7] is an initiative established to *model* the integration of information systems that support modern healthcare organizations. Its fundamental objective is to profile existing standards for practical, use case oriented (scenario specific) interoperability of health information systems. The IHE initiative is both a process and a forum for encouraging integration efforts. It defines technical frameworks for the implementation of established (messaging/service/document based) standards to achieve specific clinical goals and provides a testing process for the implementation of their frameworks. In addition, IHE organizes educational sessions and is an exhibitor at major healthcare trade-fairs and conferences, demonstrating the benefits of the IHE frameworks and encouraging their adoption.

The approach employed in the IHE initiative is not to define new integration standards, but rather to support the use of existing standards in an integrated manner and to support the definition of configuration choices when necessary. When clarifications or extensions to existing standards are necessary, IHE submits recommendations to the relevant standards bodies. IHE initially focused on HL7 and DICOM, but potentially will include other standards appropriate to specific domains.

Unfortunately, IHE has not developed a universal technical terminology for specifying their technical frameworks [4]. Instead, it has adopted the terminology used by the underlying standard for each technical framework it has assimilated. Even within a given technical domain (e.g., HL7 v2.x), concepts are not interpreted and applied consistently. More troublesome is the fact that IHE has created conformance constructs not in alignment with the underlying standards it is using (e.g., the usage indicator "R2" for HL7 v2.x). As a consequence, the technical frameworks must be read and interpreted within the context of each standard, thus preventing a common understanding of concepts across the technical domains.

---

[6]In HL7 v2.x a methodology is provided for documenting constraints on a message. In other standards no such methodology is provided; authors are left to ad hoc solutions.

[7]IHE and other organizations most relevant to healthcare are introduced in greater depth in Chap. 3 (Healthcare Standards Landscape).

Regrettably, the same issues also exist in other SDOs and initiatives, such as HL7, CDC[8] standards for public health, and the referenced standards in the ONC[9] Healthcare Information Technology (HIT) Certification Program associated with EHR Meaningful Use (MU). Consistency in the specification of standards and their common understanding are helpful for implementers and for expediting progress towards achieving interoperable systems. This premise serves as a key theme and motivation of this book.

1.2 Information Cycle

What is the primary purpose for data exchange? Why do we need communication?

Healthcare delivery is a complex undertaking that requires healthcare professionals—and also other types of actors, such as applications, devices, etc.—to act in a cooperative fashion for the good of the patient. As a consequence, team members must interact with each other, perhaps even across enterprises. Such cooperation requires communication and the precise and timely exchange of relevant information. Historically, this exchange of information has been primarily between the involved professionals directly, but is increasingly becoming supported and facilitated by information systems.

This communication, as illustrated in Fig. 1.1, is a cyclical process; that is, it is repeated until the patient's care is completed or the intended goal is achieved. It usually starts with the exchange of observations represented as data. Transformation of these data into information requires knowledge. This knowledge,[10] and also the context of the conveyed data, must be shared a priori or communicated during the data exchange transaction to correctly interpret the data, to enable making the right decisions, and, finally, to take appropriate patient care actions[11] while avoiding endangering patient safety. Establishing an agreed upon context normally is achieved, e.g., by pre-negotiating the observation process and conditions including the communication channel, which requires that the communication partners are identified in advance. Otherwise, all relevant contexts must be sent with the exchanged data in order to ensure correct interpretation by the receiver. This method introduces the appropriate semantics so the exchanged data become usable.

---

[8]Centers for Disease Control and Prevention in the United States.

[9]Office of the National Coordinator in the United States.

[10]The knowledge an actor such as a physician must have acquired through education and experience in the medical domain in order to participate in the information cycle is a different type of knowledge than the knowledge one can derive from receiving an appropriate amount of data (which is another topic and is certainly interesting and important).

[11]An example is the simple statement of a blood pressure measurement. An interpretation of "190/120" as "normal" is only possible if the interpreter knows that the patient is cycling on an ergometer. The simple observation value is meaningless or even misleading without the accompanying context.

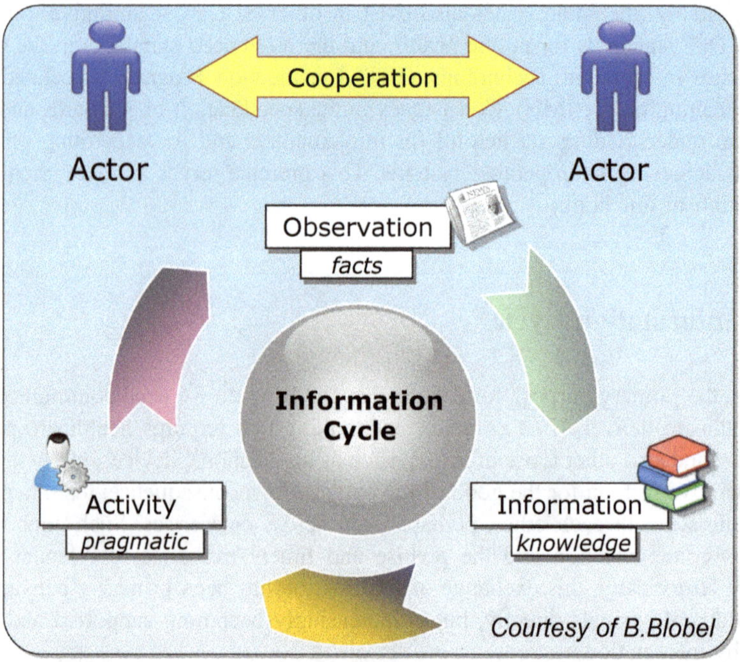

Fig. 1.1 Information cycle [5]

The interpretation of data allows for determination of additional patient care activities, which in return result in new data/information so this information cycle is continued.

1.3 Motivation for Cooperation

The communication flow in healthcare is non-trivial; it is dependent on a number of different factors as depicted in Fig. 1.2. Both the communication flow and the related factors have a direct impact on the implementation and documentation of interfaces.[12] The most obvious components of communication are the data themselves, including additional accompanying information (context or meta-data) irrespective of the particular format in which this information is sent. Usually, a message is triggered by an event, so the appeal (request) to the receiver is directly correlated with the message itself. For example, if the trigger is the admission of a patient, the appeal to the receiver is to add a new record to the database for this

[12]The term *interface* in this book refers to the software employed to exchange data between systems. Other notions of interfaces, such as a user interface, will be explicitly called out.

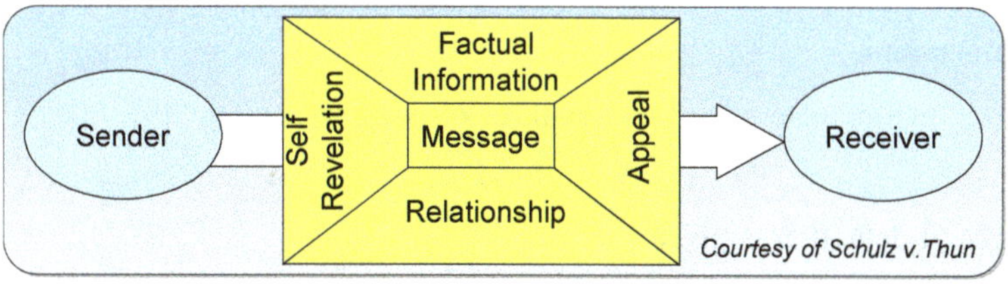

Fig. 1.2 "The four-sides of a Message" after Schulz von Thun [7, 8]

patient. Of course, in a "normal" human interaction this appeal also contains a proposition about the sender itself, which forms the relationship between the involved parties and their mutual expectations, and which can be left out of scope for computer-computer interactions [6].

The execution of communication has a goal: the triggering of a specific reaction in the receiver. To achieve this goal, different factors are necessary and must be weighed accordingly. A strong relationship among communication partners requires less data and lends itself to a well-defined appeal (request).

1.4 Definition of Key Terms and Concepts

Throughout this book, many terms and concepts will be introduced and defined. In this section, two such terms, "conformance" and "interoperability", are defined in detail. Often the definitions of given terms will have seemingly similar descriptions but with subtle differences. This issue is unavoidable; however, through applying different perspectives during analysis, the essential meanings of the concepts usually emerge and understanding is achieved. We start with conformance and interoperability since these concepts are our central theme, and we will introduce, refine, and elaborate on other terms as we proceed in this book. For some terms and concepts vagueness is tolerable, while for others exactness is a necessity. As we will see, some terms, depending on the context of their use, will have multiple meanings (e.g., compliance) or have subtle but important differences (e.g., the term *required* in HL7 v2.x versus HL7 V3).

1.4.1 Conformance

The first definition of conformance is taken from the Merriam Webster Dictionary as derived from the word conformity. Relating the term to the implementation of standards, conformance means that a system adheres to the requirements given in the standard.

Conformance

- "the fact or state of agreeing with or obeying something" [9]

A second definition is given as:

Conformance

- Conformance is defined as the fulfillment of a product, process, or service of specified requirements [10, 11].

The concept of conformance is essential for any standard to provide an objective measure of how closely implementations satisfy the requirements defined in the standard. To this end, conformance is associated with the recognition of formal testing to verify[13] adherence to the standard.

The terms compliance and conformance are often misused in practice. Compliance[14] to a standard informally indicates that the system provides support for a given standard (e.g., HL7 v2.x) or a specific version of the standard (e.g., HL7 v2.5.1). Vendors usually declare their compliance to a standard on a very high level, but a declaration at this level of granularity is not very useful for achieving interoperability. What does it take to make such a declaration truly usable? A description of refinements (e.g., constraints) to the standard (profiles), documentation of specific support, and claims of conformance are necessary for a meaningful declaration. Conformance to such documentation and claims provides the path to interoperability. How to achieve this state is explained in Chaps. 6 and 7.

1.4.2 Interoperability

Formally, two definitions of interoperability are usually cited, and both are important to include here. The first is taken from the Merriam Webster Dictionary:

[13]For a non-trivial interface, proof of conformance is unattainable even with exhaustive testing. Thus, typically a tester will declare "a system is conformant with respect to a given set of tests". Conformance testing strives to establish a degree of confidence in the conformity of a given entity based on the quantity and the quality of the tests performed.

[14]Compliance in this context has a different meaning as used in Sect. 1.9.

Interoperability

- "Ability of a system (as a weapons system) **to work with** or **use** the parts or equipment of another system." [9]

Although this definition references military systems, it conveys the correct intent by referring to more than one system and showing their specific relationship to each other. Hence, interoperability always concerns two or more systems as we will see next.

The second definition, from the IEEE Standard Computer Glossary, is the more formal and directed at information systems:

Interoperability

- "... is the ability of two or more systems or components to **exchange information** and to **use the information** that has been exchanged." [12]

The IEEE definition explicitly refers to two aspects: first of all, information must be exchanged, which refers to the functional/syntactical characteristic; but the more important part is the correct semantic interpretation allowing for use of the exchanged information.

A distinction between syntactic interoperability and semantic interoperability can be made and is given below:

Syntactic Interoperability: If two or more systems are capable of communicating and exchanging data, they are exhibiting syntactic interoperability. On this level, the systems exchanging data do not know or care about the meaning of what is exchanged [13]. No domain specific knowledge is necessary then. It allows for exchanging messages and documents without any further consideration of their contents. Syntactic conventions help to identify the data items within the exchanged data but no specific actions on the data can take place without more information. Take for example the string "20151224" which can be identified either as a number, a code (for what?) or perhaps as a date (considering the format "YYYYMMDD"), but nothing beyond that. Or, to use another example, "4548-4" represents a code, but without any other identifying information it is meaningless.

Syntactical interoperability is required for any attempts of further interoperability [12].

Semantic Interoperability: Beyond the ability of two or more computer systems to exchange information, semantic interoperability is the ability to automatically communicate information and have that information correctly interpreted by the receiving system. To achieve semantic interoperability, both sides must defer to a common information exchange reference model [12]. Continuing with the previous example of "20151224", it could be identified as the date of birth of a patient. This interpretation is a necessary precondition to store it correctly in a database or to use it meaningfully. As for the second example, when an association of the data "4548-4" is made with the LOINC[15] code system specific meaning is derived; i.e., "*Hemoglobin A1c/Hemoglobin.total in Blood*". If this code is conveyed within an order to laboratory, a receiver may initiate a specific action.

Nowadays, interoperability is frequently only achieved by negotiating data exchange interface setups; i.e., relevant information is explicitly defined and configured in the interfaces. Thus, most of the real world systems are still on a syntactical interoperability level, compared to the interoperability levels listed above (and expanded upon in Sect. 1.5), doing nothing more than exchanging special character sequences. Before proceeding to higher levels of interoperability, some essential problems must be solved. Some of these problems are caused directly by the application architecture and by a missing encapsulation of necessary transactions within the ISO/OSI stack (see Sect. 1.7).

In later chapters of this book, essential prerequisites and a strategy for overcoming these problems are explained in detail.

1.5 Interoperability Levels

Interoperability requires competence and willingness for collaboration. Interoperability depends on establishing the quality and quantity of knowledge and skills shared among the actors involved to enable intended communication and cooperation to achieve the common business objectives. This can be done a priori by education and training so that clarifying personal discussions are obsolete or at least can be performed effectively. Emergency medical technicians (EMT) demonstrate this ability when transferring patients to physicians, e.g., from an ambulance to an emergency department. EMTs summarize the status and condition of the patient including all relevant actions performed and observed outcomes. This is only possible among trained persons. Electronic data exchange has a gap between the data themselves and the necessary knowledge to process them. The shorter the communication, the bigger the gap, and thus more information and knowledge must be infused into the process to compensate for this gap. An approach to overcome this gap is to provide the missing pieces regarding quantity and quality of required knowledge and skills at runtime, i.e., during the communication and cooperation process. The system would, therefore, automatically close the gaps for the unknowledgeable or under-skilled actors to enable and complete the aforementioned information cycle, but this ability requires a higher interoperability level.

[15]Logical Observations Identifiers Names and Codes; See https://loinc.org.

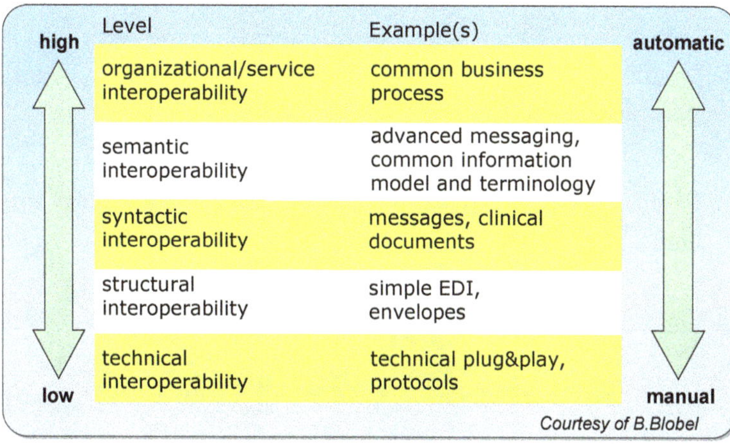

Fig. 1.3 Interoperability levels [14]

Hence, interoperability with regard to information exchange can be discussed on different levels. What counts in the end is the amount of work necessary to make the information available so it can be used. As illustrated in Fig. 1.3 and explained before, data exchange on a low technical level requires a great deal of manual intervention to establish semantic interoperability because the complete exchange is not fully defined and agreed upon; much work is still needed to configure the interfaces appropriately (i.e., because no attempts at the *higher* levels of interoperability are made).

Climbing up the levels, more and more meta-data are agreed upon that can be used to improve the communication process. This is what we mean by standardization. Nevertheless, on the highest level of communication the data themselves must be accompanied by additional information that is used to steer and control the processing of data exchange, leading to more automation. Improving the automation of data exchange requires a more sophisticated provision of meta-data so that interfaces are capable of interpreting the data without any manual interventions in the end. This state has not yet been fully achieved and remains a future challenge.

1.6 Standards Development Life-Cycle

Practical interoperability (working interoperability) can ultimately be demonstrated only in operational systems/applications. Demonstration of interoperability must be accomplished based on (more or less completely) developed interfaces,[16] because this is what is encountered in the real world.

[16]Indeed, this waterfall process model allows for repeating and updating every step, but to keep the figure simple, these aspects of the process are not made explicit.

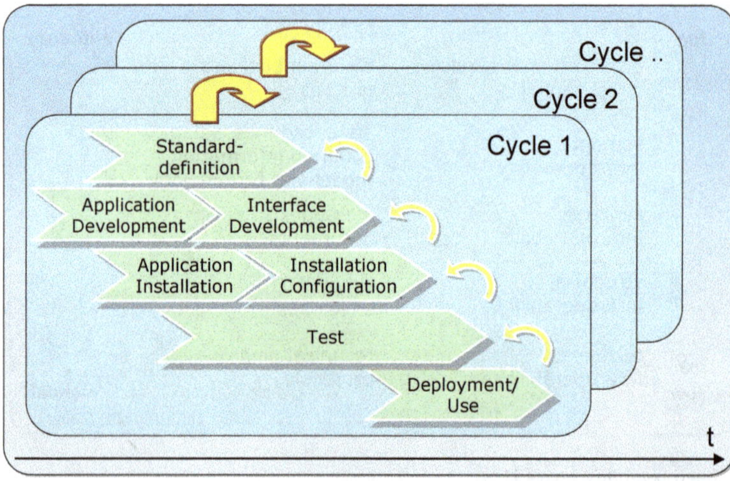

Fig. 1.4 Standards development life-cycle timeline

The typical software life-cycle models usually consist of requirements analysis, design, implementation, testing, deployment and ultimately the maintenance of software. This "typical life-cycle of software development" only considers the development of a single stand-alone application. All implementers perform this process independently from other implementers because they want to design an application that is best-suited for their customers. This independency results in a number of different applications that use different or similar approaches and architectures for the intended purpose.

The development of data exchange standards also undergoes such a life-cycle, starting with requirements analysis, design, etc. A data exchange standard tries to specify a format (and other details that are explored in this book) allowing for conveying the information needed for a specific use case. Figure 1.4 illustrates the dependencies among application development, interface development and data exchange standardization. Not surprisingly, application development starts before, and in most cases independent from, the definition of data exchange standards. The need for data exchange standards arises if different but already existing applications want to (or must) exchange data.

In a *perfect world* a complete requirements analysis is performed and a data exchange standard developed accordingly. However, this is rarely done and often is impractical, because it is difficult at the onset to definitively define the requirements and the landscape is constantly changing. Therefore, data exchange standards development is typically an incremental process. However, it is important that with each cycle the standards specify a desired state and not merely document existing practice.

As described in subsequent parts of this book, interoperable exchange of data requires that some preconditions are met within the applications, so an application may need to change its internal architecture in order to be conformant with a data exchange standard. For example, HL7 version 2.x accommodates only inpatient and outpatient visits, therefore, this simple distinction within an application is sufficient. HL7 Version 3 additionally makes use of emergency and home health visits, however, and in order to support the appropriate messages an enhancement of the application becomes necessary, perhaps resulting in a change of its internal architecture and/or vocabulary. This situation, however, can be a significant barrier to implementers, because their requirements go beyond the needs of a given interoperability specification, legacy systems and data, and support of multiple standard and non-standard interfaces. That being said, implementers should be willing to modify their application and interface and not insist on changes to standards to solely suit their needs. Additionally, any functional requirements placed on the application should be the product of analysis and collaboration between healthcare professionals (what they need and why), application implementers and developers (what the application needs to do beyond exchange data) and interoperability specialists (how to manage the needs of all parties and still be able to transfer data in a meaningful way).

As we will see, an adequate application architecture is an important prerequisite for interoperability. Specific requirements stemming from a data exchange standard can only be provided if the internal architecture is prepared and adjusted to it. In Chap. 2, we use an illustrative application to explain the impact on an interoperable data exchange. As will be shown, whatever we do may have positive and/or negative effects. The earlier and more precisely standardization is used, the more effective the activities are in aligning an application. In addition to the primary time axis, the standard used for the introduction of improvements is essential. In other words, competing or contradictory standards will not help to enforce interoperable solutions.

1.7 ISO/OSI Stack

Another important aspect related to interoperability is the so-called ISO/OSI stack (model) [15], the International Standardization Organization/Open Systems Interconnection model, which is the process of transforming and transporting information from one application to another, as illustrated in Fig. 1.5. In order to send data, an application has to collect each unit of the data in combination with its semantics and to encode it according to the rules of the underlying data exchange standard. The result is then sent to the other system, which in return has to unwrap this encapsulation and to interpret the data accordingly.

This process is explained in detail in Chaps. 2 and 5.

Most of the implemented interfaces perform all necessary steps of layers 5 ("session layer"), 6 ("syntactic:layer"), and 7 ("semantic layer") in a "single operation", that is, without clear delineation of function. The reason is the fact that the exchanged character sequence is simple. In HL7 v2.x, for example, the resulting

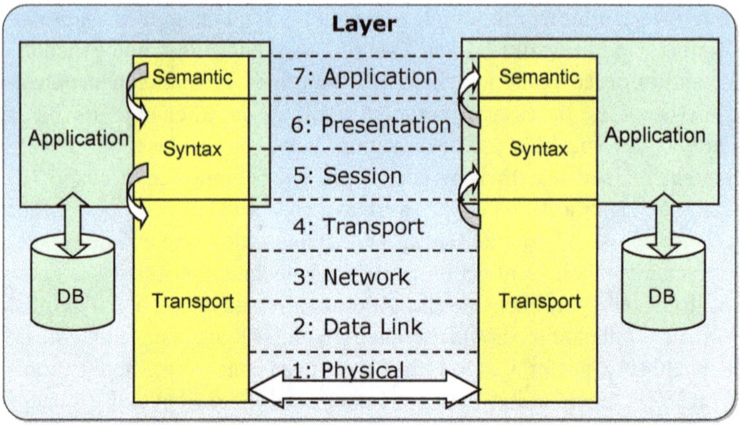

Fig. 1.5 ISO/OSI stack [15]

string has many vertical bars (field delimiters in this case), where every data element has a predefined position. (The fact that these delimiters may be subject to change is either not known or at least not considered by most of the developers.) It should be clear, however, that the encoded data (i.e., the data represented in a message) are not necessarily equal to the real data taken from a database's record set, given the separation character may change to any arbitrary printable character as with HL7 v2. If we take the standard XML encoding as another example, it is common knowledge that the character "<" must be represented by "<". Another good example is the management of different character sets, because the binary sequence to represent something may differ (the bit sequence for "ö" is not always the same). Encoding of data and an appropriate character set management are different aspects that should be handled separately when moving through the different layers of the ISO/OSI stack. Further details on this topic can be found in the "Encoding" section in Chap. 5.

Clinical data are highly structured and analogous to a tree with a lot of crotches, branches and leaves. For data exchange, this structure must be preserved by serializing and representing it in a way that can be deterministically reversed on the receiving side. A valid implementation should be agnostic to the data themselves; in other words, specific characters within the data should not prohibit a correct understanding on the receiving side.

A significant number of problems encountered at installation sites have their origin in how the different layers are managed within an interface. A relevant conformance aspect for an interface and a necessary precondition for interoperability is the correct realization of those layers.

1.8 Reference Model for Open Distributed Processing (RM-ODP)

As previously shown in Fig. 1.4, the creation of interfaces is a multi-step process that can be aligned with various viewpoints in the reference model for open distributed processing (RM-ODP), as illustrated in Fig. 1.6. RM-ODP can be applied to any communication among different systems. Hence, it also fits and helps in explaining human to human communication.

The first aspect of the model shows the purpose, scope and policies of a system that are identified as the "Enterprise View". The data, structure and content associated with the business processes are then described in the "Information View". The "Computational View" represents how the data are used for computation and their functional decomposition. The "Engineering View" expresses how the relevant components are deployed. (The latter two are less important for the standardization process.) Up to the final viewpoint, the different aspects are modeled platform independently. So, the "Technology Viewpoint" establishes a platform-dependent and technology-specific binding allowing for real implementations. For example, at this point a specific technology such as XML could come into play.

It is good practice to follow the RM-ODP when designing interoperability standards by working through this model left-to-right (as illustrated) and thus providing a solid technology-based specification.

Notably, a continuous and consistent development process can work only if the granularity of the managed artifacts in the different viewpoints is on the same level. In other words, the data must be formalized with an equivalent level of detail so they match the descriptions of the business processes.

Furthermore, different topics (i.e., domains) must not be mixed together. The generic component model, shown in Fig. 1.7, takes into account the consideration of different domains and their relationships, but also different granularity levels of the components.

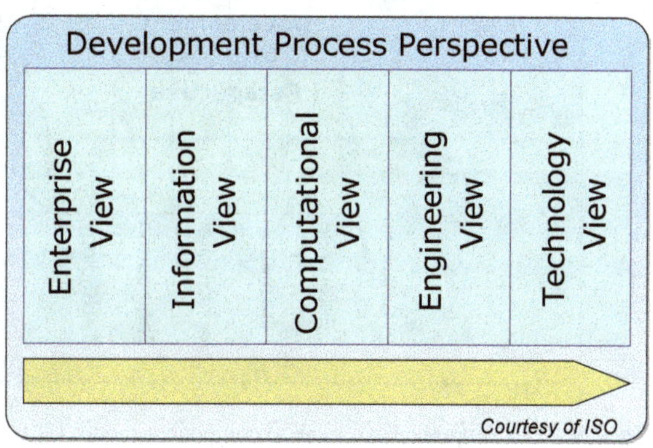

Fig. 1.6 RM-ODP (Simplified and Enhanced, [16])

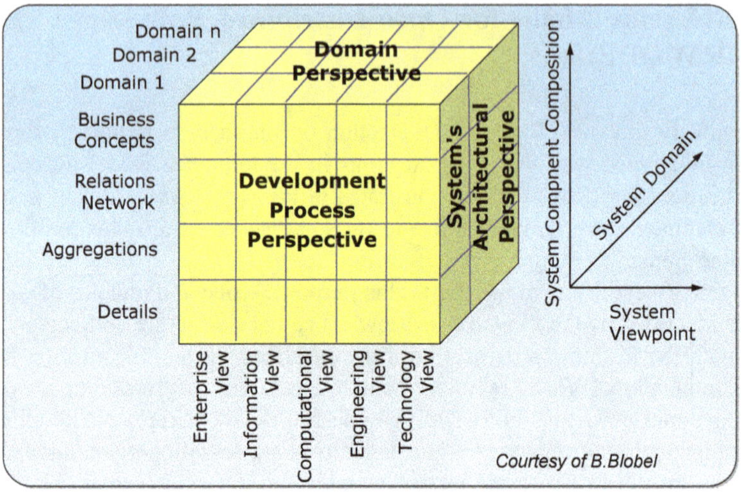

Fig. 1.7 The (comprehensive) generic component model [17, 18, 19, 20, 21]

The generic component model (GCM), shown in Fig. 1.7, adds two additional dimensions to the concepts of the RM-ODP viewpoints. On one axis, this model addresses the separation of domains. Quite often, the requirements coming from different (content) domains are mixed with each other in the presentation. A clear separation of these domains helps one understand the differences, especially when the same terms are used in multiple domains. A good example is the term "case", which has an entirely different meaning when applied in the administrative domain

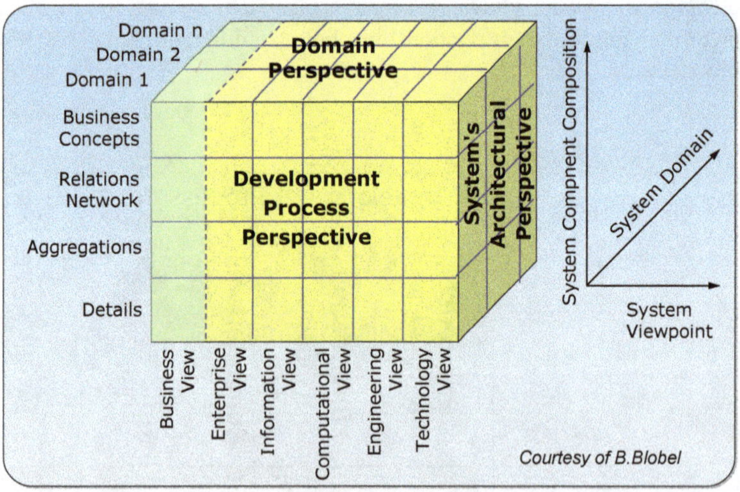

Fig. 1.8 The comprehensive generic component model [22]

compared to its use in a billing context. On the other axis, the granularity of the artifacts is taken into account. These elements are shown decomposed so their alignment becomes easier to see [21].

Here we should keep in mind that the RM-ODP and its inclusion into the GCM, as shown in Fig. 1.7, are limited to the scope of the Information and Communication Technology (ICT). The ICT world should not be realized as art for art's sake but should support real world processes, which have to be derived from real world scenarios usually described by domain experts using their domain-specific terminologies/ontologies as well as methodologies. Therefore, the complete GCM also representing the real world (business) view point looks like Fig. 1.8.

1.9 Concept Relationships

Applying the models mentioned above allows for a deeper analysis of the terms "compliance", "conformance", "compatibility", and "interoperability"(see Fig. 1.9). A more detailed examination of the terms and their implications in healthcare information systems will follow in subsequent chapters of this book.

To the point, "compliance" is the degree to which a derived specification[17] adheres to the requirements defined in the foundational specification (standard); in other words, are the rules for adding constraints faithfully followed? "Conformance" is the same in principle, but it applies to an implementation; that is, does the software implement the requirements as stated in the specification? The term "Compatibility" declares whether two specifications define sets of requirements that are harmonized with each other, allowing systems that implement them

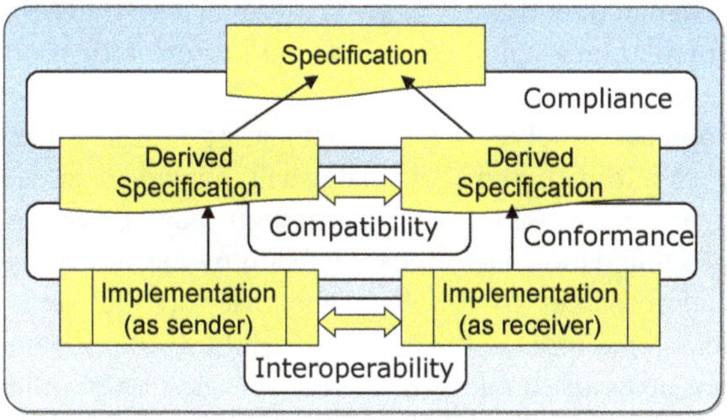

Fig. 1.9 Specification and implementation relationships

[17]We use the term "derived specification" to denote a technical documentation that is based on another technical document or set of technical documents. Often the derived specification places constraints on the base specification.

to *work* together, i.e., interoperate. Having said the above, two implementations are declared as interoperable if they can *use* the information they exchange with each other. As such, in theory, compatibility is a prerequisite for interoperability.[18]

It is clear that these terms are related, but orthogonal; no conclusion about the assessment of one can be used to deduce *definitive* information about another.[19] For example, two implementations may be interoperable and able to exchange data and *understand* the exchanged data even though neither is conformant to a given specification. The opposite of this case is that two implementations will not interoperate even if they are said to be *conformant.*[20] Both conditions are common in practice and are a source of confusion, exhaustive discussion, and unfulfilled expectations.

1.10 Approaches to Standards Development

When developing a data exchange standard, the general design approach is to create a framework of concepts and data elements that address a set of targeted use cases. This framework establishes the scope, presents the set of implementation choices, and provides a foundation that is expected to be constrained and/or extended (i.e., details are added) to meet the needs of specific domains. The creators of the standard determine what is to be included in the initial set of concepts and data elements, and this set can grow over time to include additional or expanded use cases. Elements that are not included in the set, but are needed for a use case, are manifested as extensions. In addition, elements that comprise the set can be constrained or excluded for a particular use. As such, a continuum emerges that delineates the degree to which these two methods are applied to standards development; on one end of the spectrum a comprehensive framework is developed, while on the other end only an essential core framework is provided. Although both approaches employ constraints and extensions, the former relies heavily on constraints while the latter approach relies more on extensions. The constraint favored approach involves the development of extensive data element definitions or reference information models that usually include extraneous concepts not necessary for a given use case (e.g., some elements may be very specific to a realm). This results in a foundational specification that provides broad support but takes significant time and resources to develop. The extension favored approach provides what are thought to be essential or core capabilities, and it requires significantly less time and resources to develop; however, the addition of non-core capabilities and locally

[18]Often systems will implement to the same specification, and in such cases compatibility is not of concern.

[19]Even in the case of compatibility and interoperability, it can't be assumed that the system implemented the specification correctly.

[20]Conformance is not a concept that can be proven except for the most simplistic specifications; see Chap. 11 for an in-depth discussion on this topic.

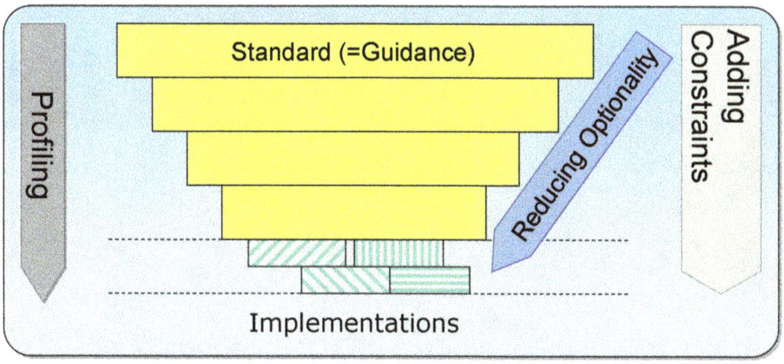

Fig. 1.10 Constraint favored approach

defined elements depends on extensions that have to be managed outside the bounds of the standard. Both approaches have advantages and disadvantages.

As illustrated previously in Fig. 1.9, to facilitate various implementations to interoperate it is advantageous that each one be developed based on a standard specification. For this purpose, a base specification is created that is the foundation for all derivations and specializations, and this foundation should cover all circumstances that the applications may have to support. As a consequence, this comprehensive foundational specification contains significantly more details than would seem to be necessary, and this constraint favored framework results in a considerable number of optional elements.

By further defining the details associated with these optional elements e.g., making them required (or mandatory[21]) or not permitting them, the original available optionality is eliminated, or at least reduced. Such a refinement is called "adding constraints". The allowable scope within which each developer may build their application is reduced by these constraints, hopefully resulting in overlapping implementations (Fig. 1.10). This overlap is illustrated above to enable visualization of the compatibility among implementations. The process of constraining a foundation standard (framework) is called profiling. Chapter 7 addresses this topic in detail.

As mentioned previously, reaching agreement on a constraint favored common specification consumes significant time and resources, because element definitions that are necessary for the scope of more use cases must be formulated and negotiated than are necessary for just one specific use case. The contrasting approach, extension favored, accelerates specification, because only core element definitions are specified. The Extension Favored Approach is depicted in Fig. 1.11.

---

[21]The terms "required" and "mandatory" are used in most of the standards, but not always with the same meaning. The differences are explained in chapters that follow. An overview of different standards is provided in Chap. 4.

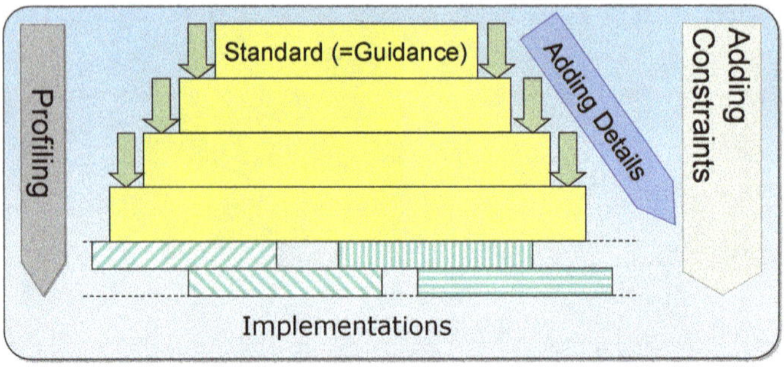

Fig. 1.11 Extension favored approach

Of course, this approach does not cover all use cases fully nor provide the details for all implementers. Adding those details is left to the individual implementations through the means of extensions, which is illustrated by the small olive arrows in Fig. 1.11. Consequently, with the extension approach the overlap of compatibility is much smaller while covering a broader spectrum of details than the constraint favored approach covers. Note, if some base requirements are specified, they still must be constrained in derived specifications (same as in the constraint favored approach).

Both approaches are valid, but the advantages and disadvantages of each one must be weighed. The time invested in developing a more detailed specification up front pays off through providing better guidance for implementers, whereas the time saved in developing a simpler specification requires investment of a significant amount of effort for defining customized extensions later on.

HL7 v2.x, with over 2500 data elements defined, and HL7 V3, with a comprehensive reference information model (the RIM), correlate more closely with the constraint favored approach, while FHIR (Fast Healthcare Interoperability Resources) as a general rule of thumb relies on extensions to address non-core capabilities and edge cases.

1.11 Testing

Conformance testing and interoperability testing are critical aspects of developing a *quality* standard, but they often are overlooked in the standards development life-cycle process. SDOs understand the importance of standards specification, piloting, and testing, and yet they fail to include these aspects into their processes. There are clear benefits for requiring pilots, reference implementations, and conformance test tools as part of the standards development process, and not publishing the (normative) standard[22] until these steps are successfully completed.

[22]Meaning the final normative standard; certainly draft standards are necessary as part of the standards development life-cycle.

Unfortunately, often there are strong barriers that inhibit this approach, including lack of resources for all parties involved and competing priorities. Part 3 of this book describes the concepts of conformance and interoperability, and how testing is critical to the standards development life-cycle discussed earlier.

An important principle in standards development is to integrate testing early in the process in order for feedback to be provided to the authors of the standard. Conformance testing is a process that determines if an entity (message, document, application, system, etc.) adheres to the requirements stated in a specification. Practically speaking, conformance (of non-trivial objects) cannot be proven. Only non-conformance can be determined, because the test space needed for proving conformance typically is so large and the number of tests so numerous[23] as to be unattainable[24]; and proving that all needed tests have been created (and performed) would be extremely difficult. In addition, there is no certainty that the created tests are correct. Therefore, conformance testing strives to establish a degree of confidence in the conformity of a given entity based on the quantity and the quality of the tests performed.

Interoperability testing assesses whether applications (or software systems) can communicate with one another effectively and correctly, and whether they can provide the expected services in accordance with defined requirements. Such testing is critical, since many modern system architectures are designed as distributed systems and rely on seamless operation. The levels of interoperability testing include transport, syntax and data format compatibility, encoding mechanisms, and a common understanding and use of the data exchanged (semantic). Chapter 11 elaborates on these subjects.

As previously mentioned, conformance and testing have a close relationship, in that testing is a method that can determine conformance. Conformance tests and tools are naturally essential to the process. Chapter 14 provides a sampling of conformance and interoperability test tools, such as those developed by the National Institute of Standards and Technology (NIST) and that are used in the ONC HIT certification program for EHR Meaningful Use [23, 24]. Chapter 11 describes the methods testers employ to assess applications/systems for conformance.

1.12 Scope and Purpose

This book explains the technical terms in sufficient depth on an abstract level to enable the reader to understand the underlying technical concepts and their differences. Given this knowledge, such concepts can be compared and relationships

[23]The different conformance constructs span a multi-dimensional test space where each point within must be tested individually, which is practically impossible.

[24]Automated test generation can help; however, in the opinion of the authors, this technology has not been proven to be reliable and comprehensive beyond a limited set of trials.

can be drawn. Therefore, our approach in this book is to explain each concept individually and independently.

Some standards are explained at a high level, and the addressed concepts are examined within the context of each standard. Table 1.1 lists selected standards, which are used to illustrate that all standards have certain commonalities, as is explained in Chap. 5.

This book uses HL7 v2.x extensively for discussion points and examples. Two factors contribute to this bias. HL7 v2.x is the most widely used healthcare data exchange standard and therefore is the most applicable to the intended audience. Additionally, the authors have extensive experience with HL7 v2.x and have contributed significantly to the standard, built and deployed production interfaces, and designed and built conformance and interoperability test tools used in various testing programs, including those in the US for the ONC HIT Certification Program. That being said, many of the principles described apply equally to other healthcare data exchange standards and data exchange standards in general.

Vocabulary standards are used extensively in data exchange standards. The principles, purpose, and use of vocabulary standards are explained in this book, however, the details of the vocabulary standards themselves are not included. Table 1.2 lists some of the most widely used vocabularies along with links to Web sites where more details and explanations about them can be found.

Table 1.1 Covered communication standards

Standard	Country	Standards body
ASTM	USA	ASTM
ClaML	International	ISO
CTS2	International	HL7
DICOM	International	RSNA
EDIFACT	Europe	CEN
FHIR	International	HL7
HL7 Version 2.x	International	HL7
HL7 Version 3, CDA	International	HL7
H.PR.I.M.	France	Interop Santé
PN13	France	PHAST
SCRIPT	USA	NCPDP
xDT	Germany	KBV

Table 1.2 Widely-used vocabulary standards

Standard	Content/domain	Standards body	Link
LOINC	Originally laboratory, later expanded	Regenstrief Institute	www.loinc.org
ICD	International classification of diseases	WHO	www.who.org
ICF	International classification of functioning, disability and health	WHO	www.who.org
UCUM	Unit of measurements	Regenstrief Instititue	www.regenstrief.org
NANDA	Nursing	NANDA International, Inc.	www.nanda.org
NDC	National drug codes in the US	Food and Drug Administration (FDA)	www.fda.gov
SNOMED CT	Clinical terms	IHTSDO	www.ihtsdo.org
CCC System	Nursing/patient care	SabaCare Inc.	www.sabacare.com

1.13 Commonly Used Terms and Definitions

One issue common across the data exchange standards landscape is that there is no one, authoritative set of terms and definitions. The definitions for the existing terms are not universally accepted, so the terms are used inconsistently within and across SDO deliberations or documents. Throughout this book terms and concepts will be defined by the authors and related to the corresponding terms in the various standards. To help the reader understand the discussions that follow, an introduction to the use of the terms is provided here. The terms and definitions presented are not uniformly agreed upon within the healthcare interoperability community, and other terms may be equally appropriate and used in various other writings.

Figure 1.12 provides an assortment of terms and various relationships for which they might be used. Note, this diagram is not intended to represent any real entity and shows a mixture of architecture and specification, but it provides a "map" for certain terms. An **Application** is software that runs on a computer and that is designed to provide specific functions for an end-user. A **Developer** is one who creates the application by means of software development. An **Installation**[25] is an instantiation of an application at a site. An **Implementer** is one who does this instantiation (e.g., an EHR vendor). An application may consist of one or more actors (note, only one is shown in the diagram). An **Actor** has a specific role, performs a specific function, and is defined in an abstract manner. The functions to

[25]Implementation is also a suitable term; however, a narrower focus is sought here.

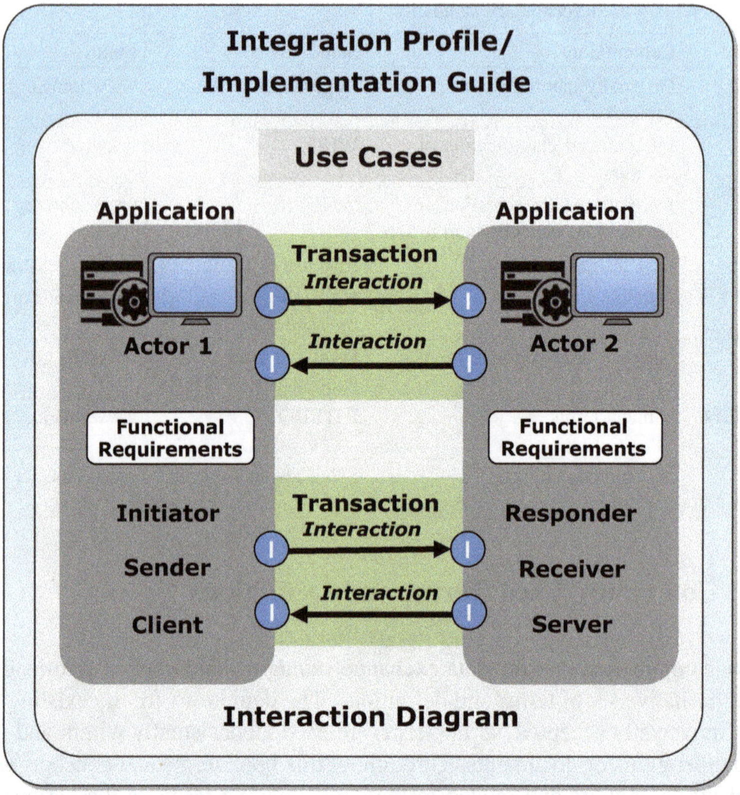

Fig. 1.12 Representative "Map" of architecture and specification

be performed by an actor or application are defined by the **Functional Requirements**—a specification of desired capabilities. An application or actor can be an initiator or a responder. An **Initiator** is an entity that starts an action and is also referred to as a **Sender** or **Client**. A **Responder** is an entity that is reacting to the action of the Initiator. A responder is also referred to as a **Receiver** or **Server**. An **Interface** (denoted as ) is a mechanism (like a socket or port) by which data are imported and exported (i.e., exchanged) between two applications. An interface normally only refers to either a sending or receiving application, but in order to exchange data both end points are needed. A single exchange of data between the two applications is referred to as an **Interaction**. A **Transaction** is an exchange of data (usually roundtrip) between two applications consisting of one, two (typical), or more interactions. A **Use Case** describes a real-world scenario that defines the actors' roles and actions along with the associated interactions and transactions. An **Interaction Diagram** is a graphical representation of the use case expressing the interaction between the actors.

An **Implementation Guide** is a document that specifies the use cases and the requirements that must be supported to satisfy the use cases using a specific standard. An alternative term for implementation guide, and one that is used in IHE, is **Integration Profile**. An implementation guide may or may not include detailed functional requirements for the actors.

Specification, standard, and implementation guide are some of the terms used to describe documents that define implementation requirements for a specific purpose. Depending on the context, one term may be used instead of another. Most often the differences between these terms are subtle, but there are important distinctions. **Specification** is a very generic name for a requirements document. **Standard** is used when referring to a base requirements document (e.g., the HL7 V3 Standard). Standard is also referred to as a **Base Standard**, especially in the context of profiling. Implementation Guide (or Integration Profile) is used when referring to a targeted use case requirements document.

A **Conformance Profile** (or **Profile**) is a set of constraints applied to a base standard that describes the requirements for a single interaction of a use case. An Integration Profile (Implementation Guide) organizes the collection of profiles to address the use case. In Fig. 1.12, a profile is defined for each interaction. For example, in the case of an immunization transaction, one profile is created for the send immunization event interaction and another profile is created for the acknowledgement. Profiling is hierarchical in nature; a specification that is created by constraining another specification is called a **Derived Specification**. Likewise, a profile that is created by constraining another profile is called a **Derived Profile**. The profiling mechanism has to follow certain rules in order to avoid logical conflicts.

An **Interoperability Solution** is a set of specifications that identifies requirements for a workflow scenario targeting specific use cases. The specifications can include transport, interoperability, and functional aspects. A **Transport Specification** stipulates the transport protocol requirements, such as SOAP based on a particular WSDL. An **Interoperability Specification** defines the data exchange requirements at the upper layers in the OSI/ISO stack. A **Functional Requirements** specification defines the desired capabilities of an application. Typically, the specifications are defined independently, because different applications could employ a different transport or data exchange specification for their solution.

1.14 Intended Audience

The intended audience of this book is:

- Technical staff of vendors participating in the standardization process or profiling initiatives,
- Information technology departments of healthcare institutions,

- Experts involved in standards development,
- Informatics professionals who design conformance testing tools,
- Informatics professionals who perform conformance testing,
- Anyone interested in the technical aspects of integrating healthcare information systems,
- University students studying healthcare information technology,
- Providers seeking a better understanding of conformance, interoperability, and certification processes,
- and last, but not least, implementers and developers.

1.15 Keywords for Use

The key words "MUST", "MUST NOT", "REQUIRED", "SHALL", "SHALL NOT", "SHOULD", "SHOULD NOT", "RECOMMENDED", "MAY", and "OPTIONAL" in this book are to be interpreted as described in RFC 2119 [25]. Expanded definitions of these key words and descriptions of how they should be used in the specification of standards are provided in Chap. 6.

1.16 Summary

This chapter provides the foundation for discussing interoperability between systems that are communicating via interfaces. The case is made for the need for information exchange and for the reaction that should be triggered in the receiver. A successful communication will occur only if the involved parties have a mutual interest in the exchange of data. The exchange of patient care data is driven by the need to improve the quality and efficiency in providing healthcare services to patients, however the desire for financial compensation is always present.

Whatever the motivation, data exchange among a set of participants will benefit from specifications in order for implementations to work together. An argument is made that the development and use of quality standards are imperative for making progress towards *out-of-the-box* interoperability (or at least for reducing the amount of translation needed). Important advances towards reaching this goal can be made but probably are unattainable for complex standards; however, whatever advances are made could reduce the effort involved in trading-partner negotiations, which could make implementations easier and reduce the cost of realizing interoperability. To achieve quality standards, the complete standards development life-cycle needs to be followed faithfully. *Standards need to be written to meet a desired state, and not merely document the current state.* Furthermore, standards must be unambiguous and specific to a targeted use case as a prerequisite to interoperability.

This chapter emphasizes the importance of defining key terms and promoting the understanding of those terms such that stakeholders can converse with each other effectively. Lack of this understanding has precipitated exhaustive debates during standards and application development discussions. Providing the reader with a clear explanation of the terms and concepts, how they are used in context, and relevant case studies based on the authors' experiences are central objectives for this book.

References

1. Object Management Group. http://www.omg.org/
2. Stecklein, J, et al.: Error Cost Escalation Through the Project Life Cycle, International Council on Systems Engineering (INCOSE) Foundation14th Annual International Symposium; 19-24 Jun. 2004; Toulouse; France, http://ntrs.nasa.gov/search.jsp?R=20100036670, June 2004.
3. Digital Imaging and COmmunication in Medicine. The DICOM Standard 2013. http://medical.nema.org/standard.html, last accessed June 18th, 2014.
4. Oemig F. IHE internal technical terminology, v0.6. http://www.ihe.net, http://groups.google.com/group/iheterminology/attach/7804505ee72e6ed9/IHE+Terminology+v07.zip?hl=en&part=2, last accessed Feb. 14 2010. http://www.hl7.org/documentcenter/public/wg/ictc/IHE%20Terminology%20v06.zip, last accessed Feb. 14 2014.
5. Blobel B. Educational Challenge of Health Information Systems Interoperability. Methods Inf Med 2007, 46, S. 52-56.
6. Oemig F, Platter W: Semantische Interoperabilitat - Kommunikation im Gesundheitswesen, in Proceedings "Prozessoptimierung, eHealth und Vernetzung im Gesundheitswesen", Jahrbuch Gesundheitswirtschaft 2007, 5.Dez. 2006, Berlin, S.162ff, ISBN: 3-932661-57-5
7. Schulz von Thun, F. Kommunikationsquadrat. http://www.schulz-von-thun.de/mod-komquad.html, last accessed April 22, 2008.
8. Schulz von Thun, F. Four-Sides Model. http://en.wikipedia.org/wiki/Four_sides_model, last accessed June 18th, 2014.
9. Merriam Webster Dictionary, derived on the term Conformity. http://www.merriam-webster.com/dictionary/, 1970.
10. ISO Reference - ISO/IEC 17000 Conformity assessment - Vocabulary and general principles, first edition 2004-11-02.
11. Glossary of Conformance Terminology, Interoperability and Conformance Technical Committee, OASIS. http://www.oasis-open.org/committees/ioc/glossary.htm
12. Institute of Electrical and Electronics Engineers. IEEE Standard Computer Dictionary: A Compilation of IEEE Standard Computer Glossaries. New York, NY: 1990.
13. Benson T. Principles of Health Interoperability HL7 and SNOMED. Health Informatics Series, Springer-Verlag, London Limited 2010.
14. Blobel B. Introduction into Advanced eHealth - The Personal Health Challenge. In: Blobel B, Pharow P, Nerlich M (Edrs.): eHealth: Combining Health Telematics, Telemedicine, Biomedical Engineering and Bio-informatics to the Edge - Global Experts Summit Textbook, pp. 3-14. Series "Studies in Health Technology and Informatics", 2007, Vol. 134. IOS Press, Amsterdam, Berlin, New York, Tokyo. ISBN-978-1-58603-835-9.
15. DIN ISO 7498. Informationsverarbeitung Kommunikation Offener Systeme, Basis-Referenzmodell. DIN EN ISO 7498-1 ISO/OSI-Modell, Beuth Verlag, 1982.
16. International Organization for Standardization (1996) ISO/IEC 10746 - 2. Information technology - Reference Model for Open Distributed Processing: Foundations. Geneva.

ISO/IEC IS 10746 / ITU-T x.901, ISO/IEC IS 10746/ITU-T x.901, http://www.rm-odp.net, last accessed 17.3.09.
17. Blobel B: Assessment of Middleware Concepts Using a Generic Component Model. Proceedings of the Conference "Toward An Electronic Health Record Europe '97", 1997, pp. 221-228. London.
18. Blobel B: Application of the Component Paradigm for Analysis and Design of Advanced Health System Architectures, International Journal of Medical Informatics 2000, 60, 3: pp. 281-301.
19. Blobel B. Analysis and Evaluation of EHR Approaches. Methods Inf Med 2009; 48, 2: pp 162-169.
20. Blobel B, Oemig F. Ontology-driven health information systems architectures. In: Adlassnig K-P, Blobel B, Mantas J, Masic I (Edrs.) Medical Informatics in a United and Healthy Europe - Proceedings of MIE 2009, pp 195-199. Series Studies in Health Technology and Informatics, Vol. 150. IOS Press, Amsterdam, Berlin, Oxford, Tokyo, Washington, IOS Press, ISBN: 978-1-60750-044-5.
21. Blobel B. Architectural approach to eHealth for enabling paradigm changes in health. Methods Inf Med 2010; 49, 2: 123-134.
22. Blobel B, Goossen W, Brochhausen M. Clinical modeling - A critical analysis. Int J Med Inform 2014; 83, 1: 57-69.
23. Snelick R, Taylor S. Understanding Meaningful Use with a Focus on Testing the HL7 V2 Messaging Standards. HL7 May 2013 Newsletter. http://www.hl7.org/documentcenter/public_temp_46CE1189-1C23-BA17-0C847B8B1C5ED33F/newsletters/HL7_NEWS_20130506.pdf.
24. National Institute of Standards and Technology (NIST) Meaningful Use Tools Portal. http://healthcare.nist.gov/NIST-TOOLS/MU/index.html
25. Network Working Group. Key words for use in RFCs to Indicate Requirement Levels. March 1997. http://tools.ietf.org/html/rfc2119.

Chapter 2
Architecture

Although the various data exchange standards address the communication between different information systems, certain assumptions must be made concerning the capability and architecture of the connected systems in order to ensure interoperability. These assumptions are discussed in this chapter.

2.1 Interface

An interface is a mechanism (like a socket or port) by which data are imported and exported (i.e., exchanged) between two applications. An interface normally only refers to either a sending or receiving application, but in order to exchange data both end points are needed. (There must be some "thing" that provides the data, and another "thing" that consumes the data.) Analysis to distinguish between the different types of interfaces is not necessary here. An integration consists of an interface for a sending application endpoint (that assembles and prepares the data for export), an interface for a receiving application endpoint (that processes the data for import in a suitable manner), and a method for moving data between the endpoints (the transport). The content that is exchanged can vary significantly and is defined by (communication) protocols such as HL7 v2.x[1] or EDIFACT. Interfaces can support exchange of simple objects (e.g., an HL7 v2.x ADT message) or a set of transactions associated with an integration profile (a complex use case). For the former, the interface is dedicated to a single interaction (e.g., an HL7 v2 A04 message). For the latter, an implementation may choose, in a single interface (via a single module), to support multiple message events such as HL7 v2 A01, A04, and A05.

[1]HL7 v2.x and other data exchange standards are communication protocols at the higher level of the ISO/OSI stack. Other communication protocols, such as TCP/IP, are at the lower level.

F. Oemig and R. Snelick, *Healthcare Interoperability Standards Compliance Handbook*, DOI 10.1007/978-3-319-44839-8_2

The communication interface is distinguishable from a technical interface within programming languages (e.g., Pascal, C, etc.); from object oriented approaches that deal with objects consisting of properties (attributes) and methods invoking activities/functions within these objects; and from links between libraries and executables, which, in a broader context and in a sense, are also interfaces. Different types and paradigms of interfaces are presented in this section, including an analysis of the procedures and the background knowledge necessary for implementing interfaces.

2.1.1 Types of Interfaces

First, a brief explanation of the different types of interfaces is presented. Regardless of which type is utilized, from a conformance perspective all interfaces share the same concepts and challenges [1–3].

2.1.1.1 Functional (Local + Remote)

Most likely, the oldest type of interface for data exchange among disparate systems is the client/server relationship, i.e., a client system that uses common functionalities provided by a server. The client/server type of interface is based on simple functional libraries where a client makes use of the published services, e.g., to display data or to calculate certain results. The client has to know how the published services can be used, which is indicated by the function names and the required parameters, including the structure of returned results.

Typically, the client and the server reside on the same computer. In the "old days of computing", the functionality was directly (statically) linked into the binary executable code, resulting in a single executable file. Later on, the functionality was separated into distinct files to separate algorithms from data thus enabling reuse, but all of the functionality was still part of a single executable file. Then, shared libraries were established to allow for reuse across applications, but these libraries were still located on the same machine.

Currently, client and server (Fig. 2.1) can be located on different machines. This approach is known as RPC—remote procedure calls. The latest technology used for supporting the RPC approach is called Web Services, which is an even further abstraction from specific programming languages and development environments and enables the combination of different solutions and products. In addition, with Web Services different clients may use the same server.

The client/server type of interface is used when an immediate response is desired with regard to a computed result or some other outcome on the server side. A key advantage of this type of interface is that it enables the response to be returned quickly.

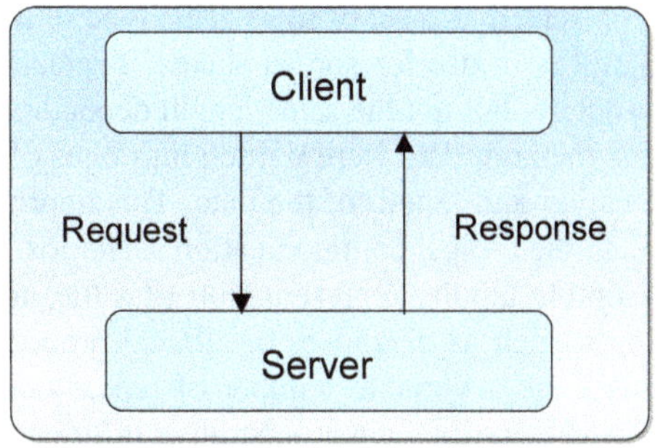

Fig. 2.1 Function calls

2.1.1.2 Message-Based Data Exchange

Another type of interface involves connecting different systems to each other, typically systems that are located on different machines. This type of interface is normally used to transfer data from one system to another (see Fig. 2.2). The relevant data are collected and encoded into a message by the sender and then are transmitted to the recipient. After the data are processed by the recipient, the message may be discarded if all relevant data have been consumed; however, often (in the healthcare domain) the message is maintained for logging and auditing purposes for a specified period of time.

In the case of a simple unidirectional data exchange (e.g., data upload), the function call is sufficient. For an on-going communication or a more complex scenario, however, a response in the form of an acknowledgment becomes important. A more thorough analysis of the different types of acknowledgments is discussed later in this chapter (see the Sect. 2.4.1).

The exchange of messages requires a definition of the data format and of the method by which the data are transported. In the early days of data exchange, the encoding was accomplished by writing the data into simple files, separating discrete data elements by a specific character. Several records with equivalent structure are

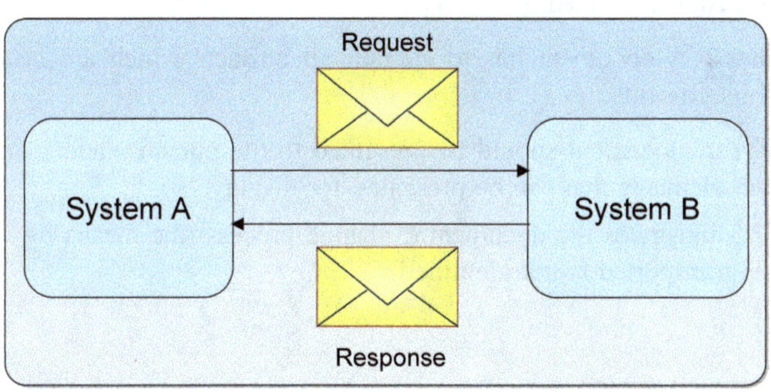

Fig. 2.2 Message exchange

represented as a set of rows. This type of file is called "comma separated file",[2] and it still is in use for spread sheets. Typically, all lines in such a file have the same structure, but not the same length depending on the data. Prior to the deployment of this method, data were written into lines of the same length that specified the exact location and length of the data. This approach was also called "fixed length files".

In the typical communication scenarios, most of the data are too complicated for a simple tabular representation (flat file) to be sufficient. For example, some concepts, such as diagnoses or clinical procedures, may repeat for a given patient. In this case, a variable number of repeat occurrences must be transmitted for these concepts while the administrative information for the patient is sent only once. For such a case, a repetition-based and/or hierarchical message structure must be defined, requiring an encoding system that allows for them. (HL7 v2, for example, provides this capability in a line-oriented format.)

In the end, the structural composition of messages can become very complex and must be managed hierarchically by appropriate separators.

2.1.1.3 Document Exchange

The same notion applies for messages and for the exchange of documents, in that document standards are necessary to define the content and format of the documents to be exchanged.

In principle, similar rules apply, i.e., documents are created by one system and sent to another. In contrast to simple messages, documents have a set of specific characteristics leading to a slightly different handling:

Persistence: The document is kept and stored after transmission. Normally both systems will have a copy of it.

Stewardship: A person or institution is responsible for maintaining it.

Accountability: A document can be signed (by a person).

Context: The context explains the environment to which the document belongs and why it has been created.

Completeness: A document has to contain all artifacts which are necessary to understand its contents.

Readability: A document should be presented to the human reader; therefore, it must contain elements that can be presented for display.

Figure 2.3 illustrates the document exchange process (the means by which the document is transported is not identified).

[2]The normal abbreviation is "CSV" which stands for "comma separated values", rarely declared as "character separated values".

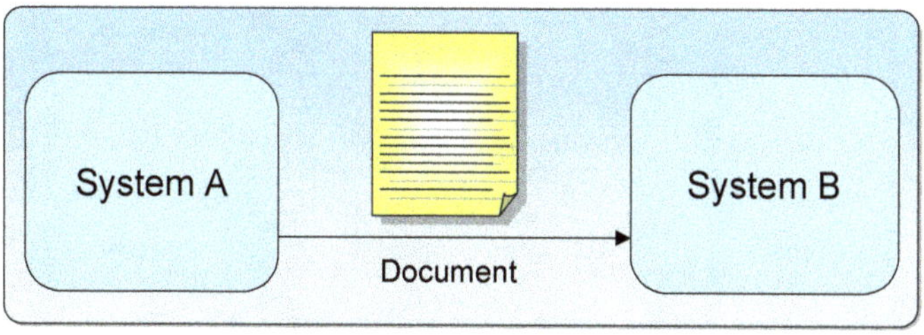

Fig. 2.3 Document exchange

2.1.2 *Communication Paradigms*

The exchange of information is normally triggered by one of the following situations:

Declarative: An event has occurred in the sending application and the sending system is used to inform one or more other systems about the current (changed) status and the associated data. A common example is the admission or transfer of a patient.

Interrogative: A system is used to obtain data from another system. In order to acquire the data, a simple request (query) is sent to the system that is assumed to have the data. The queried system will send a response. An example is the query to provide the demographic data for an identified patient.

Imperative: A system is used to trigger a specific transaction (command), such as when it is used to send an appropriate request. Orders to perform a certain task, like a lab test or radiology test, are the most prevalent kinds of requests in the healthcare domain.

Figure 2.4 highlights the different paradigms described above from a client/server perspective.[3]

The client is the system interested in the data/request and the server is the system that can provide the data/request.

The commonly used publish/subscribe mechanism is a combination of a request for information (subscribe) with the declarative notification (publish).

[3]At this point it must be noted that the systems are not interconnected in a traditional client/server architecture. The term "Server" in Fig. 2.4 indicates the availability of data, whereas the "Client" is seeking this data.

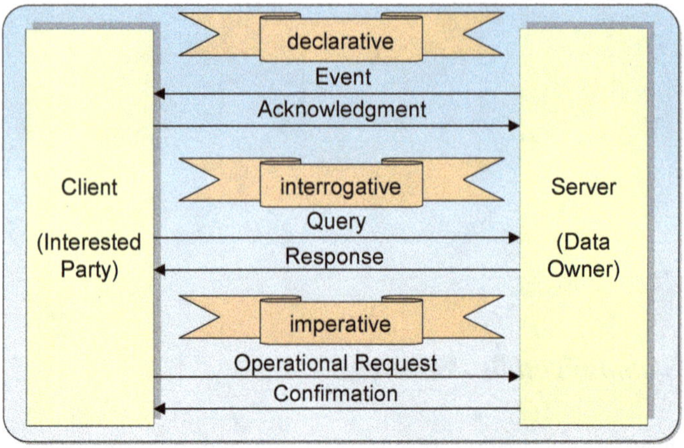

Fig. 2.4 Communication paradigms

2.1.3 *Protocol Layer*

Establishing interoperability requires a protocol stack supporting data exchange in a flexible and efficient way. On the lowest level is a simple technical interoperability that allows the simplest transmission protocols to be reused. Good examples are the hardware connections for TCP/IP. One may switch between twisted-pair connections, DSL or ISDN, while still using TCP/IP on a higher ISO level. Instead of just looking down to the IP in the ISO stack, one can also go into higher levels. As the lowest level protocol, IP is agnostic to the higher level contents. Consequently, two different higher level transport protocols exist that are incompatible with each other: TCP and UDP. Both provide different properties supporting data exchange in different ways.

The layers of the protocol that stack on top of TCP/IP and UDP/IP mediate among the technical and physical data exchange on the one side and the reuse of data as the foundation of interoperability on the other.

2.1.4 *Levels for Interoperability*

Interfaces can be established on different interoperability levels according to the layer of abstraction, as illustrated in Fig. 1.3 (Sect. 1.5).

The principle of the ISO stack applies in the same way on the application (processing) level with structural, syntactical, and semantic interoperability. For example, a syntactic understanding of what has been exchanged does not necessarily produce a correct interpretation of the contents. This interpretation must be applied manually.

With the increased interest in semantic interoperability, data will be accompanied by meta data, which will facilitate a correct understanding of the data. For example, a code such as "M" is not only placed in a certain location within the exchanged data, indicating that the correct interpretation is "married", but the code is associated with a specific code system allowing it to be distinguished from the interpretation "male", which might also be coded as "M" in another code system.

On the highest interoperability level we talk about organizational or service interoperability, which allows for direct calls of foreign services. This capability will become possible when real semantic interoperability is achieved.

2.2 Interfacing

When it comes to exchanging data between two different systems[4] (see Fig. 2.5), normally two interfaces are communicating with each other (see point 1 in the diagram). One system is sending data, and the other is receiving the data. In doing

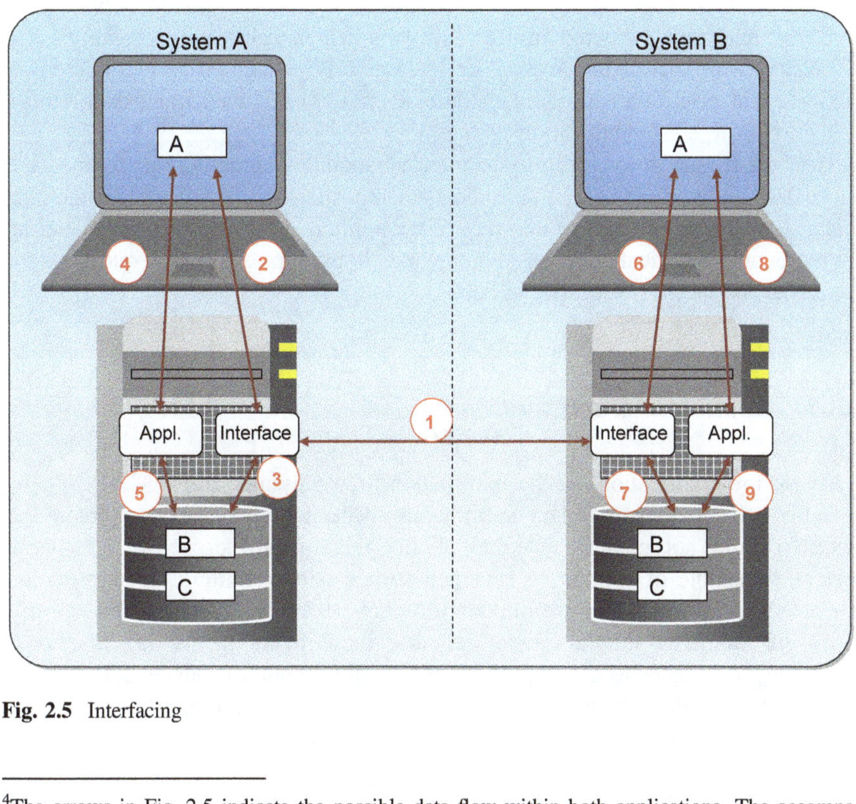

Fig. 2.5 Interfacing

[4]The arrows in Fig. 2.5 indicate the possible data flow within both applications. The accompanying numbers show the route of the data in the systems.

so, both are using the same specification, which is essential for interoperability. It is probably easy to understand that if two systems are not speaking the same language (i.e., implementing the same specification) they cannot share their data; but, as we will see later on, this prerequisite (using the same specification) is necessary, though not sufficient on its own because the appropriate understanding must be conveyed as well.

The sending system has to collect the data and convert it into the "language of the agreed upon protocol". Normally, this task is accomplished by the sending system accessing a data repository (3). The receiving system extracts the data out of the transmitted message and stores it within its own internal data repository (7).

In most cases, the interface modules are not concerned with what the application program for the graphical user interface (GUI) is doing (4, 5, 8 and 9). Furthermore, it is quite unusual for the interface module to take the data from the screen (2) or to present it directly to the screen (6). However, the latter (6) is perhaps possible for display messages, i.e., messages sent as a request do provide the information directly from a message instance to the screen to alert the end-user. In most cases, directly providing the information from a message instance to the screen is achieved by simply showing a message box that the user has to acknowledge.

What induces a sending system to send data? Data transmission is often triggered by data being entered into the system—which could mean the trigger is associated with a real-time event—or by regularly scheduled services (cron or at-jobs[5]) that prompt an interface module at pre-defined times when data require transmission to a communication partner.

How the trigger is conveyed to the interface module—directly (e.g., by message queues) or indirectly (e.g., by specific data repository tables)—and whether the trigger is managed in the user interface of the application or interface module at all are reasonable technical questions; but they are, in principle, irrelevant questions for this book and are not discussed in detail.

2.2.1 *Impact on Interfaces*

What are the ramifications of the information flow presented in Fig. 2.5?

When talking about interface specifications, the underlying architecture of the system should not matter; nevertheless, interrelationships do exist. Whether a system is capable of supporting specific features or transmitting the information requested using a standard are important aspects to know. Therefore, the specification of standards should clearly delineate these requirements: (a) whether a system must be capable of supporting specific information (relevant for a developer), and (b) under which circumstances this information is present in a message

[5]These are services that are provided by different operating systems and that run at scheduled times to perform a certain task.

instance (at runtime). This separate delineation is typically described as implementation requirements and operational requirements. (The differences for sender versus receiver are discussed separately in this chapter.)

In a standard, implementation requirements concerning the handling of a specific element can be indicated with a simple yes/no flag. If the flag is set to "yes", a developer has to write lines of code for the requirement. In derived specifications (i.e., profiles, see Chap. 7), this flag can only be switched from "no" to "yes". How this indicator is realized in data exchange standards varies—Chap. 5 provides examples. How this manifests for operational requirements is a bit more complex and is explained in the next section.

2.3 Serving Interfaces with Data

A totally different question pertains to the use of a general capability of a system in combination with its interface behavior. It is usually thought to be true that specific information that is, in principle, available within the data repository of a system (e.g., data elements B or C in Fig. 2.5) can also be exchanged with a foreign system (points 3 and 1 in Fig. 2.5). Of course, this supposition is not true. This capability is determined by the (internal) directives of the corresponding system.

From an interface perspective, it makes no difference whether specific data are hidden from an interface module, whether the data are not implemented at all, or if (data privacy/security/protection) policies prohibit making use of the data. A system functioning under these constraints must be treated as though it is not capable of handling the data (for a particular use) even if another interface within the same system may very well support the data.

2.3.1 General "Capability" of a System

The capability of a system (see Fig. 2.6) acting as an information partner within a given use case is directly influenced by how the information is obtained and subsequently handled internally. Potentially, three different situations might occur:

(1) The system's user interface offers a field to enter or to present specific information that is not stored internally.[6] This capability, represented as point

[6]When talking about "data repository", we have in mind any means to store information internally, regardless of how it is achieved or whether the data are used at all. Typically, one thinks of (relational) databases, but other mechanisms (e.g. files, USB-sticks, flash memory) are possible as well. From the perspective of this book, these distinctions are not relevant.

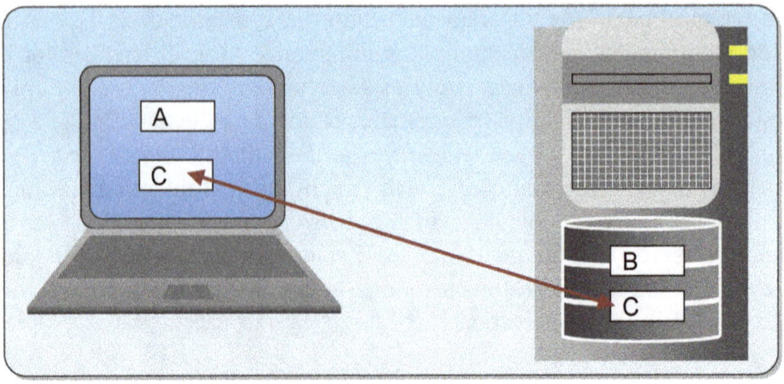

Fig. 2.6 General system capability

A in Fig. 2.6, is provided for handling temporary information and is rarely used.

(2) The system stores specific information internally, but does not present it through the user interface.[7] Here we do have persistent information present, represented as point B in Fig. 2.6.

(3) The system's user interface offers a field to enter or to present specific information that is also stored internally.[8] The arrow in the following drawing exemplifies the correlation, represented as point C in Fig. 2.6.

For interfacing, options (2) and (3) are essential in order for the system to be capable of providing specific information, given that an interface is referring to persistent information. Of course, a system may take information from an interface and provide it for display, which is also a means of meeting the requirement, but we want to abstract from this situation.

Although systems are typically implemented following option 3, the fact that a field entry mechanism is presented via the user interface does not necessarily imply that information is also entered, stored, and communicated to another system. In order to ensure accurate data entry, the user interface may contain mandatory fields that the user must complete before they can continue on with the application's workflow (e.g., name and date of birth of a patient). However, some fields are not required (e.g., address), i.e., completion is dependent on the user knowing or being able to obtain the data, and then entering the data before the system subsequently stores them. Hence, even if a system is capable of supporting the data, nothing can be communicated if the fields are not populated.

[7]System timestamps or internal identifiers are candidates for this kind of information.

[8]So whatever is typed into a certain field will be transferred—in more or less the same way—into a field of the data repository. Whether it is taken directly or indirectly, combined with other information, or separated into different data repository fields does not matter at this point.

However, in the medical domain, binary logic, meaning a piece of information is either present or absent, is sometimes not sufficient. In many situations the information cannot be provided to the user (e.g., due to the patient being unconscious) or simply is not obtainable for various reasons. Highly sophisticated applications provide some means to enter pertinent details that explain why the data were not entered, e.g., the patient was asked but was unable to answer, the patient was asked but refused to answer, or the patient was not asked at all. In some instances, knowing this information at this level of granularity is important for making informed medical decisions. Another option is to mask the information, i.e., to send something to the receiver indicating that the information is available but is not provided due to privacy policies, for example. In reality, applications allowing for such a distinction are very rare, because more sophisticated capabilities are required of the system, which will be explained later (see Sect. 2.9).

2.3.2 Relevance for Interfaces

As a consequence of the variety of legitimate reasons that certain data cannot be entered and a particular field in a message cannot be populated, in order to verify the general capability from an interface perspective, a system must create a message where such a data element is populated (disregarding policy issues and other regulations). If a system processes specific information, the situation must exist where this information is made available via an interface, otherwise, the system is declared not capable of conformance to this requirement. At this point, we have to remind the reader that such a statement is made based on the experiences gained during actual testing. Determining a system's ability to support a capability is easily handled during testing; see Chap. 11 for more information. Operational factors, such as regulatory requirements related to data privacy that prevent a system from sending (populating) the data, are not considered. Testing for capabilities is often in controlled environments where real patient and clinical information are not used.

As explained previously, this discussion focuses on capabilities required by an interface, which is one targeted use case of this book. A distinction has to be made between what a system can handle in general, and what the interface can convey or allows. Before an interface can handle the data, the application must be capable in general. But the opposite is not true. If the data is not made available for the interface (for whatever reasons), the application is declared as not capable even if it can handle the data internally. The "capability of a system" is decided from the communication partner's point of view. In other words, an interface behaves like a firewall, because only defined data elements are allowed to pass through.

2.4 Dynamic Behavior

Besides the static aspect of messages, i.e., how the messages are structured, the dynamic behavior is of interest as well. Dynamic behavior refers to the interaction specification for an exchange between two or more systems.

2.4.1 Message Pairs

As explained in the discussion about interfaces, information is typically exchanged between systems in both directions; a message is sent and a response is returned (see Fig. 2.7).

Most of the systems are implemented to support a simple (and single) message as a response to their initial message ("payload" in Fig. 2.7). In most cases this response indicates that the message has been accepted by the receiving application. Such a response is commonly referred to as a transport acknowledgement (ACK) in which a 1:1 message exchange is performed. However, a transport ACK does not indicate whether the message has been processed according to the rules established by the receiver; it simply indicates that the message was received. If the message can be processed and consumed, then an application ACK may be sent (note that not all use cases include the possibility of an application level acknowledgement). An acknowledgement response may not be sent at all, so a sending system may receive zero, one, or two messages in return.

Most data exchange standards limit acknowledgements to one or none at all. More explicit standard definitions support specific conditions under which a response should be returned, they include:

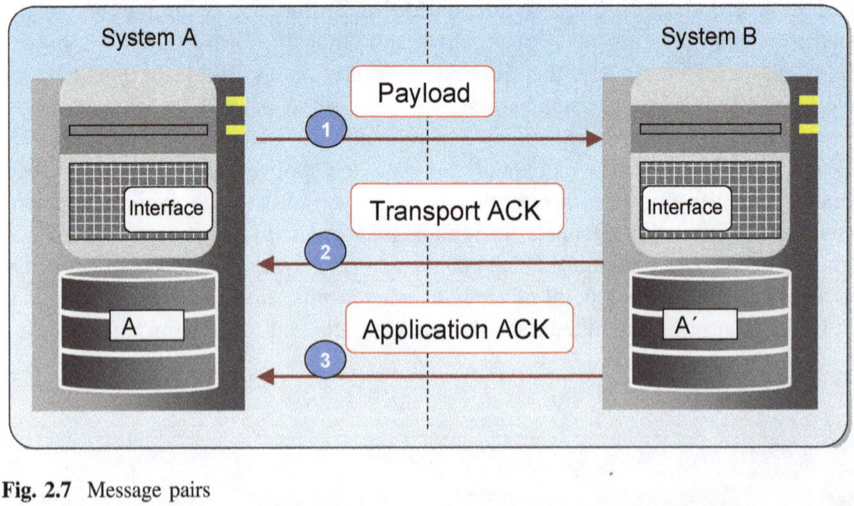

Fig. 2.7 Message pairs

- always
- in case of an error
- after successful processing only
- never

As a consequence, the sender should keep track of all messages sent and the expected responses, so in case of an unexpected behavior an appropriate notification is sent to the system administrator.

As we will see later, the situation where various recipients respond to a sender's message differently (positively and negatively) requires special treatment.

2.4.2 Timing

Implementers need to know about the timing of the messages, i.e., the relationship between a message and its response with regard to time interval. Some standards specify that a (single) response should be sent immediately, others state that no response is to be sent, while others, such as HL7 base standards, are silent on this aspect.

When the standard is silent, some implementers believe—or interpret it to mean—that a single response message should be sent immediately, and then they agree on this behavior with their communication partners. Of course, although this simplification is pragmatic, it leads to no support for zero response or two response messages as explained in the previous section, because a single response is made required. Such a solution also goes hand in hand with certain architectural decisions when developing the interfaces prohibiting enhancements.

As Fig. 2.8 demonstrates, this approach is then combined with a specific dynamic behavior: the transmission of a given message is repeated several times (1a, 1b and so forth) if no transport ACK is received within a certain period of time (timeout). This process continues until a response (1) is received or a maximum number of repetitions have been reached. When a data transmission fails, it is good practice to notify the system administrator immediately, because most likely the reason will influence real-life workflows.

The sequence diagram in Fig. 2.9 shows that several messages can be sent before a single response is received. Although rarely used, this behavior has to be accounted for in the design of the system architecture.

2.4.3 Message Identification

There are two common paradigms used in message exchange. In synchronous communication, the sending application waits for the corresponding receive (acknowledgement) before proceeding with the next message. In asynchronous

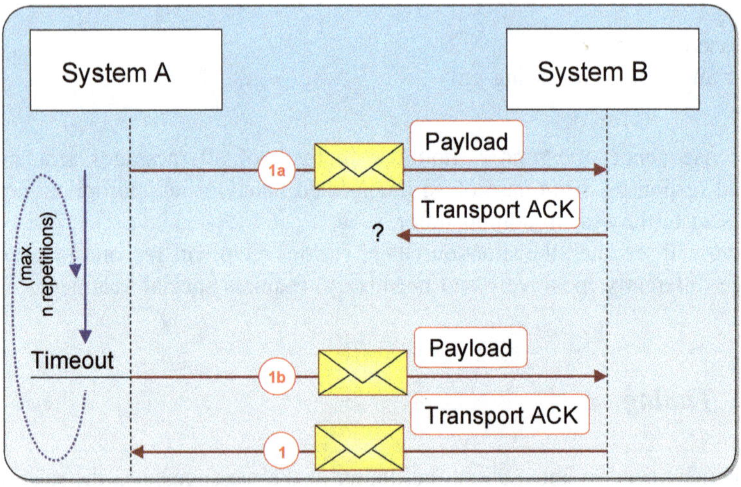

Fig. 2.8 Timeout in sending messages

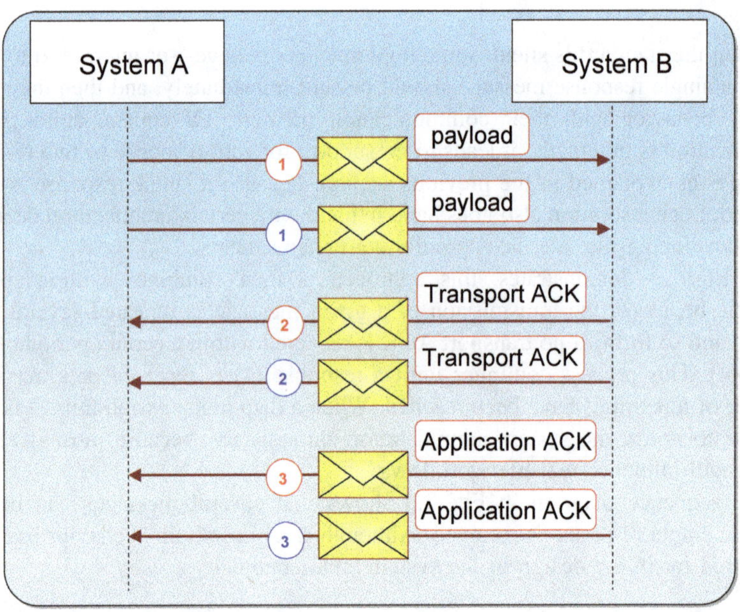

Fig. 2.9 Timing of messages

communication the sending application does not wait for the response (acknowledgement). The former has a "tight binding", and the latter has a "loose binding" and hence the need for a message ID. A response in the form of an acknowledgment must clearly indicate to which originating message it belongs. Therefore, some means to identify each message uniquely is required. The most common mechanism is to create a unique identifier for each message and to keep track of all messages sent. The response has to include the identifier of the originating message to which it is a response. In HL7 v2 the message header (MSH segment) contains this unique identifier, whereas the response references this identifier with the MSA segment.

2.4.4 Routing to Multiple Destinations

In the case of the declarative communication paradigm (see Fig. 2.4), the messages are sent concurrently to a set of recipients that have coordinated the need for the data. The ADT[9] messages are a typical example. A set of systems managing patient information needs to be informed about new patients and updates to existing patient information (Fig. 2.10).

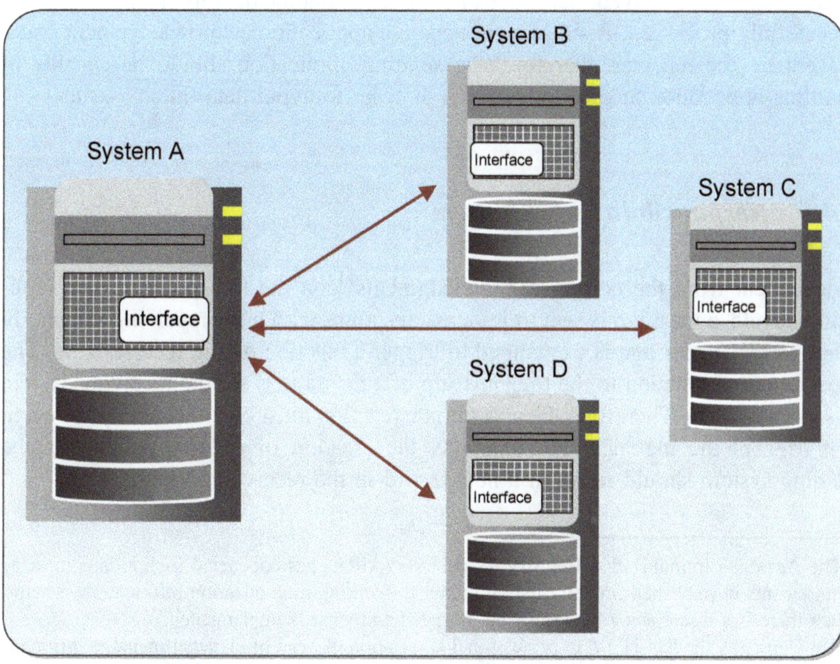

Fig. 2.10 Message routing to a set of recipients

---

[9]*ADT* is a typical abbreviation in English speaking countries and denotes "admission, discharge and transfer". More precisely, this is taken from HL7 version 2.x and Version 3. In Germany, *ADT* has a different meaning and refers to a family of standards created by KBV and ZI.

Even if the internal architectures of systems are more or less identical and their ability to process the transmitted messages is comparable, there is still no guarantee that all connected systems will respond in the same manner. As such, it is important to analyze the behavior of each connected system to determine the capabilities for processing a message, i.e., will none, some, or all of the systems accept the message? This type of probing is necessary even when a system publishes a statement of capabilities, because, in practice, often what is stated and what is implemented are different.[10]

Some systems will accept the transmitted messages while others will not, in which case the connected systems may be operating on different internal states. When a receiving system does not accept the message, the sending system has to react by notifying the receiver's system administrator (i.e., usually through a human-mediated manual process). This notification can happen only if the sending system is aware of differing results on the application level.

This use case demonstrates the important differences between a transport acknowledgment (receipt of the message) and an application acknowledgement (processing of the message). A positive transport acknowledgement indicates that the message was received, but it does not indicate that the data in the message were successfully processed. A subsequent negative application acknowledgement could be sent by the receiver, therefore, the sending application should be capable of handling application acknowledgements in order to avoid data fidelity issues.

2.4.5 *Responsibility of a System*

Independent from the correct acknowledgments[11] on the transport and the application levels, a message is sent to initiate a response within the receiving system. In other words, a message is exchanged to trigger a reaction on the receiver side. The most common reaction to the transmission of a message is for the receiving system to store new data. Therefore, the appropriate reaction must be indicated by the event that triggers the message. For example, the creation of a "new patient" in the sending system should result in a new record in the receiving system.

---

[10]The American Immunization Registry Association (AIRA) has conducted such tests comparing requirements in published implementation guides to working immunization information systems. Often there is a discrepancy between what is stated and what is implemented.

In Germany, the KH-IT [4] (a professional association of head of IT departments in hospitals) has conducted studies and created a detailed workflow description about ADT messages and the corresponding expected acknowledgements and corresponding result statuses. This summary is an excellent starting point to verify test cases regarding their correctness and completeness.

[11]In practice, integration engines are used to eliminate problems in the interpretation of the data exchange standards. These engines facilitate the use of transport acknowledgments that are sent synchronously, i.e., in an immediate 1:1 response to the initiating message. This capability hides (a) the fact that users cannot rely on an immediate response and (b) the existence and awareness of application acknowledgments.

To summarize, two different systems (as a sender/receiver pair) should operate in the same way on a user interaction by the means of exchanging an appropriate set of messages to stay in sync. For example, if the receiving system does not allow for merging of records, the internal state of the interoperating systems will be different when such an event occurs. If the sending system is capable of communicating a request to merge two records (and the trading partners are expected to do so), then the merge capability is a requirement for the set of receiving systems with which the sender interoperates. The receiving systems have the responsibility to process the messages accordingly.

2.4.6 Event Handling

As described above in Sect. 2.3.1 (Fig. 2.6), systems provide a set of forms (dialogs/windows) used to interact with the application, i.e., a user works with a set of forms for entering information. Upon acceptance by the user, the content of the form is stored by transferring the information into a set of data records. The structure and contents of the records depend on the application. The conventional and quite common behavior of an application is to store information about the actions a user has performed with the application. This logging is then used to trigger, i.e., create and exchange, the appropriate set of messages. The best way to handle those events is the decoupling of foreground editing (data input) from the background asynchronous processing (sending of messages).

Of course, depending on the application, the set of internal events (e.g., the various aspects within an admission process) differ from those being defined by a data exchange standard. In other words, even if an application supports a set of events, this set may intersect only with the standard-defined events (i.e., different coverage) and have a diverging granularity. In addition, the set of events to be supported is diverging between the different data exchange standards.[12] One of the most important steps in developing an interface for a specific data exchange standard is the mapping of the internal events to the events defined by the data exchange standard. The more closely the internal structure of the application mirrors the structure defined by the data exchange standard—or, in other words, the more aligned these structures are—the easier the mapping is to accomplish. (But it is not advisable to align an application with a specific single interoperability specification, because competing standards exist that must be supported.) The more finely grained the set of internal events is the easier the mapping will be. But in some circumstances, the mapping may be difficult and potentially not achievable, because of non-mendable, incompatible structures, in which case system redesign needs to be

[12] This can be observed in the administrative domain with HL7 version 2.x and Version 3: In HL7 v2.x the ADT messages cover in- and outpatient management, whereas in HL7 Version 3 home health and emergency admissions must be managed as well. Therefore, HL7 V3 has a more matured set of events with a finer granularity.

considered. In the case where an application needs to support multiple data exchange standards (e.g., HL7 v2.x, HL7 V3, and HL7 CDA® for sending lab results), an internal sophisticated information model that is agnostic to a particular protocol may be more advantageous.

2.4.7 Delayed Message Handling (Sender)

Certain data fidelity issues can arise as the result of delayed message handling. For example, data may be entered and collected, and then subsequently updated. In such a scenario, multiple events have occurred that affect the patient record and that need to be communicated to one or more receivers. The sender may implement message creation and transport in a number of different ways. Two common approaches for creating the message are to (1) construct the message instance immediately upon data capture from the input source, and (2) store the data in the data repository and create the message instance at a later time. Each approach has its pros and cons, and certain events that occur during the process must be accounted for in order to ensure data tracking is handled correctly (if there is a need or desire for data tracking).

A typical system architecture will separate data input (e.g., use of input forms in the user interface) and data persistence (e.g., preservation of the entered data in a data repository). In this context, the data input aspect can be thought of as the client and the data repository as the central application server. Two approaches are examined for dealing with delayed message handling that would occur when initial data are entered into a record, and then these data are updated.

In the first approach, data (e.g., a patient address, which we will call PA-1) are recorded about a patient. Upon completion of the data capture, the data are extracted from the input form and saved into the data repository, and a message instance is immediately created (i.e., close to the timing of the edits). Note that in this approach the message instance is created directly from the data that were captured. A short time later the patient record is updated to correct the patient address (PA-2). Again, after completion of the data capture the data are saved into the data repository, and another message instance is created. Sometime later (typically, the sender will send each individual message that was created immediately if possible), the messages are sent in the sequence in which they were created. The first message will contain PA-1 and the second will contain PA-2. In this case, the sender will have handled the state of the data correctly and provided the historical trace of the data to the receiver.

In the second approach, the data are stored in the data repository, but no message instance is immediately created. An indicator that the event occurred is recorded for later processing. When the update to the data is made, PA-1 is replaced by PA-2 in the data repository. Upon creation of the messages, both will contain PA-2. After the messages are processed, the state of the receiver will be the same with the first approach as with the second approach; however, a historical trace of the data is not provided to the receiver with the second approach. In order to track the data changes, a shadow data repository could be used in the sender to store PA-1. The importance of data tracking varies depending on the use case and the data.

The first approach described above eliminates the problem of delayed message handling at the cost of decentralizing all interface issues, because support for different data exchange standards must be implemented several times. The second approach results in event-handling as a separate procedure, so that a trigger event can be stored immediately after a user interaction, but is not processed immediately. So it can happen that several subsequent edits on a single record are executed before the associated events are processed accordingly.

2.4.8 Handling of Outdated Data (Receiver)

The usual paradigm of data exchange is to send the most recent data such that recipients can maintain the correct state of the data. An implementer has the choice of supporting only the most recent data or establishing a historical trace of all data. In the case of the former, the application overwrites the data currently maintained in the system (data repository) without regard to historical data preservation.

A sending application that always sends the most recent data enables a receiving application to establish a historical trace of data. Of course, the extent of this history is tied directly to the number of events that are triggered in reaction to modifications made to the initial data that were sent. The more details (i.e., more data elements) that are maintained about a data record the better the chance of updates. Consider a scenario where a patient is admitted to hospital unit "A" on day 1, transferred to unit "B" on day 2, and finally to unit "C" on day 3. When this sequence of transactions transpired, however, an error was made. The patient was actually transferred to hospital unit "F" on Day 2. Another example would be the case of a caregiver entering a diagnosis that later was found to be erroneous and subsequently was updated. How does the receiving system recognize the *outdated* (*invalid*) data and what steps does it need to take to correct the data?

Some receiving applications do not track the history and always expect to get the most recent data, while other applications maintain a historical trace for the data. Therefore, it is imperative that a mechanism exists that clearly indicates whether a message contains the most recent data or *outdated* (*invalid*) data. Different solutions exist (or should exist) in each of the current standards to account for this situation.

One method that has been specified by the IHE Patient Administration Management (PAM) integration profile is to provide a separate customized event (a Z99 event). IHE adopted this approach because they thought that implementation of the A08 (update) event may ignore the subtlety of an *outdated* (*invalid*) data indicator in the message. Some of the impetus of this reasoning was that many legacy systems would not be updated (to account for the subtlety of the outdated data indicator) and thus processing of an A08 message would lead to erroneous destruction of data. Use of the special trigger event increases the possibility of correct implementation, because a clear distinction can be made between data included in the most recent data event ("A08") and data in the *outdated* data event ("Z99"). Systems that don't support tracking of historical data will ignore the outdated data event ("Z99") to maintain data fidelity. Evaluating this distinction at the event level may raise the awareness of implementers, allowing them to determine quickly (and, hopefully, unambiguously) the timeliness of received data before processing them so that a misunderstanding and destruction of the most recent data are prevented. This example illustrates one documented solution; other solutions are equally plausible.

2.5 Intermediate Message Handling

Another topic worth discussing is the forwarding of messages by a receiving system (System B in Fig. 2.11) to other systems. This section explores the impact on the data, but it does not define the target system or any receiver responsibilities in the case of misrouted messages or error handling. The correct handling of received information becomes important if the data are used as input to other applications.

What happens if information received from System A via (1) should be sent to System C via (5)? The easiest approach to use is for the intermediate application (System B) to act as a 'pass through', routing the message without consuming the incoming message and recreating a new outgoing message. This solution is quite uncommon and not recommended, because the routed information should be consumed and stored by the intermediate application (System B)[13] (otherwise, no

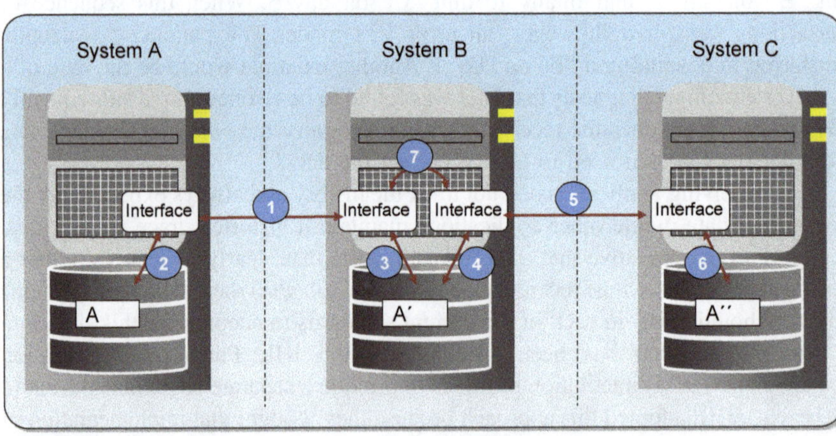

Fig. 2.11 Message routing

[13]This even applies to, and is common practice of, integration engines, although they do not act upon the data in any meaningful way.

real bridging to other data exchange standards or re-use for other use cases is possible). Therefore, the receiving interface (System B) stores the information within the data repository (3), and the sending interface extracts the data from the data repository upon request (4). Another option is the internal routing between both interfaces (7), which is also an uncommon implementation.

But even if data are sent from System A via System B to System C, it is not necessarily true that the information stays the same after it is stored in the various data repositories (A, A′ and A″ in Fig. 2.11). The different interfaced modules may translate the information received in the message from the protocols required by the interface message standard into an internal format/value/code.

As has been explained in Sect. 2.3.1, storing this information internally can be defined as “being capable”. A distinction between (B) and (C), as shown in Fig. 2.6, is not necessary here. [Note: (C) would present this value to the user; (B) will keep it hidden].

2.6 Message Population

Achieving semantic interoperability requires some means of identifying misinterpretations when creating or consuming a message. However, one cannot detect whether there is a (semantic) mismatch of information on the sending side (Fields 2 and 3) or the receiving side (Fields 1 and 2) by using a given standard (represented by the cross-overs in Fig. 2.12).

Therefore, the different parties have to trust that the information populating the fields in a messages is accurate, i.e., whether a date in the field for the patient date of birth really represents the date of birth and not some other date. This issue is important, but it requires an abstract means of expressing the semantics of a field

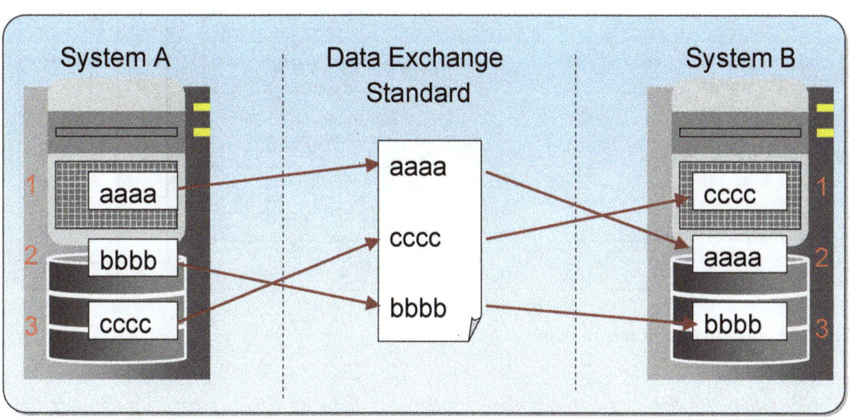

Fig. 2.12 Message population

according to the processing of the data within the application to avoid misinterpretation of data element. As explained in Chap. 1, this feature is introduced on higher interoperability levels by semantically annotating data elements. Until this feature is available, trust in the data is essential, and misusing fields for other purposes is strongly discouraged and should be prohibited.

2.7 Information Transmission

The most conventional method for data exchange is initiation of an appropriate event in response to data being imported into an application (e.g., a patient is registered). Figure 2.13 demonstrates this process with artificial elements and data, where data are provided, collected, and packaged in System A (on the left side) and sent as a message to System B (in the middle). System B incorporates the data (right hand side). The table associated with System B indicates the known state of System B after each transaction.

As can be seen in transactions 1, 2, and 3, as long as valid data are communicated by System A, the data in System B are as they are expected to be. An issue arises when data are deleted without being replaced by new data, as shown in the transaction 4.[14] Element Y is deleted from System A's data repository (as indicated

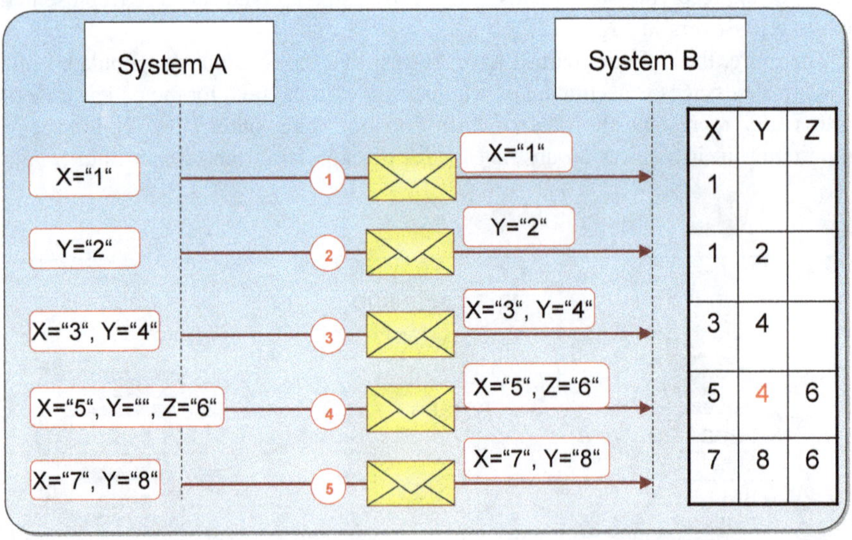

Fig. 2.13 Information transmission

[14]Assuming that the intent of the workflow is that the systems have matching data.

by Y = "" on the left hand side)[15] because the data are no longer valid (see Sect. 2.4.6). However, since no data, nor any notification about the deleted data, are sent, the receiver does not have any indication that something has changed, and, therefore, cannot delete the erroneous data. This situation is denoted by the red "4" in the table summarizing the current values in System B. At this point in operation of these applications, Element Y should be empty in both systems so their data are synchronized.

There are different solutions for indicating to the receiver that data are no longer valid. The first option is to send a "placeholder" indicating that the data must be deleted (to be explained in the next section). Other solutions include the snapshot and update modes, which are covered near the end of this chapter.

In transaction 5 shown in Fig. 2.13, new data are sent and both applications are in sync again.

2.8 Delete Indication

HL7 Version 2.x has the notion of a "delete" indicator,[16] which is two double quotes ("").[17] This indicator notifies a trading partner that specific data are to be deleted from their system because the data are no longer valid. To facilitate implementation, the sending system must be capable of recognizing the need for data to be deleted when an event is being processed. The easiest way for the sending system to meet this requirement is by maintaining the history of previous (i.e., "out-of-date") data. The most common method for persisting historical data is the use of a "shadow table".[18] Figures 2.14, 2.15 and 2.16 illustrate the shadow table concept.

Figure 2.14 illustrates the status of a value after the initial data entry. The value is stored in the data repository, the shadow table is empty (white box), and the value is presented to the user on the screen.

Now the user enters new data ("B" in Fig. 2.15) for this particular data element, which should be stored, thus overwriting the old value ("A" in Fig. 2.15). The

[15]HL7 v2.x provides a notation to use for explicitly indicating that the data for a specific element must be deleted. The notation consists of two double quotes ("" ""). Most other standards do not handle deletion at all or provide an explicit transaction for this purpose. Furthermore, it must be noted that not sending information is different from sending a delete request, and both of these actions are different from sending null values. Each of these circumstances is explained in this book.

[16]HL7 v2.x is the only standard the authors are aware of that supports a delete indicator.

[17]Quite often, the concept of a delete indicator is misinterpreted as a null value! Also, some systems erroneously send two double quotes to indicate that the field is empty, which triggers an incorrect action by the receiver. This is especially important in case the receiver is collecting information from different sending systems.

[18]There are additional methods for storing historical data (e.g. SQL stored procedures) that have their advantages and disadvantages, but these methods are left to the reader to explore.

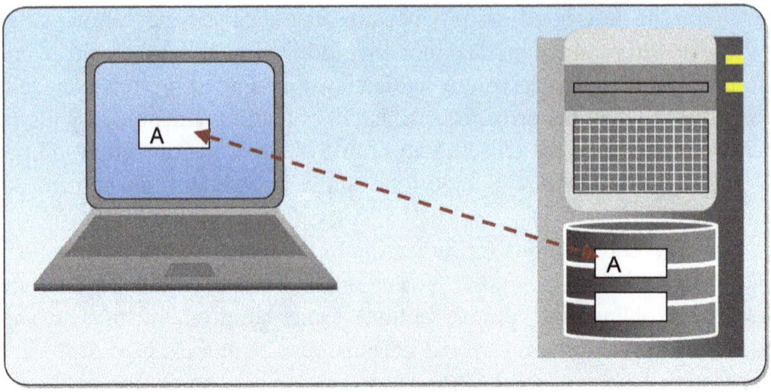

Fig. 2.14 Shadow table concept (after first data entry)

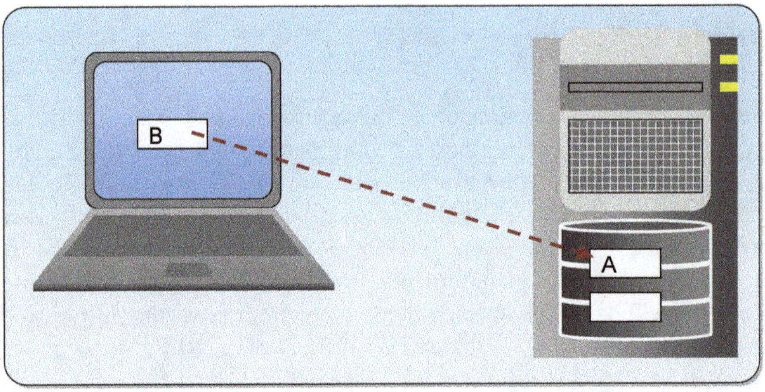

Fig. 2.15 Shadow table concept (before data update)

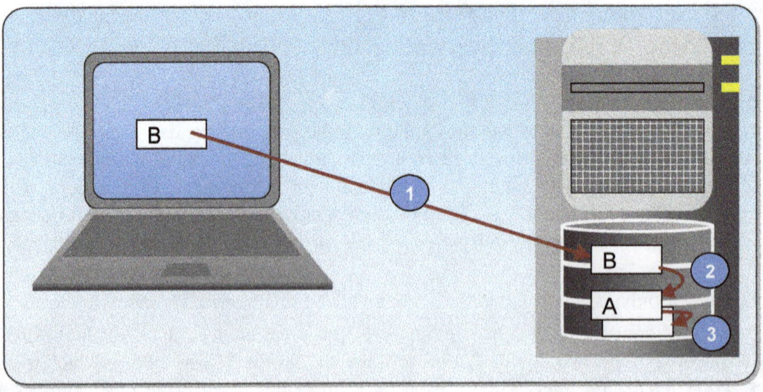

Fig. 2.16 Shadow table concept (after data update)

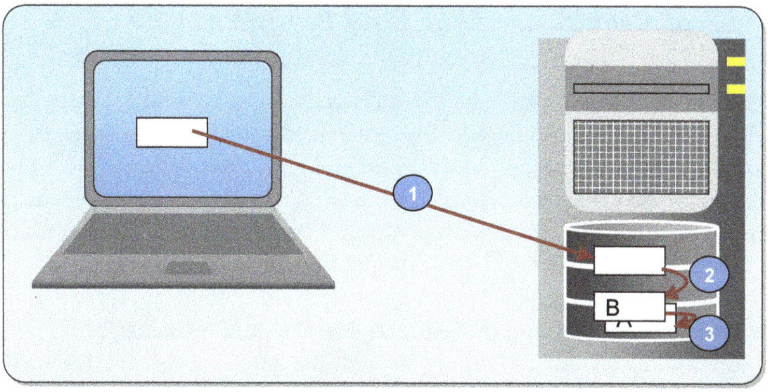

Fig. 2.17 Shadow table concept (delete data)

system becomes aware (e.g., user enters data) of an updated value ("A" in Fig. 2.15) for a particular data element (indicated by the white box on the screen containing "A"). When saving this information in the data repository (arrow 1 in Fig. 2.17), the following transactions must occur as an atomic process[19]: the previous value "A" for this element is transferred internally into the shadow table [as designated by arrow 2 (Fig. 2.17)], moving the old value "A" to the shadow table; the current ("new") value ("B") is transferred to the "active" location for the element, replacing the old value; and if previous data existed in the shadow table, then another layer of tracking data is employed as shown by arrow 3 in Fig. 2.16. Hence, the trigger of the whole transaction is arrow 1, but the processing sequence is 3, 2, and, finally, 1, so data loss is prevented.

Note that this set of events also can be applied when the data are to be deleted. In this case, "B" is written to the shadow table and the "active" element location becomes empty as is demonstrated with Fig. 2.17.

Without such a mechanism,[20] an interface module is unable to distinguish between a simple missing (empty) value and a deleted value, because the internal appearance as a record set value is identical. There is a precondition, however, on the sending side. Having the shadow table capability allows a system to identify data that are to be deleted and to send the two double quotes in the message, notifying the receiving system to execute the deletion. The receiving system can process the deletion request without having the data history and can simply react to the delete indicator.

---

[19]A quite common method employed to accomplish this process is to use stored procedures in the data repository.

[20]The concept of a shadow table is not the only way to achieve a delete indication. Another option, for example, is to use stored procedures in common DBMS where old and new data are available simultaneously. This method allows for detecting of a deletion and storing of this information for the interface module, because in this case the old data are not necessary.

2.8.1 Legal Requirements for Data Persistence

Deleting information must be handled with care. In most settings, legal requirements (e.g., accountability and liability issues) oblige entities to keep track of a subset of data and any changes made to previously stored data.

A physician may be called upon to show the information upon which their treatment of a patient is based. As such, any change in the information must be tracked along with relevant dates and times of updates, especially in the case where the data were no longer applicable[21] and were deleted.[22] Relevant information must not simply disappear from the patient record in the data repository.

This topic is discussed in more depth with the snapshot and update modes for transactions.

2.8.2 Receiver Responsibility

Receiving applications are expected to be able to process the delete indicator in accordance with the prescribed semantics. In operation, the receiver is informed that the data sent previously by the sender are no longer applicable and that the sender is requesting they be deleted.[23]

An example of data for which a sender might request a deletion is a patient address. The clerk at the front desk realizes that he typed in a wrong address and eliminates it from the input form. The form is submitted, which causes the system to move the current data to a shadow table and to remove that data from the "active" data repository. The interface module compares the empty value in the "active" element location with the value in the shadow table and concludes that data have been deleted. As a consequence, the interface module inserts the delete indicator ("") into the message location corresponding to the address element where a value has been deleted. The receiver interprets the two double quotes ("") as an indication to delete the address from its data repository. If the receiver wants to maintain historical records, then its "shadow table" is updated.

[21] This may include incorrect data or outdated data that are no longer pertinent.

[22] A distinction must be made between logical and physical deletion of data, but this is not addressed here.

[23] This arrangement is based on prior agreement between the sender and receiver; in most cases the data are deemed to be incorrect, and the receiver will delete the data. It may be, however, that the receiver system also obtains data transmissions from other sources, and that it may have stored an update already, in which case the receiver can ignore this delete request.

2.8.3 Data Granularity

Data are normally transmitted with varying levels of detail. An address may consist of a street, house number, city, ZIP code, and state. Deleting of the address data may occur at a high level, resulting in the deletion of the complete address, or at specific level, for example, the street or house number. The delete indicator can trigger deletion at either of these levels; i.e., when positioned on a high level (e.g., a field in HL7 v2.x), the indicator denotes the deletion of the complete address, whereas, when positioned at a more detailed level (e.g., a component in HL7 v2.x), the indicator denotes deletion of a specific component only.

2.8.4 Impact of Order of Messages

If two parties are exchanging information, the result in the receiving system is easy to determine,[24] because there is only one sender. If more than one party is sending the same type of information, the result depends on the sequence in which the messages were sent (Fig. 2.18).

The following table provides an interaction scenario with concrete values for a single data element. It is assumed that in System A or System C (both are sending systems in this context) the appropriate change has been applied and the information is sent via the appropriate transaction (1 or 2) immediately afterward. Table 2.1 presents a hypothetical sequence of transactions, data or lack of data sent, and the resulting state of the receiving system. The notation "<empty>" is used to indicate the absence of data in the transaction. The "<delete>" notation represents active communication of the delete indicator.

As one can see, empty information versus an explicit delete indication will have different results. Not sending any data causes the previous/old information to be maintained as is on the receiving side, whereas a processed delete indication will result in deleted data. (In combination with handling outdated data, the systems will be aware of the data history if necessary.)

---

[24] Only if each message is a complete "transaction" on its own—which is the case for HL7 but not for DICOM. For example, the sequencing of image transmission (storage), MPPS and Storage Commitment is undefined for an IHE Modality actor, and so is the mapping between transactions and DICOM network associations (TCP connections). Therefore, the result is not always easy to determine, and, of course, with more than two systems, the results are even more complex.

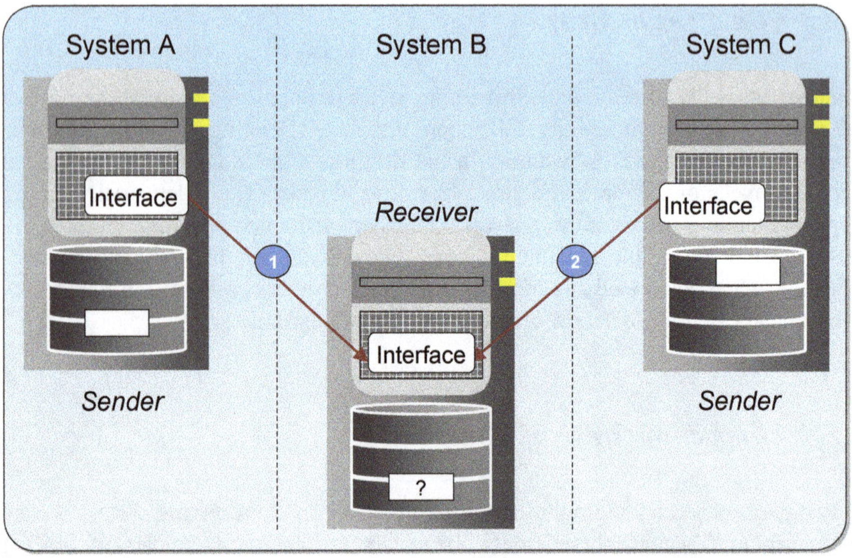

Fig. 2.18 Receiver responsibility

Table 2.1 Order of messages

Seq		Information	Comment	Result in system		
				A	B	C
1	1	"x"		"x"	"x"	<empty>
2	2	"y"		"x"	"y"	"y"
3	1	<empty>	Deleted in System A	<empty>	"y"	"y"
4	2	<empty>	Deleted in System C (without history)	<empty>	"y"	<empty>
5	1	"z"		"z"	"z"	<empty>
6	2	"x"		"z"	"x"	"x"
7	2	<delete>	Deleted in System C with history	"z"	<empty>	<empty>

2.8.5 Sender Responsibility: Impact to System Design

For a receiver, it is relatively easy to take care of the delete indication that is sent on a segment, field, or component level within a message. As indicated before, for the sending system to detect the need for a deletion is much more complicated, because each field must be checked against a previous value. There are different methods for implementing the delete capability:

- stored procedures to update values
- shadow tables with a history of the data
- special encoding of deleted information.

The interested reader is invited to think about additional means for realizing this requirement.

To summarize briefly, implementers must be aware of and implement the delete indicator, otherwise data fidelity issues likely will occur among the communicating entities. This is especially true if the delete indicator is treated as normal data and is stored as such.

2.9 Null Flavors

An oddly "similar", but distinctly different, concept to the delete indicator is the so-called null-flavor that indicates why certain information is not available (e.g., "asked but not known").

HL7 Version 3 provides a very detailed explanation about the different concepts associated with null flavor. Table 2.2 provides an excerpt, and the complete definition can be found in Chap. 5.

Table 2.2 HK7® Null Flavors [5 MB 2013]

Concept code	Print name	Level[a]
NI	No information	0
INV	Invalid	1
DER	Derived	2
OTH	Other	2
NINF	Negative infinity	3
PINF	Positive infinity	3
UNC	Un-encoded	2
MSK	Masked	1
NA	Not applicable	1
UNK	Unknown	1
ASKU	Asked but unknown	2
NAV	Temporarily unavailable	3
NASK	Not asked	2
QS	Sufficient quantity	2
TRC	Trace	2

[a]"Level" indicates the nesting of the listed codes

Some of the values listed in Table 2.2 are clear indications of why information is not provided ("ASKU"), whereas others are a matter of representation, e.g., negative or positive infinity or quantity measures.

The most common way of providing null-flavors is in the form of explicit values, as is shown in Table 2.3 ("O" and "U").

If null-flavor code values (e.g., "O"—"Other") are handled in the same way as individual concepts (e.g., "M"—"Male"), then, typically, within various tables different codes are defined to express the same concept (e.g., if no code matches using the values "O" or "OTH" ("other"), or the information is unknown using the values "U" or "UNK" ("unknown"), etc.). The approach very much depends on the author of the code system and/or other codes in the code system and other dependencies. The three letter code "UNK" is typically selected for "unknown" if the other codes are longer than a single character.

The way null flavors are managed correlates closely with the way the data exchange standard is designed. Introducing a separate set of concepts to be used is permissible only if an appropriate methodology is provided, as can be seen with HL7 version 3 in contrast to HL7 version 2.x.

Providing the null-flavor as a code in each code system (and, therefore, value set) where applicable is—from an implementer's perspective—considered the easiest method, because the null-flavor code is treated the same as any other code. This method also facilitates easy implementation, because the null-flavors are maintained and updated directly in the given value set. However, this approach does not ensure conformity of the codes across different code systems, so a specific null flavor may be represented by different codes (e.g., "U" or "UNK" for "unknown").

The described concept of null flavors is a general methodology to convey information about why certain data are missing. This methodology should be available and applicable for all data elements independent from their data type (also including non-coded data types such as String). Therefore, the first method discussed is limited to coded information when a code must be selected from a drop-down list. Introducing a methodology—as in HL7 V3—to provide null-flavors for all data types is a sophisticated approach, but it requires an appropriate enhancement of the application in general. In most cases—if not in all—there is no

Table 2.3 Table 0001—administrative gender[a] (HL7 v2.7)

Value	Description	
F	Female	
M	Male	
O	Other	⇐
U	Unknown	⇐
A	Ambiguous	
N	Not applicable	

[a]In HL7 v2, the element is referred to as "Sex" and not "Gender"; however, gender better represents the concept and is used in V3 and FHIR. In this book we will refer to as Gender

means to enter (coded) null-flavor information into a conventional text field, such as fields used for entry of names and addresses. ("I have asked the patient for his name, but he did not tell me.")

Managing null flavors for all data elements of an application implies a significant architectural enhancement that is hard to realize and therefore not realistic. From an interoperability perspective, changing one application alone is not sufficient, as the example application at the end of this chapter will demonstrate. Therefore, necessary support of null flavors for certain (un-coded) data elements shall be indicated explicitly in the implementation guides in order for a special treatment to be developed individually for the requested data elements.

Chapter 5 explains methods for creating, managing, and applying value sets and code systems effectively. One such method is to combine the null flavor code system with the code system (containing the concept codes needed for the element) into a single value set. This approach is generally, from a maintenance and management perspective, superior, because it ensures conformity of the "null" concepts. Otherwise, it is not possible to detect that "U" and "UNK" are both codes for the same concept.

2.10 Snapshot Mode Versus Update Mode

The most common interaction users have with an application is that of entering new data. As explained previously, a "new data" event may trigger an exchange of data from one system to another. All needed data could be known and entered into the system together, or bits of data may become known and entered over time as they are available. The latter scenario is typical with laboratory test results. For simple lab tests all result data components likely become available simultaneously; however, for panels, often only partial results are available initially, and the remainder of the data for the lab panel test are available later.

In the case of partial data availability, how should these data be transmitted? One option is to repeat the transmission of all the data as soon as they become available, i.e., including data already sent for this event. This method mandates for every known result component to be sent at the time the message is created regardless of when the data became known. This method is called snapshot mode. Another option is to convey in the transmitted message only the data that are new or that have changed. This option is referred to as update mode.

Before continuing with the explanation, it is worth noting that the distinction between these two modes is only necessary in case of multiple values for the same concept, for example, a set of result values providing the details to an order, or a set of diagnoses (e.g., admission or treatment, or primary and secondary). If only a single value is possible, such a distinction is not necessary. Transmitting the current marital status does not require such a determination, but if the history of marital statuses should be sent it becomes important.

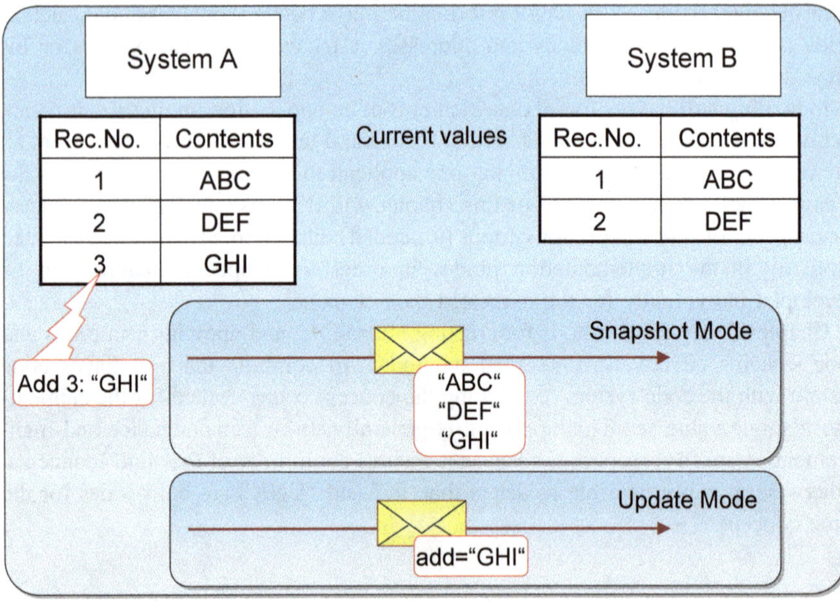

Fig. 2.19 Snapshot mode versus update mode

The decision as to which method is preferable is implementation-dependent and typically is influenced by the particular interaction. A trade-off exists between the ease of processing and the ease of messaging. Figure 2.19 illustrates the contrasting approaches.

Systems A and B have participated in a previous data exchange resulting in two synchronized records 1 ("ABC") and 2 ("DEF"). Now a user enters data "GHI" as the 3rd record into system A. In snapshot mode, all three records are communicated, and system B replaces the existing data in the records with these new data. In update mode, system A only sends the new data "GHI" with instructions to add it to the already stored set of records. In both modes, system B will have the same data as system A.

Two requirements must be met for the update mode to work. As depicted in Fig. 2.19, the update mode requires an indicator ("add", in this example) to signal the change. There are a variety of methods for implementing update mode indicators, and action codes are one method. Table 2.4 provides the segment action codes for HL7 v2.7.

The second requirement for using update mode is the capability to identify the data of concern. If the status of a result value should be updated, the correct data entry must be identified. The code or value of the data (e.g., "hematocrit" lab result value) or any of its attributes (e.g., the status "preliminary") is not sufficient, because these items are subject to change. To provide another example using identifiers: For managing patients or visits, the update mode is the most common

Table 2.4 Table 0206—segment action code (HL7 v2.7)

Value	Description	Explanation
A	Add/insert	The transmitted data are new and should be added as a new record into the system
D	Delete	The referenced data should be deleted. Therefore, an identification of the data is sufficient
U	Update	The transmitted data indicates the updated information, therefore the original data must be uniquely identified
X	No change	This action code just references the data and indicates no change. Such a transmission makes sense in the case where a requirement exists that enforces the presence of data. Therefore, this requirement can be met while optimizing data processing

choice, because only a few attributes (like the address etc.) should be altered. Here, the patient or visit identifier is used, and not the name, address or any other demographic data. Each data item must have a unique and persistent identifier that will not change over time. Inserting new data or using the snapshot mode can be done without any reference to existing data; but, in case of updates or deletes, the referenced information must be clearly identified, which can, of course, not be done based on the data and its attributes. So, even when inserting new data for later updates, an identifier is required.

In principle, both modes allow for adding, updating, and deleting data. The advantages and disadvantages of each mode primarily depend on the frequency of changes or additions to the data, the message size, and the receiver's responsibilities.

If most of the data are entered at once, then snapshot mode is generally the best approach. If a single record contains a lot of details, then the update mode is more suitable. On the other hand, snapshot mode is simpler to implement given that the data referenced in the snapshot are easy to identify.

The most common processing method used with snapshot mode is to delete all the existing stored data and to add the newly received data afterwards. This approach is easier, but it may lead to a loss of relevant data in case the new submission does not cover previous information. The shadow data repository mentioned earlier only supports keeping track of the overall changes. Therefore, for update mode, the burden to identify the changes is on the sender, whereas in snapshot mode the receiver has to identify the delta.

In circumstances where the receiver is collecting data from multiple sources, using snapshot mode is risky, because one sender is unaware of the data another sender has provided. Deleting all data received previously from all senders just because new data are received from a single sender most likely will lead to a loss of important data. Therefore, in these cases the snapshot mode should be implemented to affect only data exchange among each sender/receiver pairing. In other words, in snapshot mode the receiver should only update the data received from this specific sender and leave the remainder of the data from other senders untouched, otherwise, assurance must be provided that all possible senders are aware of the same data.

Laboratory results are a bad example here, because the results are always order specific and, by this means, are clearly indicated. Better examples are procedures, diagnoses, and allergy codes, because multiple systems will collect and communicate these data.

2.11 Considerations in Application Development

The following example is used to discuss how design decisions can impact interoperability. To demonstrate this point, contrived requirements are introduced, resulting in the development of a demonstrative data repository schema (because this is an illustrative example, the scope is limited). The reader can relate this scenario to an application they are familiar with.

The requirements introduced are somewhat arbitrary, but are selected to enforce specific changes in order to exemplify different stages in developing an application.

The example shows how the schema evolves, with new requirements (shown in boxes in italics) being incorporated into design changes, which are analyzed in the Conformance Discussion section following the scenario. The evolution of the schema does not consider any practical impacts that may result in additional problems when deploying this example application or problems that may occur when converting data from an old schema to a new schema. It is intended to be an example to explain and compare the different steps of the evolution (phases) with respect to the data exchange requirements. Additionally, it highlights the impact of changes to interoperability specifications on internal application design. Such changes may not be easy for implementers, and authors of specifications should fully understand the implications when changes are sought; however, this consideration does not justify excluding needed capabilities.

2.11.1 Introducing Functional Requirements

We start with a very simple set of requirements:

Functional Requirement 1
The application shall be capable of managing (storing) demographic information about a person. This includes the person's given name, family name, date of birth, and gender.

The application shall be capable of managing (storing) two allergies for this person.

One implementation approach is to create a single (simple) schema without a primary key and using simple data types (see Fig. 2.20).

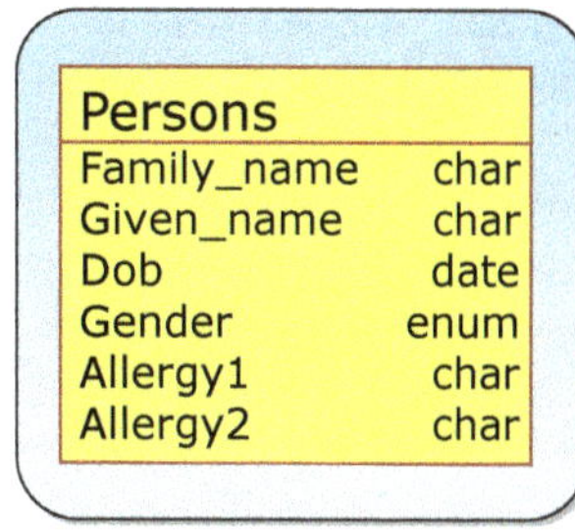

Fig. 2.20 Sample schema for requirement 1

A second approach is to add the use of a primary key. This approach is not derived from the original requirement, but it does not violate it. Therefore, enforcing an additional requirement is introduced.

Functional Requirement 2
The application shall provide a primary key that is independent from any other information.

Figure 2.21 illustrates the revised data repository schema that includes the primary key Id (identifier). (In the figures that follow, primary keys are marked in bold).

Next, a country-specific requirement is introduced.

Functional Requirement 3
The application shall be capable of managing (storing) information about the birthname in accordance with German law.

To understand this requirement, it must be understood that in Germany the birthname is only referring to the family name. Official registration of a newborn must be completed within 3 days after birth and is permanent (i.e., birthname). Changes to the given name are (normally) not allowed. Figure 2.22 illustrates the data repository schema that includes the birthname.

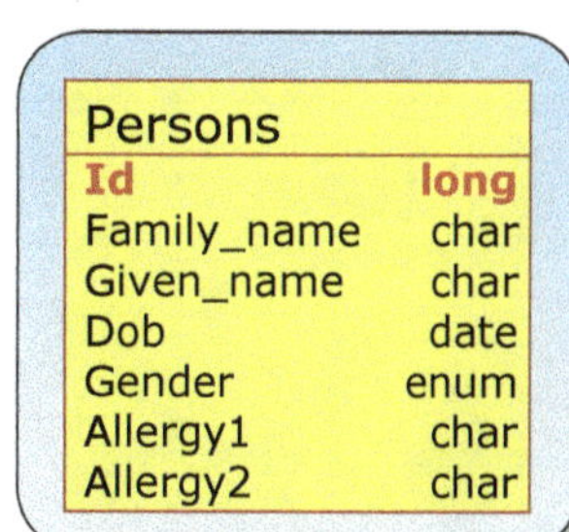

Fig. 2.21 Sample schema for requirement 2

Fig. 2.22 Sample schema for requirement 3

Persons	
Id	**long**
Family_name	char
Given_name	char
Name_at_birth	char
Dob	date
Gender	enum
Allergy1	char
Allergy2	char

Now, we introduce the United States-specific requirement to manage birthnames (in addition to the German requirement).

Functional Requirement 4
The application shall be capable of managing (storing) information about the birthname in accordance with American law.

Within the United States, it is possible to change the given (first) name within a certain time frame, a rule that varies among the different US jurisdictions. The introduction of this requirement leads to a revision of the data element *Name_at_birth* to *Family_name_at_birth* and *Given_name_at_birth*. Caution must be taken when converting the data. Typically, the old attribute name *Name_at_birth* is changed to *Family_name_at_birth*, and a new attribute *Given_name_at_birth* is added. If the original attribute was used erroneously to capture the full name at birth, this information will reside in the wrong field after converting the data repository schema (Fig. 2.23).

Fig. 2.23 Sample schema for requirement 4

Persons	
Id	**long**
Family_name	char
Given_name	char
Family_name_at_birth	char
Given_name_at_birth	char
Dob	date
Gender	enum
Allergy1	char
Allergy2	char

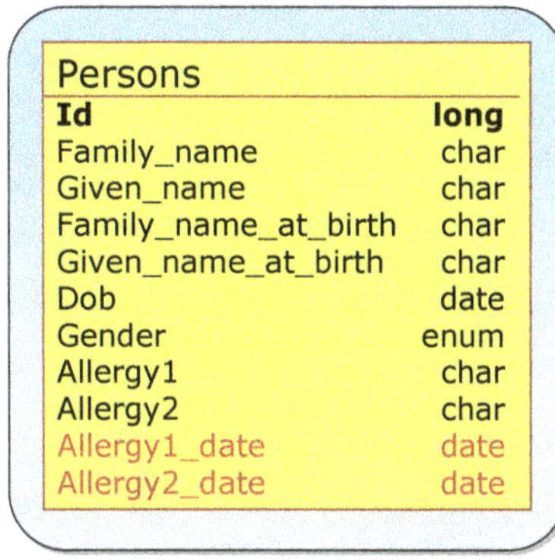

Fig. 2.24 Sample schema for requirement 5

For the next version, a minor new feature is added:

Functional Requirement 5
For both allergies, the associated date of onset shall be managed.

This request results in the schema as shown in Fig. 2.24. In the next step, we introduce some flexibility:

Functional Requirement 6
The application shall be capable of managing (storing) multiple names and identifiers. The management of those data shall be supported by name and identifier types.

This new requirement is included on purpose to show the information being divided between two additional schemas, which are introduced in Fig. 2.25. Some of the original data items are moved to the new schemas, and an additional type attribute is introduced to create the primary key of the sub-schemas. The primary key is used to link those schemas.

As can be seen in Fig. 2.25, both the given and family names for persons are migrated to *PersonNames*. The distinction between the current name and the birth name is indicated by the *Name_Type*. To support the previously introduced requirements, at least two name types must be provided: legal name and birth name.

The external identifier for the person is managed as part of the primary key in table *PersonIdentifiers*.

This schema supports the functional requirement, as multiple names can be used, but its utility is limited to names of different types. To solve this problem, the schema must be enhanced even further, as is shown in Fig. 2.26.

The sequence number as part of the primary key allows for storing multiple names comprised of given and family names of the same type. (Populating this field

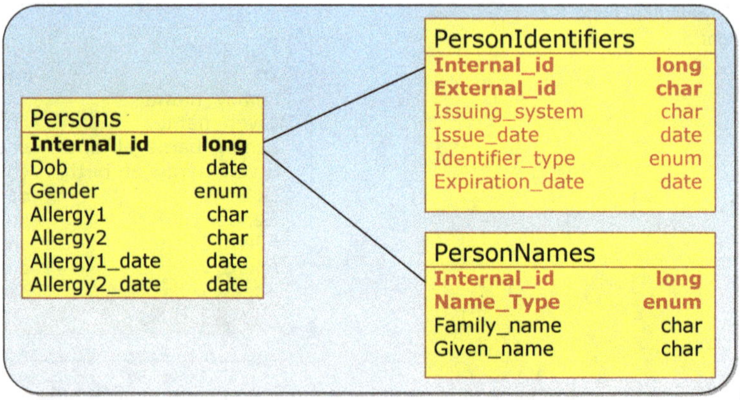

Fig. 2.25 Sample schema for requirement 6

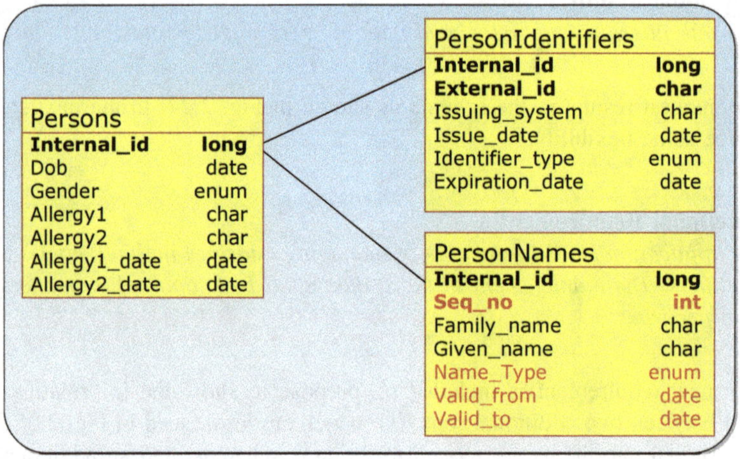

Fig. 2.26 Enhanced sample schema for requirement 6

correctly is delegated to the application.) To help with deciding which name to select, a validity range has been added. This feature is not mentioned in the requirement, but it supports proper use.

The next step should eliminate the restrictions for the maintenance of the allergies:

Functional Requirement 7
The application shall be capable of managing (storing) an unlimited number of allergies.

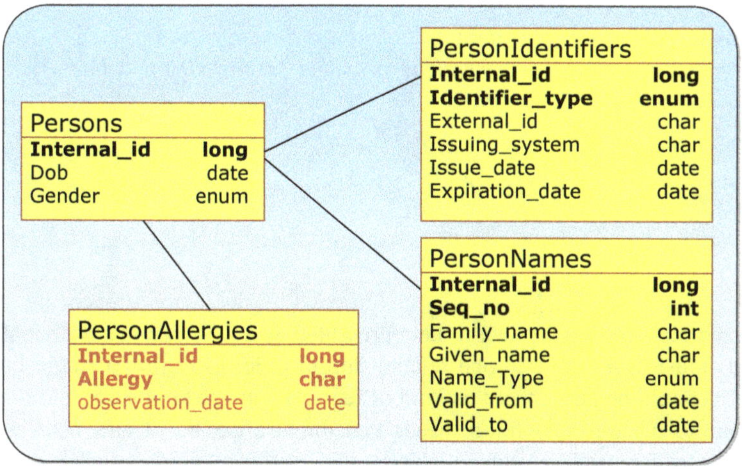

Fig. 2.27 Sample schema for requirement 7

Now the allergy information is migrated to another schema. Assuming that a person will not have the same allergy listed twice, this data element is made part of the primary key. This approach allows for maintaining an up-to-date set of the person's allergies without including the same allergy twice in that set, which makes sense in this simple use case (Fig. 2.27).

We could continue on with development of example data repository schema, however, the versions presented thus far are sufficient for a thorough discussion of implementation and conformance implications.

2.11.2 Conformance Discussion

In the previous subsection, a simple data repository schema was developed on behalf of the application it supports. The complexity of the resulting schema structure increased with the insertion of each new requirement, reflecting typical changes and stages in application development.

An analysis of the different data repository schemas compared with their ability to fulfill requirements for data exchange is provided next. These requirements are presented in a very simple format. Interoperability aspects are also considered in this analysis. The requirements are examined with respect to the seven example data repository schemas. The check marks simply indicate the fulfillment of the requirement.

Let's start with a simple requirement:

Data Exchange Requirement 1

The following information shall be provided (exported) on a line-oriented basis in form of a CSV file:

family name
given name
allergy 1
allergy 2

The requirement for the data to be represented as a CSV file means that all data elements must have a one-to-one relationship in order to fit into a single line. Of course, it should be noted that this kind of requirement is bad practice and does not contribute to meeting any future needs that might arise, but it aids here in comparing the different development phases with different kinds of data exchange requirements (Table 2.5).

The last data repository schema—and the most sophisticated one—can cause problems under certain circumstances (for example, if the schema is used when the ability to designate allergy 1 vs. 2 is needed) if the data exchange requirements are kept too simple (select only 2 allergies).

Data Exchange Requirement 2

(2a) A timestamp for marking the export shall be provided.
(2b) The export function shall support re-identification of the person to update previously transmitted information.
(2c) A date for each allergy shall be supported.

Table 2.5 Conformance assessment for (export) requirement 1

Schema	1	2	3	4	5	6	7
Assessment (explanation)	√	√	√	√	√	√	√ This data repository schema allows for an unlimited number of allergies to be listed; therefore, a choice must be made, e.g., to arrange the list starting with the oldest or newest allergies Another enhancement of the data repository schema could be assigning of a sequence number to manage the order of the allergies. This method of organizing these elements can guarantee that the first two entries represent the most important allergies

Table 2.6 Conformance assessment for data exchange requirement 2

Schema	1	2	3	4	5	6	7
(2b) Re-identification of person	Not supported	√	√	√	√	√	√
(2c) Allergy date	Not supported	Not supported	Not supported	Not supported	√	√	√

The first part (2a) of this requirement that deals with the export date can be solved very easily by using the creation date attribute of the filesystem for the export file. However, the most common way (although, maybe not the best way) this requirement is handled is by incorporating this information into the filename. Adding the information to the data itself does not make sense, because it is duplicate information and, therefore, misleading. An alternative approach would be to convey the information by adding meta-data into the file, but the CSV format does not allow this addition without duplicating the information. This alternative works best with other representation formats such as XML.

Table 2.6 provides a summary of application support for the other two requirements.

The next requirement deals with export and import of information.

Data Exchange Requirement 3

The following information shall be provided (in export and import direction) on a line-oriented basis in form of a CSV file:

identifier
family name
given name
allergy
allergy observation date

The allergy and allergy observation date shall be appended to the line for as many occurrences as present in the data set.

The CSV format can be used as long as repeating information is appended at the end of the line. This simple approach allows for appending tuples of data, but its use is strongly discouraged given that more suitable approaches exist. Of course, data with more complex structures, e.g., repeat occurrences of allergies and medications, require additional control information.

The conformance assessment evaluates the third requirement against the data repository schemas for export and import support (Table 2.7).

If the data exchange requirements are expanded, simple applications may not be able to support the requirements satisfactorily.

Table 2.7 Conformance assessment for requirement 3

Schema	1	2	3	4	5	6	7
Export	Identifier not available	No allergy observation data element			√	√	√
Import	No Identification possible, i.e., this information is ignored, possibly leading to duplicate records	No allergy observation data element					√
	Unable to handle more than two allergies						

The step-by-step development of an example application, along with the evaluation of the appropriate data repository schema needed to support data exchange requirements, leads to a very simple conclusion: an application is not always conformant to given requirements, at least not without further organizational directives!

The data repository schema represents the different maturity levels of an application. The complexity of the schema depends on the set of requirements, and usually this complexity is increased over time. Each level added to the schema to support a specific requirement may prove to be too simple/immature, suitable, or too complex/powerful.

2.12 Summary

This chapter explains basic architectural components and elements that are directly related to interfaces and their behavior. All data exchange requirements are closely tied to the underlying architecture of the application.

A key point identified by the authors is that the development of an interface is not independent from the underlying application. All relevant terms, and their implications for and interrelations with an application, have been defined and explained. An example of the steps involved in application development (represented as a data repository schema) is given to illustrate the challenges of establishing an interface while dealing with changing requirements. Furthermore, this example also demonstrates that, without additional guidance and implementation and/or organizational directives, each combination of functional and data exchange requirements may lead to problematic situations.

The primary purpose of an application is to support a user in their workflow. Therefore, an application typically is not designed to match a single data exchange standard. The example presented demonstrates the difficulties of matching a single set of requirements, depending on how these requirements are formulated. Having an application match a set of distinct interoperability specifications is unlikely for a variety of reasons including

The application has to meet other requirements beyond interoperability, and they may conflict with the interoperability requirements.

There is no guarantee that multiple interoperability specs won't conflict with each other, thus making it impossible for an application to be structured in accordance with both.

Legacy data within live instances of the application may make it difficult to change the underlying structure.

Interoperability standards developers must understand the application needs of the systems that are likely to implement the standards and then work to develop standards that are compatible with these needs. Vendors should support this process by providing information about their applications' functionality to the standards developers. This collaboration will help ensure that the applications will be more in line with the end user needs relative to using the data while also supporting interoperable data exchange. Standards developers must keep in mind, however, that, while this collaboration is needed, new and evolving standards must drive the industry toward the desired state for health IT interoperability and not merely document requirements based on applications' existing capabilities.

References

1. Blobel B, Holena M: *Comparing middleware concepts for advanced healthcare system architectures*. International Journal of Medical Informatics 1997;46:69-85.
2. Blobel B, Holena M: *Comparison, Evaluation, and Possible Harmonisation of the HL7, DHE, and CORBA Middleware*. In: Dudeck J, Blobel B, Lordieck W, Bürkle T (Edrs.): New Technologies in Hospital Information Systems, pp. 40-47. Series Studies in Health Technology and Informatics, Vol. 45. IOS Press, Amsterdam; 1997.
3. Blobel B: *Analysis, Design and Implementation of Secure and Interoperable Distributed Health Information Systems*. Series Studies in Health Technology and Informatics, Vol. 89. IOS Press, Amsterdam; 2002, pages 12-31.
4. Bundesverband der Krankenhaus-IT-Leiterinnen/Leiter e.V., http://www.kh-it.de, last accessed August, 13 2015.
5. HL7 V3 Product Suite, http://www.hl7.org/implement/standards/product_brief.cfm?product_id=186, last accessed December 14, 2015.
6. HL7 V2 Product Suite, http://www.hl7.org/implement/standards/product_brief.cfm?product_id=185, last accessed December 14, 2015.

Chapter 3
Healthcare Standards Landscape

At the heart of healthcare information technology interoperability are the data exchange standards. This chapter provides background about the organizations that create assemble these standards that create solutions for given use cases. In addition the chapter provides an overview of relevant worldwide standards. An introduction of the most widely used standards such as the suite provided by HL7 is also presented.

3.1 Introduction

If a vendor has to implement a specific data exchange with another communication partner and the partner is not using a common data exchange (communication) standard,[1] this vendor has to develop customized software to convert the information received from the communication partner into their own internal data format. If the vendor has multiple communication partners, this situation unnecessarily results in substantial expenditures, because different data formats must be implemented for each partner; therefore, market forces will provide the impetus for the vendors to agree on a few uniform standards.

The outcome is that, over the years, a variety of communication standards have been developed in healthcare specified by a number of organizations and institutions. In some cases, the standards are complementary, while in other cases they are competing. The most relevant data exchange standards in healthcare are HL7 v2.x and V3. As of this writing, HL7 FHIR® (Fast Healthcare Interoperability Resources) is progressing very quickly and is attracting a lot of interest, so readers should monitor its development.

Electronic Data Interchange (EDI) is the generic term for "intervention-free" exchange of messages for controlling business processes. "Intervention-free" means

[1]The term *data exchange standard* is used interchangeably with *communication standard.*

F. Oemig and R. Snelick, *Healthcare Interoperability Standards Compliance Handbook*, DOI 10.1007/978-3-319-44839-8_3

that only computer programs are involved in the exchange of structured data and that no manual (human) intervention is necessary. In the early days of EDI, only data were transmitted, for example, the data used in orders or invoices. Over time, the use of EDI was extended to documents and other structured information. The data exchange standards described in this book are a specialization of EDI.

EDI standards are specified by official bodies commonly referred to as Standards Developing Organizations (SDO) and are published in the form of specifications. Each SDO has established its own set of rules for specification of data exchange standards. Both the SDOs and the rules vary by country, region, industry, and initiator.

While no formal requirements are generated by authors of data exchange standards, it is important for these authors to include expertise from both information technology (IT) or information and communication technology (ICT) oriented organizations, as well domain content organizations (e.g., cancer registries, public health agencies or professional associations), in the process. Typically, collaborative efforts yield improved specifications in terms of maturity and quality.

Consensus based standards are developed by a community of stakeholders and usually include industry participants and government agencies. Agreement is achieved by an incremental and recursive process that is time consuming, especially when new participants join and cause topics to be revisited. Prolonged delays sometimes cause industry organizations with significant market influence to develop and use their proprietary solution. Such instruments are referred to as de facto standards, and, if they are not universally adopted, which is often the case, hinder interoperability.

3.2 Standards Developing Organizations

The following information provides an overview of some of the major SDOs and their most popular data exchange standards, some of which will be explained in detail in subsequent sections of this chapter.

3.2.1 UNECE

The independent industry-standard EDI UN/EDIFACT [1, 2, 3] was developed by the United Nations (UN) through the *United Nations Economic Commission for Europe* (UNECE) and was published as ISO standard 9735 in 1987. This particular standard is in widespread use in Europe; for example, it forms the basis for the reimbursement declaration pursuant to German §301 SGB V [4] and the technical appendix 3 (TA-3) [5], and 4 (TA-4) for pharmacy data [5].

As mentioned already, EDIFACT is one EDI standard. It is the abbreviation for *United Nations Electronic Data Interchange For Administration, Commerce and Transport,* and its primary purpose is to simplify ordering of items/goods as well as billing among trading partners.

The United Nations' *Centre for Trade Facilitation and Electronic Business* (CEFACT) is associated with the UNECE and is the department responsible for defining the standard.

EDIFACT represents a family of standards using the same basic data exchange mechanism. Numerous domain-specific subsets have been created based on EDIFACT:

• CEFIC—Chemical Industry	• EDILIBE—Bookstore
• EANCOM—Consumer Products	• EDITEC—Sanitary
• EDIBDB—Construction Materials	• EDITEX—Textile
• EDIFICE—High Tech Industry	• EDITRANS—Transport
• EDIFOR—Trucking	• EDIWHEEL—Tires
• EDIFURN—Furniture	• ODA/ODIF—Document Formats
• EDIGAS—Gas	• ODETTE—Automotive
• EDILEKTRO—Electricity	• RINET—Insurance

Within the European Union (EU), several libraries for the healthcare sector have been defined as well.

- MEDPID—Person Identification
- MEDPRE—Medical Prescriptions
- MEDREQ—Medical Service Request
- MEDRRT—Medical Service Report
- MEDRUQ—Medical Resource Usage and Cost

With the emergence of the HL7 standards, however, *Comité Européen de Normalisation* (CEN), which is the European institution for standards and norms, has decided not to use EDIFACT any longer. Some countries have followed the guidance not to use EDIFACT while others have not. As an example, Germany is still using a specific EDIFACT based communication protocol for §301 SGB V (billing). This decision was originally influenced by the use of EDIFACT in the United Kingdom (UK), but the UK has subsequently moved to HL7.

3.2.2 ASC (US)

In the US and Canada, the *Accredited Standards Committee* (ASC) is the prevailing SDO. This organization recently published ANSI X.12, which is a logistic standard that supports orders, deliveries, goods receipts, invoices, and payments [X.12] within and beyond the healthcare domain.

3.2.3 ASTM (US)

The *American Society for Testing and Materials* (ASTM) [6], founded in 1898 as the *American Section* of the *International Association for Testing and Materials* (IATM), claims to be the largest community for developing standards. Several thousand of their committees are working on more than 12,000 standards. ASTM annually publishes a book that covers the 15 sections of interest listed below plus a master index.

• Iron and Steel Products • Nonferrous Metal Products • Construction • Textiles • Plastics • Rubber • Medical Devices and Services • Electrical Insulation and Electronics	• Metals Test Methods and Analytical Procedures • Petroleum Products, Lubricants, and Fossil Fuels • Paints, Related Coatings, and Aromatics • Water and Environmental Technology • Nuclear, Solar, and Geothermal Energy • General Methods and Instrumentation • General Products, Chemical Specialties, and End Use Products • Index to all sections and volumes

Some of the ASTM standards are used as the foundation for other standards, as will be explained in the following sub-sections.

3.2.4 HL7

Health Level Seven (HL7®) originated in 1987 as a group of companies that came together in Palo Alto, California, to collaborate on standardizing healthcare data exchange, specifically between applications within a hospital. A whitepaper is available that summarizes a vast amount of material on the early history of HL7 [7].

Shortly after the HL7 organization was formed, the first version of the HL7 standard (HL7 1.0, [8]) was developed based on the *American Society for Testing and Materials* (ASTM) standards [6]. After HL7's accreditation by the *American National Standards Institute* (ANSI), the subsequent publications (the family of the HL7 2.x versions also known as "v2") became widely used and are an ANSI standard.

The family of 2.x versions started with the rudimentary HL7 version 2.1, which was quickly replaced by version 2.2. The focus of use was a hospital's internal communications. Even today, "HL7 v2" is often associated with inpatient types of communications, although this HL7 family of standards now covers much more than just intra-hospital data exchange.

HL7 [9] was originally designed purely to communicate patient-related administrative data. Since that time, however, this standard has been expanded to include the exchange of medical data that captures the whole spectrum of healthcare and social services. Communication is the purpose of the entire event-oriented HL7 message exchange.

HL7 now consists of a family of standards that are cited here, and they all deal with the exchange of data:

- HL7 version 2.x
- HL7 Version 3
- Clinical Document Architecture (CDA) Release 1, 1999 (independent of HL7 V3)
- CDA Release 2, 2005 (being based on HL7 V3)
- Clinical Context Object Working Group (CCOW)
- Guideline Interchange Format (GLIF)
- GELLO, an expression language
- Arden Syntax for knowledge representation
- Fast Healthcare Interoperability Resources (FHIR).

3.2.4.1 Affiliates

In 1993, some countries began to form groups of local representatives associated with the HL7 organization. Germany [10] and the Netherlands [11] were the first two affiliates that tried to adopt the standards. Especially in Germany, a small group of activists has interpreted (translated) the v2.x standard into German to support national extensions and has released an adaptation (extension) to national requirements.

Now more than 35 affiliates have been formed around the world. The most relevant parts of the HL7 standard have been translated into other languages, such as Japanese and Spanish; and educational materials and e-learning courses have been developed globally to teach users about the standard.

3.2.5 *DICOM*

In 1985, the *American College of Radiologists* (ACR) started an initiative to connect imaging devices/equipment used in the healthcare setting. At the time, implementers used a proprietary protocol to provide a communication solution, which was mostly based on a 50-pin connector using the OSI model. With the introduction of Internet technology, this communication protocol has moved to ISO using TCP/IP, and the overall design has been improved and has stabilized. In 1988 the second version of the standard was published as *ACR-NEMA Standards Publication No. 300-1988.*

Today, this protocol is known as *Digital Imaging and Communication in Medicine* (DICOM) and is available as Version 3.0. Instead of providing new releases/versions, different supplements and change proposals have been incorporated into it. As a result, an update is published every two years. Due to a liaison with ISO, the DICOM standards are also labeled as ISO specifications; a bundle of those specifications as an ISO spec is underway.

3.2.6 KBV, ZI and QMS (Germany)

In the 1980s and 90s, the German *Kassenärztliche Bundesvereinigung* (KBV) [12], the statutory healthcare organization for ambulatory healthcare, defined a standard for transferring billing data from *General Practitioners* offices to the responsible *Kassenärztliche Vereinigung* (KV). This standard was called *Abrechnungsdatentransfer*[2] (ADT).

In the early 90s the KBV wanted to prevent General Practitioners in Germany from losing all their patients' healthcare data if they change a software provider. Therefore, the *Zentralinstitut für die kassenärztliche Versorgung* (ZI) defined a first version of a standard that enables the exchange of a basic data set for patients. The outcome supports and promotes data migration from one system to another. This format is known as the *Behandlungsdatentransfer* (BDT).

Subsequently, the same data exchange foundation has been used to provide different specifications for different purposes/domains. The so-called *Datentransfer* (xDT)-family was born, which mainly was developed and maintained by KBV in cooperation with the ZI and with scientific institutes such as the Institute for Medical Informatics of the University Gießen. Since 2011, the *Qualitätsring Medizinische Software* (QMS) [13], a consortium of software vendors and healthcare providers, has been maintaining all standards of the xDT family that are outside of billing purposes (for which the KBV is responsible). Meanwhile, the following set of standards for different domains has been released (Table 3.1).

Today, the (xDT)-family allows for the exchange of physician letters (*eArztbrief*) or medication schemes using, for example, BDT. The main focus of the further development of the xDT-family standards is not on syntax aspects (XML could be used) but on describing all semantic aspects of all data used in ambulatory healthcare in Germany.

3.2.7 KV-Telematik (Germany)

The KV Telematik GmbH is a subsidiary of the KBV and is responsible for managing IT related topics. This organization is currently working on establishing a

[2]The first documentation uses the term *Abrechnungsdatenträger*, because the standard ADT was originally defined for floppy disks.

Table 3.1 xDT family of standards

Standard	German description	Domain	First developed by	Maintained by
ADT	Abrechnungsdatentransfer	Billing	KBV	KBV
BDT	Behandlungsdatentransfer	Administration/Medical documentation	ZI	QMS
GDT	Gerätedatentransfer	Devices	QMS	QMS
KADT	Kurärztliche Abrechnungsdaten	Billing	KBV	KBV
KVDT	Kassenärztliche Vereinigungen Datentransfer	Billing	KBV	KBV
LDT	Labordatentransfer	Laboratory	KBV	QMS
SADT	Abrechnungsdaten zum Schwangerschaftsabbruch NRW	Billing on induced abortion	KBV	KBV
WDT	Wissenschaftsdatentransfer	Research	Universities of Hannover and Göttingen	QMS

secure communication infrastructure to allow for data exchange among physician offices. This infrastructure is called *KV connect* and is based on proprietary protocols.

KV Telematik offers certain content specifications for defining the payloads that are exchanged. One of their projects is the *eArztbrief* specification, which refers to the official specification of the German "Arztbrief 2014" implementation guide that is based on CDA.

3.2.8 NCPDP (USA)

The National Council for Prescription Drug Programs (NCPDP) is an ANSI accredited SDO working on standards for the pharmacy industry [14]. NCPDP uses a consensus-building process to create national standards for real-time, electronic exchange of healthcare information. NCPDP's primary focus is on information exchange for prescribing, dispensing, monitoring, managing and paying for medications and pharmacy services crucial to quality healthcare.

NCPDP standards are named in federal legislation, including HIPAA, MMA, HITECH, and Meaningful Use (MU). NCPDP advises regulatory agencies, actively participates in the rule-making process, educates legislators about NCPDP's problem-solving forum and consensus-based solutions, and serves as a resource to policy makers.

NCPDP's list of standards includes:

• Audit Standard • Batch Transaction • Billing Unit • Data Dictionary • External Code List • Functional Profiles for Electronic Health Record (EHR) Systems • Financial Information Reporting • Formulary and Benefit • Manufacturer Rebates • Operating Rules for Connectivity • Medicaid Subrogation • Medical Rebates Data Submission	• Pharmacy and/or Combination ID Card • Post Adjudication • Prescription File Transfer • Retiree Drug Subsidy Standard Implementation Guide • Prior Authorization Transfer • SCRIPT • Specialized • Structured and Codified Sig Format • Telecommunication • Uniform Healthcare Payer Data Standard Implementation Guide • XML Standard Implementation • Universal Claim Forms

SCRIPT is the most relevant NCPDP standard for the context of this book and is explained in more detail in Appendix. SCRIPT was developed for transmitting prescription information electronically between prescribers, providers, and other entities.

3.2.9 OASIS

Organization for the Advancement of Structured Information Standards (OASIS) is a non-profit consortium that drives the development, convergence, and adoption of open standards for the global information society [15].

OASIS was founded under the name "SGML Open" in 1993. It began as a consortium of vendors and users devoted to developing guidelines for interoperability among products that support the Standard Generalized Markup Language (SGML). The consortium changed its name to "OASIS" in 1998 to reflect an expanded scope of technical work.

OASIS promotes industry consensus and produces worldwide standards for security, cloud computing, SOA, web-services, the smart grid, electronic publishing, emergency management, and other areas. OASIS open standards offer the potential to lower cost, stimulate innovation, grow global markets, and protect the right of free choice of technology.

OASIS members broadly represent the marketplace of public and private sector technology leaders, users, and influencers. The consortium has more than 5,000 participants representing over 600 organizations and individual members in more than 65 countries.

Some relevant and popular standards developed and released by OASIS are:

- Darwin Information Typing Architecture (DITA)
- DocBook
- ebXML[3]: Registry Information Model, Message Service Specification
- eXtensible Access Control Markup Language (XACML)
- Open Document Format for Office Applications (OpenDocument)
- Security Assertion Markup Language (SAML)
- Universal Description, Discovery and Integration (UDDI)
- Web Service Security (WS-Security).

3.3 Profile Development Organizations

Besides the set of SDOs already presented in Sect. 3.2 of this chapter, several other organizations exist that do not develop standards themselves but re-use and constrain the standards developed by other groups for application to a certain use case. These organizations are called *Profile Development Organizations* (PDO). The most prominent ones are introduced in the sub-sections to follow.

It is important to note that the term "profile" has different meanings depending on the context in which it is used. A distinction must be made regarding its use and granularity. At a single specification level, profile is used to describe a set of constrained requirements of a broader specification. Profile is also used to define requirements for a collection of specifications for a specific use case or workflow. The former is often referred to as a conformance profile and the latter as an integration profile. PDOs often address both types of profiles. The different ways of using the term profile are expanded in chapters to follow.

3.3.1 IHE

Integrating the Healthcare Enterprise (IHE) is the most prominent global initiative acting as a PDO in the healthcare domain. IHE was founded in 1998 originally to harmonize the discrepancies among HL7 version 2.x and DICOM. Hence, IHE started in the radiology domain, but subsequently it has been expanded to other domains.

A very important aspect of IHE is the separation of its supporting community into two roles: (1) users who provide requirements and details for a specific workflow or use case; and (2) vendors who specify how they are fulfilling those requirements in the form of technical specifications. The scope of the use cases is

[3]This is the basis for IHE ITI XDS.

limited, enabling a complete cycle to be performed in a single year and preventing endless discussions.

The specifications are implemented by vendors and subsequently tested and, thus, verified during a connect-a-thon. Finally, the specifications are published in the form of Technical Frameworks. Figure 3.1 illustrates the IHE annual cycle for creating Technical Frameworks starting in the upper left corner with the documentation of the user requirements.

As of this writing, IHE has created a set of such specifications, which are called Technical Frameworks, for the following domains:

• Anatomic Pathology	• Patient Care Coordination
• Cardiology	• Patient Care Devices
• Dental	• Pharmacy
• Eye Care	• Quality, Research and Public Health
• IT Infrastructure	• Radiation Oncology
• Laboratory	• Radiology (including mammography and nuclear medicine)

For each of the domains listed above, a Technical Framework (TF) is provided that is publicly available for download. Each TF consists of at least two, and sometimes four, Volumes.

- Volume 1: Integration Profiles
- Volume 2: Transactions
- Volume 3: Cross-Transaction Specifications, Content and other details
- Volume 4: National Extensions.

In Volume 1, all the integration profiles for a certain domain are listed and described in detail.

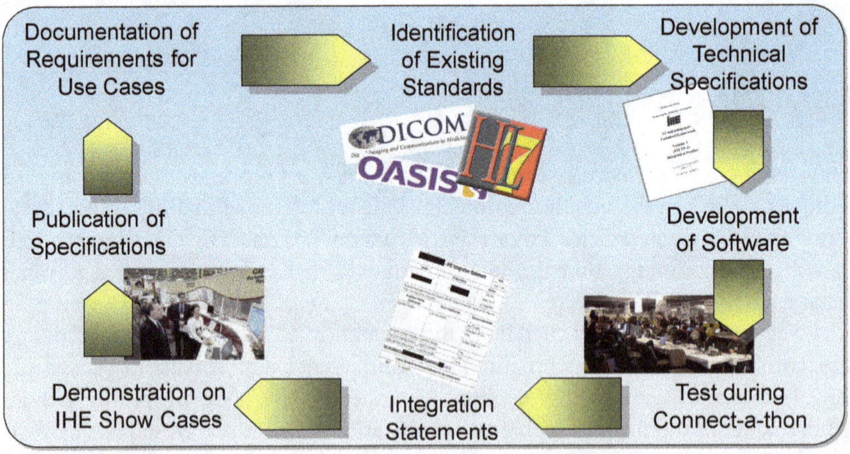

Fig. 3.1 IHE annual cycle

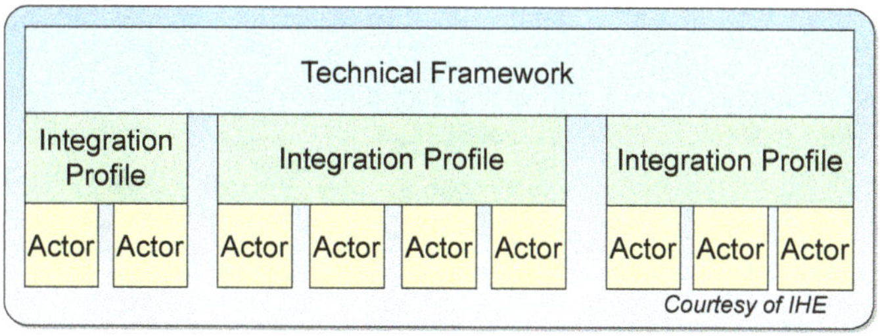

Fig. 3.2 IHE Technical Framework

As illustrated in Fig. 3.2, a Technical Framework is a collection of integration profiles. An integration profile is a set of sequenced interactions among different actors. A very simple example thereof is the Patient Administration Management (PAM) integration profile, which consists of four different actors as is shown in Fig. 3.3.

Two of the actors are the senders of information and the other two actors are receivers of information. The integration profiles are designed to allow for maximum flexibility so that they are applicable in most situations. Taking PAM as an example, the presented actors can be combined in different ways. The most common two ways are shown in Fig. 3.4. It must be noted that real world systems are, in the end, playing the roles as presented in the form of actors in the different profiles. So the hospital information system (HIS) will act as the source, sending the patient's demographics and encounter information to the various subsystems that are acting as the consumer.

According to the way IHE works, the integration profiles must be treated as a global directive for all countries. (Most of the specifications are not restricted to certain countries but are used as is.)

The process IHE is using to specify and publish the TFs includes providing an official ISO standard and an antetype for other communities and bodies to use to profile existing standards for their own needs. Countries have the opportunity to issue country-specific additions to those technical frameworks, and the so-called "national extensions" are published as volume 4.

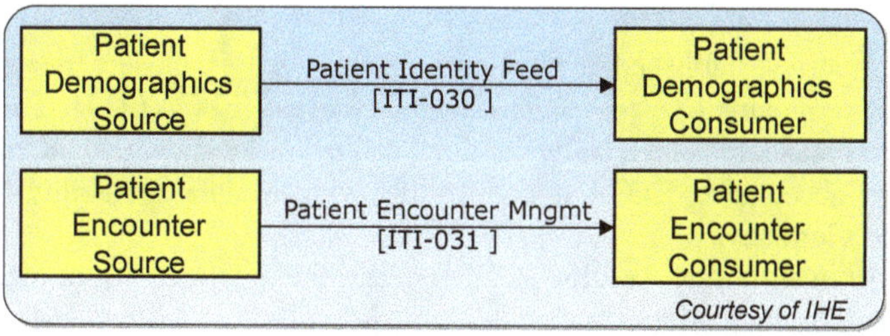

Fig. 3.3 IHE ITI PAM transaction (as an example)

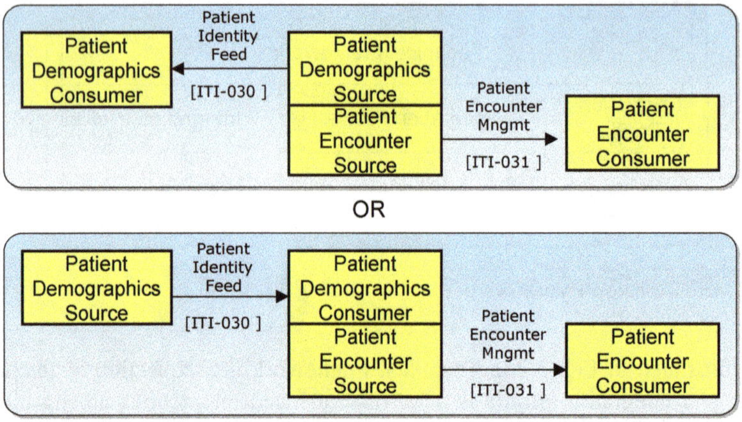

Fig. 3.4 IHE ITI PAM grouping of transactions (as an example)

IHE also promotes and organizes "connect-a-thons". This name is a combination of the two words "connection" and "marathon". The first part of the name symbolizes that systems are connected, while the last part introduces the notion of intensive testing of the participating systems. IHE testing employs a number of incremental testing methods. First, vendors conduct conformance testing of their products. This task involves testing in isolation to determine if the system implements the requirements specified in the TFs correctly; these tests are called pre-connect-a-thon tests. Interoperability testing (peer-to-peer testing) is conducted at the connect-a-thon in which scores of vendors bring their products to a central site and live-monitored tests are performed over a period of a week [16]. Such concentrated events are useful as vendors can interact with many other vendors in a short period of time, and they currently are held once a year in the United States, Europe, and Asia. Connect-a-thons are receiving increasing interest, because they provide a convenient environment where vendors have the opportunity for testing their prototypes and final products to ensure working interoperability.

3.3.2 ELGA (Austria)

In 2009, Austria established a new organization that is closely related to the Austrian government: *ELektronische GesundheitsAkte* (ELGA) [17]. This organization selects standards and IHE integration profiles for local use. To facilitate more wide-spread acceptance, ELGA is cooperating with the interoperability forums in Austria and Germany.

The most well-known results of ELGA are the publications of CDA-based implementation guides, including:

- physician discharge letter (from hospital)
- rehabilitation discharge letter
- laboratory reports
- image reports.

3.3.3 eHealth Suisse (Switzerland)

In Switzerland, the government has formed an agreement with the different cantons—aka federal states—to establish a national institution for ehealth. It is funded by the government and the Swiss conference of regional directors for healthcare. The primary goal is to provide some guidance to ensure reliability for planning and financing ehealth [18].

Their strategy is to provide a set of foundational specifications—like modules in a toolbox—which can then be combined in a flexible way (Fig. 3.5). The most prominent is the CDA-CH family of implementation guides. The first version was published in 2008, facilitating the German, French, and Italian languages. In 2011, it was enhanced by a guideline describing how to provide new modules to this set of implementation guides.

This set of documents specifies the fundamentals for exchanging clinical documents in Switzerland, facilitating use of CDA Release 2. Figure 3.5 demonstrates how the different exchange formats (aka, documents types) are assembled from different modules. Currently the set of documents cover the following topics:

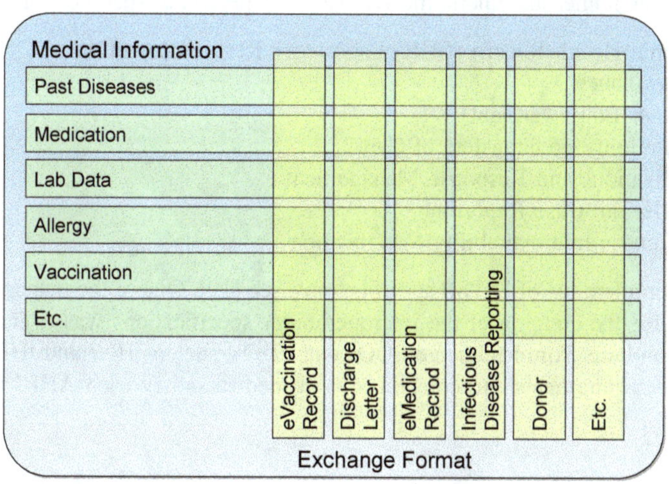

Fig. 3.5 Exchange formats defined by eHealth Suisse

- lab reports
- transplantation
- infectious diseases
- vaccination.

To foster the process of establishing interoperability specifications, Switzerland has joined IHTSDO as an affiliate to enable SNOMED CT codes to be used in their national IGs.

These implementation guides—and also the Austrian and German ones—are permanently harmonized and are being developed further, thus improving the national specifications through sharing of others' experiences.

3.3.4 HITSP (US)

The Healthcare Information Technology Standards Panel (HITSP) was an organization created to harmonize and integrate standards that meet the clinical and business needs for sharing information among organizations and systems [19]. This effort was a cooperative partnership between caregivers, developers, government agencies, and end users, and it also included international experts. The initiative was founded in October, 2005, under contract from the United States Department of Health and Human Services, and it ended in April, 2010. The harmonized standards targeted the priority use cases identified by the American Health Information Community (AHIC) recommendations. Although HITSP is no longer in operation, many of the outcomes, lessons learned, and processes, as well as much of the knowledge, have been leveraged in other efforts, such as the S&I Framework.

As well as numerous others, the HITSP interoperability specifications include:

- Electronic Health Record (EHR) Laboratory Results Reporting
- Biosurveillance
- Consumer Empowerment
- Consultations and Transfers of Care
- Immunizations and Response Management
- Public Health Case Reporting
- EHR-Centric Interoperability Specification

For a complete list of HITSP specifications, see [19]. One of the mandates given to HITSP for the creation of the interoperability specifications was to incorporate existing standards from healthcare SDOs and PDOs, such as HL7 and IHE. HITSP added new requirements and constructs as needed to satisfy each AHIC use case.

3.3.5 S&I Framework (US)

One responsibility of the Office of the National Coordinator (ONC) is to curate the set of standards and specifications that support interoperability, ensuring that they can be assembled into solutions for a variety of health information exchange scenarios [20]. ONC established the *Standards and Interoperability (S&I) Framework* in January, 2011, to develop standards and implementation guidance to support national health outcomes and healthcare priorities [21]. This initiative is United States-centric and provides a community-led open forum to work on harmonized interoperability specifications collaboratively. A key focus is to ensure that all resulting specifications align with The Centers for Medicare and Medicaid (CMS) EHR Meaningful Use (MU) requirements and support the Nationwide Health Information Network (NwHIN) [22].

The S&I effort employs activities that support the complete standards development life-cycle process as depicted in Fig. 3.6 [22]. Building on a foundation that promotes reuse and harmonization, the S&I Framework includes the following elements for addressing the interoperability challenge:

- Use cases and health information standards
- Tools to support the adoption and use of standards
- Process to evaluate, test, and refine the standards exchange
- Certified products that meet security and interoperability standards
- Policies and governance structures for the Nationwide Health Information Network
- Technical infrastructure (directories and certificate authority) for the Nationwide Health Information Network.

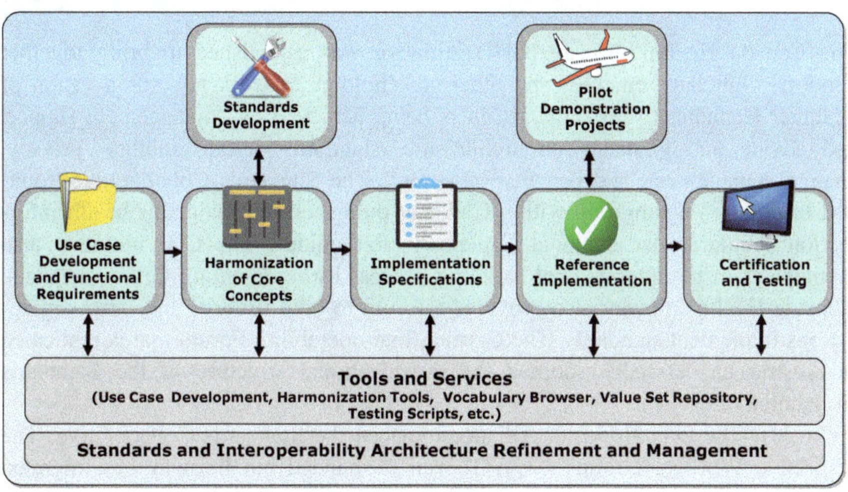

Fig. 3.6 S&I framework standards development process [21]

The S&I Framework works closely with HL7, IHE, and NIST in this process. If an existing standard is available, it is leveraged as much as possible; in many cases it provides the starting point for the development of a new standard or a profile for an existing standard. Many of the specifications created by the S&I Framework are published by HL7 and, therefore, go through the HL7 ballot process (as US-realm specifications). Many of the HL7 working group participants also participate in the S&I Framework forum, which enables alignment with and updates to the HL7 standards to be maintained. For some initiatives, NIST builds conformance test tools while the standards are still in development in order to provide feedback before final publication.

As well as numerous others, the S&I Framework initiatives include:

- Structured Data Capture
- Data Access Framework
- Blue Button Plus (allows patient access to their personal health information)
- Lab Results Interface
- Lab Orders Interface
- Clinical Quality Framework
- Data Provenance
- Transition of Care.

Some of the activities are heavily supported and driven by ONC, while others leverage the S&I Framework platform. Initiatives are fluid; new ones are added as needed (and often directed by MU needs), and others are completed or become inactive.

3.3.6 Standards Collaborative (Canada)

The Canada Health Infoway (CHI) initiative was established to bring together vendors, clinicians, citizens, and other stakeholders to work towards a vision of healthier Canadians [23]. This vision is being achieved by "management support and advice and guidance on architecture, standards, interoperability, privacy, change management, and benefit evaluation". The Standards Collaborative, founded in 2006, is a subgroup within CHI that publishes and maintains health information standards and national implementation guides. The CHI initiative also participates in the international balloting process by representing CHI's members. (Canada Health Infoway also provides a forum to help vendors and other organizations implement standards. The German Interoperability Forum that is replicated in Austria has partially adopted the organizational structure of the Standards Collaborative.

In 2016 the Digital Health Alliance replaced the Standards Collaborative. The respective Working Groups (SCWG) were disbanded but Infoway has migrated many of the working groups into collaborative communities on InfoCentral - communication and collaboration platform.

3.3.7 Interop'Santé (France)

In 1990, the laboratory information system vendors that were active in the French market, together with the major reference labs, established the non-profit association H.PR.I.M. (hereafter referred to as Hprim in this book) for the purpose of producing an interoperability standard for the exchange of orders and results between clinical laboratories. The ASTM standard E1238 (one of the ancestors of HL7 v2) was selected, adapted, translated into French, and released as the first Hprim recommendation, named "Hprim Labo". Two years later in 1992, the Hprim association opened its membership to vendors of clinic EMR systems and vendors of ambulatory EHR systems. Together with these additional contributors, the association produced a new recommendation called "Hprim Médecins" for messaging lab results to ambulatory physicians' EHR systems and also broadened the scope of the former "Hprim Labo" to include ADT messages and order messages from clinics to labs, as well as invoice and results messages from labs to clinics. The recommendation became "Hprim Santé", and from that point on kept evolving regularly until 2004. During that period the association incorporated "user" members, such as hospitals, labs, physicians.

In 1999, the association started to build a new recommendation, based on an XML syntax called "Hprim XML", carrying the same set of functional messages (patient demographics, orders, results, invoices), and adding a new set of messages to support the French Diagnosis Related Group (DRG) in hospitals and clinics.

In 2001, the public institution GMSIH played an active role in importing the IHE initiative into Europe in general, and France in particular, through the organization of a first European connect-a-thon in Paris. From 2001 to its dissolution in 2008, IHE France was a subsidiary to GMSIH.

In 2004, the H.PR.I.M association became the French affiliate of HL7 and changed its name to "HL7 France H.PR.I.M.", with a new status and internal rules.

At that point, the decision was made to stop the maintenance of "Hprim Santé" and "Hprim Médecins" and to promote instead the migration to HL7 standards embedded in IHE profiles. Only evolution of the "Hprim xml" recommendation was continued, reduced to its set of DRG messages, which had no alternative international standard.

In 2009, the GMSIH was disbanded. At that time the HL7 France H.PR.I.M association took over the "IHE France" activity, in combination with the "HL7 France" and "Hprim xml" activities, and became "Interop'Santé". During the same period the "interoperability" activities of GMSIH were transferred to the newly established public institution called ASIP Santé.

3.3.8 ASIP Santé (France)

The *Agence des systèmes d'information partagés de santé* (ASIP Santé) was created in 2009 to drive national-level competence for eHealth. This public agency set up a national interoperability framework first released in October, 2009, in close cooperation with Interop'Santé and Health IT vendor associations. This framework was focused on sharing of electronic health documents and was more than 95 % based on IHE profiles (the XDS family), with the HL7 CDAr2 standard being made mandatory for content in that framework.

The agency is in charge of the production of smart cards and certificates for health providers as well as the related Public Key Infrastructure (PKI). Its first big project was to set up the *Dossier Médical Personnel* (DMP), started by the government in order to provide each French citizen with an EHR/PHR composed of the whole history of past illnesses. The healthcare providers are requested to follow the patient's wishes by submitting the appropriate medical documentation (discharge letters, results, consultation notes, patient summaries, etc.) to the DMP [24].

In 2011, ASIP Santé provided functional and technical specifications for the DMP interfaces of health IT systems (Dossier de spécifications fonctionnelles et techniques des interfaces DMP des Logiciels de Professionnels de Santé). This specification was entirely based on the national interoperability framework released two years earlier.

From 2011 to 2015, the government agency ASIP Santé sponsored four domains in IHE: IT-Infrastructure (ITI); Patient Care Coordination (PCC); Laboratory (LAB); and Quality, Research and Public Health (QRPH). During that period, it organized yearly face-to-face meetings for the committees of these domains. In 2016, the agency gave up sponsoring LAB, which was merged into the new domain PaLM, and the sponsorship was taken over by Phast, which is discussed in the next section of this chapter.

ASIP Santé has built and maintains the interoperability framework for France health IT systems. This process is driven in close cooperation with Interop'Santé. This interoperability framework contains the French extension of the XD* family of profiles as well as the French extensions for some CDA content profiles from IHE PCC, LAB, AP.

ASIP Santé works closely with Interop'Santé on the French extensions of IHE profiles.

3.3.9 Phast (France)

Phast is a non-profit standard services organization created in 1989. Its primary goal is to develop Healthcare Information Technology Standards for the French market.

Phast started with standardizing intra-hospital medication management workflows (with a PN13[4] set of messages for prescribing medicine), and then, for the deployment of the PN13 messages, developed the appropriate semantic resource for the content (CIOsp). Then the scope was extended to medical devices, with the development and provision of the appropriate semantic resource (CIOdm). At this point, Phast generalized the experience it gained from providing semantic resources and began contributing actively to the building of the new standard CTS2, first in HL7 for the functional specification and then in OMG for the technical specification. Along with that CTS2 standardization process, Phast built a terminology server named STS (Standard Terminology Services), which is a conformant implementation of CTS2-FM. This terminology server provides the stakeholders (software vendors, hospitals, and others) with the semantic resources maintained by Phast. Taking advantage of this asset, Phast now intends to provide Systemized Nomenclature of Medicine Clinical Terms (SNOMED CT) on this terminology server. For that purpose, Phast recently signed an affiliate license with IHTSDO as well as a contract with IHTSDO, which entitles Phast to be a translator of a subset of SNOMED CT into French with the consent of the health ministry. Phast is also implementing the HL7 V3 Structured Product Labeling (SPL) standard on its terminology server.

Phast is extending the interface of STS to include a FHIR interface.

Phast is HIBCC France, and Phast also provides the location for the headquarters of Interop'Santé.

3.3.10 eSanté (Luxembourg)

Luxembourg is pursuing the same approach as Austria by creating a governmental organization called eSanté that establishes IHE integration profiles.

They are working on an interoperability specification by defining an architecture detailing how the different components should work together. The first edition addresses the most common and core integration profiles, e.g., XDS, CDA with header templates, and PIX/PDQ.

3.3.11 Interoperability Forum (Germany)

Interoperability is a topic no one group can solve alone. Based on this premise, the following major organizations in Germany that are working on the establishment of

[4]PN13 is a French standard for prescribing, dispensing, and administering medicine in hospitals. PN13 is still in use in French hospitals today. A detailed explanation can be found in Appendix.

interoperable solutions decided to merge their resources and work together collaboratively:

- HL7 Germany
- IHE Germany
- DIN
- bvitg (German vendors association)
- GMDS
- and others

The work is accomplished through various projects, the results of which can be found in the German HL7 wiki [25]. The most important projects are the IHE Cookbook, the German National Extensions for IHE ITI PAM, and a set of document specifications based on CDA. The most important task is updating the VHitG-Arztbrief (discharge letter) from 2005/2006 to the state-of-the-art knowledge as "Arztbrief 2014/15" with some detailed modules (templates) in 2016.

Some organizations and projects are built on top of the results produced from the German Interoperability Forum (Fig. 3.7). Good examples are the electronic Case Record/elektronische Fallakte (eCR/EFA), the eBPG project [26], and InfoPat project [27], all of which are creating different kinds of EHR-S on top of the same foundational specification.

Most of the other institutions and organizations are creating specifications that do not have anything to do with the overarching specifications from HL7 and IHE, but are totally proprietary. In the best case, those specifications are built based on XML.

The eHealth Planning Study ("Planungsstudie") provides a very detailed overview about the current situation in Germany and presents a possible solution to overcome the issues [PlanStud]. This proposed solution should result in a new eHealth law in Germany (end of 2015) that is intended to overcome the identified problems. Experts in this field, however, still claim they do not understand the real underlying causes for interoperability problems, resulting in a statement being made that this new law will not achieve the intended goal. In contrast to other countries' strategies of enforcing international standards, Germany will provide a registry of (interoperability) standards instead of listing and evaluating the required and

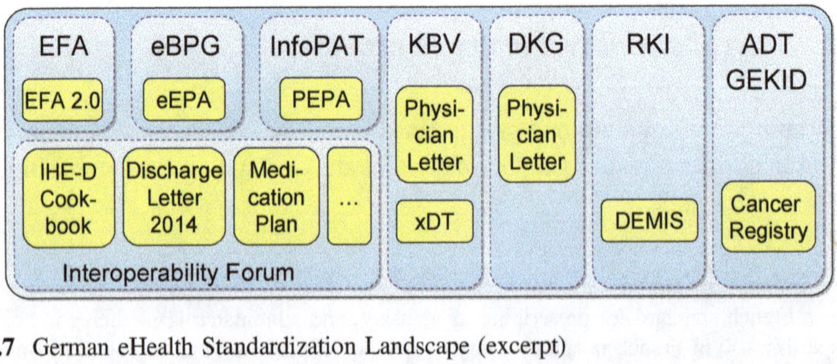

Fig. 3.7 German eHealth Standardization Landscape (excerpt)

accepted standards. The law does not provide any guidance for the quality criteria that "standards" must meet in order to become registered. The main concern is that all standards will be entered into the registry regardless of quality, thus limiting the usefulness of the registry. Another aspect of this new law is a paragraph enforcing "open interfaces", allowing patients to switch from one general practitioner (GP) to another or GPs to migrate their data from one vendor's system to another. The large number of interfaces among systems transmitting real-time data are not mentioned.

3.3.12 NHS (UK)

The *National Health Service* (NHS) is national organization managing and providing the publicly funded healthcare system for United Kingdom (UK). It is the largest and the oldest single-payer healthcare system in the world. Primarily funded through the general taxation system, the NHS provides healthcare to every legal resident in the United Kingdom, with most services being provided for free[5] at the point of use.

The NHS delivers the majority of healthcare in UK, including primary care, in-patient care, long-term healthcare, ophthalmology, and dentistry. The National Health Service Act of 1946 came into effect on 5 July 1948. Private health care has continued parallel to the NHS, paid for largely by private insurance. It is used by about 8 % of the population, generally as an add-on to NHS services. In the first decade of the 21st century, the private sector started to be used more by the NHS to increase its capacity.

The NHS is largely funded from general taxation with a small amount being contributed by National Insurance payments. The UK government department responsible for the NHS is the Department of Health, headed by the Secretary of State for Health. Most of the expenditures of the Department of Health (£98.7 billion in 2008–2009) are for the NHS [28].

Several years ago, the NHS decided to use EDIFACT as its primary communication standard for healthcare; but this decision was revised with the introduction of HL7 Version 3 and its modern methodology. NHS became a sponsor of this approach by working on a toolset, which today is known as model driven health tools (MDHT). Using MDHT, NHS started to work in parallel on its own

[5]Free healthcare at the point of use comes from the core principles at the founding of the National Health Service by the United Kingdom Labor government in 1948. In practice, "free at the point of use" normally means that anyone legitimately fully registered with the system (i.e., in possession of an NHS number), including UK citizens and legal immigrants, can access the full breadth of critical and non-critical medical care without any out-of-pocket payment. Some specific NHS services do, however, require a financial contribution from the patient. Since 1948, patients have been charged for some services such as eye tests, dental care, prescriptions, and aspects of long-term care. These charges are often lower than equivalent services offered by a private health care provider.

information models based on HL7 Version 3. Unfortunately, this approach did not earn acceptance and, therefore, can be said to be unsuccessful. To overcome this problem, NHS has migrated their communication infrastructure to HL7 version 2.4, facilitated by a new toolset called the Interoperability Tool Kit (ITK).

3.3.13 SMART Health IT on FHIR® (US)

When the SMART[6] Health IT initiative was started in 2009, the main idea behind it was to foster the development of mobile applications. A standardized interface between mobile app[7] clients and centralized EHR systems was expected to stimulate app development to enable competition and better quality. Ideally, a mobile app can be used with any EHR system as long as the interfaces are designed as specified by the profiles. Due to the latest improvements in and increasing acceptance of HL7 FHIR®, SMART Health IT is migrating to FHIR and OAuth as its base standards for its mobile app development [29].

The US government initially funded this project. By 2015, a number of large vendors had joined SMART via the Argonaut project.

The SMART app gallery provides an impressive overview about the mobile apps that are currently available.

3.3.13.1 Profiles

The SMART initiative provides profiles for the following FHIR® resources:

- Patient Demographics
- Allergy or Intolerance
- Immunizations
- Conditions
- Procedures
- Family History
- Smoking Status
- Medication Prescription
- Medication Dispense
- Vital Signs
- Lab Results

Unfortunately, the profiles are not yet provided on a central server using the profile mechanism FHIR® describes, but this most likely will be offered in the near

[6]SMART is neither an acronym nor abbreviation.

[7]With mobile apps, small software components run on smart devices such as mobile phones and tablet computers. The primary purpose is ubiquitous use, everywhere, anytime.

future once FHIR® has become stabilized. Each profile is currently listed with its corresponding requirements and using its own binding syntax. As an example, for patient demographics the following requirements are listed:

- 1 or more medical record numbers in Patient.identifier
- 1 or more names in Patient.name
- 1 administrative gender in Patient.gender

For more details, we refer the reader to the explanation about FHIR in Chap. 4.

3.4 Overview of Widely Used Standards

The aforementioned institutions and organizations (SDOs and PEOs) use more or less the same communication standards, which are briefly presented in this section along with their essential characteristics. To a certain extent, the standard fundamentals and constituent components are key elements in determining how useful the standard is for achieving interoperability. How these aspects play a role will become apparent and will be discussed later in the next chapter.

3.4.1 HL7

As mentioned already, HL7 International provides a set of standards that are used for different purposes, each of which will be discussed in detail in the following sub-sections.

3.4.1.1 Version 2.x and 3.0

HL7 version 2.x (v2.x®) and HL7 version 3.0 (V3®) are designed for the exchange of patient-related administrative and clinical data in the form of messages.

Version 2.x has been released in the form of different versions with individual numbers, e.g., v2.1, v2.2, etc., at irregular intervals.

Version 3.0 is an HL7 standard that was developed beginning in 1995. It is based on its own methodology called *Message Development Framework* (MDF) [30]; MDF was further developed as the *HL7 Development Framework* (HDF) [31]). Due to the underlying methodology, updates of Version 3 are released each year by combining the newest results of the different components, such as data types, domain models, and vocabularies, that comprise this standard.

It is not always possible to predict which "family" of standards will overshadow the others. Most likely, all of the standards will play a role in targeted areas for which they are best suited. From a standards organization perspective, V3 was anticipated to make in-roads into and eventually replace v2; however, in practice, the large installed base of v2 will prevent this from occurring in the foreseeable future, and possibly forever. Therefore, the focus for version 3 will be in new domains that are not covered with v2.x.

Both the v2.x and V3 standards are explained in greater depth in the next chapter.

3.4.1.2 CDA

The Clinical Document Architecture (CDA®) [32, 33] specifies the structure of clinical documents. Unlike a message-based standard, such as v2.x or V3, with CDA a persistent document is transmitted where the emphasis is upon human readable text, while at the same time providing the relationships between the data items, context, and external references, as well as accountability and justification information. CDA attempts to create a framework for the medical context in which a clinical document of any type (doctor's letter, findings, notes, etc.) can be implemented. The aim is to format any document so that it is both readable by humans and by the computer. Hence, structuring and encoding of the text is necessary based on a markup language. This encoding is achieved using the eXtensible Markup Language (XML) [34] that can contain any text, including known markups for semantic information.[8]

The CDA document is divided into two parts: the header and the body. The accompanying information (e.g., patient, author) is placed in the header as meta-data, and the body contains the text and additional clinical data. The body may contain a complete document in display-oriented form such as PDF (Portable Data Format) or RTF (Rich Text Format), and then the header is only used for the transmission of additional information (meta-data). It is assumed that at least (ASCII) text with corresponding XML markup is submitted. A CDA document can be prepared with the help of so-called XML style sheets to make the text easily readable by the user. In addition, the text can be enriched with further markup, and a computer program can extract these details in a structured way and re-use them.

It is important to note that there are different releases of CDA (Release 1 and Release 2) that are based on different versions (0098 and 0207 respectively) of the HL7 RIM (*Reference Information Model*) [HL7-RIM]. Release 3 and a more general format, called *Structured Document Architecture* (SDA), are currently being developed. Furthermore, different levels can be defined that use the aforementioned markup in the body for various use cases.

[8]The beginning of the CDA specification goes back before the availability of XML, so the work was based on the Standard Generalized Markup Language (SGML) [SGML].

3.4.1.3 CCOW

Bringing object- and service-orientation to HL7, the Clinical Context Object Working Group (CCOW®) [CCOW] deals with so-called "visual integration", meaning that different applications share their work context. The individual applications exchange context information via a special Context Manager, i.e., a special software component that is running as a service in the background and keeping track of the current context. The context is about patient and/or user-related information, i.e., the patient data currently being processed or the user logging into or off of the system. Synchronizing a workstation's desktop applications eliminates time-consuming steps for the user. The CCOW® specification also enables a context to be interrupted (broken), for example, allowing a user to be able to stop and search for another patient's data while a document about the currently selected patient is being finalized. The patient context can then be picked up by re-synchronization mechanisms to allow the user to continue working with the document. This type of integration requires a working-data integration as well as master data on the patient-level so patients or users can be recognized by their corresponding identifiers.

3.4.1.4 FHIR

One of the newest activities in HL7 is the development of *Fast Healthcare Interoperability Resources* (FHIR). FHIR® takes a pragmatic approach that defines simple structures for a service-oriented, REST-based information exchange. (REST is an acronym for *representational state transfer* and refers to a syntax that defines how to call stateless web-services.) The methodology used in FHIR is more closely related to HL7 v2 than to HL7 V3. A key design principle of FHIR is to only specify data elements that are applicable in at least 80 % of the use cases. This simplifies implementations and allows implementers to achieve a core set of common elements quickly, "out of the box", without the clutter of peripheral elements. In circumstances where this subset is not sufficient, trading partners have to extend the standard as needed. FHIR provides a standardized mechanism for extensions. The 2nd DSTU as the basis for Version 1.0 was published in September 2015, minor updates to DSTU 2.1, and major changes to DSTU 3 are in progress.

3.4.1.5 More HL7 Family Members

In addition to the main standards, a number of "smaller standards" that deal with communication and knowledge representation have been added to the HL7 family of standards, including *Arden Syntax*, an OCL-like common expression language

Table 3.2 Healthcare data exchange standards (in alphabetical order)

Standard	Content	Organization	Country
Arden Syntax	Knowledge Representation (primarily for decision support)	HL7	Global
CDA®	Clinical documents	HL7	Global
ClaML	Classification Markup Language	ISO	Global
DICOM	Clinical images	RSNA	Global
ebRIM	Electronic business reference information model	OASIS	Global
EDIFACT	Different domains	CEN	Europe
FHIR®	RESTful web-services for different domains, supporting different communication paradigms (services, messaging, documents)	HL7	Global
GLIF®	Guideline Interchange Format	HL7	Global
GELLO®	An OCL-like common expression language	HL7	Global
Hprim	Messaging for different domains	eSanté	France
PN13	Pharmacy	PHAST	France
SCRIPT	Pharmacy	NCPDP	USA
Version 2.x	Messaging for different domains	HL7	Global
Version 3	Messaging for different domains	HL7	Global
X.12	Logistics	ASC	US
xDT	Family of communication standards for the ambulatory sector	KBV, ZI, QMS	Germany

called GELLO®,[9] *Guideline Interchange Format* (GLIF®), and Claims Attachments.

3.4.2 Other Standards

Besides the standards that are widely-known, several countries have developed a set of their own specifications that still are in use today. Table 3.2 lists some of these standards.

More in-depth information about the various standards is provided in Chap. 4 and Appendix.

[9]For GELLO no long-form exists which explains the acronym.

3.5 Summary

The organizations that create or use data exchange standards fall into one of two categories. They are either creators of new standards or users of existing standards who modify an interoperability specification for a specific purpose. The first group of users are called Standards Developing Organizations (SDO), the latter are called Profile Development Organizations (PDO). It does not matter what or who authorizes the work, nor whether this work is performed by domain or IT/ICT oriented organizations. What counts is the outcome of the work. A prerequisite for general (perhaps "world-wide") acceptance of any particular standard is that it be derived from an international base standard. More and more organizations have recognized these facts and considered them in their decisions when developing specifications.

References

1. EDIFACTORY. http://www.edifactory.de, last accessed May 5 2008
2. UN/EDIFACT. United Nations Directories for Electronic Data Interchange for Administration, Commerce and Transport. http://www.unece.org/trade/untdid/welcome.htm
3. UN/EDIFACT: D.04A (Batch), Syntax version 3, http://www.gefeg.com/edifact/Index.htm
4. §301 SGB V. Sozialgesetzbuch Fünftes Buch, Gesetzliche Krankenversicherung: §301 Krankenhäuser. http://www.sozialgesetzbuch.de/gesetze/05/index.php?norm_ID=0530100, last accessed May 5 2008
5. Technische Anlage 3 zur Datenübermittlung nach §300 SGB V. http://www.gkv-datenaustausch.de/media/dokumente/leistungserbringer_1/apotheken/technische_anlagen_archiv/ta3/TA3_027_20120228.pdf
6. American Society for Testing and Materials. http://www.astm.org
7. Spronk R. The early History of HL7. Whitepaper, 2013, www.ringholm.com
8. An Application Protocol for Electronic Data Interchange in Healthcare Environment. HL7 Inc., Sept.1987, scanned version, http://www.hl7.org/documentcenter/private/standards/v2xIG/HL7v1_specification_19870928.pdf
9. Health Level Seven International. http://www.hl7.org
10. HL7 Deutschland (Germany). http://www.hl7.de/
11. HL7 Netherlands http://www.hl7.nl
12. Kassenärztliche Bundesvereinigung. www.kbv.de/html/ita.php, last accessed July 14th, 2015.
13. Qualitätsring Medizinische Software, http://www.qms-standards.de/
14. National Council for Prescription Drug Programs, http://www.ncpdp.org
15. Organization for the Advancement of Structured Information Standards, http://www.oasis-open.org
16. http://www.ihe.net/connectathon/
17. ELGA vernetzte Gesundheit. http://www.elga.gv.at/
18. eHealth Suisse. http://www.e-health-suisse.ch
19. Healthcare Information Technology Standards Panel. http://www.hitsp.org/
20. Standards and Interoperability (S&I) Framework Overview Homepage http://www.healthit.gov/policy-researchers-implementers/standards-interoperability-si-framework

21. Standards and Interoperability (S&I) Framework Overview Document (PDF) http://www.healthit.gov/sites/default/files/pdf/fact-sheets/standards-and-interoperability-framework.pdf
22. Standards and Interoperability (S&I) Framework Homepage http://www.siframework.org/
23. Canada Health Infoway, http://www.infoway-inforoute.ca, http://www.infoway-inforoute.ca/index.php/progams-services/standards-collaborative/membership, last accessed November 17th, 2015
24. Dossier Médical Personnel. http://www.dmp.gouv.fr/
25. Collaboration Platform for the German interoperability forum: http://wiki.hl7.de
26. Electronic Business Plattform im Gesundheitswesen. http://www.ebpg-nrw.de/
27. InfoPAT Rhein Neckar, INFOPAT e.V., http://www.infopat.eu/
28. National Health Service, http://en.wikipedia.org, http://en.wikipedia.org/wiki/National_Health_Service_(England)
29. This is a shortcut to the following references: SMART Homepage, http://smarthealthit.org/. SMART on FHIR Documentation, https://github.com/smart-on-fhir/smart-on-fhir.github.io. SMART Profiles: https://github.com/smart-on-fhir/smart-on-fhir.github.io/blob/master/profiles/index.md. SMART Example Profile for Patient Demographics: https://fhir-open-api.smarthealthit.org/Patient/1032702
30. HL7 Message Development Framework
31. HL7 Development Framework
32. Clinical Document Architecture, Normative Edition, May 2005, http://www.hl7.org
33. Boone K. The CDA Book. Springer, 2011, ISBN 978-0857293350
34. Extensible Markup Language. http://www.w3c.org
35. ASN1. Standard. http://www.itu.int/ITU-T/studygroups/com17/languages/
36. Binary XML, www.w3.org/XML/Binary
37. eHealthOntario, http://www.ehealthblueprint.com, last accessed November 17th, 2015
38. Booch G, Rumbaugh J, Jacobson I. Das UML-Benutzerhandbuch: Aktuell zur Version 2.0. Addison-Wesley, 2006, ISBN 978-3827325709,
39. Booch G, Rumbaugh J,.Jacobson I. The Unified Modeling Language User Guide. Addison-Wesley, 2007, ISBN 0321267974
40. UN Centre for Trade Facilitation and E-business (UN/CEFACT)
41. DICOM. Digital Images and Communication in Medicine. http://www.rsna.org/Technology/DICOM/index.cfm
42. ebXML Reference Information Model. http://www.oasis-open.org/committees/regrep/documents/2.0/specs/ebRIM.pdf
43. Introducing UN/EDIFACT. http://www.unece.org/trade/untdid/welcome.html
44. ASIP Santé, France, http://esante.gouv.fr, http://esante.gouv.fr/en, http://www.asipsante.fr
45. Gesellschaft für Telematik im Gesundheitswesen. http://www.gematik.de
46. Fast Healthcare Interoperability Resources. http://www.hl7.org/fhir
47. HL7 proposal database http://www.hl7.org/memonly/dbsub.cfm?
48. HL7 Version 3 Reference Information Model http://www.hl7.org
49. Health Level 7 (HL7) Standard Version 2.5, ANSI/HL7 V2.5-2003, June 26, 2003, http://www.hl7.org.
50. HL7 Version 2. XML Encoding Syntax, Release 1. ANSI/HL7 V2 XML-2003; June 4, 2003; Release 2. ANSI/HL7 V2 XML-2012; 2012.
51. Health Level 7 (HL7) Standard Version 3, http://www.hl7.org.
52. Integrating the Healthcare Enterprise (IHE). IHE Technical Framework Volume II Transactions (Scheduled Workflow); http://www.ihe.net/tf/.
53. http://www.interopsante.org/
54. Object Management Group. http://www.omg.org
55. Planungsstudie (Planning Study), https://publicwiki-01.fraunhofer.de/Planungsstudie_Interoperabilitaet/index.php/Hauptseite/

56. Standardized General Markup Language
57. Unified Modeling Language. ISO/IEC 19501:2005, http://www.uml.org
58. UNECE: United Nations Economic Commission for Europe: http://www.unece.org/trade/untdid/d05b/
59. Zentralinstitut für die kassenärztliche Versorgung in der Bundesrepublik Deutschland (central institute for public insurances), http://www.zi.de/

Chapter 4
Healthcare Data Exchange Standards

The standards landscape from an organizational and scope perspective was presented in Chap. 3. In this chapter we will examine data exchange standards from a technical viewpoint, with a focus on the conformance approach that is used for each standard. This chapter presents a sampling of the most commonly used and well-known healthcare data exchange standards from a variety of categories. It begins with an overview of Version 2.x®, and FHIR® (Fast Healthcare Interoperability Resources) from the family of products specified by HL7 International. This chapter continues with EDIFACT as a European data exchange standard that is also employed in healthcare. ebXML as the foundation for the IHE (Integrating the Healthcare Enterprise) ITI (Information Technology Infrastructure) XDS integration profile is described next. To complete this sampling, details about the HL7 CTS2 (Common Terminology Services, Rel.2) and ISO/FDIS 13120 ClaML (Classification Markup Language) are presented.

Some additional healthcare data exchange standards are presented in Appendix. Those standards include (among others) HL7 Version 3®, HL7 CDA® (Clinical Document Architecture), ASTM (American Society for Testing and Materials), DICOM (Digital Imaging and Communications in Medicine), and the German xDT family of standards used in the ambulatory sector. To complete this overview, details about Hprim Santé, PN13 being used in France are presented as well.

Some of the standards presented are still under development, and therefore the information provided about them cannot be guaranteed to be up-to-date. The reader is kindly asked to use the overviews about the data exchange standards provided in this chapter as introductory materials and combine them with the original documentation, which may be located using the references at the end of this chapter.

F. Oemig and R. Snelick, *Healthcare Interoperability Standards Compliance Handbook*, DOI 10.1007/978-3-319-44839-8_4

4.1 Introduction

As part of the overview for each data exchange standard, a brief discussion is provided about the conformance constructs employed by the standard. Readers wishing to have a better understanding of the conformance constructs can go to Chap. 5 and read it concurrently with this chapter. Each overview concludes with a short analysis of the conformance methodology the standard uses. The chapter concludes with a comparison matrix showing the conformance constructs that are utilized by each standard (including the standards from the appendix), which should help the reader grasp the subtle differences among the various standards.

4.2 HL7 Version 2.X

HL7 Version 2.x is the most well-known and widely used data exchange standard in healthcare worldwide. It is employed for the transmission of messages to support data exchange within hospitals, between providers and hospitals, and between providers and registries.

The first version of HL7 (Version 1.0) was produced in 1987 by agreement among several HIT companies with the goal of enabling information exchange in a "standardized" ASTM-derived format. The second version of the standard was developed in 1990 and became the basis of the widely deployed family of HL7 Version 2.x standards. HL7 v2.x continues to evolve; at the time of this book's publication, Version 2.8 has been completed and v2.9 is being developed. Subsequent versions can be anticipated to be released over the coming years.

HL7 v2.x defines messages using an abstract notion. Rules for building an abstract message definition are specified in the HL7 message framework, which is hierarchical in nature and consists of building blocks generically called *elements*. These elements are *segment groups*, *segments*, *fields*, *components*, and *sub-components*, as shown in Figs. 4.3 and 4.4. Each element has associated attributes that further define the element and include optionality, cardinality, table, length, and data type.

Encoding rules are then applied to convert this formal specification into a specific representation allowing for an instantiation of messages. Currently, two different encodings are defined. The first is called "Encoding Rules Seven" (ER7), which uses the well-known pipe-delimited message format (please see Fig. 4.2 for an example). The second representation uses XML and is named "HL7 v2.xml".

In the early days of HL7, the length of the exchanged messages was important because of the limited capacity of the systems being used at that time. The need to use storage space efficiently was one reason for the pragmatic selection of the delimited exchange format for HL7 messages. The default encoding, with the use of five hierarchically oriented separators (for segments, field, components,

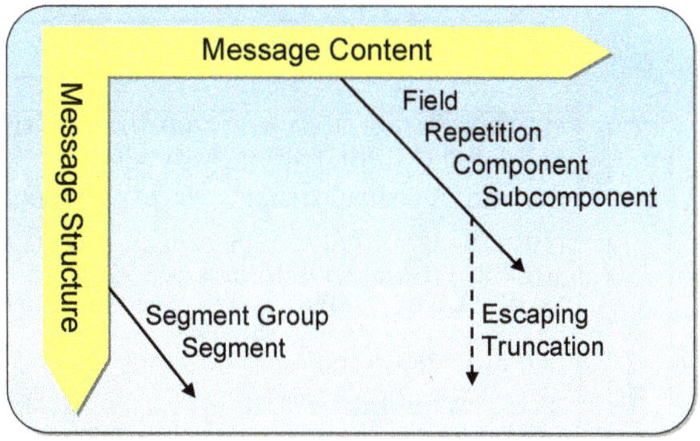

Fig. 4.1 Two-dimensional parsing HL7 v2.x messages

subcomponents and repetitions) plus two special indicators (for escaping and truncation), allows for the construction of structured messages. This method is called *Encoding Rules Seven* (ER7) and will be described in detail later in this chapter. The delimiter on the segment level enables a two-dimensional approach for sharing the message content, as is illustrated in Fig. 4.1.

The most significant delimiter, the carriage return (CR), separates the individual segments and permits the segment-oriented message structure to be expressed in coherent message units. This capability allows for a top-level determination as to whether a segment or segment group (i.e., information unit) can be processed or not. (In Fig. 4.1, this approach is represented by the vertical arrow.) For this determination to be made, the structure of the message must be known. Furthermore, when parsing the appropriate hierarchy structure of the message, a determination can be made as to whether processing of the segment or segment group is possible and whether the contents of this segment must be "taken care of" or can be discarded.

A segment, which is represented by a three letter acronym (e.g., PID represents Patient IDentification), consists of fields that hold the data content. As a segment is being processed, the decoding takes place in the second dimension (represented by the horizontal arrow in Fig. 4.1), during which the discrete data elements are extracted in accordance to the processing rules of the five other delimiters.

Figure 4.2 provides an example of an HL7 admission message. The segment delimiter (CR) is shown as "<CR>" at the end of each row, and the other delimiters are highlighted via colors. The first two fields in the message header specify the delimiters to be used within the message. The background colors correspond to the font color within the message.

4.2.1 Versions

The first version of HL7 v2.x was released more than 20 years ago. Since that time, a significant number of enhancements have been applied to v2.x, including a

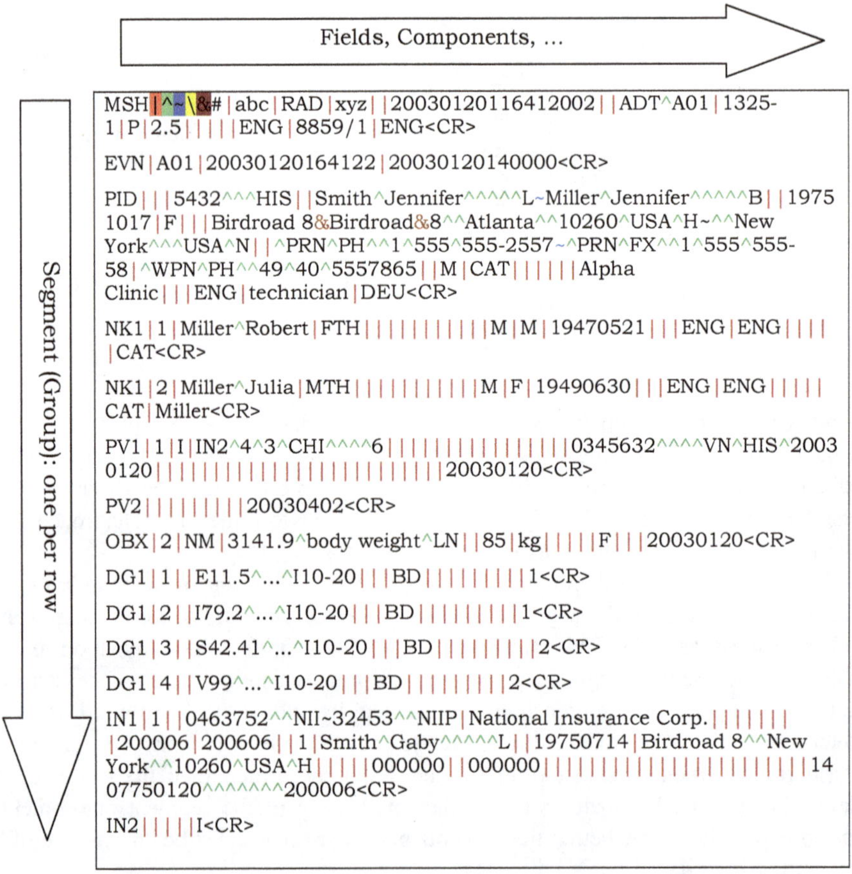

Fig. 4.2 Example HL7 v2.x message in ER7 format

component model for data types, conformance profiles, specifying conditions, message structures, segment grouping, and handling of lengths, to name a few. In principle, HL7 v2.x is backward-compatible. The different releases represent milestones in the development of the standard; however, in some cases, problems are introduced related to processing messages that are based on requirements defined in an earlier version. One of these problems involves the deprecation of existing data elements in a new version, requiring content that previously populated these data elements in an HL7 message to be relocated to other fields (data elements). Installed interfaces typically do not account for specific contents (values) having been moved to other fields, leading to a loss of data in the receiving system even though the content is included in the message, albeit in an unaccounted for location. Another problem involves changes or improvements in data types, which may lead to the addition of more components or subcomponents to the message structure. HL7 "rules for the recipient" require receiving systems to "ignore segments, fields, components, subcomponents, and extra repetitions of a field that are present but were not expected". Thus, a robust implementation may not be able to support the use of new components or subcomponents, but it would be able to prevent a total "crash" and, in most cases, would allow the processing of at least minimal data provided in the HL7 message.

4.2.2 Information Model

The overall information model[1] for HL7 v2.x, which was created by reverse-engineering the HL7 v2 standard, is shown in Fig. 4.3. This information model includes all essential components and, by that means, includes those components related to conformance.

The elements contained within this model that are relevant for a conformance discussion are explained in detail in the next subsections.

4.2.3 Message Structure

HL7 Version 2.x is a message-oriented data exchange standard, i.e., the primary purpose is the exchange of messages. Figure 4.3 contains a formal representation of HL7 v2.x. If the message-oriented classes are removed from Fig. 4.3, simplifying it to show only relevant classes that cover messaging, the result is the diagram shown in Fig. 4.4.

A message is represented by a message structure. A message structure consists of a sequence of segments and group of segments. Each segment is composed of a set of sequentially ordered fields, each of which has a data type specifying the components and, iteratively, subcomponents.

HL7 v2.x uses the optionality (usage), length, repetitions (cardinality), and tables conformance constructs. According to the construct rules, not all conformance constructs apply to all of the elements shown in Fig. 4.4. Optionality can be used with all elements; therefore, segments, segment groups, fields, components and subcomponents have an attribute specifying the optionality. Cardinality, often also called repetitions in HL7 v2.x, can only be used on the segment and field levels, since only occurrences of segments, segment groups, and fields can repeat. Components and subcomponents are defined by means of the data types and,

---

[1]The diagram, in certain aspects, is simplified; some classes in the model should be shown as properties of the corresponding relations and not as separate classes. A good example is the set of conformance elements that are defined by the standard. Furthermore, the associated data types in the diagram are in most cases reduced to strings, although enumerations or other data types are more appropriate.

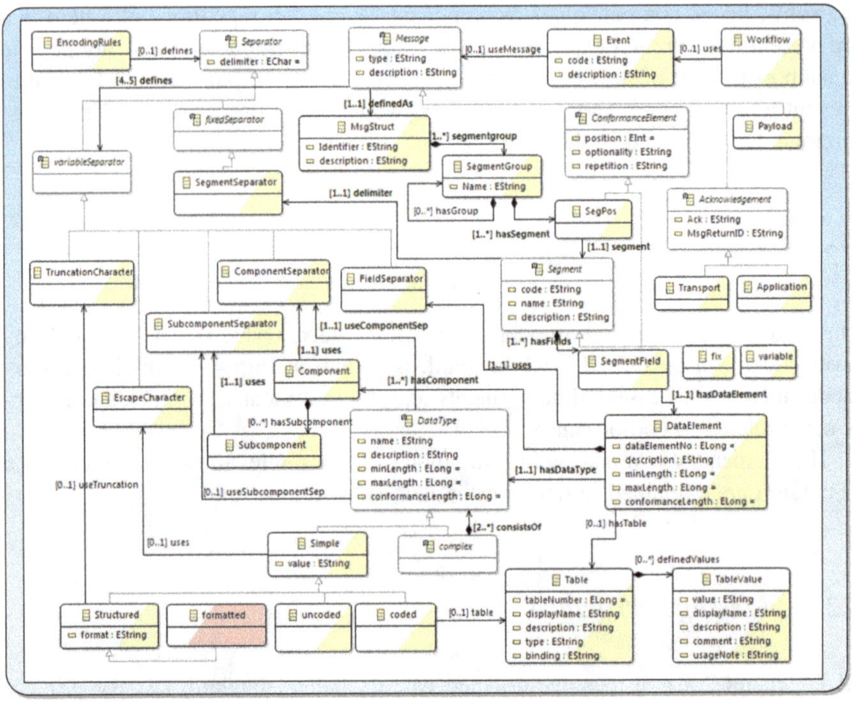

Fig. 4.3 HL7 v2.x information model

Fig. 4.4 HL7 v2.x (simplified) message structure

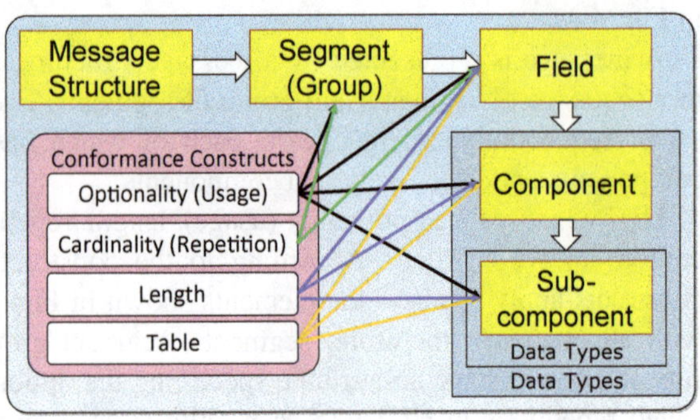

therefore, are not allowed to repeat. Finally, tables can be assigned to fields, components, and subcomponents.

HL7 v2.x does not provide an architecture that controls how messages, segments, or fields are defined. The necessary elements are created upon request to fulfill a specific need.

4.2.4 Optionality

HL7 v2.x uses the optionality (usage) concepts listed in Table 4.1 for segment (groups), fields, components and subcomponents.

Most of the codes listed in Table 4.1 are self-explanatory. An element marked as "R" (required) must appear in a message and must have a valid value. The presence of a conditional element ("C") in a message depends on a specified condition that can be evaluated using values that are present in other elements in the same message. "RE" (required but may be empty) usage, however, has been the cause of an on-going dispute focused on what "available" means regarding the content for an element. The section "Serving Interfaces with Data" in Chap. 2 (Architecture) explains the prerequisites that must be met in order to support the presence of a certain element in a message. The notion that not implementing an element with RE usage and, therefore, not providing any support for it such that this element is simply never present in a message would not distinguish it from *optional* ("O") elements that are not being supported or do *not implement* ("X") elements in derived specifications. An "RE" element therefore requires fundamental support, but allows a minimal cardinality of zero ("0"). In summary, an element with "RE" usage must be supported by the implementation but in a message instance, data may or may not be present based on data available or appropriateness. Placing additional requirements onto an "RE" element would mean making it "R" (required).

Since HL7 v2.x is a position-oriented data exchange standard, data elements cannot be deleted from the message structure. Their position must remain in the message structure even if the position is not used for data exchange any more. "B" (backward) and "W" (withdrawn) are used to support the process of deprecating

Table 4.1 HL7 v2.x optionality (usage)

Code	Description	Constrainable to	Comment
R	Required	R	This element must appear in a message
RE	Required but may be empty	R	This element must appear in a message if values are available
C	Conditional	C, R	
CE	Conditional but may be empty	C, CE, R, RE	Introduced into the base standard with v2.7
C (a/b)	Conditional	C(a'/b')[a]	Introduced with v2.7.1, replaces C and CE
O	Optional	O, R, RE, C, CE, C(a/b), X	
B	Backward compatibility only	R, RE, O, C, CE, C(a/b), X	
W	Withdrawn	X	
X	Forbidden/not allowed/Not supported	X	

[a]See Chap. 8 for details on allowable constraints

elements. The field descriptions for such elements refer the implementer to newer alternatives. PID-4 (Alternate Patient Identifier) is one example of this situation; the reader is referred to PID-3 (Patient Identifier List) instead. PID-3, meanwhile, has been enhanced to become a repeating element, thus replacing PID-2 and PID-4 and allowing the conveying of a set of patient identifiers in a message.

4.2.5 Encoding

HL7 v2.x messages utilize a set of delimiters and special handling indicators/characters that are applied in a hierarchical manner. The message must be separated into its parts using the delimiters (and special characters) in the order[2] presented below:

• Segment	Fixed to Carriage Return[a], therefore it defines a line-oriented format.
• Field	Defined by MSH-1 and denotes how fields are separated from each other within a segment
• Repetition	Although defined by MSH-2 <2>[b], this is the next highest relevant delimiter, because fields can only be repeated as a whole
• Component	Declares, as defined by MSH-2 <1>, how the components of a field are separated
• Subcomponent	Separates subcomponents within components, defined by MSH-2 <4
• Escape	No delimiter is allowed to be represented as itself. The escape character is defined by MSH-2 <3>. The way the escape character is used for escaping is very specific, as will be explained in Chap. 5
• Truncation	New with v2.7 and defined by MSH-2 <5>; represents a character that can be used to indicate that certain data are truncated

[a]Quite a few systems erroneously use Carriage Return + Line Feed instead
[b]This notation indicates this is the second character in the MSH-2 field. The notation for MSH-2 differs from the notation of elements that consist of data types

The first five concepts in the list above are delimiters and must be used for separating the parts of the message. The sixth concept is a delimiter used to declare the character that introduces a special sequence when a character must be represented that is itself a delimiter.

The last element in the above list is not a delimiter but, rather, a special character. It can be used at the end of a value to indicate that the value was truncated either when it was stored in the sender's database or when creating the message. As such, this delimiter helps to identify in a round-trip data exchange that the data stored in the original sender's database may be more precise than the data currently being returned from the original receiver.

---

[2]This sequence is not the same as the order in which they are defined in MSH-2.

Table 4.2 Notation to refer to fields in HL7 v2.x

Notation equivalence	Description	Example
SEG-FLD SEG-FLD[1].1	Field: This is equal to the first component of the first repetition[a] of the field	PID-3 PID-3[1].1
SEG-FLD[REP] SEG-FLD[REP].1	Specific repetition of a field: This is equal to first component of this specific repetition	PID-3[2] PID-3[2].1
SEG-FLD.COMP SEG-FLD[1].COMP.1	Component of a field: This is equal to the first subcomponent of this component. If no repetition is given, the first repetition is meant	PID-3.5 PID-3[1].5
SEG-FLD[REP].COMP SEG-FLD[REP].COMP.1	Component of specific repetition of a field: This is equal to the first subcomponent of this component	PID-3[2].4 PID-3[2].4.1
SEG-FLD.COMP.SUB SEG-FLD[1].COMP.SUB	Subcomponent of a component: If no repetition is given this is equal to the subcomponent of the first repetition	PID-3.4.1 PID-3[1].4.1
SEG-FLD[REP].COMP.SUB None	Specific subcomponent of a specific component of a specific repetition of a field There is not an equivalent shorthand alternative to represent this element	PID-3[2].5.1

[a]HL7 v2.x often uses the term "repetition" when occurrence or cardinality is meant. In this case, the [1] is referring to the first occurrence, not the first repetition

This truncation character can also be used to indicate that the sender has data that are longer[3] than allowed by the standard. The truncation character is an indication to the receiver that more data are available.

The common way of referring to a specific data element is shown in Table 4.2. The upper case acronyms denote the following: SEG = segment, FLD = field, COMP = component, and SUB = subcomponent. In order to comply with the encoding rules, access to data should be accomplished according to the logic explained in Table 4.2.

As shown in Table 4.2, an ER7 conformant implementation expands access to data until no further expansion (last row) is possible. Accessing the data by using this approach it is ensured that unknown or unexpected (sub)components are detected and handled correctly. Therefore, a value like "abc^def" in a field that is officially[4] defined as a single component will not result in "abc^def" but "abc". In essence, a direct access is made to known and valid locations of the data being agnostic to allowed modifications based on the abstract message definition.

[3]As in a "character array", i.e., the number of bytes to represent the data, and not repetitions of the data ("data array").

[4]Note: HL7 v2 officially allows for adding components and subcomponents where necessary.

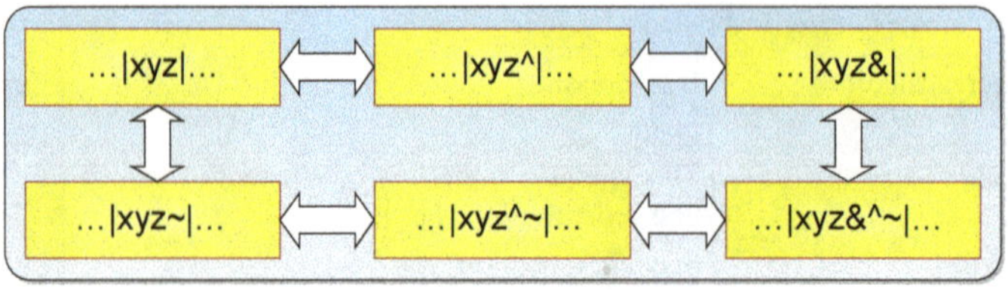

Fig. 4.5 Equivalence of data representation for a single component field

Accordingly, as shown in Fig. 4.5, each of the different representations for a field as a whole, (i.e., fields having only a single component) are equivalent and must be used when accessing the data. It should be noted that each equivalence shown is only valid for the whole field, but equivalent representations for fields with more than one component and subcomponent can be identified as well.

4.2.6 Delimiters

The left-hand side of the information model presented in Fig. 4.3 shows the use of delimiters that are important for correct encoding. As can be seen, most of the delimiters allow for variable characters. This was originally introduced to help legacy systems that were unable to support the default delimiters; the segment delimiter is the only fixed one bound to Carriage Return.[5] The HL7 v2.x default delimiters are "^ ~\&#" but could equally be "abcde" or "01234".

As this variability is part of the base encoding, adhering to it is essential for a conformant implementation. Adherence to this variability enforces special treatment of data during encoding and prevents, for example, line breaks within normal field data.

4.2.7 Delete Requests

The HL7 version 2.x includes only three "types of data" (see [1]):

- existing data
- non-existing data
- data to be deleted

[5]The standard explicitly states to use Carriage Return as the segment delimiter; however, many systems use Carriage Return + Line Feed instead, because it is easier to implement and not immediately visible without carefully reading the specification. Although this approach is not conformant, it is good practice to allow for it.

The first two types are relatively easy to understand: a value for an element is sent when available, otherwise, the element remains unvalued.

In the event that information is to be deleted, the double quote ("") is the special character sequence designated to activate this behavior.[6] This feature places some burden on the sending application, because the implementation of this behavior requires the application to recognize when previously communicated data has been deleted (See Chap. 2, section on Delete Indication) [1]. Most applications do not track the history of the specific data for an item, so the interface can't detect that this item previously contained some data that are no longer valid. Typically, "no information" is transferred, leaving the target system with the old information until a new value is transmitted. The introduction of the double quote special character solves this problem.

Difficulties arise when a receiver processes information from different sources, because the sequence in which the information is received affects the state of the associated data. Without broad notification to all interested parties regarding the changes made to the data, the integrity of the data cannot be guaranteed.

The delete feature is specific to HL7 version 2.x. Further details and background information about this feature are presented in Chap. 2.

4.2.8 Null-Flavors

HL7 version 2.x does not support the notion of a null flavor, which is a concept used to indicate the reason data are not present in an element (e.g., unknown). A work-around method in which coded values are used to represent a null flavor has been employed since the initial version for the standard was published. Unfortunately, the solution has been applied irregularly and in an inconsistent manner. A proposal to support null flavors has been submitted, but backward compatibility concerns have prevented its adoption.

4.2.9 Data Types

Data types impose additional message content structure within the message hierarchy. The data types define the division of the fields into components and the division of components into sub-components. The first version of the v2.x family had only one generic compound data type (data type CM). In the course of the

[6]It is important to note that the delete indicator is a "request to delete data" based on what the sender knows. However, the receiver may have other sources for that data; therefore, the receiver determines whether or not to remove data for that element.

Table 4.3 HL7 XPN data type specification (nesting resolved)

<table>
<tr><th>SEQ</th><th>LEN</th><th>DT</th><th>OPT</th><th>TBL#</th><th>COMPONENT NAME</th><th></th></tr>
<tr><td>1</td><td>194</td><td>FN</td><td>C</td><td></td><td>Family Name</td><td>
<table>
<tr><th>SEQ</th><th>LEN</th><th>DT</th><th>OPT</th><th>TBL #</th><th>COMPONENT NAME</th></tr>
<tr><td>1</td><td>50</td><td>ST</td><td>R</td><td></td><td>Surname</td></tr>
<tr><td>2</td><td>20</td><td>ST</td><td>O</td><td></td><td>Own Surname Prefix</td></tr>
<tr><td>3</td><td>50</td><td>ST</td><td>O</td><td></td><td>Own Surname</td></tr>
<tr><td>4</td><td>20</td><td>ST</td><td>O</td><td></td><td>Surname Prefix From Partner/Spouse</td></tr>
<tr><td>5</td><td>50</td><td>ST</td><td>O</td><td></td><td>Surname From Partner/Spouse</td></tr>
</table>
</td></tr>
<tr><td>2</td><td>30</td><td>ST</td><td>O</td><td></td><td>Given Name</td><td></td></tr>
<tr><td>3</td><td>30</td><td>ST</td><td>O</td><td></td><td>Second and Further Given Names or Initials Thereof</td><td></td></tr>
<tr><td>4</td><td>20</td><td>ST</td><td>O</td><td></td><td>Suffix (e.g., JR or III)</td><td></td></tr>
<tr><td>5</td><td>20</td><td>ST</td><td>O</td><td></td><td>Prefix (e.g., DR)</td><td></td></tr>
<tr><td>6</td><td>6</td><td>IS</td><td>B</td><td>0360</td><td>Degree (e.g., MD)</td><td></td></tr>
<tr><td>7</td><td>1</td><td>ID</td><td>O</td><td>0200</td><td>Name Type Code</td><td></td></tr>
<tr><td>8</td><td>1</td><td>ID</td><td>O</td><td>0465</td><td>Name Representation Code</td><td></td></tr>
<tr><td>9</td><td>705</td><td>CWE</td><td>O</td><td>0448</td><td>Name Context</td><td></td></tr>
<tr><td>10</td><td>49</td><td>DR</td><td>B</td><td></td><td>Name Validity Range</td><td>
<table>
<tr><th>SEQ</th><th>LEN</th><th>DT</th><th>OPT</th><th>TBL #</th><th>COMPONENT NAME</th></tr>
<tr><td>1</td><td>24</td><td>DTM</td><td>O</td><td></td><td>Range Start Date/ Time</td></tr>
<tr><td>2</td><td>24</td><td>DTM</td><td>O</td><td></td><td>Range End Date/ Time</td></tr>
</table>
</td></tr>
<tr><td>11</td><td>1</td><td>ID</td><td>O</td><td>0444</td><td>Name Assembly Order</td><td></td></tr>
<tr><td>12</td><td>24</td><td>DTM</td><td>O</td><td></td><td>Effective Date</td><td></td></tr>
<tr><td>13</td><td>24</td><td>DTM</td><td>O</td><td></td><td>Expiration Date</td><td></td></tr>
<tr><td>14</td><td>199</td><td>ST</td><td>O</td><td></td><td>Professional Suffix</td><td></td></tr>
</table>

development of the model, the data types have been further refined. In version 2.6, more than 90 data types are available.

Unlike typical programming languages, HL7 v2.x data types are defined based on the content they are intended to represent. Examples include:

- Person names
- Addresses
- Time range

The limitation on the number of delimiters imposes a two-level structure (components and sub-components) on data types. The length of a field is the sum of the components plus the necessary delimiters. Table 4.3 demonstrates the makeup of the *Extended Person Name* (XPN) data type in which two data types, *Family Name* (FN) and *Date Range* (DR), are nested. For further details, please refer to [2]. The columns are explained in Table 4.4.

In the first renderings of the v2.x standard, additional information for the different parts of a field was described in natural language sentences so the user could figure out where this information belonged. An example thereof is the designation of a table of values to be used for a specific component of a field. With v2.5, a so-called component model was officially introduced, which provided a table (Table 4.3 is an example) that had columns for the different attributes, such as optionality, length and tables, and had rows for each component of a field.

Using this component model has eliminated many of the ambiguities within the standard specification.

4.2.10 Events

An event in the real world, for example the admission of a patient or the creation of a new order, may be the trigger that establishes communication between trading partners. The information that should be exchanged depends on the use case. The associated message is built from different segments; HL7 v2.x defines a set of predefined message structures (templates) that models a real-world event.

Originally with HL7 v2.1, the event could be derived from the type of message, and the type of message provided sufficient information to determine the content of the message. Further details about the underlying event were then conveyed in a particular field in another message segment. In the administration domain (*Admission Discharge and Transfer*, ADT), this field was the first field in the event segment (EVN-1); and for order and result messages (ORM), this field was the first field of the order control segment (ORC-1). In the course of HL7 evolution, the messages became more comprehensive, and they could not be built identically for all events of the same message type. For this reason, the event field was moved into the message header (MSH) segment. Unfortunately, the various HL7 working groups (WGs) have implemented this change in different ways. The ADT working

Table 4.4 Columns for HL7 data type specifications

Column	Description	Explanation
SEQ	Sequence number	
LEN	Length of the (sub)component	(Minimum and) maximum length
C.LEN	(not shown above)	Conformance length (introduced in version 2.7)
DT	Data	Type (recursive definition)
OPT	Optionality	
TBL#	Table number	Four digit number referencing a table with values
COMPONENT NAME	Name of the component	Short description, a longer explanation is given in a subsequent section
COMMENTS	(not shown above)	Additional comments for the component
SEC.REF.	(not shown above)	Reference to a section in Chap. 2A

group has developed many similar message types (actually, there are three basic message structures that support many ADT events); and the Orders and Observations (OO) working group has decided on a very small set of message structures in ORM, but has developed many *sub-events* in the form of the Order Control Code (ORC-1).

The introduction of an identifier (ID) for the message structure (Message Structure Identifier, e.g., ADT_A01) should alleviate this design flaw. Initially, all messages were compared in order to determine such an ID. The message structure identifier and the event mapping should be used to determine the parsing processes. Some messages can be parsed easily due to their internal structure, and different message structures exist that use the same event code. In Version 2.5, the concept of a message profile was introduced along with a message profile identifier that precisely indicates the composition of a message when used correctly. A detailed explanation of this topic is explored in Chap. 7.

The standard is written using a popular text processing software tool and is not developed based on a database [SchoOem2001]. For reasons of convenience, different elements are repeated in different sections in the standard. A good example is the message structure, where the same message structure is associated with different events and is repeated in the specification document with each of these events. When the next version of the standard is published, such a message structure may be shown to be enhanced for some segments, but, unfortunately, not all messages with the same structure (and ID) are enhanced identically—the messages have become inconsistent. As a consequence, different structures with the same ID are presented in the HL7 ballot process. An example thereof is the addition of the SFT (software) or ARV (access restriction) segments in the ADT domain. A thorough inspection during the ballot process reveals these kinds of issues so they can be corrected. In cases when these editorial errors are not detected, they are published "as is", which often leads to exhaustive discussions about which version of the standard is correct.

Additionally, a cleanup of the standard is difficult to perform because of objections from stakeholders insisting on backward compatibility of the specification. This situation leads to duplication in a standard's definitions of messages, which in turn complicates or prevents consistent definitions. As a remedy, there remains only the systematic collection and review of appeals during the ballot phase (see "The HL7 database" [HL7-DB] on the website).

4.2.11 Dynamic Behavior

In addition to the previously described static message structure, there is a dynamic behavior that determines how two applications interact with regard to a single message. When the initiating application sends a message, this application needs to get an indication as to whether the receiving application received the message or not. For this reason, the receiving application is expected to respond with a receipt, which is called acknowledgement.

This acknowledgement can be provided on two different levels,[7] as shown in Fig. 4.6:

- transport[8] and
- application

The acknowledgement on the transport level, also called transport acknowledgement, indicates that the receiving application has gotten the message successfully and will take care of it. This indication releases the sending application from pursuing any further attempts to resend this message; however, this kind of acknowledgement does not provide any indication as to whether the receiving application was able to process this message successfully. This information is provided when the receiving application sends an appropriate application (processing) acknowledgment.

Hence, each message that is sent may be responded to with zero, one, or two messages by the recipient. The number of acknowledgement messages that are generated depends on the sending application, which can indicate what kind of response is desired. The message header provides the relevant information, as depicted in Fig. 4.7.

The condition of the acknowledgment requirement for transport and processing is defined in a message instance with MSH-15/16 and determines whether a receipt should be sent and under what conditions. If no requirement is specified, the default behavior is to send an application acknowledgement. In return, a sending application may already expect zero, one, or two responses (i.e., no acknowledgement, a transport acknowledgement, or a transport acknowledgement and an application

[7]These two levels have been introduced into HL7 v2 with v2.2 in form of an enhanced acknowledgement mode.

[8]Sometimes a transport acknowledgement is also known as accept or system acknowledgement.

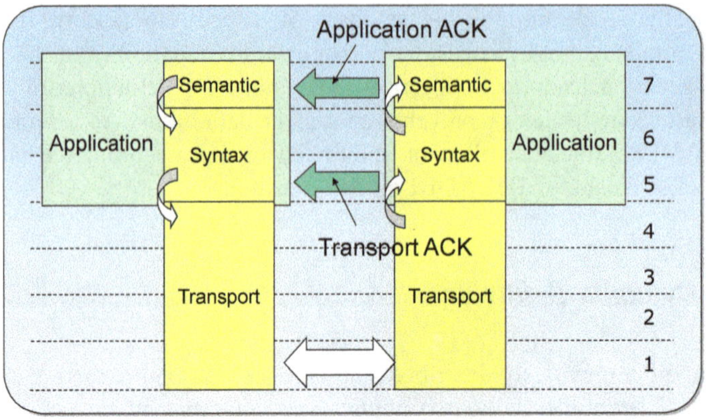

Fig. 4.6 Application and transport acknowledgements

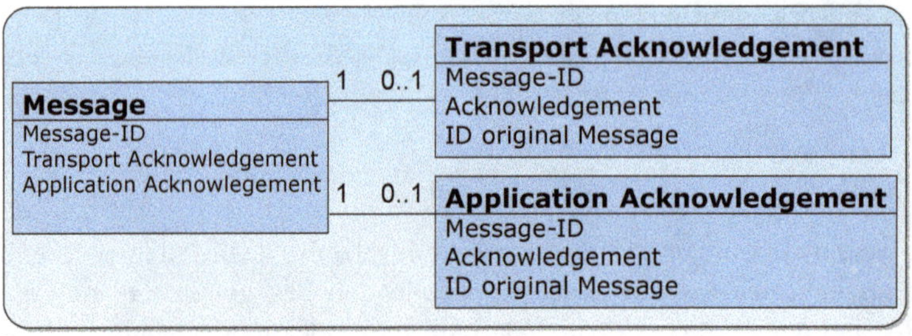

Fig. 4.7 Dynamic behavior in HL7 v2.x messages

acknowledgement) to each message sent. In the case of "broadcast" messages (e.g., ADT), this expectation is multiplied by the number of recipients, which raises a problem that must be dealt with on a case by case basis when conflicting responses are returned from the various trading partners. For example, what is the remedy when two of eight receiving applications reject the message and refuse to process a transfer of a patient?

Currently, the most common implemented standard behavior related to this issue is the simple return of a transport acknowledgment, which is, however, not really evaluated by the receiving application. This response message only serves to fulfill the requirement to send an acknowledgement. But the transport acknowledgement simply indicates that the message was received and nothing more. It does not indicate, that the message wasn't processed appropriately.

Strictly speaking, several messages can be sent by the sending application before a single response (acknowledgement) may occur, if a response is requested at all.

A response message references the original message by the message identifier. This identifier can have any format, but it must be a string recognizable to the original sending application. To correctly assign/identify errors and be able to correct them, a sending application must maintain a log of all messages. Unfortunately, most installations do not maintain this log, thus preventing a continuous pro-active system for monitoring, detecting, and reporting errors.

Another problem associated with the dynamic behavior occurs when messages are *forwarded* to a recipient or recipients. The HL7 standard itself does not state how the messages are to be propagated, that is, whether the sending application itself is responsible for delivery. A communication server (in many circles referred to as an integration or interface engine) can be entrusted with the message delivery. In return, the communication server guarantees the transfer and directly provides a transport acknowledgement. Hence, the question arises as to how different application acknowledgements should be handled if, for example, two of eight target systems do not process the message?

Ultimately, only manual intervention will solve this problem, assuming the administrator or someone else is notified so the participating systems can be synchronized.

4.2.12 Transmission Protocols

As previously mentioned, ASTM [ASTM] is used as the basis for defining the HL7 v2.x transmission protocols, but improvements have been introduced; for example, segment names are limited to three letters. Some short-comings still remain [HL7 v1], however, such as the lack of inclusion of a message end (or message trailer) segment. This oversight leads to problems with certain transmission protocols, in particular the socket-based communication. For a file-based transmission, the messages are simply written sequentially into a file. When transferring a file,[9] additional safeguards (files acting as semaphores, locking, or renaming) are required to ensure completeness of the messages.

For a socket-based communication, an additional framing must be used so an interruption of the transmission can be detected.

4.2.13 Tables and Table Values

HL7 v2.x supports the notion of coded data, which is accomplished by defining a table of values (or a placeholder for values) and then binding that table to a particular message element. With the latest release of HL7 v2.x, more than 500 tables have been defined, some of which also provide a list of values. Figure 4.8

[9]The easiest and most reliable mechanism for exchanging files is the use of renaming, because this process is supported at the file level by all operating systems as an atomic action. For unexplained reasons, however, semaphore files are preferred for solving the problem, although two files must be handled when using this approach.

provides a good example thereof and demonstrates the diverging nature of the values for such a table.

The tables use four-digit numbers for their primary identification. The numbers are repeated within fields and/or components indicating that the values of those tables should be used to convey the appropriate information.

Some tables are declared as *HL7-defined*. The codes for the listed values in these tables must be used if the specific concept that is needed is represented by one of those codes, but extending the table with additional coded values that are needed for local processing is allowed. On the other hand, *user-defined tables* only provide a list of suggested values that can be used. A vendor is allowed to replace a user-defined table with a different set of values. Tables in the HL7 v2.x context represent a starting set of allowable values for creating value sets. The use and understanding of HL7 v2.x tables has been problematic historically; recent proposals have been submitted to address the issue and to align use of the tables more closely with HL7 core principles. The intended result is the definition of code systems and value sets that are in alignment with other HL7 standards, especially V3 and FHIR.

In Version 2.x, the tables are used in four different ways, which are presented in Fig. 4.8. Although the term "tables" is commonly used, tables should not be confused with "code systems".

"Standard-defined" or "HL7-defined" tables provide a universal list of coded values that are required to be used in conjunction with the datatypes ID and CNE. "User-defined" tables list values that are provided for convenience so that a user of a health information technology (HIT) vendor's product may select them, and it does not violate the standard to create one's own list of values. The user-defined tables are used with the data types IS and CWE. In some rare cases the community has decided to reference or import "tables" from other SDOs such as ISO. Good examples are the language and country codes. Finally, there are the "locally-defined" or site-specific tables, which are designed to enable the use of coded values, but do not provide guidance or list any suggested values.

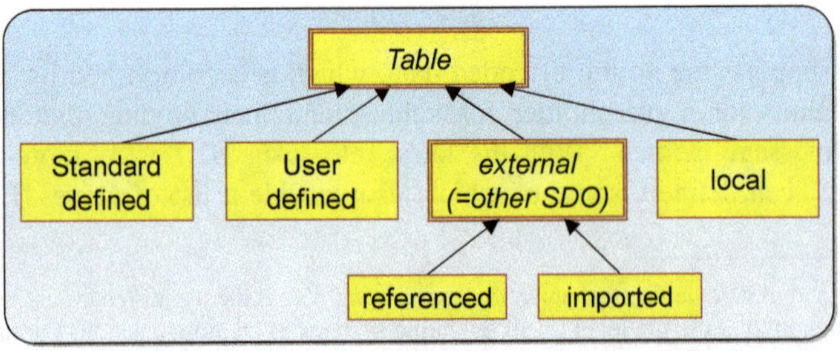

Fig. 4.8 Different kinds of tables

4.2.14 *Conformance Methodology*

With HL7 v2.5, profiles were introduced as part of the official standard. Profiles are comprised of a constraint methodology applied to the available conformance constructs, and they provide a formal representation that allows for precisely expressing the introduced constraints.

4.3 FHIR (HL7)

Ideas generated within the HL7 community about how to improve and leverage data exchange standards led to an initiative called FHIR® (pronounced "fire")—Fast Healthcare Interoperability Resources—that seeks to simplify and modernize interface specifications for use among disparate systems. Furthermore, FHIR is anticipated to leverage and promote the use of RESTful web technology.

4.3.1 *Introduction and Overview*

As stated in the FHIR® [FHIR] specification, this health care information exchange standard attempts to take advantage of the successful aspects of v2.x, V3, and CDA family of HL7 standards, facilitated by web technologies. FHIR makes use of models but limits them to a core set of common functionality. This core set of common functionality is guided by the principle that "80 % of the applications will need it". Everything else not included in the base model will be added as needed by a standardized extension methodology. The goal of limiting the core functionality is to allow implementers to concentrate on the important aspects of a resource and to arrive at solutions quickly.

The primary building blocks in FHIR are *resources*. Figure 4.9 illustrates an example XML instance for a specific patient resource.

The same example can also be shown in the alternative representation form JSON as shown in Fig. 4.10.

Figure 4.11 depicts the model for the patient resource in the UML representation. The data for the resources are organized into classes and attributes. Attributes use simple or complex data types (Figs. 4.17, 4.18, 4.19) in combination with cardinality.

FHIR® provides a set of pre-defined resources, delineated by categories, for specifying various services (Fig. 4.12). The resources are taken from FHIR version 1..1, published in September, 2015.

The model for each resource (Fig. 4.11 shows an example) defines the structure of the data elements.

XML	Explanation
<Patient xmlns="http://hl7.org/fhir">	Main Resource
<id value="cda"/>	• internal identifier
<text>	Human Readable Summary
<status value="generated"/>	
<div xmlns="http://www.w3.org/1999/xhtml">	
<p>Henry LEVIN the 7th, DOB 24-Sept 1932</p>	
<p>MRN: 123456</p>	
</div>	
</text>	
<extension url="http://hl7.org/fhir/StructureDefinition/us-core-race">	Extension with reference to its definition
<valueCodeableConcept>	
<coding>	
<system value="http://hl7.org/fhir/v3/Race"/>	
<code value="1096-7"/>	
</coding>	
</valueCodeableConcept>	
</extension>	
<identifier>	Standard Data Content:
<use value="usual"/>	
<type>	• Medical Record Number
<coding>	
<system value="http://hl7.org/fhir/v2/0203"/>	
<code value="MR"/>	
</coding>	
</type>	
<system value="urn:oid:2.16.840.1.113883.19.5"/>	
<value value="12345MR"/>	
</identifier>	
<active value="true"/>	
<name>	From Demographics:
<family value="Levin"/>	
<given value="Henry"/>	• Name
<suffix value="The 7th"/>	• Gender
</name>	• Date of Birth
<gender value="male"/>	
<birthDate value="1932-09-24"/>	
<careProvider>	• Provider
<type value="Organization/1"/>	
<display value="Good Health Clinic"/>	
</careProvider>	
</Patient>	

Fig. 4.9 XML example instance for a FHIR patient resource

JSON | **Explanation**

```
{
  "resourceType": "Patient",
  "id": "xcda",
```

Main Resource

- internal identifier

```
  "text": {
    "status": "generated",
    "div": "<div><p> Henry LEVIN the 7th, DOB 24-Sept
1932</p><p>MRN: 123456</p></div>"
  },
```

Human Readable Summary

```
  "extension": [
    {
      "url": "http://hl7.org/fhir/
                    StructureDefinition/us-core-race",
      "valueCodeableConcept": {
        "coding": [
          {
            "system": "http://hl7.org/fhir/v3/Race",
            "code": "1096-7"
          }
        ]
      }
    },
```

Extension with reference to its definition

```
  "identifier": [
    {
      "use": "usual",
      "type": {
        "coding": [
          {
            "system": "http://hl7.org/fhir/v2/0203",
            "code": "MR"
          }
        ]
      },
      "system": "urn:oid:2.16.840.1.113883.19.5",
      "value": "12345"
    }
  ],
```

Standard Data Content:

- Medical Record Number

```
  "active": true,
  "name": [
    {
      "family": [
        "Levin"
      ],
      "given": [
        "Henry"
      ]
    }
  ],
  "gender": "male",
  "birthDate": "1932-09-24",
```

From Demographics:

- Name
- Gender
- Date of Birth

```
  "careProvider": {
    "reference":
              "Organization/2.16.840.1.113883.19.5",
    "display": "Good Health Clinic"
  }
}
```

- Provider

Fig. 4.10 JSON example instance for a FHIR patient resource

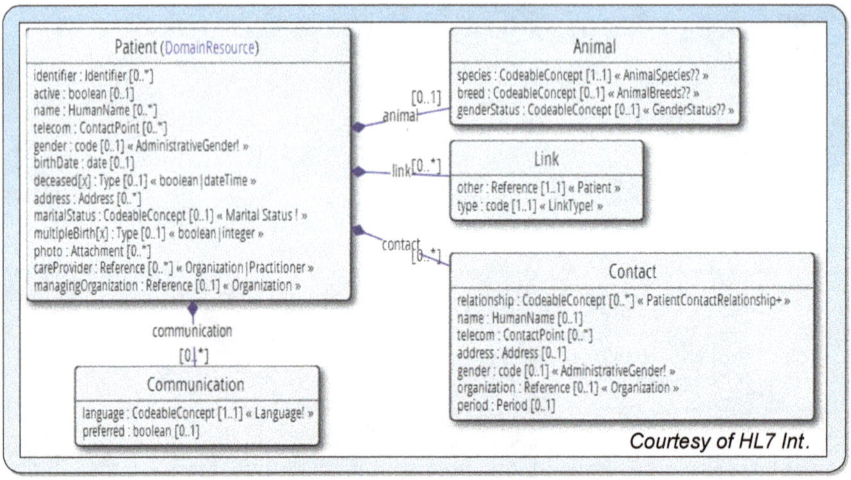

Fig. 4.11 UML model for the patient resource

4.3.2 Element Hierarchy

In FHIR®, all defined artifacts are derived from a common root element, as shown in Fig. 4.13. (The figure does not provide a complete overview, only a few examples are given that help to explain the hierarchy.) The root element itself provides the means to ensure that all derived artifacts **allow** for extensions. This includes the data types as well. In the left half of the figure the data types are represented with some example specializations. The complex data types are used as well as the primitive ones.

Utilizable resources like *Patient* and *Encounter* are specializations of an abstract *domain resource,* which is itself based on an abstract *resource* specification. This ensures that each resource optionally is composed of a textual description of the resource, and it allows for using an internal identification of the resource and attaching additional metadata.

The attributes of a resource are either associated with another resource by reference, or are the base for further attributes (as a backbone element), or are directly associated with a specific data type. However, some attributes of a resource allow for different data types, for example, the attribute *deceased* that can be a *Boolean* or *DateTime* data type. Such optionality is then a candidate for further constraints in derived profiles.

Each attribute does have an initial cardinality (Table 4.5). Each attribute is also combined with one or more of the flags listed in Table 4.6 that controls or indicates their behavior.

Table 4.5 FHIR® cardinality

Card.	Description
0..1	This attribute may optionally occur only once
0..*	This attribute may optionally occur
1..1	This attribute must occur exactly once
1..*	This attribute must occur, but may repeat

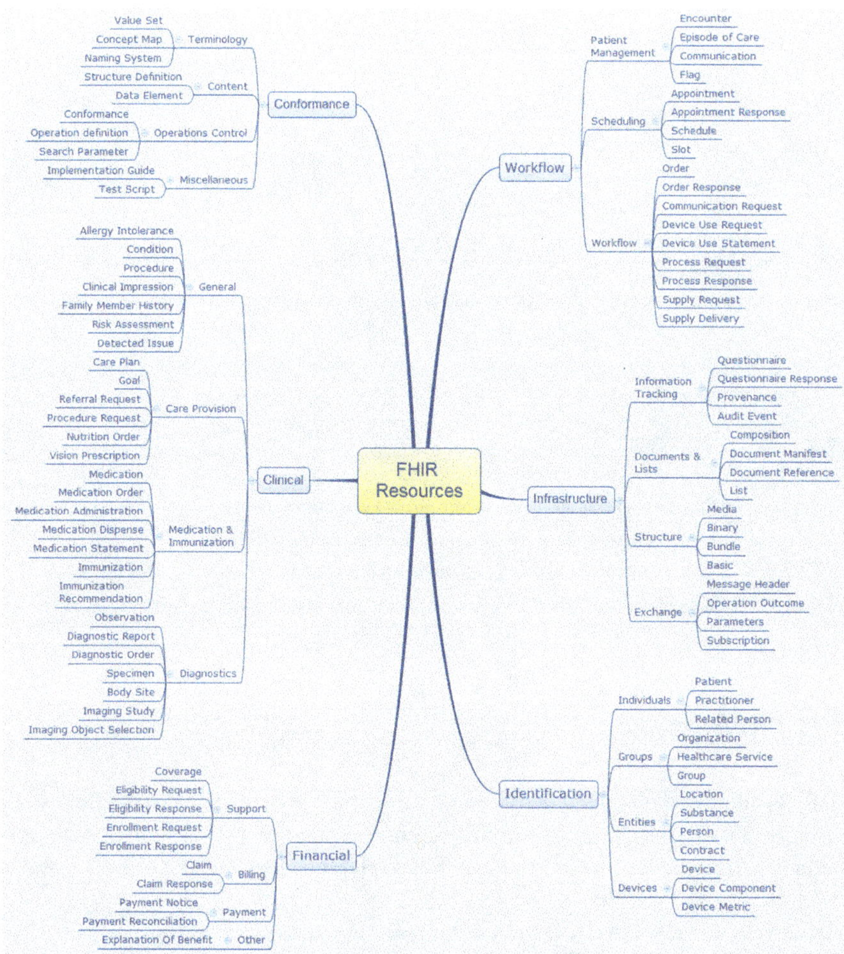

Fig. 4.12 Pre-defined FHIR resources (v1.0. 2-7202)

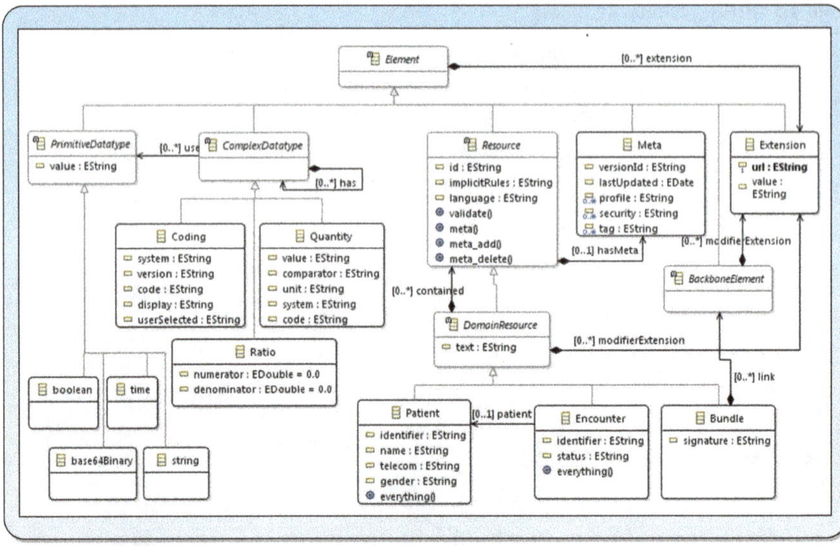

Fig. 4.13 HL7 FHIR® element hierarchy (derived from the specification)

Table 4.6 FHIR® flags

Flags	Description
?!	This element is a modifying element
S	This element is an element that must be supported
Σ	This element is an element that is part of the summary set
I	This element defines or is affected by constraints
NE	This element cannot have extensions (some infrastructural elements only)

4.3.3 References

FHIR facilitates web technology on a fundamental level. As such almost all resources provide attributes in form of references. Figure 4.14 demonstrates some references from the Procedure resource. Each reference may consist of a URL and a textual description for display (Fig. 4.15).

Figure 4.15 shows an example how a reference is represented in XML.

References can be provided as an absolute reference targeting resources somewhere in the web, relatively to the resource from which it is referenced, or internal to the bundle. By that means a web of resources can be established spanning multiple organizations.

Interfaces should be capable to deal with the different types of references and query the resources if necessary.

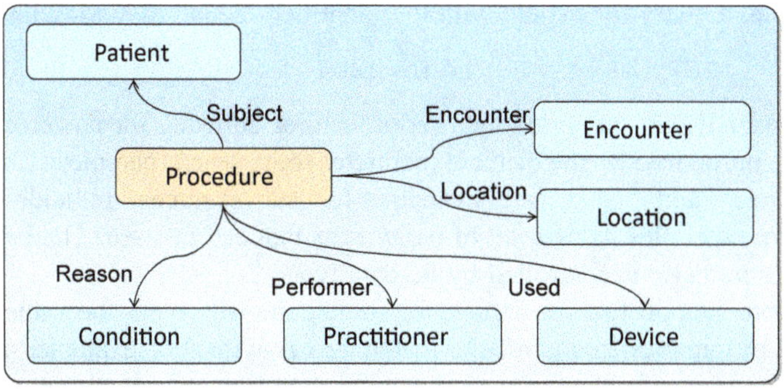

Fig. 4.14 References

```
<performer>
  <actor>
    <reference value="Practitioner/example"/>
    <display value="Dr Cecil Surgeon"/>
  </actor>
</performer>
```

Fig. 4.15 Example reference [3]

4.3.4 Bundling

The primary building block in FHIR is a resource. Each resource may be sent either as a reference or containing the appropriate details. But conveying a single resource alone is only sufficient in simple contexts. In most cases several resources will be grouped together to establish a specific context. This may be used to query a list, e.g. a list of patients. Or it can be used to query the history for a specific resource, e.g. the data sets for a specific patient at different points in time. Another option is to aggregate specific data, e.g. the medication for a specific patient including the conditions or a composition of sections providing a document. Such sets of resources are encompassed by a resource called Bundle.

4.3.5 Retrieval and Queries

Resources are searched and retrieved by RESTful operations:

```
GET [base]/[resourcetype]?name = value&...
```

For example, a query for patient with the identifier "2234" may look like this:

```
GET [base]/Patient/2234
```

Searches in FHIR are supported by a set of features allowing for powerful queries. First of all, introduced by the element hierarchy some search parameters like "_id", "_lastUpdated" and "_text" are available for all resources. In addition, each resource type specifies its own set of parameters that can be used. The behavior of the search parameter is controlled by its data type.

In order to support fuzzy searches, for some parameter types the values may be prepended by prefixes to control the matching behavior. For example, a numeric value may be prepended by "gt" to indicate the searched value is greater or equal to the provided value.

Another feature is the use of modifiers to negate the matching (":not"), or to search for absent values (":missing = true"). The latter is a kind of null flavor that is at least available in queries.

As a short summary, the FHIR query mechanics is in its functional power equivalent to an SQL query to a relational database.

4.3.6 *Extensibility*

Since the central design principle of FHIR is to include only core resource attributes in the base model guided by the 80:20 rule, extensions become an important part of the standard to account for elements not considered when the base model is developed. Given the high number of optional elements in other standard families introduced by individual requirements, the likelihood for extensions is very high. In other words, extensions are necessary to account for non-core requirements. The use of registries comes to mind as they would allow existing extensions to be copied, thereby avoiding creation of a large number of distinct solutions for the same problem. In fact, the current FHIR specification already contains a set of extensions especially for the US market. Other countries are currently working on their own set of initial extensions.

Because an extension is a built-in paradigm to FHIR and part of the topmost element, adding a specific extension to a resource can, therefore, be seen as a specific constraint on the possible extension for this resource.

4.3.7 *Use of Vocabulary*

Like all other data exchange standards, FHIR® has to support coded information as well. The specification of resources is based on value sets incorporating code systems and codes.

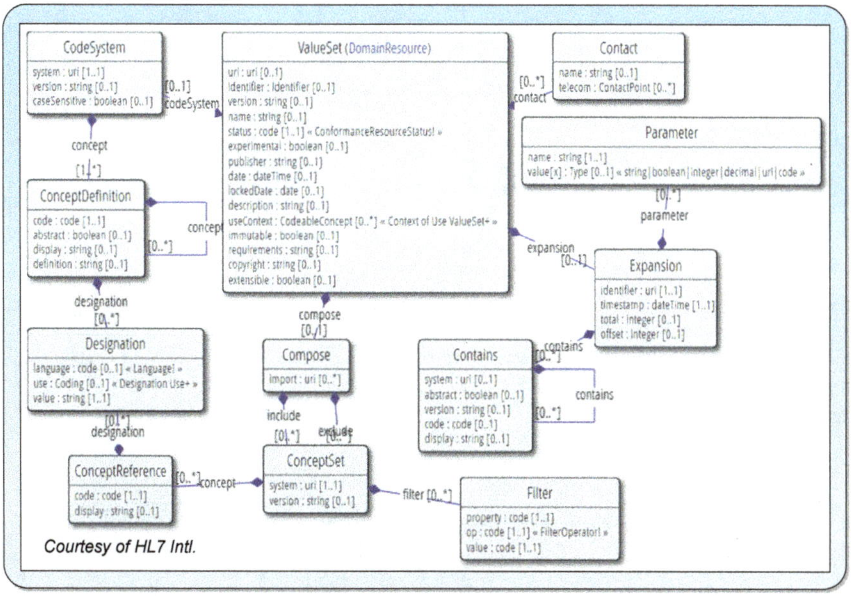

Fig. 4.16 "Value set" resource

In FHIR, this specification of resources is accomplished based on one of four data types:

- Code
- Coding
- CodeableConcept
- Quantity

The vocabulary binding is set for each element in a resource definition.

The use of human readable URLs instead of cryptic OIDs is an improvement offered by FHIR. Those URLs should point to the value content so that implementers may download them from the site (Fig. 4.16).

4.3.8 Data Types

FHIR®'s primitive data types are aligned as closely as possible with the underlying XML standard. The primitive data types are shown in Fig. 4.17. They all have the attribute *value* in common. This attribute is quite helpful when extensions are needed, because they can be nested inside primitive data types as well. Good examples for extensions are translations, null flavors, precision (for numeric values), and masking information.

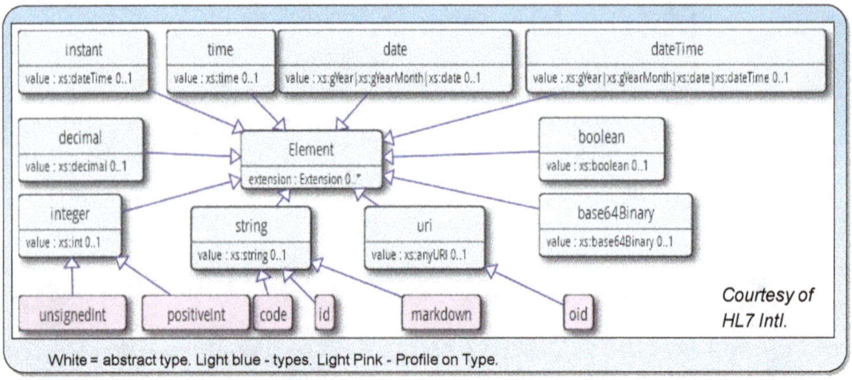

Fig. 4.17 FHIR primitive data types

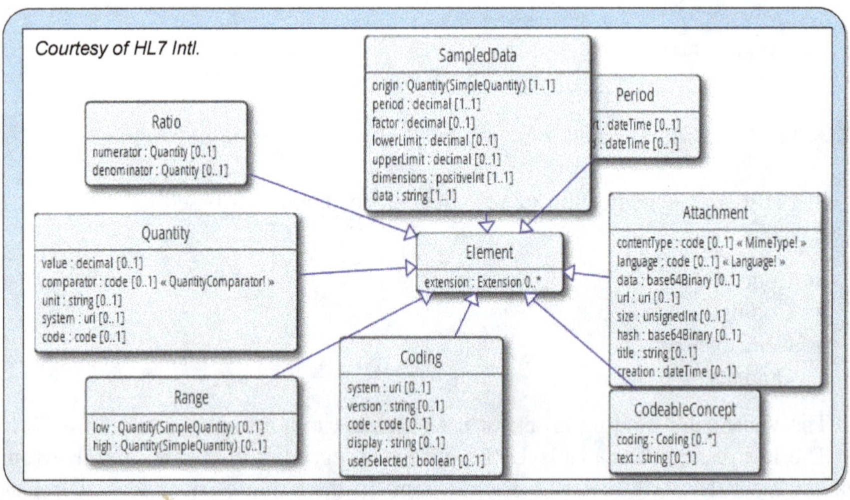

Fig. 4.18 FHIR complex data types (part 1)

FHIR® also provides complex data types, as shown in Figs. 4.18 and 4.19. These data types represent logical structures, which are comparable to those provided in HL7 version 2.x and V3, and FHIR® consolidates them into a new set.

Figure 4.18 part 1 lists a set of more "technical" data types, whereas part 2 in Fig. 4.19 is more user- and application-oriented.

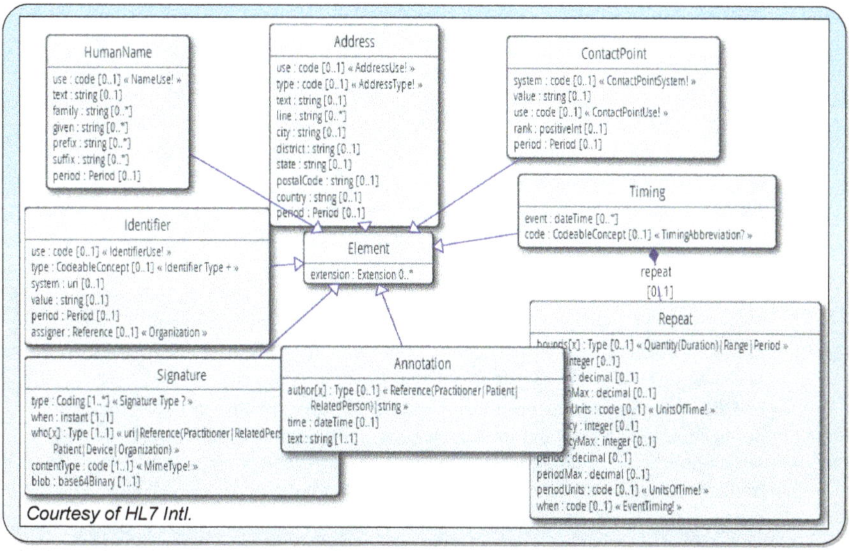

Fig. 4.19 FHIR complex data types (part 2)

4.3.9 *Representation/Encoding*

FHIR® provides two different kinds of encodings based on either XML or the *Java Script Object Notation* (JSON). Figures 4.9 and 4.10 demonstrate how the same set of data is represented in both encodings respectively (Table 4.7).

4.3.10 *Maturity Model*

A new mechanism has been introduced in FHIR for ranking the stability or maturity of resources. The Maturity Model is a measurement for the inverse probability that changes will be applied. Table 4.8 lists the different maturity levels according to the FHIR® specification.

Table 4.7 Attributes for a FHIR value set definition

Concept	Description
Path	A simple path reference to the element in question
Definition	Short description of the value set
Type	Binding strength of the element: • Required: the given codes shall be used • Extensible: the given codes shall be used, but additional codes are allowed • Preferred: the given codes should be used Example: the codes are listed for demonstration purposes only
Reference	Link to the value set itself

Table 4.8 FHIR® maturity model (v1.0.2)

FMM	Description
0	The resource or profile (artifact) has been published on the current build
1	FMM0 + the artifact produces no warnings during the build process and the responsible WG has indicated that they consider the artifact substantially complete and ready for implementation
2	FMM1 + the artifact has been tested and successfully exchanged between at least three independently developed systems at a connect-a-thon whose results have been reported to the FHIR Management Group
3	FMM2 + the artifact has been verified by the work group as meeting the Standard for Trial Use (STU) Quality Guidelines and has been subject to a round of formal balloting with at least 10 implementer comments drawn from at least 3 organizations resulting in at least one substantive change
4	FMM3 + the artifact has been tested across its scope, published in a formal publication (e.g. STU), and implemented in multiple prototype projects. As well, the responsible work group agrees the resource is sufficiently stable to require implementer consensus for subsequent non-backward compatible changes
5	FMM4 + the artifact has been published in two formal publication release cycles at FMM1 + (i.e. STU level) and has been implemented in at least 5 independent production systems in more than one country

To ensure backward compatibility, the FHIR community has to take great care in applying changes to a resource that has been assigned a high maturity level. Only resources with a certain maturity are made normative.

4.3.11 Versions

FHIR® has been a work in progress over the past few years. After a first draft was released as STU 1, a major revision was provided in response to the experiences gained through use of STU 1 as listed in Table 4.9.

Table 4.9 FHIR® versions

STU	Description
1	First draft for comments, provided in 2013 and 2014
2	Major revisions to the framework and the resource definitions, increased and improved set of resources, released September 2015 as v1..1
2.1	Minor corrections without substantial changes
3	New version as a response to implementations of STU 2

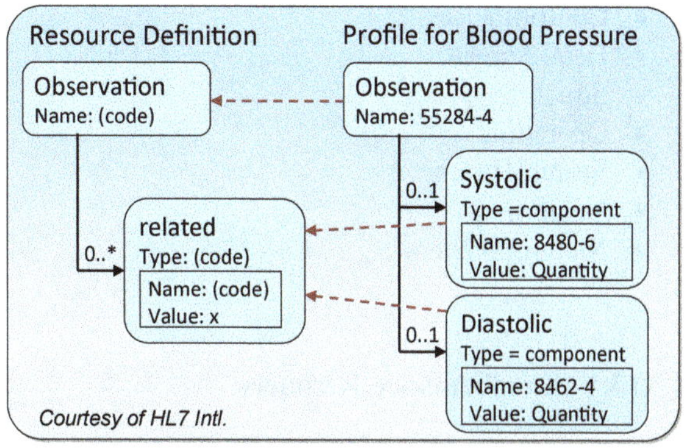

Fig. 4.20 "Slicing"

4.3.12 *Profiling by "Slicing"*

The mechanism for adding further precision (constraints) to a recursive element in FHIR® is called "slicing". Slicing results in a more specialized profile, as demonstrated in Fig. 4.20, and is comparable to unfolding recursive relationships in HL7 Version 3:

In our example, the generic component allowing for multiple repetitions is constrained to exactly two optional, but not repeating, components of a specific type.

FHIR's slicing capability, in conjunction with the creation of extensions, will then lead to more and more sets of profiles, which become necessary to solve a certain requirement.

4.3.13 *Conformance*

As mentioned above, FHIR® only takes care of the most relevant data elements, i.e., those items that are commonly used in at least 80 % of use cases. The consequence of this rule is a relatively large set of profiles. In the worst case, each FHIR server will support a multitude of extensions managed by profiles. A methodology for handling them automatically is essential. Each FHIR server must (SHALL) provide all profiles in a computable form in order to be FHIR-conformant. These profiles are themselves FHIR resources, which simplifies their processing.

For a patient, for example, the items include the name, the gender, and date of birth. Less relevant items like the religion are not specified. FHIR® provides a methodology that should allow vendors the flexibility to define the less relevant items for themselves. In order to control those self-defined modifications, a vendor has to declare what their interface supports and expects. This declaration is made through conformance statements. FHIR® has defined a set of resources for this purpose, including the following list of resources, each of which is explained briefly in the subsections below:

- Conformance
- DataElement
- Structure
- Operation
- Search Parameters
- Value Set
- Naming System

4.3.13.1 Conformance Resource

The conformance resource is used to describe the system's capabilities with regard to the actual (as implemented) (Fig. 4.21), expected (what is the necessary behavior), or desired (what someone is looking for) implementation, and it is linked to the profile resource.

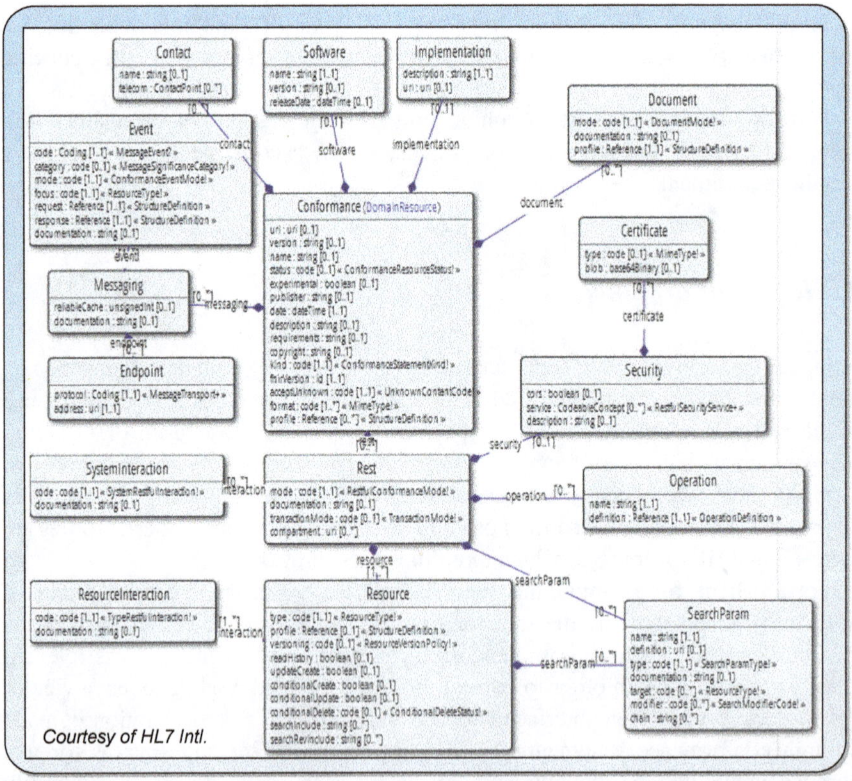

Fig. 4.21 FHIR® "conformance" resource

Table 4.10 Important FHIR conformance concepts

Concept	Description
Definition	A short description of this element.
Note	Personal notes of the implementer or public notes of the vendor.
Control (Min.. Max)	Minimum and Maximum cardinality of this element
Type	Data type
Requirements	Additional constraints
Summary	This element is part of a summary set.
Comments	Other additional information
Invariants	Fixed requirements and assurances for this element.
Condition	A set of computable statements (commonly in XPath) that allow you to formulate more complex constraints on the data in the instance
Alternate names	Other common names this element is known by.

Table 4.10 is an extract of the most important concepts for our conformance analysis:

4.3.13.2 DataElement Resource

This resource helps with defining a single piece of information that may be used in other specifications. In contrast to Structure Definition, these formal descriptions can also be used outside the scope of FHIR.

4.3.13.3 Structure Definition Resource

This resource is used to describe the content in the FHIR specification itself, i.e., the resources, data types, infrastructural types, and extensions. This computable documentation helps in publishing, sharing, and comparing of FHIR specifications, and also in generating code, reports, and user interfaces. The basic structure is shown in Fig. 4.22.

The structured definition resource is used by the conformance resource instances to describe how resources are used. It also is combined ("bundled") with value sets to introduce the use of coded concepts.

4.3.13.4 Operation Definition Resource

This resource is used to formally describe what additional functions can be invoked by a resource for data in a FHIR server. This includes the necessary parameters and the return value.

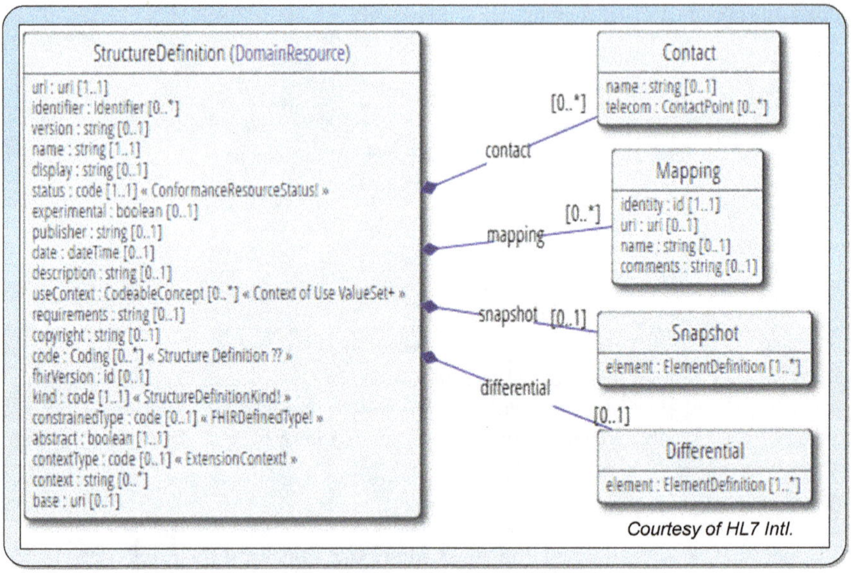

Fig. 4.22 FHIR® “structure definition” resource

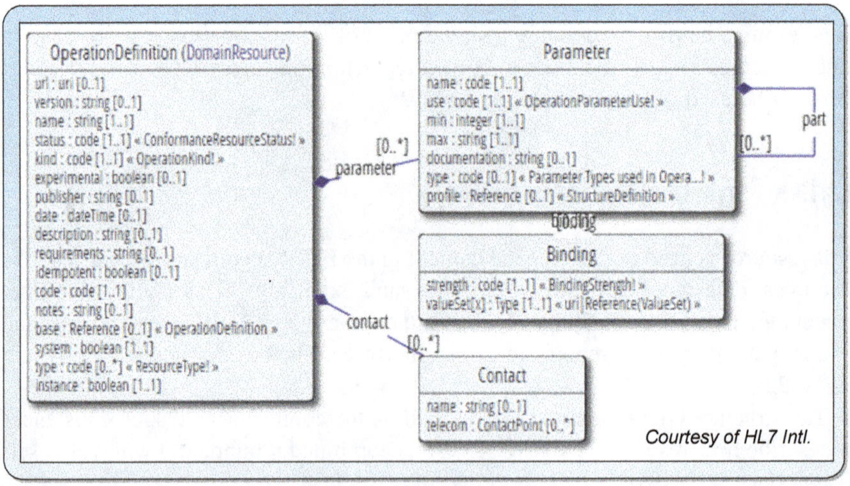

Fig. 4.23 FHIR® “operation definition” resource

By this means new operations can be defined for a resource, which expands the overall functionality (Fig. 4.23).

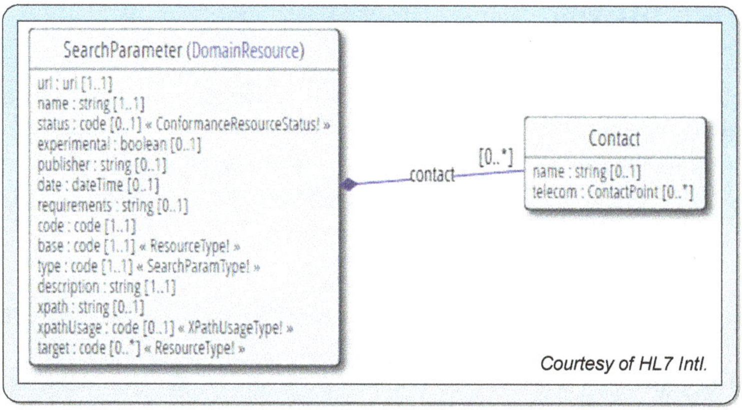

Fig. 4.24 FHIR® "search parameter" resource

4.3.13.5 Search Parameter Resource

This resource (Fig. 4.24) specifies the meta data to describe the name of a search function and the associated parameters that can be used when querying or filtering for specific resources.

4.3.14 Conformance Methodology

The HL7 Conformance Work Group was able to ensure that providing profiles and conformance resources is made mandatory for vendors. Using specific resources for this purpose would help in establishing the provision. Even better, these declarations should be made available online in order for users to resolve profile and conformance resources problems more easily and independently.

The Conformance resources then could control how the server implements searches, resource elements, and extensions, but this capability would not be required.

Besides the explicit use of conformance resources, implementations may vary in their support of specific FHIR features, such as inclusion of related resources versus references to them, and whether and which (modifier) extensions are being used.

4.4 UN/EDIFACT

UN/CEFACT (as part of UN/ECE) has defined UN/EDIFACT [4] as a family of EDI standards to support data exchange among trading partners within different domains. The common construct is the *United Nations Standards Message* (UNSM), which can be regarded as a framework to define domain specific message types.

4.4.1 Introduction and Overview

Table 4.11 provides a schematic overview of the UN/EDIFACT message envelope. Square brackets denote optional elements, and curly brackets indicate structures that can have multiple occurrences.

Within the boundaries of UNB and UNZ, a set of individual messages can be conveyed. Hence, those two segments can be treated as batch headers and trailers for messages.

Figure 4.25 provides an example of a single message instance in EDIFACT.

4.4.2 Message Structure

Table 4.12 shows a complete message structure as it appears in the original EDIFACT specification for the medical domain. It consists of segments and segment groups. To indicate the starting of a new group the first segment of a group is made mandatory/required.

Table 4.11 EDIFACT message structure

Segments	Description
[UNA]	Service string advice
UNB	Interchange header
{	
[UNG]	Functional group header
UNH	Message header
<Data Segment>	User data segments
UNT	Message trailer
[UNE]	Functional group trailer
}	
UNZ	Interchange trailer

```
UNA:+. ?'
UNB+UNOC:3+Senderkennung+Empfaengerkennung+060620:0931+1++1234567'
UNH+1+ORDERS:D:96A:UN'
BGM+220+B10001'
DTM+4:20060620:102'
NAD+BY+++Seller+Street+City++23436+xx'
LIN+1++Product Screws:SA'
QTY+1:1000'
UNS+S'
CNT+2:1'
UNT+9+1'
UNZ+1+1234567'
```

Fig. 4.25 EDIFACT example message

The segment status ("S" column in the table above) denotes whether a segment is mandatory ("M") or dependent on certain conditions ("C") that are either specified or negotiated between trading partners. The same status indicators apply for data elements within segments.

Segments may repeat individually, and groups of segments may repeat as well. The allowed number of repetitions is indicated under the "R" column.

As an example, the PDI segment, which contains a person's demographic information, is defined as shown in Table 4.13. If a given element in the segment contains additional components, these sub-components are listed with that element. Each of these entities has an assigned data type (alphanumeric and numeric) and maximum allowable length.

4.4.3 Delimiter

EDIFACT is a delimited format and as such makes use of special characters to represent those delimiters that are assigned a default value. In case a sender wants to deviate from those defaults the UNA segment as listed in Table 4.14 can be used at the beginning of the message.

EDIFACT does not support repetitions of data elements. Instead, the whole segment must be repeated. To support this approach, segments are quite small and normally consists only of a few elements. Consequently, the data for a specific person like a patient is spread over a set of distinct segments.

Table 4.12 EDIFACT MEDPID message structure

```
Pos    Tag Name                                   S   R

0010   UNH Message header                         M   1
0020   BGM Beginning of message                   M   1
0030   DTM Date/time/period                       C   9
0040   RFF Reference                              C   9
0050   FTX Free text                              C   99

0060       ----- Segment group 1 ---------------- M   99----------+
0070   PNA Party identification                   M   1           |
0080   ADR Address                                C   9           |
0090   CTA Contact information                    C   9           |
0100   COM Communication contact                  C   9           |
0110   RFF Reference                              C   99          |
0120   LAN Language                               C   9-----------+

0130       ----- Segment group 2 ---------------- M   9999--------+
0140   GEI Processing information                 M   1           |
0150   PNA Party identification                   C   1           |
0160   ADR Address                                C   9           |
0170   RFF Reference                              C   99          |
0180   DTM Date/time/period                       C   9           |
0190   IHC Person characteristic                  C   9           |
0200   NAT Nationality                            C   9           |
0210   FTX Free text                              C   9           |
0220   LAN Language                               C   9           |
0230   HAN Handling instructions                  C   9           |
0240   LOC Place/location identification          C   9           |
0250   FII Financial institution information      C   9           |
0260   CTA Contact information                    C   9           |
                                                                  |
0270       ----- Segment group 3 ---------------- C   9----------+|
0280   PDI Person demographic information         M   1          ||
0290   DTM Date/time/period                       C   9----------+|
                                                                  |
0300       ----- Segment group 4 ---------------- C   9----------+|
0310   COM Communication contact                  M   1          ||
0320   CTA Contact information                    C   9----------+|
                                                                  |
0330       ----- Segment group 5 ---------------- C   99---------+|
0340   REL Relationship                           M   1          ||
0350   PNA Party identification                   C   1          ||
0360   ADR Address                                C   9          ||
0370   RFF Reference                              C   9          ||
0380   DTM Date/time/period                       C   9          ||
0390   PDI Person demographic information         C   1          ||
0400   IHC Person characteristic                  C   9          ||
0410   NAT Nationality                            C   9          ||
0420   LAN Language                               C   9----------++

0430       ----- Segment group 6 ---------------- C   9-----------+
0440   AUT Authentication result                  M   1           |
0450   DTM Date/time/period                       C   9-----------+
0460   UNT Message trailer                        M   1
```

Table 4.13 EDIFACT PDI (person demographic information)

```
010    3499 GENDER CODE                                 C   1  an..3

020    C085 MARITAL STATUS DETAILS                      C   1
       3479  Marital status description code            C      an..3
       1131  Code list identification code              C      an..17
       3055  Code list responsible agency code          C      an..3
       3478  Marital status description                 C      an..35

030    C101 RELIGION DETAILS                            C   1
       3483  Religion name code                         C      an..3
       1131  Code list identification code              C      an..17
       3055  Code list responsible agency code          C      an..3
       3482  Religion name                              C      an..35
```

Table 4.14 EDIFACT UNA segment

Position	Element	Description	Default
1	Component data element separator	This delimiter separates the components of an element	:
2	Data element separator	This delimiter separates the elements (fields) within a segment	+
3	Decimal notification	This delimiter specifies the character that is used as a decimal point	.
4	Release indicator	This delimiter is used to indicate that the next character is not used as separator	?
5	Reserved for future use	This place is reserved and contains a space	
6	Segment terminator	This delimiter indicates the end of the segment	'

4.4.4 Data Types Format Notation

A specific notation is used in the EDIFACT standard to denote the data types for each element, as shown and explained in Table 4.15.

Because of the small segment sizes, no specific data structures are defined in the EDIFACT standard; specific segments are used instead. Other aspects, such as the formatting of dates, are indicated via additional information in the specification of the data elements. Table 4.16 illustrates this approach using the date/time/period segment as an example; and Tables 4.17 and 4.18 augment this information.

Table 4.15 EDIFACT data type format notation

Standard	Description	Comment
a3	3 alphabetic characters, fixed length	
n6	numeric characters (numbers), fixed length	A minus sign and a decimal mark are not counted as characters
an5	5 alphanumeric characters, fixed length	
a..6	up to 6 alphabetic characters	
an..35	up to 35 alphanumeric characters	
n..9	up to 9 numeric characters (number)	

Table 4.16 EDIFACT DTM segment

```
0010  C507 DATE/TIME/PERIOD                                   M   1
      2005  Date or time or period function code qualifier    M       an..3
      2380  Date or time or period text                       C       an..35
      2379  Date or time or period format code                C       an..3
```

Table 4.17 EDIFACT data element 2005

Code	Description	Explanation
1	Service completion date/time, actual	Actual date/time on which the service was completed
2	Delivery date/time, requested	Date on which buyer requests goods to be delivered
3	Invoice date/time	[2376] Date when a Commercial Invoice is issued
4	Order date/time	[2010] Date when an order is issued
.....		

4.4.5 *Tables*

EDIFACT does not provide a notation for tables. Data elements function as anchors instead, as can be seen with data element 2005 (Table 4.17) and 2379 (Table 4.18). The data element numbers can be seen as tables then.

Table 4.18 EDIFACT data element 2379

Code	Description	Explanation
2	DDMMYY	Calendar date: D = Day; M = Month; Y = Year
3	MMDDYY	Calendar date: M = Month; D = Day; Y = Year
4	DDMMCCYY	Calendar date: C = Century; Y = Year; M = Month; D = Day
5	DDMMCCYYHHMM	Calendar date and time: C = Century; Y = Year; M = Month; D = Day; H = Hour; M = Minute
6	CCYYMMB	Half-month: CC = century, YY = year, MM = month, B = 1:first half month, B = 2: second half month
…		

4.4.6 Conformance Methodology

EDIFACT only specifies the mandatory/required elements, and it does so by marking these elements with an "M". Analyzing a message structure, one can see that only a few elements are marked as mandatory, and that the message has a flat structure (a lot of segments); therefore, most elements are designated as optional in the standard, and their usage is left to be determined through trading partner negotiation, allowing for and facilitating a wide adoption of this standard.

4.5 ebXML

ebXML is an abbreviation for *electronic business XML.* Its primary purpose is to enable and facilitate business to business (B2B) partnerships by providing a means for persistent storage of information in a standardized registry or database. This capability is achieved by using web-based services to access the stored objects (content).

IHE ITI has based their Cross-Enterprise Document Sharing (XDS) Integration Profile on ebXML by constraining the available classes to a set suitable for the use case of this profile [5].

4.5.1 ebRIM

The ebRIM, *electronic business registry information model*, is a blueprint for the B2B registry itself. ebRIM provides a guideline for developers to organize their database structure for storing the information and its associated meta-data. It abstracts from concrete details by using generic classes that can be assigned attributes according to specific requirements. Figure 4.26 provides a high-level overview of the ebRIM:

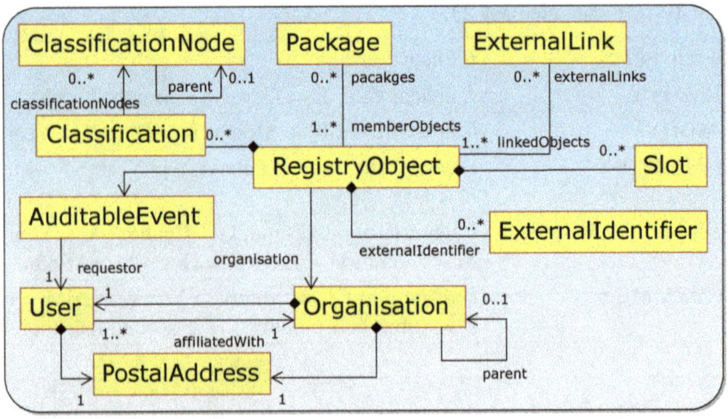

Fig. 4.26 ebXML registry information model (simplified after OASIS)

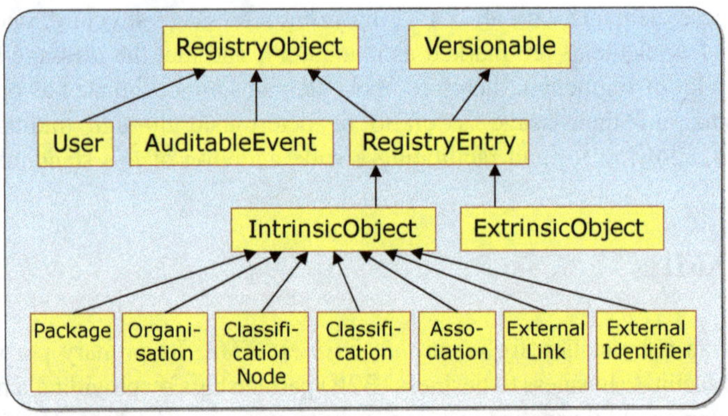

Fig. 4.27 ebXML information model inheritance (after OASIS)

The classes in Fig. 4.26 are organized in a hierarchical way, i.e., via the inherited properties. Through use of ebRIM, developers may benefit from a simplified architecture for their software solution (Fig. 4.27).

4.5.2 Data Types

In order to provide an uncomplicated approach for constructing and maintaining an ebRIM database, only a few basic data types are used in assigning the data type attribute to the generic classes, making these classes domain-independent. As depicted in Table 4.19, some of the data types only differ from each other in their lengths:

Table 4.19 ebRIM data types

Data type	XML schema data type	Description	Length
Boolean	boolean	Used for a true or false value	
String4	string	Used for strings that are 4 characters long	4 characters
String8	string	Used for strings that are 8 characters long	8 characters
String16	string	Used for strings that are 16 characters long	16 characters
String32	string	Used for strings that are 32 characters long	32 characters
ShortName	string	Used for a short text string	64 characters
LongName	string	Used for a long text string	128 characters
FreeFormText	string	Used for a very long text string in freeform text	256 characters
UUID	string	DCE 128 Bit Universally unique IDs used for referencing another object	64 characters
URI	string	Used for URL and URN values	256 characters
Integer	integer	Used for integer values	4 bytes
DateTime	dateTime	Used for a timestamp value such as Date	

Table 4.20 Explanation of ebRIM class parameters

Column headers	Description
Attribute	The name of the attribute being assigned for a particular class
Data type	Specifies the data type for the attribute assigned to the class
Required	Specifies whether the attribute is required to be specified
Default value	Specifies the default value in case the attribute is omitted
Specified by	Indicates whether the attribute's values are specified by the client or specified by the registry. In some cases both are listed
Mutable	Specifies whether an attribute (or the values assigned to the attribute) may be changed once it has been set to a certain value

4.5.3 Classes and Attributes

The classes defined in the registry information model are by the parameters as listed in Table 4.20. Table 4.21 illustrates an example specification for the RegistryObject class.

4.5.4 Methods

In addition to the attributes, the methods for a class are specified as well. The methods are specified in Table 4.22.

Table 4.21 ebRIM class attributes for registry object (example)

Attribute	Data type	Required	Default value	Specified by	Mutable
AccessControlPolicy	UUID	No		Registry	No
Description	International-String	No		Client	Yes
Id	UUID	Yes		Client or registry	No
Name	International-String	No		Client	Yes
Object type	LongName	Yes		Registry	No

Table 4.22 ebRIM class methods (example)

Return type	Method	Explanation
Collection	getOrganizations (String type)	Returns a list of organizations which are associated with this object. The query can be constrained by a specific type of object
...	...	...

4.5.5 *Conformance Methodology*

ebXML does not declare any specific conformance methodology. Conformance is condensed to the requirement to support all elements marked as required (Required = "Yes"). Derived specifications like IHE ITI XDS instantiate use case-specific models, introducing only those classes that are necessary to support and realize the underlying use case.

4.6 CTS2 (HL7)

"*The goal of the Common Terminology Services 2 (CTS 2) specification stack is to provide a standardized interface for the usage and management of terminologies. Terminologies provide the atomic building blocks of shared semantics, concepts. In a shared semantics environment, CTS2 provides a modular, common and universally deployable set of behaviors which can be used to deal with a set of terminologies chosen by the users of the service in their deployment environment. The service will contribute to interoperability by supporting an easy access to the foundational elements of shared semantics. It will also foster the authoring of high-quality terminologies* via *its authoring profile. This goal is realized* via *the expansion of the original functionality outlined in HL7's Common Terminology Service (CTS) Specification. CTS 2 defines the functional requirements of a set of service interfaces to allow the representation, access, and maintenance of terminology content either locally, or across a federation of terminology service nodes."* [6].

With the transition to a normative standard, several enhancements have been applied to the specification. With regard to conformance issues, the most prominent change is the introduction of profiles, a kind of related function intended to support a specific functionality.

4.6.1 Information Model

Figure 4.28 provides the official CTS2 functional model.

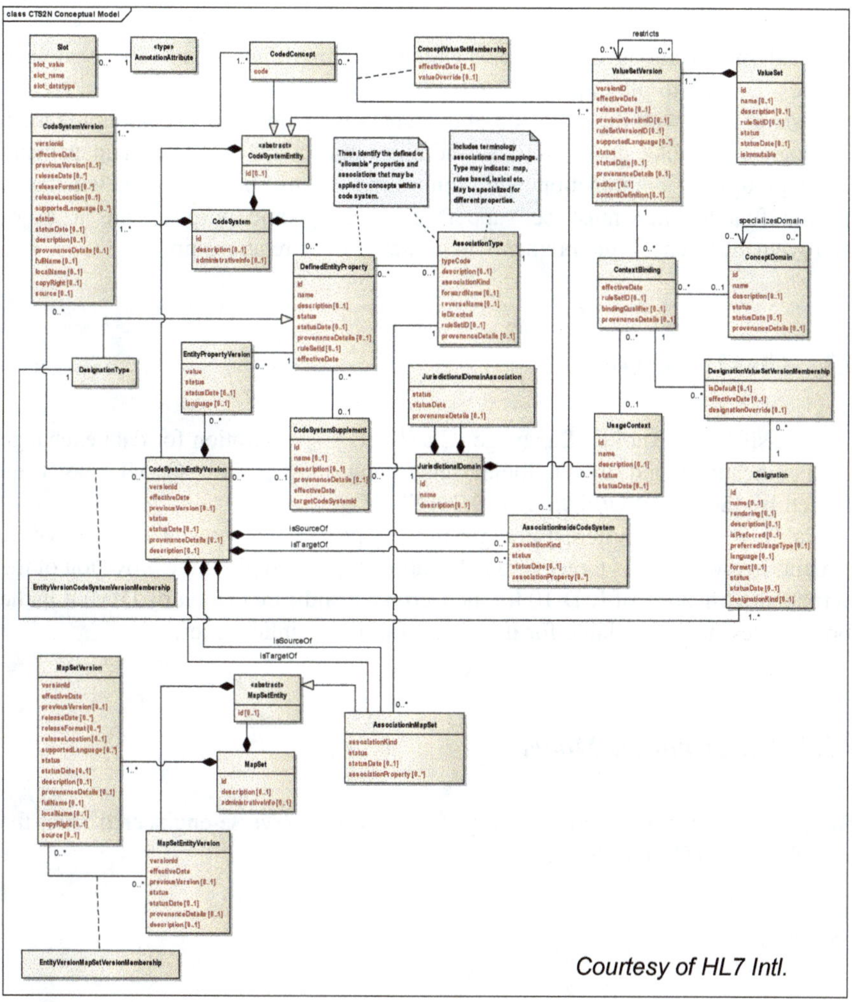

Fig. 4.28 HL7® CTS2 information model

4.6.2 Conformance Methodology

As mentioned earlier, CTS2 provides functional requirements, but on an abstract level only; therefore, it does not provide definitive guidance on specific implementations and the use of certain technologies. Vendors are free to decide on their own how they apply this functionality. Consequently, several implementations exist that claim conformance to CTS2-FM with the intention of indicating that they have implemented the functional model. The terminology server itself should be accessed then by employing appropriate services defined by the vendor. Without any further guidance, each service definition is disparate so that plug&play in the sense of switching URLs does not work.

To overcome this problem, the Object Management Group (OMG) has undertaken an initiative to transform the functional model into a set of concrete web-services based on WSDL and WADL. Vendors are now invited to use these technical specifications when implementing and providing their CTS2-compliant services, leading to plug&play.

Another issue with the provision of the functional requirements is grouping them into logical sets like query&retrieve, administration, and value set management. These groups, in combination with some kind of information about whether a specific functionality must be supported for a specific purpose, are a major improvement to check requirements in a client/server relationship.

4.7 ClaML (ISO)

The Classification Markup Language (ClaML) is a specification for data exchange of classifications and terminologies underlying master files. ClaML has been defined by ISO as "ISO/FDIS 13120:2012" [7].

ClaML is used by different organizations to provide the vocabulary for specific domains in a way that is targeted to publication. One example is the provision of the German modification of ICD-10 for the German healthcare market by DIMDI in the form of files made available for download from its public server.

4.7.1 Information Model

The information model shown in Fig. 4.29 has been reverse-engineered from the official XML DTD for ClaML.

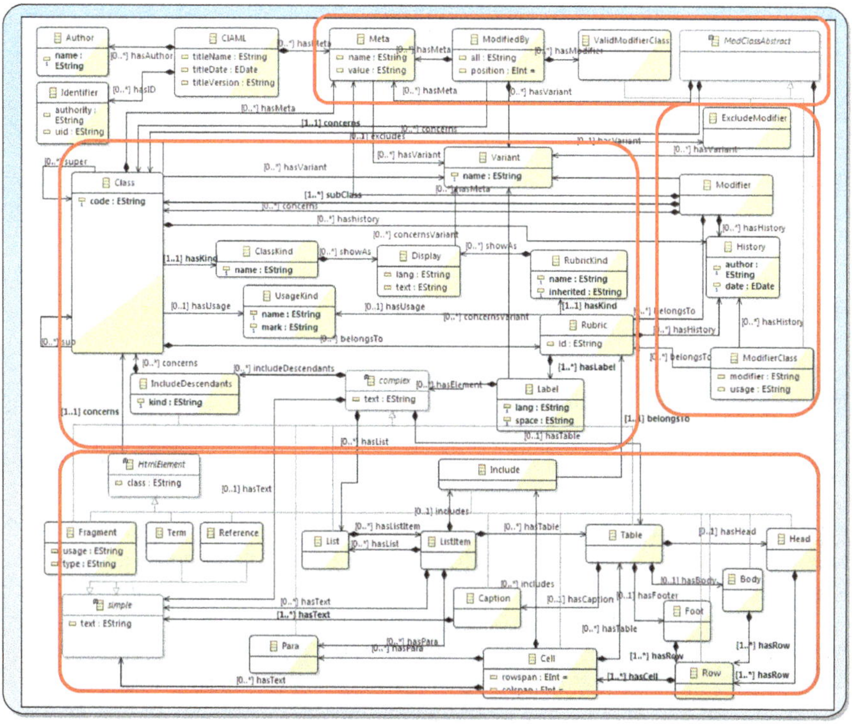

Fig. 4.29 ClaML information model

Besides some versioning information, the information model for ClaML can be divided into four main parts. The first part, shown in the left-hand side of the figure, refers to the codes being defined and their associated description. The second part describes the options for formatting and laying out the textual information, which is shown in the lower half of the figure. The codes can be described by additional meta-information in form of attribute value tags. This capability is shown at the top marked section of the figure. The last part reflects so-called modifiers that help to expand the available codes into subordinated hierarchies.

4.7.2 Conformance Methodology

ClaML does not provide any explicit conformance methodology nor any details in this regard. However, experience and feedback from real implementations demonstrate that the use of the specification results in individual interpretations of the available classes, which lead to incompatibilities in processing the files.

One possible option for declaring conformance is to specify the level to which text formatting is supported. Most ClaML files are limited to very simple representations like paragraphs, perhaps extended to simple lists. However, ClaML allows complex structures like tables, references, and lists that can be nested in arbitrary ways. Due to XML being an encoding without explicit semantics, textual descriptions provided in this way may not be processed from received files.

Another option for implementers is to support modifiers, which are intended to generate new codes.

The third option for implementers of ClaML is the use of meta-data. The tags can be used to mark a specific item for a specific purpose. An example thereof is the use of the meta-data "infectiousDisease" to indicate those codes in the German ICD modification that require notification of public health agencies in Germany. This markup clearly indicates some kind of semantics that need specific treatment during processing ClaML files.

Also, multi-language support may cause additional requirements on implementers.

This analysis leads to the conclusion that metadata should be used on a high level to introduce the levels of details (or features) that are used within a ClaML file so a parser (recipient of this information) is aware of possible import oversights. The meta-data may replace a conformance statement.

4.8 Technical Compatibility Matrix

As mentioned earlier in this chapter, the presented healthcare data exchange standards use various conformance constructs. These standards have different names for those concepts, and each concept may represent a pre-coordination of other concepts. Not every standard supports each construct. The different conformance constructs in use are described and grouped according to their attributes, and are listed in the left-hand column of Table 4.23 to facilitate comparing them. The data exchange standards are listed across the top of the table, and the standards used by each construct are marked with a checkmark in the row for the construct. Note, some of the standards listed are covered in this chapter, others are covered in Appendix, and others are referred to in this book but not described.

4.9 Summary

In this chapter, we have presented a set of established communication standards. Although they are or have been in use in different countries and their specification facilitates different languages (English, German, French), they all introduce the same overall concepts with or without consistent definitions:

Table 4.23 Technical comparison matrix of conformance constructs

Attributes	HL7 v2.x	HL7 V3/ CDA	HL7 FHIR	ebXML	EDIFACT	DICOM	xDT	H. PR. I.M.	PN13	CTS2	ClAML
Reference Model		✓		✓						✓	✓
Optionality										✓	✓
Required w/o mentioning null values[14]	✓					✓			✓		
Required w/o null value		✓ 15		✓	✓		✓				
Required w/ null value		✓ 16									
Required but may be empty	✓										
Optional	✓	✓	✓	✓	✓	✓	✓	✓	✓		
Forbidden/not permitted	✓	✓									
For backward compatibility reasons, about to be deprecated	✓										
Conditions	✓	✓			✓		✓				
Null Values											
Null Flavor			✓ 17								
Different specializations of null flavors		✓									
Delete Indication[18]	✓										
Cardinality/ repetition											
Min	✓	✓									
Max	✓	✓			✓		✓	✓			
Unlimited repetitions	✓	✓									
Length											
Min	✓										
Max	✓	✓	✓		✓	✓	✓				
Conformance	✓										
Other Concepts											

(continued)

Table 4.23 (continued)

Attributes	HL7 v2.x	HL7 V3/ CDA	HL7 FHIR	ebXML	EDIFACT	DICOM	xDT	H. PR. I.M.	PN13	CTS2	ClAML
Mutable		✓[1]		✓							
Must Support[2]	✓		✓		✓		✓				
Vocabulary											
Coding strength/extensible	✓	✓	✓								
Binding			✓								
Binding: example	✓	✓	✓								
Vocabulary Domain		✓									
Value sets		✓	✓								
Code systems		✓	✓								
Values	✓			✓			✓	✓	✓		
Data Structures			✓	✓			✓	✓			
Simple	✓	✓	✓			✓		✓			
Complex	✓	✓	✓			✓		✓			
Hierarchical Definition		✓									
Unspecified (varies, ANY)	✓	✓									
Choice (defined alternatives)			✓								
Data Types			✓	✓			✓	✓			
Technical (numeric, alpha, ..)	✓			✓		✓	✓		✓		
Extensions											
Foundationally built-in	✓		✓			✓		✓			
Allows for		✓									
As constraints			✓								
Arbitrary	✓							✓			
Other											
Delimiter	✓				✓			✓			
Backward Compatibility	✓					✓					

[a]This attribute is marked in cases where no separation is made between the different specializations

[b]Mandatory

[c]Required

[d]FHIR allows for querying empty fields

[f]This is introduced with the structural attributes like *classCode* and *moodCode* but not referenced explicitly

[g]Required elements implicitly introduce this concept because some kind of support is needed in order to provide or consume this element

- structural information for messages and segments (although this information may be called by different names)
- optionality, sometimes combined with conditions
- cardinality, sometimes as repetitions
- length information
- data types
- vocabulary, mostly as a list of values

Some of the standards also provide models for their constituent elements and associations.

Each standard differs in the way it represents concepts. In some cases, the representation is very intuitive, while in other cases the representation makes it very difficult to discern and understand the overall structure.

In the subsequent chapters, we will concentrate on the features HL7 v2.x provides, because this standard is very mature in its definition of conformance constructs and the methodology for dealing with conformance. As shown in this chapter, the specifications of the data exchange standards are fairly similar; therefore, the concepts that are explained for HL7 v2 in the chapters to follow will be easy to apply to other standards.

References

1. Oemig F: IHE internal technical terminology, v0.6, http://www.ihe.net. http://groups.google.com/group/iheterminology/attach/7804505ee72e6ed9/IHE+Terminology+v07.zip?hl=en&part=2. Last accessed Feb. 14 2010, http://www.hl7.org/documentcenter/public/wg/ictc/IHE%20Terminology%20v06.zip. Last accessed Feb. 14 2014.
2. Health Level 7 (HL7) Standard Version 2.5. ANSI/HL7 V2.5-2003. June 26, 2003. http://www.hl7.org.
3. Fast Healthcare Interoperability Resources. http://www.hl7.org/fhir.
4. UN/EDIFACT. United Nations Directories for Electronic Data Interchange for Administration, Commerce and Transport. http://www.unece.org/trade/untdid/welcome.htm. UN/EDIFACT: Directory, D.15.B, Message Type Directory Batch (EDMD). http://www.unece.org/tradewelcome/un-centre-for-trade-facilitation-and-e-business-uncefact/outputs/standards/unedifact/directories/2011-present.html.
5. IHE IT-Infrastructure Technical Framework. http://www.ihe.net.
6. HL7 Common Terminology Services, Release 2. Draft Standard for Trial Use. http://www.hl7.org/documentcenter/public/standards/dstu/2009may/V3_CTS_R2_DSTU_2009OCT.pdf. Last accessed February 26th, 2016.
7. Health informatics - Syntax to represent the content of healthcare classification systems - Classification Markup Language (ClaML). ISO/FDIS 13120:2012.
8. UN Centre for Trade Facilitation and E-business (UN/CEFACT)
9. ebXML Reference Information Model. http://www.oasis-open.org/committees/regrep/documents/2.0/specs/ebRIM.pdf.
10. ebXML Registry Services
11. "Introducing UN/EDIFACT". http://www.unece.org/trade/untdid/welcome.html.
12. EDIFACTORY. http://www.edifactory.de. Last accessed December 28 2015.

13. HL7 Common Terminology Services, Release 2. Normative Edition. http://www.hl7.org/implement/standards/product_brief.cfm?product_id=384. Last accessed February 26th, 2016.
14. HL7 Version 3 Reference Information Model. http://www.hl7.org.
15. Organization for the Advancement of Structured Information Standards. http://www.oasis-open.org.
16. UNECE: United Nations Economic Commission for Europe: http://www.unece.org/trade/untdid/d09b/trmd/medpid_c.htm. Last accessed February 12, 2016.

Part II
Conformance (and Tools)

Chapter 5
Conformance Constructs

5.1 Overview

Specifications state requirements for applications and systems. In order to specify these requirements precisely and consistently, conformance constructs are employed. Unfortunately, the set of conformance constructs are not defined sufficiently and uniformly across the spectrum of data exchange standards. A generic concept-level definition of common conformance constructs is presented in this chapter. More detailed definitions related to this information, including comparing and contrasting the variations of the conformance constructs across the assorted standards, also are discussed. The in-depth analysis will help the reader understand the salient facets of these constructs.

Conformance constructs can be viewed as a shorthand notation for expressing explicit statements of requirements. For example, if the desire is to make an element required, a conformance construct can be employed, such as Usage with an indicator of "R" (for required). The meaning of the indicator is defined in the standard. Use of conformance constructs reduces the instances of exhaustive and repetitive statements such as "The Element PID-8 is required." More details on this subject can be found in Chap. 6. Using conformance constructs, a table can be created that lists the elements in rows and requirement categories in columns. The requirement categories are defined by the conformance constructs and are the focus of this chapter.

Figure 5.1 provides a summary of conformance constructs commonly used to specify requirements in data exchanged standards. Additionally, the figure provides related conformance concepts that can't quite be classified as conformance constructs, but are important enough to include, and indicates how they are related. Between the constructs and concepts shown in this diagram, a solid line indicates a direct relationship, whereas a dashed line indicates an indirect relationship.

F. Oemig and R. Snelick, *Healthcare Interoperability Standards Compliance Handbook*, DOI 10.1007/978-3-319-44839-8_5

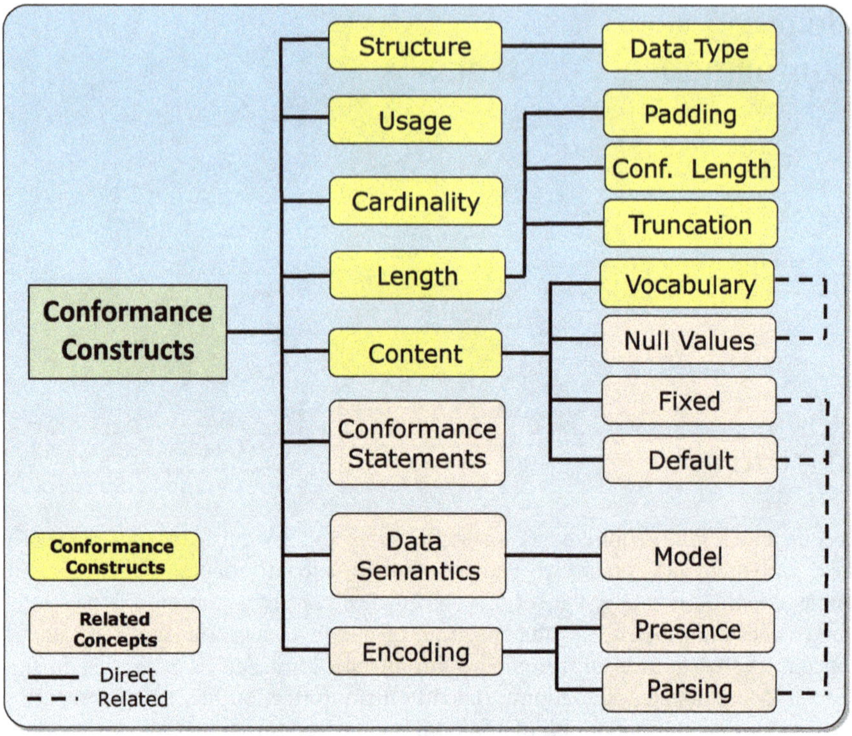

Fig. 5.1 Conformance constructs

The sub-sections that follow give a brief overview of the identified conformance constructs, their synonyms, and concept definitions, each of which will be expanded on in the remainder of the chapter.

The use of conformance constructs is a key mechanism used for constraining a standard for a specific use case. This concept is called profiling and is described in Chap. 7. The conformance constructs provide a foundation that facilitates profiling.

5.1.1 Conformance Constructs Overview

Structure: Defines a predefined sequence of elements. More sophisticated standards contain hierarchical structures. Examples include a document, resource, or message structure.

Less sophisticated standards only specify simple constraints on the element level, like alphanumeric or numeric values. The more sophisticated a data exchange standard is, the more hierarchies are introduced reusing previously defined structures. At the bottom level, the definition starts with (obvious) data types like (person or organization) names and addresses as building blocks, and the handling of identifiers and coded information is specified as well.

A common sub-structure is **Data Type,** which defines the data element structure and, at the primitive level, the type of data it may contain. Constraints include type substitution and specialization (when combined with other constraint types). String, Date, Time, Address, Numeric, and Coded Element are examples of Data Types.

Usage: Indicates requirements for the way an element must be supported by an application; commonly expressed as the presence (appearance) of this element. The presence requirement usually is expressed as "shall be present", "may be present", or "is not allowed to appear". Usage also is referred to as Appearance or Optionality indicator. An example of a usage indicator is R-Required. In HL7 v2.x, "R" is interpreted to mean that the element must be supported and valid data must be present in every message instance. The Usage construct in some data exchange standards has interdependencies with cardinality, which is addressed later in this chapter.

Cardinality: Identifies the minimum and maximum number of occurrences that must be supported for an element. Cardinalities are expressed as a minimum-maximum pair of non-negative integers. Cardinality is also referred to as repetition and occurrence.

Cardinality controls the number of occurrences of an element appearing in a message or document. Some elements shall always be present (e.g., cardinality [1..1], [1..n]); others shall never be present (i.e., cardinality [0..0]); and others may or may not appear, with zero or more occurrences specified (e.g., cardinality [0..n]). A conformant message or document must always contain at least the minimum number of occurrences, and shall not contain more than the maximum number of occurrences [1]. An example is [0..1], which indicates that the element may be omitted and can have at most one occurrence.

Length: Defines a constraint on the number of characters that may be present in one occurrence of an element. The length indicator can specify a maximum or the minimum and maximum bounds. The length controls the number of characters that are allowed for the value of a specific element. Some of the data exchange standards define a restriction on the length of an element's value, but most standards only support the restriction of the maximum length. Examples include 80, which means the value for this element must have at most 80 characters, and [2..4], which means the element must have at minimum 2 and at most 4 characters.

Care must be taken to determine whether the characters themselves or the bytes that represent them are to be counted. The details about this topic are explained in the Encoding section.

Data that are exchanged among different systems must be stored in some way. In most cases the storage of data for the elements is limited in length, typically caused by the length of each element's field in the database table that holds these data. If the length of an element value maintained in an application differs from the length as specified in the data exchange standard, a special treatment becomes necessary. The primary question when this situation arises is whether the value for the element is allowed to be truncated or not, and if not, how should the user interface behave?

Most data exchange standards are silent about special length considerations and leave the issue to the developer of an application, who in most cases is not even aware of this fundamental problem. More sophisticated standards have an explicit indicator as to whether truncation of the value for an element is permitted or not.

Content: Defines a mechanism to specify content (value) requirements of an element. Typically, it defines the allowable values for a coded element in the form of a list of values. As illustrated in Fig. 5.1, the content construct has four types, with the most important and most extensively used being vocabulary.

A vocabulary binding specifies a computable set of coded concepts for a data element, with additional useful parameters to support their use. An example is the administrative gender element that could be constrained to allow only the values M, F, U, and O. Vocabulary[1] is the term used in general (high-level) to express the idea of defining and using codes to constrain the content of an element. The primary reason for using codes for concepts is to have universally used computationally tractable identifiers for concepts across languages, cultures, and linguistic variants, and to avoid the inaccuracies of natural language processing. Additionally, the use of codes is an effective method to avoid sending lengthy strings or repeating the same information, or just to enable a reference to additional details by sending a short placeholder in a message or document. The use of codes facilitates processing and data mining. The different data exchange standards use different terms to address and support coding of data elements. These terms differ in their meaning and use:

- table and table values
- code systems and codes
- value sets and values

There also are coded methods for expressing "unknown content", i.e., to provide information as to the reason there may be no valid data.

Much confusion regarding the definition and specification of vocabulary exists in standards and implementation guides. This subject is explored later in this chapter and in Chap. 7 (for profiling of vocabulary).

The use of "null flavors (values)" is related to vocabulary. A null flavor is a concept for representing "unknown" content. Depending on the standard, a null flavor can be part of a value set (HL7 v2.x) or can be represented independently (e.g., HL7 V3). Some standards do not support the concept at all.

[1]The term vocabulary has a much broader context than stated here.

A fixed value constrains the content to a single value, e.g., "A08" that indicates an update event type in v2.x ADT messages. The more detailed and specific a certain data exchange standard is, especially in the case of specific use cases, the fewer possible options are valid for a data element. In some cases, the options for an element are reduced to a single value, thus providing a constant (fixed) value.

A default value is a pre-determined value assigned to an element. If the value is not present in the message or document, the recipient processes the element as though it is populated with the pre-determined value. Unlike a constant, the default value is overridden if the value is present in the message or document. The use of a default value is a common means of saving space by omitting data from a transmitted message or document. This approach requires the recipient to know what value should be used by default when a value is omitted. The use of default values is not recommended.

5.1.2 Related Conformance Concepts

In addition to the conformance constructs described in the section above, the following related concepts play an important role in specifying requirements for applications and systems.

Conformance Statement (Predicate Constraint): Provides an explicit normative statement expressed in text or a testable expression that defines a constraint. A conformance statement is used when a conformance construct is insufficient to specify a requirement or the conformance construct is not defined by the standard.

Patterns can be established to categorize conformance statements, such as a simple constant (e.g., element ABC = "15"). An example of a conformance statement would be "OBR-8 (Observation End Date/Time) SHALL be equal to or later than OBR-7 (Observation Date/Time)". A conformance statement is sometimes referred to as a "Predicate Constraint".

Data Semantics: Defines a concept (semantic) binding to a data element, that is, the sort of data the element is carrying. The "Patient Identifier" element provides information for identifying a patient, the definition of which provides the meaning of the data. A model can be developed to define the semantics and the related concepts (data elements).

Encoding: Data conform to suitable models and normally are organized in hierarchies. Encoding is a set of rules specifying how these data must be serialized and represented in a bijective fashion (i.e., in a one-to-one correspondence), so the recipient can decode this encoding to gather the original data.

5.1.3 Example Specifications

Conformance constructs are manifested in a number of different ways depending on the standard. Standards initiated in the late 1980s were based on EDI encoding and typically used tables to specify requirements, whereas later standards using XML encoding use model representations.

Table 5.1 shows a representative specification of requirements in a table format. The example is for fields in an HL7 v2.x RXA (Pharmacy Treatment Administration) Segment that can be used to message information about immunizations. The structure is indicated in the "SEQ" (Sequence) column and defines a specific order of data elements. The Element Name indicates the name of the data element; the concept (data semantics) that the element represents is typically defined in the standard in a separate element definition in the form of a description or potentially further in a constrained specification. Usage determines the appearance (presence) of the element. The table shows conditional usage (to be discussed later in this chapter). Cardinality indicates how many times the element may occur, and length gives the range for the number of characters that can be in the value for the element. Data Type defines the sub-structure of the data element, which is either complex or primitive. Value Set indicates the vocabulary binding.

Conformance statements (if there were any) and the condition predicate (for the conditional usage) would also be specified, either in additional columns or shown below the table because of space limitations. Length is not particularly meaningful for complex data types and, therefore, is not indicated in this example.

Figure 5.2 illustrates an example of requirement expressions using conformance constructs in CDA that facilitate the HL7 Templates specification. This particular statement expresses that the code attribute must be present with a specific fixed value. Figure 5.3 provides another example for constraining the attribute "string" in FHIR. This example is self-explanatory, because it also contains the definition. Although, the representations are different, the principle of using conformance constructs to express requirements is the same.

Table 5.1 Representative specification of requirements in a table format

SEQ	Element name	Usage	Card	Len	Data type	Value set
…						
RXA-5	Administered code	R	[1..1]		CE	CVX
RXA-6	Administered amount	R	[1..1]	[1..20]	NM	
RXA-7	Administered units	C(R/X)	[0..1]		CE	UCUM
RXA-8	Administration dosage	O	[0..1]		CE	
RXA-9	Administration notes	C(R/O)	[0..*]		CE	NIP001
…						

```
<element conformance="R"
         datatype="CE"
         Id="2.16.840.1.113883.3.1937.777.1.9.275"
         isMandatory="true"
         maximumMultiplicity="1"
         minimumMultiplicity="1"
         name="hl7:code">
  <vocabulary code="39135-9"
              codeSystem="2.16.840.1.113883.6.1"
              codeSystemName="LOINC"
              displayName="WoundAssessmentPanel"/>
</element>
```

Fig. 5.2 Conformance construct expressed as CDA template (excerpt)

```
<element>
  <path value="string"/>
  <short value="Primitive Type code"/>
  <definition value="A string which has at least one character
         and no leading or trailing whitespace and where there is
         no whitespace other than single spaces in the contents"/>
  <min value="0"/>
  <max value="*"/>
  <base>
    <path value="string"/>
    <min value="0"/>
    <max value="*"/>
  </base>
  <type>
    <code value="Element"/>
  </type>
</element>
```

Fig. 5.3 Conformance construct expressed as a FHIR code profile (excerpt)

5.1.4 Summary

The conformance constructs are foundational components that are used to define requirements in a structured approach. Since the conformance constructs are used to define requirements, and such use has implications for implementers, the constructs must be well understood by both the authors and readers of the specifications. That is, a common understanding of the requirements relies on a common understanding of the constructs that are used to define the requirements. The structured approach also provides short-hand notations (e.g., in a table format) for expressing the requirements. This approach allows the reader to view such requirements quickly without having to sift through extensive text. The structured approach also promotes automated processing of requirements and inclusion in models. All requirements should be easily viewable by readers; the use of conformance constructs promotes this practice.

The above list provided an overview of the general conformance concepts used to specify requirements in data exchange standards. The sections that follow elaborate on each concept and, when necessary, point out the subtle differences in definitions and interpretations in the various standards. Detailed examples of each construct are given to help the reader understand the concepts.

5.2 Data Structures and Data Types

Data exchange standards realize data types in different ways. In some standards, data types that are created by aggregating components are utilized in order to manage what normally is called a data structure ("struct" in C/C++ or "class" in Java). This approach is explained in the sub-sections below using atomic versus complex data as an example. In other standards, a data type is both the indirect association of a storage space for information and the way the information is represented ("char/int" in C/C++ or "strings/int" in Java). This representation and formatting approach also is explained in the sub-sections below.

5.2.1 Binding to Elements

The data structure construct is used in specifications to express further details about and the expectations associated with a data element. The data structure is bound to an element. Depending on the design of the standard, this binding can be established on field level and/or component and subcomponent level. HL7 v2.x provides all three levels, where the higher level (starting with a field) dictates the next level (i.e., field to component; or component to subcomponent). In HL7 V3, the binding is accomplished using the attributes of the classes. The German xDT family only provides "fields" that allow for binding to alphanumeric or numeric data. Data structures are not provided in xDT.

Most data exchange standards require an explicit and unambiguous data type binding to a data element to allow no other choices. HL7® FHIR® allows for binding of a set of data types to an element. A person's deceased date (attribute "deceased") is an example thereof, allowing for a Boolean value ("yes" or "no" in "deceasedBoolean") or a specific date ("died on July 1st 2013") up to a point in time (in "deceasedDateTime"). A profile must be created to constrain this element to a single data type.

5.2.2 *Atomic Versus Complex Information*

More sophisticated standards allow for the specification of structured information—or higher level data types. A precondition thereof is the availability of substructures and further delimiters to keep the related information together. XML-based standards have an arbitrary number of options to support this capability. Other standards—like DICOM—borrow the required delimiters from "friends" like HL7 v2. "Old standards", like the German xDT, do not allow for complex data types at all. As a result, more sophisticated standards provide higher level aggregations like the ones listed in the Table 5.2.

Complex data types typically are created out of other data types, possibly resulting in an endless nesting. In the end, this capability is limited by the expressivity of the associated encoding. For the HL7 v2.x family, a field is limited to components and subcomponents, i.e., two levels, simply because of the self-imposed limit of delimiters. Table 5.3 is used to clarify this point.

Table 5.2 Common complex data types

Complex data type	Explanation
Name	Names (including the appropriate parts) for persons and organizations
Address	Addresses (and the related details) for locations
Contact information	Telecom information and email addresses
Coded information	A concept is always combined with other details like description, code system, etc.
Identification	Instances of something (e.g., persons, organization, or specific person-related diagnosis) require a means for unique identification
...	

Table 5.3 Example data structure for address

Component	Explanation	Data structure	Data type	Remark
Street	Name of the street		String	
House number	Number of the house		Integer	Does not allow for number in combination with a character, e.g. "1010b"
ZIP	Postal code	Code		A list of codes must be defined; most probably in the form of strings because some countries use alphanumeric codes
City	Name of the city		String	
Country	Country code	Code		See remark for ZIP

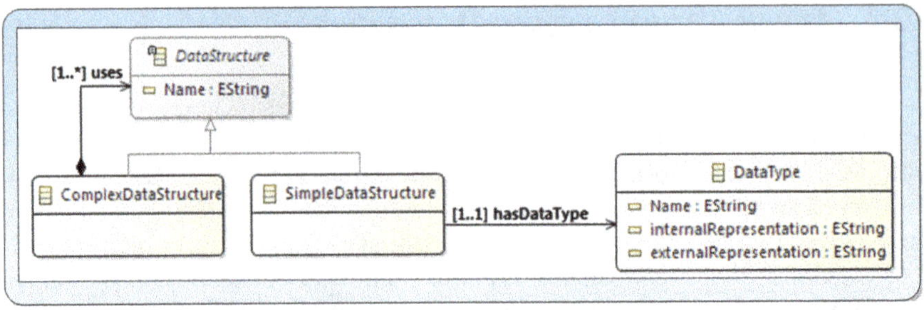

Fig. 5.4 Data structures and data types

The assignment of a data type, as illustrated in Fig. 5.4, only makes sense on an atomic level, i.e., when there is no further refinement; therefore, the two components that are using codes are refined by another data structure definition.

Another point to note is that, typically, the ZIP code and country information for addresses are specified as normal text fields, i.e., strings, which allows for ease-of-use. In some circumstances, those two fields must be treated as codes, in which case the correct accompanying information about value sets and code systems is necessary. For example, ZIP codes are assumed to use the set of values that are valid in the country of use. For country codes, the ISO table can be used. The sets of values to use for either of these address-related codes are rarely mentioned explicitly in a standard.

5.2.3 Representation/Formats

Table 5.4 provides an overview of data types usually used in data exchange standards. Most use cases only require the data types that are indicated by the "X" in the right most column.

Table 5.4 Common data types

Data type	Explanation	Common usage
String	Any combination of (printable) characters; this is the most universal use without any restrictions	X
Real	Any (decimal) number w/ or w/o fractions	X
Integer/Numeric	Integer values, sometimes restricted to positive or negative integers w/or w/o infinitive values	X
Date	A date	X
Time	A point in time (without specifying an associated date)	X
Timestamp	A point in time at a specific date	
Binary	The information is taken as a blob ("binary large object"). Additional information about the contents and an associated special interpreter (parser) are required for this format The most common usage is the transmission of files in different formats (e.g. PDF , MS-Word), HMTL, or XML	

Table 5.5 Formatting of data

Contents	Format(s)	Comment/Remarks
Date	dd/mm/yyyy mm/dd/yyyy dd.mm.yyyy yyyymmdd	Different ways to express the same information, but some ways are ambiguous because the correct interpretation is not clear (please see paragraph after this table for an example)
Numbers		The character for the decimal point can be different ("." or ","), and thousands can be separated ("1.000" or "1000")? Does precision matter, i.e. is "1.100" different from "1.1"?
eMail	<account>@<domain>	
URL	<access>:<address>	
UNC name	//<base address>/<pathname>	Depending on the operating system the slash is used in conjunction with or as an alternative to a backslash
URI		UUID, GUID, OID
Telephone numbers	<country><city><base><extension>	With or w/o delimiters? How are special numbers like speed dial codes handled?
...		

The transmission of those data types usually raises the question about how associated data should be represented. This issue requires special attention in cases where different options are possible, which would allow for misinterpretations. Table 5.5 provides an overview of the formats used for various types of data.

As can be seen regarding dates, some representations of the values allow for misinterpretation. "12/24/2013" is easy to interpret as December 24th, 2013, but "5/6/2013" can either be "May 6th 2013" or "June 5th 2013". Without any additional information, a firm conclusion cannot be reached.

5.2.4 *Precision in Representation*

Another issue for discussion is the manner in which numbers with decimals are represented. When specifying numbers, the way they are presented to an end-user in a graphical user interface or on a report should not matter to the exchange specification (the display of the number is a local matter). The areas of concern are related to the separation of thousands by a comma or a decimal point (e.g., "1.000.0000" vs. "1,000,000.0" vs. "1000000"), and to leading/trailing zeros (e.g., "00123" vs. "123"). Though these issues are just focused on the formatting of a number, the quantity of digits in the number and the use of a comma versus a decimal point are important considerations. The first factor limits the precision, and the latter factor places a requirement on writing/parsing the number.

For all formats, however, a regular expression that could be used for both evaluations and validations would be helpful.

5.2.5 Precision in Meaning

Another issue rarely addressed within data exchange standards is the precision of specific information. Table 5.6 provides some examples of relevant situations.

The problem is solved using different approaches across the various standards. For example, pertaining to an imprecise date, HL7 v2 combines an arbitrary date with explicit information about the precision. Taking the 3rd example (1.1.2013) from Table 5.6, the "Y" in "20130101^Y" says that only the year is valid information, although the month and day are conveyed as well. For the same reason, other standards use numbers for dates in a way that allows only the year to be represented.

Interfaces require that some kind of intelligence, combined with an appropriate data model, be designed into the application to handle this correctly. For example, an application may not store a "year" if the implementation is built on top of a date data type that only allows for storing exact dates based on a day.

5.2.6 Collections of Data Types

As indicated previously during the discussion of the cardinality (repetition) of an element, collections of attributes can be treated as certain kinds of aggregations. Table 5.7 presents an overview of the semantics, which go beyond a simple repetition of an element, related to these aggregations. As shown by the semantics presented in Table 5.7, repetitions can be treated as simple lists, because the only

Table 5.6 Examples for precision of information

Information	Meaning	Representation
"Take a pill every 12 hours"	A pill should normally be taken approximately twice a day, but not necessarily every 12 h	"2 ea/24 h" ("ea" means "each")
	A pill should be taken as closely as possible every 12 h	"1 ea/12 h"
"He is in his thirties"	The person is between 30 and 39 years old	"30-39 a"
"1.1.2013, precision year"	Any day in the year 2013	"2013" "20130101^Y"
…		

Table 5.7 Aggregations of data types

Construct	Comments
Set	More than a single element of a certain type without any duplicates
Bag	Some elements of a certain type, but duplicates are allowed
List	The elements are ordered into a sequence. The semantics of this sequence is not directly indicated and can, therefore, vary
Interval	A range of something that is built upon another generic data type. It requires the ability to establish a sequence so that it can be determined whether a specific element belongs into this range or not The most common use is with points in time (timestamp) and numbers (integer and real) A relevant aspect is whether the two end points belong to the interval or not ("open" vs. "closed")

Table 5.8 Collections used in some standards

Construct	HL7 v2.x	HL7 V3	DICOM	xDT
Bag	Yes (*)	Yes	Yes (*)	Yes (*)
Set	Yes (*)	Yes	Yes (*)	Yes (*)
List	Yes (*)	Yes	Yes (*)	Yes (*)
Interval	Realized by specific data types	Yes	Realized by specific elements/tags	Realized by specific fields

The use of these constructs in the different standards, as indicated with "(*)", depends on the implementation guide associated with a specific use case, since the underlying standard does not provide a clear separation

ordering mechanism a list provides is a sequence. Repetitions allow for duplicate data, which is a property of a bag. Different standards use different ways to represent these aggregations, as shown in Table 5.8.

5.2.7 Promotion/Demotion (in HL7 V3)

HL7 V3 introduced an interesting concept called promotion/demotion of data types. The idea behind this concept is quite simple: within the standard, some data types used in the models are necessary to allow for a generic use. Nevertheless, under some circumstances the data types can be simplified further. A good example based on one circumstance is the reduction of an interval to a single point, which applies to time constraints and metered values. Another example is the reduction of the set of something to only a single instance, as in the reduction of a set of identifiers for a person to a single special identifier such as the social security number.

5.3 Usage (Optionality)

Data exchange standards specify data elements of interest for a specific use case. Whether this specification of elements is provided in the form of a hierarchy or linearly, e.g., for a line-oriented exchange format, does not matter. Usage (Optionality) defines the presence of an element in a message or document and is commonly expressed as "shall be present", "may be present", or "is not allowed to appear".

The expectations from using a data format specification in an application can be demonstrated using a very simple application, which is presented in the form of a database excerpt in the upper part of Fig. 5.5. (Section 5.3.1 discusses in detail the information depicted in Fig. 5.5.)

The lower part of Fig. 5.5 represents the elements that are expected to be transmitted for this interaction. The standard requires a specific sequence, i.e., the ordering of the elements (by "field numbers"). As shown, it is typical for the naming conventions between an application and the data exchange standards to differ. This fact is one reason why mapping an internal element to an external data exchange format allows for misinterpretations and possibly wrong mappings.

The optionality is intentionally not indicated yet in the diagram and is represented by the four question marks. Below is a list of possible choices for indicating the requirements related to the presence of elements.

- A value for an element must always be present; i.e., the element cannot be empty, and applications can rely on the existence of a value. The common

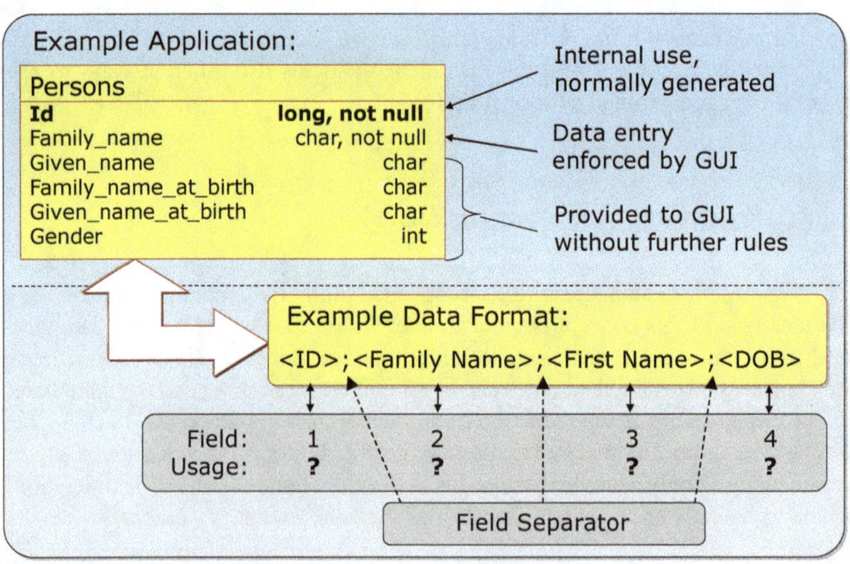

Fig. 5.5 Usage for an example application

Table 5.9 General optionality concepts

General concept	Common notations	Concepts meaning
Required	R-Required[a] M-Mandatory	The element must be present in a message or document. Different rules apply when managing null values
Optional	O-Optional	It is left for the implementer to decide what to do with an element
Forbidden	X-Not supported NP-Not permitted	The element is not allowed to be placed in a message or document

[a]The term "required" has different meanings in different standards, so it does not always mean that an element is actually present in a message instance. The same notion is valid for "RE-required but may be empty" (in HL7 v2). The minimum cardinality for an RE element is set to zero, so the element can be empty. In other words, the intent is for an application to *be able to* support an RE element, although data may not be provided for it in all cases

optionality terms used in standards to represent this concept are "Required" and "Mandatory". Quite commonly, this idea is verbally expressed by "this element shall be present".

- No statement is made for a specific element; i.e., no conclusion can be drawn regarding the existence of a value at this point in the specification. Ultimately (i.e., before implementation) a definitive statement has to be made. The optionality term used in standards to represent this concept is "Optional". As a verbal expression, "may be populated" or "can be present" are used.
- An element is forbidden[2]; i.e., the element (placeholder) shall not be valued. The optionality term used in standards to represent this concept is "Not Supported".

The above list provides the three major categories (further explained in Table 5.9) for describing the Optionality (or Usage) of an element presented at the concept level. The various standards use different notations, both to represent these concepts and to define subtle semantic differences between them.

A special case not included in Table 5.9 is the use of conditions: a certain element must be supported under specific conditions.

In the following sub-sections, the subtle differences among these concepts are explained.

5.3.1 Example Application Discussion

The example exchange specification shown in Fig. 5.5 provides two different aspects that can be examined now. First, the upper part of the diagram defines how

[2]Forbidden elements usually only appear in long-lasting standards where a better way to express certain information will be established later on, or in profiles where the element doesn't apply to the constraint use case.

our example application is implemented. Second, the lower part specifies an example data format. As a starting point, and in real life, an application is developed without necessarily considering any data exchange formats, and therefore the application typically has no relationship to the format except for an implicit, but hidden, use case.

If the first two elements ("ID" and "Family Name") are required in the data format specification, there is no problem or conflict for the implemented application; the information for those two fields stems from the appropriate fields out of the example database, and both fields prohibit null values ("not null"). (At this point it should be noted that when a table column in a database has a "not null" property, data must be entered for that element in order for the record to be committed to the database. This requirement is managed by the GUI forcing the user to enter data.) Consequently, when data are exported from the database, the data are obtained from a valid record set containing trusted, valid data. Importing and storing of trusted data into the database are supported as well. (When importing data, the unique identifier of the new record set may be in conflict with an already existing record identifier, but this problem is out of scope for this book.) Such a specification would be in sync with the application, and no special adaptation would be necessary.

The situation is different for the element "first name", which maps to "given name" in the example application, because this field can be empty when the record is stored. Normally, the table attributes (columns) are used in—or are bound to—forms allowing for their manipulation. Therefore, the presence of data in the record set is dependent on the user entering the data into the form. Table 5.10 shows the possible usages and the associated implications when data are imported into the database (inbound) or exported from the database (outbound) in the example application.

If data are used from the record set, the existence of data in the message directly depends on the data having been entered. We call this kind of behavior "required, but may be empty" in HL7® version 2.x and "required" in HL7® version 3.

The application does not support the last data element (DOB-date of birth) in the data exchange specification. The table in the example application's database does not maintain this kind of information and, therefore, the application is incapable of providing the data for outbound messages. As a consequence, this field will always be empty when the message is generated from this record set. The usual term for such a case is "not supported". When receiving a message like this, the application has to ignore this information, because there is no field for it in the application's database.

If the DOB element is indeed required in the specification and the application needs to (or must) support this specification (for whatever reason), it becomes obvious that the internal functionality of the application must be changed or enhanced. For example, if the DOB is made required, the application must first add a date field in the table to store this information, and, second, this new field must be tagged as a "not null" value, or the requirement must be enforced by other means such as at the data entry point. (The implication of this change for the application

Table 5.10 Options to handle "first name" in example

Possible usages	Inbound (import into database)	Outbound (export from database)
Required	No problem: Data will be present in the message, which can be stored	Problem: For the cases in which no data have been entered, this field cannot be populated, which results in a specification violation. Consequently, no valid message can be created
Optional[a]	No problem: In most cases the developer will decide to accept the provided data and store it in the database. The application will most likely be capable of dealing with the missing information, as the designated field in the database is allowed to be empty. This implementation behavior is called "required, but may be empty" (in HL7 v2) If the developer decides not to accept these data, this implementation is still valid for the given requirements, although it is not typical. This implementation behavior is called "ignored"	No problem: The developer can decide to populate this element with the data from the appropriate column of the database table; but the presence of valid data is dependent on the data entry design of the form, so the presence of the data cannot be guaranteed. This kind of behavior is called "required, but may be empty" (in HL7 v2) The developer also can decide not to populate this field, an implementation behavior called "ignored"
Forbidden	No problem: The message must not include the specified data, and no treatment is necessary	No problem: even if data are available, the application doesn't populate the element in the message

[a]For optional elements in a specification, no specific requirement is defined for the implementer, so the consequences for data exchange rely only on the implementers decisions

and the potential unfeasibility of performing this change are out of scope here.) The application must be adapted in order to be conformant to this specification.

5.3.2 Support for an Element

As introduced in the previous section, there are circumstances in which an element must to be supported, but it does not need to be present in a message or document instance. This usage indicator is commonly referred to as "Must Support" or "Required, but may be Empty". Not all data exchange standards include this concept.

One way to view the "Must Support" usage indicator is from the perspective of implementation and operational requirements. From the perspective of an implementation, elements with the "Must Support" usage indicator must be implemented. From an operational perspective, elements must be valued if relevant data are available. In short, an implementation must be capable of supporting these elements and supplying (or processing) the data when available.

Over the years, the interpretation of the "RE" usage indicator and the "O-optional" usage indicator has been a source of much confusion in the HL7 v2.x standard. Many implementers and other stakeholders thought that "O" and "RE" are similar implementation usage requirements, and "RE" often has been interpreted as optional. In the context of HL7 v2.x, "RE" is defined as explained above, and the element has to be supported in an application. Conformance tests can be created to verify the capability (see Chap. 11 for more details). Optional simply means that in a derived (profiled) specification, the "O" usage indicator can be replaced with another usage indicator, such as "R", "RE", or "X", and, ultimately, all "O" usage indicators must be replaced in the implementation specification.

5.3.3 Implementation Support Versus Presence in Instances

The use of optionality in specifications normally refers to the presence of data in message instances. The optionality *Required* and the verbal statement *must be present* indicate that the presence of data in an instance of a message is compulsory, i.e., data for an element must occur at least once. Very simple interface specifications that instruct different senders to convey specific information to a single recipient use only two codes for optionality: *Required* and *Optional*. This kind of specification is used predominately to collect specific data, e.g., billing information for insurance companies. Those specifications are written from the receiver's perspective to ensure that the message contains the needed information, and only those elements the receiver has an interest in are specified. The receiver supports all elements, while the sender must support the required elements and should (but is not required to) support the optional elements.

For bilateral communication, an indicator should be used to denote that a certain element should be supported, with the understanding that those data are not always present in every message. With HL7 version 2 this concept is called *Required, but may be empty* and is pre-coordinated with a minimum cardinality of zero.

Newer standards like FHIR® separate cardinality aspects from the presence of an element by calling this construct "must support", indicating that the sender and/or receiver must handle the element in an adequate way. A separate statement like "must support" is easier to understand than "Required, but may be empty", which has long caused confusion (Table 5.11).

Note that when "must support" is designated, no concrete determination can be made as to what kind of support is required, i.e., what should be done with this element definitively, because the specific use case must provide the context and further processing requirements for this element.

Table 5.11 Supporting optionality concepts

General concept	Must support	Concepts meaning	Constrainable to
Required	Yes—supported	The interface must handle it	Yes
Optional	Unspecified	The requirement for use of this element is set in a derived specification (whether it is written by a PEO, customer, or the implementer)	Yes or no
Forbidden	No—not supported	The message is not allowed to include this element	No

5.3.4 Conditional Usage

The optionality of an element often is determined by other related data in the message or document. Typically, data exchange standards provide a broad set of elements in order to support the variety of circumstances in a given use case and based on the data found in real world situations. In some instances, data in one element are dependent on the value used in another element. In immunization data exchange, for example, the message or document "template" contains elements for transmitting vaccine lot numbers and manufacturer identification codes. This information is presumed to be available for a newly administered vaccine. For an historical immunization, however, such information may not be known. The optionality/usage for the lot number and manufacturer code (qualified) elements is dependent on another element that is populated with a value indicating whether the vaccine administration is new or historical. This dependency is expressed through a conditional usage. These qualified elements can have a usage that is expressed as follows:

$$C(R/RE)$$

The "C" indicates that the element is conditional and the ultimate usage for this element is based on the data that are present in another element of the message. Conditional usage requires that an associated condition predicate be provided stating the optionality of the conditional element when the outcome is true (e.g., the immunization is new) and when the outcome is false (e.g., the immunization is historical). The first optionality value ("R") indicates the usage of the element when the condition predicate is "true", and the second value ("RE") indicates the usage when the condition predicate resolves to false. It should be noted that all usages resolve to the base usages described earlier in this section.

The basic pattern of a conditional usage is:

$$C(a/b) \text{ and a Condition Predicate}$$

Note, "a" and "b" are placeholders for the possible values of usage/optionality indicators. Not all standards support all such combinations, and some standards do

Table 5.12 Example usage codes for condition in HL7 v2.x

HL7 element	Usage	Condition predicate
PID-24: Multiple birth indicator	RE	
PID-25: Birth order	C(RE/X)	If the value of PID-24 (multiple birth indicator) is 'Y'

not support conditional usage at all. HL7 v2.x (as of version 2.7.1) supports the full combination of conditional usage in the profiling capabilities. A discussion about the information included in the base standard is provided later. Prior to version 2.7.1, HL7 v2.x only supported conditional usages of C and CE, which correspond to C(R/X) and C(RE/X) respectively.

Precisely specifying the condition predicate is an important aspect of this mechanism; however, most standards and implementation guides in use do not do so. Recent work in HL7 v2.x implementation guides named for ONC EHR certification have provided exact definitions, since such precise information is needed for consistent implementations and conformance testing (and are just good practice for development of specifications).

Table 5.12 illustrates an example of conditional usage. The "Multiple Birth Indicator", if known, must be valued (as designated by RE usage). If it is valued as "Y" for yes, then the "Birth Order", if known, must be valued. If "Multiple Birth Indicator" is not valued or is valued "N" (for No), then "Birth Order" is not to be valued. The outcome of the condition predicate determines the runtime requirement.

An observation of conditional usage is that they are not "*really*" conditional usage. A more correct statement is that conditions can only be evaluated at runtime, and that only then can a definitive usage be determined. The *conditional usage* provides a mechanism for documenting the possible circumstances and determining the actual usage. From an implementation perspective, the same requirements for usage apply. For example, for an element with a conditional usage of C(R/X), the implementer must be able to support the element. Operationally in this example, in some circumstances the implementation must provide data for this element in the message or document, whereas in other circumstances data must not be provided.

5.3.5 *Case Study: HL7 v2.x Conditional Usage*

Conditional usage in HL7 v2.x has evolved and has been used in various ways in specifications. A brief history, along with various examples, is given here. The early versions of the base standard are quite vague on how conditional usage is intended to be used; that is, the standard states little more than that the usage can be conditionally determined, and no "standard" mechanism was provided to specify it. Therefore, specifications typically were vague (only a "C" was given as the usage indicator), not only about what the condition was but also what the usage was to be under true and false outcomes of the condition.

Profiling was introduced in v2.5, and the profiling usage indicators of C and CE were introduced along with it. Note that the meaning of C in the base standard is different from the definition of C used in the profiling chapter. C and CE provided fixed conditional combinations, and technically they were more restrictive than the base standard; however, in many ways these conditional usages had little impact, since the correct way to apply them was rarely specified. C resolved to R/X for true/false, i.e., whenever a condition is met the usage is "R", and if the condition is false the usage is "X". CE resolved to RE/X. The limited set of predefined combinations was too restrictive and prevented the granularity necessary to address specific use cases. In fall of 2011, this fact became evident as the laboratory specification intended for use in ONC 2014 Edition EHR Certification was being developed, leading to the unrestricted combinations of usage described earlier (i.e., C(a/b)).

As is shown in Table 5.13, "C" and "CE", the two codes used for conditions, are not used consistently. It is worth noting that these definitions/specifications are not quite in sync or, at least, are not used consistently. The details are explained in Chap. 7.

5.3.6 "Required" Versus "Mandatory"

HL7 version v2.x and V3 use different terms for representing the concept of *Required*, i.e., the enforced presence of an element. *Required* is used in HL7 v2.x and *Mandatory* is used in HL7 V3 to denote this concept. Readers of the specifications need to be aware of the different semantics defined by these related concepts. The origin of the disparity is historical. In v2.x, the concept of null flavors does not exist; in V3, null flavor was adopted by the underlying methodology. This divergence in the concepts has caused confusion and requires understanding of the specifications by users. In V3, this concept is combined with knowledge about the absence of valid data, which is called a null-flavor. (This concept is explained in greater detail in a subsequent section of this chapter.) *Mandatory* in V3 enforces the presence of an element while disallowing the use of null-flavors. In contrast, *Required* in V3 enforces the support of this element by an implementer, even though in a given instance the element either can be empty or null flavors can be used. The concept of "RE" in v2.x is similar to *Required* in V3, but v2.x does not support null-flavors. In V3, elements with required usage can use null-flavors to value the element or can stay empty.

Table 5.13 Usage codes for condition in HL7 v2.x

<table>
<tr><th>Usage with conditions</th><th>C</th><th>CE</th></tr>
<tr><td>HL7 standard</td><td>The element is conditional on the trigger event or on some other field(s). The field definitions following the segment attribute table should specify the algorithm that defines the conditionality for this field. Therefore, any combination is allowed</td><td>This Code is only used starting with v2.8 in the standard specification</td></tr>
<tr><td rowspan="3">HL7 profiles</td><td colspan="2">This usage has an associated condition predicate (see Chap. 2 in the HL7 v2 base standard) [1]</td></tr>
<tr><td>If the predicate is satisfied, follow the rules for R usage.
If the predicate is NOT satisfied, follow the rules for X usage</td><td>If the predicate is satisfied, follow the rules for the RE usage.
If the predicate is not satisfied, follow the rules for X usage</td></tr>
<tr><td colspan="2">The predicate must be testable and be based on other values within the message</td></tr>
<tr><td rowspan="2">IHE ITI technical framework</td><td>If the predicate is satisfied:
• A compliant sending application shall populate the element
• A compliant receiving application may ignore data in the element, and it may raise an error if the element is not present</td><td>If the predicate is satisfied:
• If the conforming sending application knows the required values for the element, then the application must populate the element
• If the conforming sending application does not know the values required for this element, then the element shall be omitted
• The conforming sending application must be capable of populating the element (when the predicate is true) for all 'CE' elements
• If the element is present, the conformant receiving application may ignore the values of that element
• If the element is not present, the conformant receiving application shall not raise an error due to the presence or absence of the element</td></tr>
<tr><td>If the predicate is NOT satisfied:
• A conformant sending application shall NOT populate the element
• A conformant receiving application shall NOT raise an error if the condition predicate is false and the element is not present, though it may raise an error if the element IS present</td><td>If the predicate is NOT satisfied:
• The conformant sending application shall not populate the element
• The conformant receiving application may raise an application error if the element is present</td></tr>
</table>

5.3.7 Binding of Elements

In the example shown in Fig. 5.5, the database table attributes optimally are bound to the corresponding fields in the data exchange format. The example also explains the impact on certain requirements from the data exchange specification in combination with different options for an implementation. In such a simple environment, some usage requirements may work well while others will cause problems.

A vendor may have a reason to handle the requirements in a different way. For example, if the first name is not sent in a message, this element must be declared as "not supported" even if the data for this element could be obtained from the existing implemented application. As a consequence, the field stays empty, although the application may have a value for it. In other words, although the application is capable of handling this information, it is not supported by the interface.

In the normal procedure used to define usage, one does not start with the capabilities that an application can support but with a given data exchange specification that was created to support a particular use case. As a consequence, vendors have to determine whether they can fulfill the requirements with their application as stipulated by this data exchange specification. An application, therefore, must be capable of providing the data for all elements declared as "required", otherwise, a valid exchange record cannot be constructed from the application. (At this point, it only matters whether a requested information item is provided or not.) In other words, if the application needs to deliver a valid exchange record, a change in the implementation may become inevitable.

Although this information may seem to indicate dependencies related to how applications evolve, it is presented here only for discussion purposes. In practice, applications are designed and written irrespective of data exchange standards, and what an interface supports is independent of what an application is capable of.

5.3.8 Interface Design Choices

A number of vendors have chosen to implement configurable interfaces to deal with the multiple options they need to support. An alternative is to develop dedicated interfaces to address each specification. A trade-off exists between these approaches: is it easier to develop multi-purpose interfaces, many targeted interfaces, or a combination solution? For example, which field is responsible for conveying the visit number for a patient? Is a specific sequence to be used to check a series of fields for the visit number? This situation where multiple choices are available makes it very difficult to provide a good and precise specification (referred to as an implementable profile). In principle, these variations can be expressed by conditions that refer to an option of the interface module (e.g., information about patient's diagnoses is available in this or that way if purchased by a customer). If this approach is taken, such implementations should be documented. Profiling and profile components are effective ways to produce this documentation (See Chap. 7).

5.3.9 *Sender and Receiver Perspectives*

Verification of whether the sender has correctly populated the exchanged data string is quite easy; therefore, the requirements are normally stated for the sender and are clearly expressed.

The specification for data exchange should specify the common denominator both systems have to support, i.e., the sending **and** the receiving systems. In that way, some trust is established regarding what a sender will send and what the receiver will process out of the transmitted data. It would not make sense to make an element required for the sender if the receiver can ignore it! A common argument in favor of determining the requirements just for the sender is that this approach establishes a data set in which a receiver can have trust, i.e., a set of data elements from which a receiver can select. This raises the question, then, as to why a data set is defined by a sender if no receiver may exist. From that perspective, it would make more sense to establish a minimum data set that all systems must support, i.e., a user could trust that all systems provide the same amount of information. The additional requirement for senders to support a maximum data set can be provided on top, but this subject will be discussed as *profile hierarchies* in conjunction with the handling of profiles.

While a sender data set could be defined relatively easily, specifying what a receiver of the data set must do with it is difficult. The required receiver actions could include processing, storing, displaying, and printing the data. What's important is that the receiver takes care of the data and does not simply ignore them. Optimally, functional requirement specifications should be defined for applications and be associated with the related interoperability specifications.

5.4 Cardinality

Cardinality controls the number of occurrences of an element an implementation must support and the number of instances of an element that can appear in a message or document. Some elements shall always be present (e.g., cardinality [1..1], [1..n]). Others shall never be present (i.e., cardinality [0..0]). Still other elements may or may not appear, with zero or more occurrences (e.g., cardinality [0..n]). Cardinality identifies the minimum and maximum number of occurrences that a message (or document) element must have in a conformant message (or document). Cardinalities are expressed as a minimum-maximum pair of non-negative integers. A conformant message (or document) must always contain at least the minimum number of occurrences and shall not contain more than the maximum number of occurrences.

A data element often must occur more than once in the instance of a message or document. Cardinality is the conformance construct that is used to indicate this requirement. Cardinality boundaries apply to both "atomic" data contained in a simple data type and a collection of data contained in a complex data type.

A typical example is "patient name", which often includes several categories such as legal name and maiden name.[3] It is quite common to model this specialized element with a corresponding name element, e.g., "familyname" and "maiden-name". An alternative approach is to generically represent the concept by supporting multiple occurrences of an element. Cardinality is used to specify the allowed range of occurrences, and the element typically will provide a mechanism to distinguish the instances, e.g., a type code may be part of the element data type, one type code indicating legal name and the other maiden name.

In HL7 v2, this situation is handled by a data type, with appropriate components being used only once. The components can be repeated as a whole on the field level. In HL7 V3, the "patient name" is expressed as a "list of name parts", where each part can be repeated individually. For example, in V3 each given name has its own instantiation.

Another pertinent example is diagnosis, where each diagnosis consists of different attributes that can repeat individually. The diagnosis is a high level concept that embodies the different attributes and repeats as a group. HL7 v2 uses a segment with fields, and HL7 V3 uses a class with attributes.

5.4.1 *Limitations*

In some cases, applications don't support the full range of cardinality specified. To deal with this state, the maximum cardinality becomes relevant and must be specified—on both the sender and receiver sides. An assessment must be made to ensure the requirements of the use case can be fulfilled for these instances.

As is indicated in Chap. 12, even if an application has limited capabilities (e.g., n elements), it is not necessarily true that only the first n elements will be processed. Depending on the business needs and the provided accompanying information, the appropriate information can be selected.

Another option, which was introduced in HL7 v2.8, is to assign a specific meaning to a certain position in the set of this repeating element (referred to as profiling multiple occurrences). Using the previous example shown in Fig. 5.5, the family name could be associated with the first occurrence, while the second occurrence is reserved for the maiden name. This approach would eliminate the

[3]It must be noted, that "maiden name" is different from "mother's maiden name".

need for a specific type code within an occurrence, but it would also reduce the flexibility in using unrestricted multiple occurrences.

5.4.2 Delimiters

It is important to note that a specific delimiter is necessary to delineate and identify an individual occurrence of the data element or component. This delineation is achieved in different ways depending on the particular standard. For example, the excerpt below shows an example in HL7 v2 in which the "~" delimiter is used to denote to occurrences of a person's phone number (Home and Work).

```
|^PRN^PH^^^406^5557896~^WPN^PH^^^406^5551234|
```

5.4.3 Alternate Terms for Cardinality

Alternative names used in standards for cardinality include occurrences and repetitions. It is important to note that if the upper bound for repetition is *n* it means n occurrences and not *n* repetitions (i.e., $n + 1$ occurrences). Repetition is used in some standards (e.g., HL7 v2.x) to indicate the upper limit and not actually the number of times an element may repeat (in contrast to its well-established dictionary definition). The term occurrence is the preferred term when describing the number of times an element may appear in a message or document. Implementers should be aware of the subtle differences. Regardless of how the concept is specified, the important aspect of the conformance construct is the lower and upper bound requirement that is placed on the element.

5.4.4 Notation for Cardinality

The notation for specifying cardinality constraints varies in standards. In principle, however, the notation and interpretation convey comparable information. A common format is depicted in Table 5.14.

5.4.5 Use of Cardinality

The cardinality construct can, in principle, be applied to any data element on every level. Certain encoding mechanisms, however, do not provide a means to support this capability.

Table 5.14 Cardinality

Cardinality	Interpretation [1]
[0..0]	Element never present
[0..1]	Element may be omitted, and it can have at most one occurrence
[1..1]	Element must have exactly one occurrence
[0..n]	Element may be omitted or may have up to n occurrences
[1..n]	Element must appear at least once and may have up to n occurrences
[0..*]	Element may be omitted or may have an unlimited number of occurrences
[1..*]	Element must appear at least once and may have an unlimited number of occurrences
[m..n]	Element must have at least "m" occurrences and may have at most "n" occurrences
[m..*]	Element must have at least "m" occurrences and may have an unlimited number of occurrences

For example, in HL7 v2 the cardinality is only applied on the outermost data structures, e.g., at the field or segment level. The inner structure, such as a component, can only occur once. In other words, a component, in essence, has a cardinality of [0..1].

Other standards, like the German xDT family, do not provide detailed data types. Every data element is represented by fields in combination with their nesting in a hierarchy. Consequently, each element can have an arbitrary number of occurrences (cardinality [0..*]).

5.4.6 *Relationship of Optionality and Cardinality*

A natural relationship exists between the optionality and cardinality constructs. As introduced in the beginning of this chapter, a required element must be present in a message. Another way to express this requirement is to set the minimum cardinality to "1". Table 5.15 provides the set of allowed cardinality and optionality combinations.

Required elements must have a minimum cardinality of one, and forbidden elements must have a minimum and maximum cardinality of zero. Optional elements must have a minimum cardinality of zero and a maximum cardinality that is at least 1.

Table 5.15 Allowed cardinality and optionality combinations

Optionality	[0..0]	[0..1]	[1..1]	[0..m]	[1..m]	[0..*]	[1..*]	[n..*]	[n..m]
Required			✓		✓		✓	✓	✓
Optional		✓		✓		✓			
Forbidden	✓								

5.5 Length

The length construct defines a constraint on the number of characters that may be present in one occurrence of an element. The length indicator can specify a maximum or the minimum and maximum bounds.

A core requirement for applications is the storing of information. In most cases, storing is accomplished with relational databases, which manage all data elements in the form of tables with columns. Quite commonly, each item has its own column, allowing for storing the data up to a maximum length. (Certain management techniques and specific data types eliminate this constraint, but this point is not being considered in this discussion.)

In order to avoid issues when storing data, the length should be limited to a certain maximum, i.e., no data shall be transmitted and stored that are longer than allowed by the storage space unless truncation is permitted. Ideally, a message should be rejected rather than permitting data to be truncated in case important parts of the data would be lost; this behavior requires that advanced techniques be built into the interfaces anticipating this situation and taking appropriate actions.

In cases where all possible values are known, as with specific value sets, a minimum length can be determined and specified. Pre-testing simply on data representation is helpful without examining the data themselves. For example, a designated length of [3..4] for a specific element can be used to declare data with length 7 as invalid even without verifying the contents of the data.

The result of testing both data representation and the data themselves together is shown in Table 5.16.

Some observations that can be drawn from the information in Table 5.16 are that the length [0..0] is to be used for forbidden elements only; a minimum length of zero characters should not be used, because minimum and maximum length should refer to valid values only; without a single character no valid information can be represented; and the indicated length should refer to the number of characters itself, not the amount characters (i.e. bytes) needed to represent them. For example, UTF-32 requires four bytes to represent each character.

Table 5.16 Length

Minimum/maximum length	Explanation
[0..0]	Element does not occur, i.e., it is forbidden
[1..n]	An element has no minimal length but is limited to n characters
[1..*]	An element has no minimal length and no (theoretical) limitation
[m..n]	An element must have between m and n characters (including), with m greater than one
[m..*]	An element must have at least m characters, with m greater than one and no (theoretical) limitation

5.5.1 Sender/Receiver Role

Table 5.17 provides an overview about the consequences of a specific length when it is implemented by both the sender and receiver. Table 5.17 shows that "true" interoperability (for exchange of data back and forth) is only possible if sender and receiver have implemented the same length capabilities; otherwise, data loss will occur in some circumstances. Truncation is especially problematic if the elements convey codes (imagine if an interface shortens an ICD10 code from 6 to 5 characters!).

Nowadays, implementers rarely consider length capabilities when setting up an interface at a site. Problems are detected individually in specific runtime environments. With most of the implementations, the fields are long enough to avoid conflicts. But the risk of errors rises if the length of the stored information increases.

Good practice for data exchange standards is to define a maximum length only for those elements where specific values must be enforced.

5.5.2 Truncation

In practical terms, the application's capacity to store data for elements is limited and is often different for each element. Truncation is the process of substituting an indicator for data that exceed an application's ability to *process* or store it.

Table 5.17 Possible combinations of implementing length

	Sender	Receiver	Consequence
Implemented maximum length	10	20	Normally, this combination is fine, because the receiver can always store the transmitted information. Note: if a user changes the information on the receiving side to something with a greater length, a problem will occur if these data are returned to the original sender
	20	10	The receiver can handle this situation in two ways: (1) evaluate the data and detect the invalid length and return an error, or (2) ignore the invalid length and store the information it can. The latter can only be done by truncation. Therefore, a loss of information is—most probably—unavoidable. From a testing perspective, this kind of problem can only be detected if a data exchange is performed with information of maximum length (for each element)
	10	10	No conflict

An interface has two choices for reacting to the receipt of data that exceed the application's capability to store it: rejecting the data (i.e., message or document) entirely with an appropriate error code, or storing whatever is possible to store. The first option requires a pre-checking of the data based on the capabilities of the application, a procedure that normally is not implemented; in this case, the interface stores the data, unknowingly disregarding potential errors and warnings. As a consequence, only part of the data is consumed and stored by the application.

For a correct implementation, the interface must know the maximum length of each element an application can support. System validation is helpful in determining if the data exceed the limits, and then to verify whether the application rejects the message or keeps and stores it while accepting data loss. The latter could be accomplished with special treatment, such as providing a notification of lost information. The truncation indicator enables this capability, typically using a special character to mark the end of the data that an application was able to consume and store. In essence, the truncation character replaces the data that were lost.

When the receiver returns truncated data to the original sender, the presence of a truncation indicator allows for a comparison of the original data with the data that are returned. If the data are identical up to the truncation indicator, the original sender may decide to keep (preserve) its (original) information.

5.5.3 Padding

Padding does exactly the opposite of truncation. Padding expands data with artificial characters to a specified length. Good examples are numbers that are filled (*padded*) with zeros (to the left), or texts that are expanded with spaces (to the right). Padding has been introduced with fixed-format representations where an exchanged object is required to have a specific length. In modern systems, the use of padding is unusual.

Padding leads to the discussion of how certain characters, like spaces and zeros, should be handled in special cases. When should a sender expand data; to which side (left or right); and what should a receiver do with the data?

In the financial domain, expanding an account number to the left by filling in zeros is common practice. There is no doubt that two numbers refer to the same account if they only differ by leading zeros. In the medical domain, there may be a difference between two numbers like "1.0" or "1.000". From a mathematical perspective the two numbers are equal, but from a medical perspective they produce the impression of different precision when measuring values. Whether padded characters are kept or eliminated, and whether padding is necessary at all, must be carefully considered.

Finally, padding should not be mixed with formatting. Using spaces to format text output is quite common. Spaces are inserted to align numbers into columns, a behavior that has been used quite extensively in the laboratory domain in the past.

With the increased deployment of enhanced formatting using HTML or "printed" results in the form of PDF documents, use of padding in formatting is decreasing.

5.5.4 Conformance Length

Discussions among members of the interoperability community about the correct maximum length for an international data exchange standard has produced a conformance construct that is only available in newer versions of the HL7 v2 standard family (v2.7 and upwards). A decision was made to provide requirements in the form of a minimum and maximum length for those elements where possible values are definitely known and to delete this information for all other elements. Hence, starting with v2.7 the length information is normative. (From v1.0 up to v2.6 the length is informative.)

The conformance length should provide some guidance to implementers as to the reasonable minimum length (for the maximum length) that should be supported for elements for which a normative length is not provided. Implementers are free to select any greater length they need for their application to fulfill the requirements. The conformance length values are taken from the maximum length in HL7 v2.6.

5.6 Content

In healthcare data exchange, the information communicated can be divided into two broad categories: (1) specific information about an entity (e.g., a person's name or a lab result value) and (2) pre-defined concepts about an entity (e.g., a person's name type, e.g., legal or the type of the lab test performed). For the first category, field entry forms typically are provided in the user interface of an application where variable information can be entered. A person's first name, "Austin", is an example. The second category requires the exchange of "key indicators" that function as a placeholder or a representation on behalf of the concepts. Usually, these "key indicators" are codes, and are maintained in the form of code systems that also specify the exact meaning of each code, thus eliminating ambiguities. The appropriate set of values is known in advance; thus, when the administrative gender needs to be represented, a code "M" is used to indicate "male". The context of the code "M" and the concept it represents are defined in a code system. This mechanism is generically called vocabulary. In some circumstances, the use case can be sufficiently narrowed, and the context can be constrained to contain a single concept that is represented by a single value, which is a constant. Certain use cases allow for the assumption of a specific value in case no data are transmitted. This concept is called default value. Another content-related concept is "null flavors", which provides a method of expressing why content is not being conveyed. These four forms of specifying content using conformance constructs or related conformance concepts are the topics of this section. Of the four forms, vocabulary is the most prevalent and important.

5.6.1 Vocabulary

Vocabulary is a term used to describe, in general, the mechanics of defining, maintaining, and using codes to represent concepts in healthcare data exchange. A **Code System** is defined as a managed collection of codes that represent concepts used in a particular business or technical area, and often also have relationships between the coded concepts. In the above example, "Administrative Gender" is the concept domain, "male" is the concept, and "M" is the code representing the concept "male" within the context of the code system. Code systems are developed to provide a set of coded concepts for a particular domain, and they are designed for one or many specific or general business uses.[4] A code system may be a simple list of coded concepts, or it may be designed with one or more explicit relationships between the coded concepts (at least hierarchical, and often many other types of relationships in a multi-dimensional fashion).

A **Value Set** is defined as a collection of codes targeted for a specific use. A value set draws codes from one (usually) or more code systems; the result is a set of codes that constrains the possible content of a data element. A key distinction between a value set and a code system is that a code system is used as a reference source of coded meaning, whereas a value set is a specific constraint for a set of explicit business uses. For example, the Logical Observation Identifiers Names and Codes (LOINC) is a code system that has tens of thousands of observations and is widely used in healthcare data exchange standards to specify all existing laboratory tests in current use everywhere, and very common clinical observations. Two examples of value sets that draw from the LOINC code system are the set of codes that specify radiology study types and the set of codes that just specify laboratory observations. Another example value set that draws from the LOINC code system is the NIP003 value set that contains immunization observations such as "30963-3" for "Vaccine Funding Source". The NIP003 value set only includes a few dozen out of these tens of thousands of LOINC codes.

Note that a value set and a code system can contain the same set of codes if the situation warrants the use of the entire code system. A problem with many specifications is that value sets should be, but are not, explicitly created; instead, the entire code system is referenced, leaving it up to the implementers to select appropriate values for a specific use case, which likely results in different value sets being used by

[4]However, in practice a significant number of code systems are defined for a very limited use case, thus not allowing for re-use. Quite often code systems are invented just because of a lack of time to define appropriate value sets consisting of codes from existing code systems. On the other hand, some code systems such as LOINC and SNOMED CT have broad applicability and opportunity for reuse.

different implementers. This variation between implementations can be an interoperability and safety issue. Chap. 7 identifies additional concerns about current practice and describes the profiling methodology for creating and applying value sets.

A **Concept Domain** is an abstract notion that refers to a set of related ideas (concepts) and is essentially a named Semantic Category that serves to help define the meaning of a particular data element (over and above just the name of the data element). A concept domain does not directly define a particular set of concepts and is independent from a specific and explicit association to a particular vocabulary (code system or value set). The concept domain of postal code (ZIP code in the US) is a good example. Postal codes are, in general, a set of digits and/or letters used to identify certain geographic regions in most countries in the world, and are used to aid in the sorting and delivery of physical mail. This abstract notion of postal codes is the concept domain, and one can say that a particular data element, such as that contained in a guarantor's mailing address, must have content consistent with this concept domain. A particular set of postal codes can be defined as a code system, and may be used as the vocabulary binding for that concept domain. For example, one code system can be defined for US postal codes and a different one for German postal codes. Furthermore, a subset of postal codes can be defined as a value set for a particular use, for example, a value set of zip codes used in the state of Alaska for use in sending immunization events to public health. Concept domains (*placeholders*) or code systems typically are specified at the base standard level. Value sets are defined as the standard is constrained to make it implementable. Good practice is to manage value sets explicitly, as discussed below.

At this point, it is important to raise the related notion of a **Table**. A table sometimes acts like a code system, value set, and/or a concept domain depending on how it is used, and it is a mechanism introduced in *older* data exchange standards.[5] A very well-known and widely used set of tables are those defined in HL7 v2.x. Early standards provided a list of (short) codes that were used to replace (long) text/strings to conserve space. The list was directly bound to a certain element—no identifier was provided as a 'handle' to aid in the management of this set of codes. The German xDT standard is an example of one that used this approach. An extensive set of tables and table identifiers is provided in more recent releases of HL7 v2.x. In some cases, the tables included values that had to be used if the concept to be conveyed was contained in the table. In the HL7 v2 product family this collection of values was defined as an *HL7 Table*. A table could also be categorized as a *User Table*; this kind of table provided a list of suggested values that could be used, or, alternatively, a different set of values could be defined and used. The User Table could be empty with no values suggested, which indicated that this entire set of values must be defined at the *local* level. The HL7 v2.x tables do have a pre-defined identifier—the table number—that helps in managing the tables and in binding them to a data element. More details of HL7 v2.x tables can be found in

[5]Depending on the data exchange standard (see Chaps. 4 and Appendix), this still is common practice.

Chap. 4. As standards matured, more sophisticated vocabulary techniques emerged, as is evident in HL7 V3. As a result, the authors of the most recent versions of HL7 v2.x specifications are adopting these more sophisticated vocabulary models. This method is being implemented in the HL7 v2.x conformance profiling approach (See Chap. 7 [2, 13]). Additionally, HL7 v2 Tables[6] are being converted into vocabulary domains, code systems, or value sets in a joint project between the Vocabulary and the Conformance Working Groups [3].

The entire process of creating and applying vocabulary in data exchange standards is a complex subject and varies significantly across standards. Before proceeding further on this topic, it must be pointed out that the discussion on vocabulary is purposely being kept at a level that focuses on the core concepts without getting bogged down into all of the nuances.

5.6.1.1 Vocabulary Mechanics

Specifying the use of coded data elements and how to apply or interpret the specification correctly have been troublesome in nearly all implementation guides across the various standards families. Many users of standards do not have a good understanding of vocabulary concepts and processes, and this lack of understanding has long been a source of difficulty. The various standards specify vocabulary in a multitude of ways. Even within each SDO (e.g., HL7), the terminology and specifications are inconsistent. Through recent efforts [3–5] spearheaded by the HL7 Vocabulary Working Group, a harmonization process targeting the different standards families has begun. The effort will harmonize the structure and content of the value sets (which is a big step forward); however, the mechanics of specifying vocabulary conformance will likely only extend to the conceptual level, because the vocabulary mechanics are far too embedded in each standard to be changed significantly [5].

Given that there is no unified way to describe the concepts of specifying the constraints and representation format for coded elements, a description of the general concepts is presented here. An example that most closely resembles the newly proposed method for HL7 v2.x is used to show the process and concepts. Admittedly, some nuances have been omitted in this description in order to keep the discussion focused on the core concepts.

Now that the notions of a code system and value set have been defined, an explanation of how value sets are used in data exchange standards can be presented. Figure 5.6 provides this overview. A code system provides the universe of available standardized coded concepts in a particular field or business area. A value set is a subset of those codes or a combination of codes from different code systems for a

[6]There is a subtle difference between a table consisting of codes and associated descriptions and a code system with concepts, display names, descriptions, formal identification, and other controlling and explanatory detail.

Patient Identification (PID) Definition Excerpt					
Seq	**Data Element**	**DT**	**Usage**	**Value Set**	**Strength**
7	...	... (1)	...	(2)	(3)
8	Administrative Sex	IS	R	HL70001_EX	Required
9	Patient Alias		X		
10	Race	CE	RE	HL70005_EX	Suggested

Basic Process Summary

1. Analyze data semantics of element for use case
2. Assess code system(s) to match semantics and concept domain
3. Create value set definition including codes for use case
4. Bind the value set to the element
5. Assign the strength of the binding

Administrative Gender -Value Set Definition (4)			
Name (5)	Administrative Gender		
Identifier (6)	HL70001_EX		
Extensibility (7)	Closed		
Stability (8)	Static		
Value	**Description**	**Usage**	**Code System** (12)
A (9)	Ambiguous (10)	(11)	HL70001_v2.5.1
F	Female	✓	HL70001_v2.5.1
M	Male	✓	HL70001_v2.5.1
N	Not Applicable		HL70001_v2.5.1
O	Other		HL70001_v2.5.1
U	Unknown	✓	HL70001_v2.5.1

Point	Description
1	Coded Element Data Type - Can contain a code
2	Binding - Link the data element to a value set
3	Binding Strength - Conformance of the binding
4	Value Set Definition - Details of the value set
5	Name - Long name of the value set
6	Identifier - Used to bind data element to value set
7	Extensibility - Indicates if value set can be extended
8	Stability - Indicates if value set is static or dynamic
9	Value - Code to be used in object instance
10	Description - Describes value (code)
11	Usage - Indicates the inclusion into the value set
12	Code System - Indicates the source of the code

Fig. 5.6 Summary of vocabulary mechanics (*Note* Binding Strength in the table heading is shortened to strength for aesthetic purposes)

specific use (business purpose). The specific use is defined and associated with an element in the data exchange standard. Elements to which coded concepts are bound are generically called **Coded Elements,** and they have a data type definition that reflects this relationship. This connection is shown as point (1) in Fig. 5.6. Figure 5.7 (shown a few pages later) illustrates the general data type structures used to convey coded element information in data exchange standards. The impact of both the data type definition for a coded element and the general data type structures is discussed later.

A significant portion of the semantics carried by a coded data element are expressed at a conceptual level through an association of a concept domain and made implementable by an association to a value set. These associations are called **Binding**. Depending on the level of the specification, the binding can be to a concept domain, code system, or value set.[7] At each specification (profile) level, the binding becomes increasingly specific, refining the data semantics of the element by limiting its content to a particular set of coded values. For example, at the base standard level a concept domain may be specified, and at the profile level a value set is specified, with specific codes for an implementation.

[7]This is in conflict with some views in which a binding is only to a value set. However, in the definition of vocabulary in specifications, an association is made at all levels. Whether it is called a binding or not is not the key point, the point that an explicit association is made, is.

A **Value Set Binding**, in simple terms, refers to assigning a set of coded concepts to a particular data element in order to implement the concept domain associated with the data element. A binding is thus to a value set and is what is indicated in Fig. 5.6 as point (2).

In Fig. 5.6, the Administrative Gender data element (1) in the Patient Identification Definition is bound to the value set identified by HL70001_EX in the value set column (2). The Value Set Identifier is an attribute of the value set definition (6). The **Binding Strength** (3) indicates the conformance of the binding, that is, whether the vocabulary[8] must be used or not. There are two possible values: Required and Suggested (Recommended). All bindings are eventually required in implementations, and a suggested binding can be specified in a constrainable profile (i.e., the specification needs to be further constrained). The bound vocabulary definition with a binding strength of "Suggested" can be used, modified, or replaced by an alternative set. Bindings to concept domains and code systems[9] always have a binding strength of "Suggested".

The **Value Set Definition** (4) provides meta data and the codes.[10] Meta data shown in Fig. 5.6 include the name of the value set (5), the identifier (6), and value set properties extensibility (7) and stability (8). Extensibility and stability will be explained later. The codes (9) contained in the value set are F, M, and U, as indicated by the check marks[11] in the usage column (11). For each code (value), a description is given (10). The value set is composed of codes from the HL70001 v2.5.1 code system[12] (12). Note: a value set may include codes from multiple code systems. The value set definition shown in Fig. 5.6 shows all of the codes in the code system (A, F, M, N, O, U) and the codes selected for inclusion into the value set (F, M, U). A value set definition may or may not include the complete set of codes in the source code system. The complete set is presented in this example to show the value set in the context of the source code system. Other forms of representation are equally acceptable as long as sufficient information is provided to indicated the status of the code (See Vocabulary Profiling in Chap. 7 for more information).

In this example value set, the usage[13] is limited to inclusion or exclusion. Additional specificity can be associated with the code usage. To understand the

[8]In this context, vocabulary is used to refer to concept domain, code system, or value set.

[9]However, a value set can use an entire code system.

[10]To simplify explanation this definition includes meta data and the codes. See recent work in HL7 [5] and discussion to follow in which the Value Set Definition consists of the meta data and *information to determine* the codes. The generated list is known as the Value Set Expansion.

[11]Check marks are used for simplicity and replaced by more detailed usage concepts later on.

[12]As mentioned, HL7 v2.x tables are not yet formally code systems, and HL70001 is used here as a simple example. For convenience, HL7 v2 tables are referred to as code systems.

[13]The term "Usage" here is not related to the usage of elements (e.g., R, RE, etc.) described earlier in this chapter; See Chap. 7 for details of vocabulary usage.

concepts of code usage and its implications, however, knowledge about profiling and applying constraints is necessary. Therefore, the concept is briefly introduced here and is explained in detail in Chap. 7. Usage can represent the exclusion, definite inclusion, or possible inclusion of a code in a value set. The various standards have different vocabulary conformance models where the use and meaning of usage varies. HL7 V3 realizes this notion using the words *min/max/ignore*, whereas some standards don't explicitly deal with this idea at all.

The **Content Definition** of the value set indicates the method used to expand a value set definition into a set of codes. The example presented in Fig. 5.6 is an explicit listing (i.e., enumeration). An enumerated value set definition is called an **Extensional** definition. Other means used to expand a value set definition into a set of codes include using regular expressions, characterizing specific attributes for a specific code system (e.g., all laboratory codes in LOINC), or using hierarchical associations that include all specializations of the codes in question. By applying these kinds of mechanisms, a value set definition can be expanded to the Value Set Expansion providing all codes required for the identified business use in the implementation. This form is called an **Intensional** definition.

Extensibility indicates whether the value set definition can be extended or not in a derived (profiled) version of the specification. This concept is also linked to the profiling, so it is only introduced here and is expanded upon in Chap. 7. The extensibility of a value set definition can be either *open* or *closed*. Open means that more values can be added to the value set in a derived specification.[14] Closed means that no more values can be added to the value set in a derived specification.

In HL7 V3 and CDA, CNE (Coded, No Extensions) is used to express that only the codes in the value set are allowed to be used for HL7 V3 or CDA components to which the value set is bound. This is similar to "closed" extensibility (but not equivalent). Likewise, CWE (Coded, With Extensions) allows additional codes outside the value set if a code does not exist in the value set needed. This is similar to "open" extensibility (but not equivalent). Note, the CNE and CWE counterparts used in HL7 v2.x convey an entirely different notion.

Stability indicates whether the content of a value set[15] can change outside of the definition of the value set or the specification in which it is bound to one or more data elements. Often the value set is dependent on an external code system that may be updated or replaced after publication of the interoperability specification. Stability can have one of two values: *static* or *dynamic*. Static indicates that for this version of the specification the value set is completely fixed, both its definition and the expanded list of codes. If the value set needs to be modified, then a new value set and an updated version of the specification must be created. Dynamic means that a value set can change outside of the definition of the specification (and, thus in essence, it becomes a new value set that may be managed and referred to in various ways). In

[14]Only for concepts that don't exist; i.e., a new code can't be added for an existing concept.

[15]Referred to as a value set expansion in HL7 V3 (and as of May 2016, in all of HL7 with the publication of the Value Set Definition specification [5]).

some instances, dynamic value sets are entire code systems that periodically are updated. The CVX code system (used for immunization messaging in the US) or the German PZN (pharmaceutical central numbers) are good examples. A new vaccine may be developed or an existing one deprecated and replaced with another. Another good example is the set of codes used for diagnoses. In Germany, a new code system for this purpose is released every year (e.g., "ICD-10 German Modification Release 2016"). In order to avoid the need for an updated release of the specification each year, the binding to a value set with dynamic stability is established. Under these circumstances the latest version[16] of the value set should be used. How trading partners convey the use of the updated value set varies in practice. In some cases, it may be critical for them to be in harmony with the latest version immediately, while in others it may not be. Without prior agreement, the use of the conformance claim is useful. For example, in HL7 v2.x, the value set being used (the value set is a profile component) can be conveyed in the Message Profile Identifier element (MSH-21). Unfortunately, not all standards provide such a mechanism.

5.6.1.2 Value Set Definition and Value Set Expansion

Discussion to this point has, for the most part, treated a value set as the combination of the value set meta data and the list of codes. This is a common understanding of what a value set is in many of the healthcare standards (including HL7). However, recent work within HL7 (specifically the Value Set Definition project [5]) defines these as separate entities. The Value Set Definition provides meta data and information to determine the codes. The Value Set Expansion is the realization of the codes in a computable format, such as an enumerated list. This separation allows for better management of vocabulary. The binding is to the Value Set Definition. The notions of Value Set Definition and Value Set Expansion are beginning to be used in some new specifications. However, the majority of specifications refer to and specify a value set as both the value set definition meta data and the list of codes. See Chap. 7 for a more detailed discussion on Value Set Definition and Value Set Expansion.

5.6.1.3 Value Sets Using Multiple Code Systems

Value sets may include codes from multiple code systems. Table 5.18 presents the value set (identified by HL70001_EX2) in which the code X (for X-gender just as an arbitrary and meaningless example code) is added to value set HL70001_EX above.[17] The code X is drawn from the 99_My_Code_System code system.

---

[16]In essence a new value set has been created.

[17]Note: for this value set the choice was made to list only the included codes in the value set definition.

Table 5.18 Administrative gender value set (HL70001_EX2)

Value	Description	Code system
F	Female	HL70001 v2.5.1
M	Male	HL70001 v2.5.1
X	X-gender	99_My_Code_System
U	Unknown	HL70001 v2.5.1

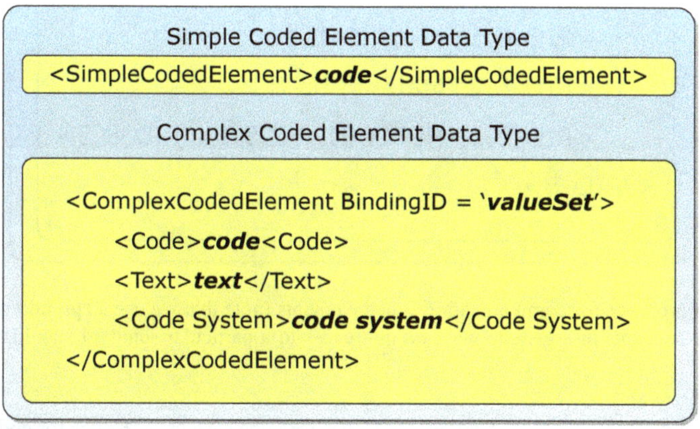

Fig. 5.7 Common data structures of coded elements

It is essential that the association between the code and the source code system is maintained. The code system provides the context for determining the meaning of the code. In standards, this connection is accomplished in two ways: directly in the object instance (e.g., message) or derived from the specification (i.e., the binding of the data element to the value set specified in the profile). The method used is determined by the complexity of the data type. If the data type is a simple coded element, then only the code is sent; in this case, the association is limited to that declared in the binding and the underlying code system can be identified from the profile. If the data type is a complex coded element, then the code and code system are sent together, making either method of interpreting the code available (see Fig. 5.7).

Figure 5.8 presents the two approaches (shown in Fig. 5.7) discussed for communicating coded elements in data exchange standards with some example data. Additional information is needed when using Approach 1. That is, knowing what "M" means is not possible until it is linked to the code system or an explicit knowledge about the contents of the data element it is bound to is available. Approach 2 provides sufficient context for understanding the meaning of the code, since the code system is given directly in the object.

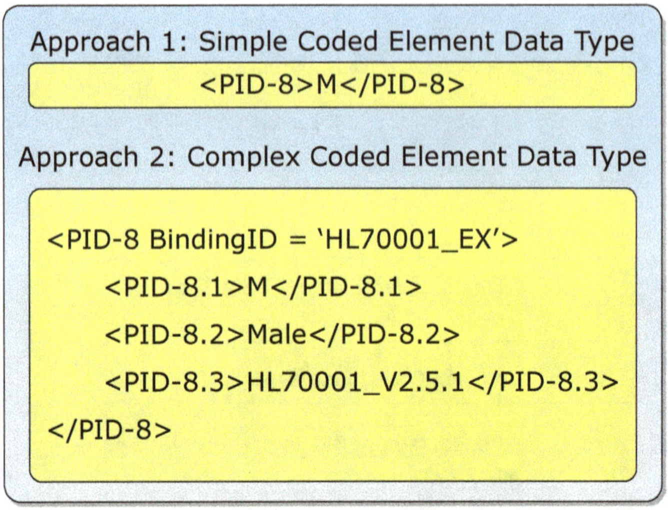

Fig. 5.8 Approaches for communicating coded elements (note that we use a "pseudo notation" to describe the concepts in a generic way; no inferences to a particular standard should be made)

Table 5.19 Example code systems

Concept	Codes for code system X	Codes for code system Y
Female	1	0
Male	2	1

Table 5.20 Example value set

Concept	Code	Code system
Female	1	X
Male	1	Y

It is important to note that value set definitions that use the same code from different code systems have to be bound to data elements with a complex coded element data type. Otherwise, it is not possible to distinguish which concept is being conveyed. Tables 5.19 and 5.20 present a contrived example to illustrate the important points of the code and code system association.

Table 5.19 shows two different (example) code systems for representing the concepts of Female and Male. For code system X the code for Female is "1" and the code for Male is "2". For code system Y the code for Female is "0" and the code for Male is "1". In Table 5.20 a value set is constructed in which the concepts of Female and Male are represented. For Female the code "1" is drawn from code system **X**, and for Male the code "1" is drawn from code system **Y**. This is a valid value set definition, albeit a poor one (aesthetically).

Even though the code "1" is used for both concepts, the meaning can be determined because of the association to the code system; however, if only the code is sent in the object (e.g., message), as is the case for a simple coded element data type, then the concept can't be determined. This example illustrates the need for clean code system management, because combining specific values from different code systems into a value set may be more reasonable than arbitrarily defining some local codes.

5.6.1.4 Coded Elements with Text Exceptions

Circumstances do arise in which it is preferred to use a coded element, but the required concept is not available in the value set for one reason or another; therefore, the specification must allow for conveying the concept as free text to support these known possibilities. Standards handle this need in various ways. Unfortunately, the most frequently chosen manner conflates the value set definition, the binding strength, and the data type definition, which unnecessarily complicates the specification and hinders understanding the intent of the requirements.

For example, the HL7 v2.x uses the notion of the CNE (Coded no-exception) and CWE (Coded with Exceptions)[18] data types that provide a structure definition combined with the binding strength; however, neither the base standard data type definition nor the associated binding strength definition is sufficient for use in specifications. That is, the data type definitions need to be constrained via profiling, and the implication of the defined binding strength is insufficient, not clear, and not well understood.

The use of coded elements with exceptions can be managed sufficiently with the complex coded element data type definition and the value set definition. A key to this management is the profiling mechanism. The figures that follow illustrate how such a mechanism can be used effectively.

Figure 5.7 provided the data type structure for a simple and complex definition. The use of each component was not specified. Figure 5.9 shows a complex data type definition where a code is required (no exceptions) for the value set specified as '*valueSet*'. *Please note that in this figure and the figures to follow, a demonstrative pseudo notation is used help the reader visualize the concept—no relationship to a particular standard or information model should be inferred.*

The specification can be interpreted as: for a data element (not indicated in diagram) with this data type definition (ComplexCodedElement), a Code is required (indicated by R usage), an associated Text is required to be supported and valued if known (indicated by the RE usage), and the Code System is required (indicated by R usage). The set of allowable codes are defined in the "*valueSet*" (indicated by BindingID = 'valueSet'). The value of ***code*** is selected from ***valueSet*** with an associated ***code system***.

[18]Note: CNE and CWE convey different concepts in v2 versus V3.

```
<ComplexCodedElement BindingID = 'valueSet'>
    <Code Usage = 'R' >code<Code>
    <Text Usage = 'RE' >text</Text>
    <CodeSystem Usage = 'R' >code system</CodeSystem>
</ComplexCodedElement>
```

Fig. 5.9 Coded with no exception specification

```
<ComplexCodedElement BindingID = 'valueSet'>
    <Code Usage = 'RE' >code<Code>
    <Text Usage = 'C(R/RE)' >text</Text>
    <CodeSystem Usage = 'C(R/X)' >code system</CodeSystem>
</ComplexCodedElement>
```

Fig. 5.10 Coded with exception specification

Figure 5.10 shows the situation where a code is desired, but, if one is not available, text can be conveyed instead. Note that the common interpretation of this construct is that if a code that conveys the desired concept exists in the value set, then the code must be used, i.e., using text instead is not an option. This requirement is indicated by the "RE" usage and the value set binding (i.e., loosely speaking, the implementation must be capable of supporting a code for this element, and if a code is available in the value set for the desired concept, then that code must be used). The use of the conditional usage requires a condition predicate. For example, in the case of the CodeSystem, the predicate would be "If Code is valued" (the predicate is not shown in Fig. 5.10).

Coded element data types are not limited to the examples provided here. Some standards include additional elements that allow for an alternative code, that is, a second set of the *code*, *text*, and *code system* tuple (commonly referred to as a "triplet"). HL7 V3, for example, allows use of an alternative coding if the preferred value set does not provide the code needed. Another common element is the "*original text*", which is used to indicate the original information provided that led to the selection of a particular code.

5.6.1.5 Explicit Binding Strength Specification

Continuing with the specification in a pseudo notation, the binding strength needs to be indicated, as is shown in Fig. 5.11 with the Binding Strength attribute. If the binding strength is defined as "Required", the code that is used must be drawn from

```
<ComplexCodedElement BindingID = 'valueSet' BindingStrength = 'Required'>
    <Code Usage = 'R' >code<Code>
    <Text Usage = 'RE' >text</Text>
    <CodeSystem Usage = 'R' >code system</CodeSystem>
</ComplexCodedElement>
```

Fig. 5.11 Required binding specification

the value set specified. If the binding is "Suggested", then it is interpreted as "a code must be used" as indicated in the data type definition; however, any value set can be specified for the concept domain in a derived specification. As mentioned previously, different standards specify these concepts in different ways, and some don't support these notions at all. In the standards that do support them, often the data type definition and binding strength are conflated (which is a source of confusion).

5.6.1.6 Types of Bindings Used in Standards

As described earlier, the binding strength can have only two practical states: "Required" and "Suggested". Required is Implementable (normative) and Suggested is Illustrative (informative). Different standards use different terms to represent these binding strengths. Many standards (unfortunately) do not specify an explicit binding strength, however, the intent is for the value set to be used, and therefore the binding is implicitly Implementable (normative). Additionally, some standards have multiple categories to represent various types of Illustrative (informative) information. This information is defined as an attribute of the vocabulary. Note: the Illustrative binding may point to a "real" value set or code system, or simply refer to a set of representative codes or an example code set indicating the "idea" behind the value set. Such codes have no standing as a requirement. For example, CDA has the notion of a preferred vocabulary, which is a strong recommendation, but it is still just a flavor of informative. Ultimately, a value set must be referenced and declared normative for an implementation (Table 5.21).

5.6.2 Null Flavors (Values)

On occasion, there are no available valid data to be carried in a data element. It has proven desirable in some business contexts to provide information to express why the content is not present in the data element. In order to do this, a content-related concept called "null flavors" has been developed. Depending on the standard, a null flavor can be an integral part of a value set (e.g., HL7 v2.x) or can be represented

Table 5.21 Vocabulary binding

Binding	Explanation	Replacement
Implementable	Definitive requirement to use the value set as provided	Not allowed
Universal	Term used with HL7 v2.x as a replacement for HL7-defined tables	
Illustrative	The value set is only a suggestion for this use case to illustrate how vocabulary may be chosen for implementation	Allowed
Preferred	Preferred (or recommended) is an indication that the authors strongly suggest use of this vocabulary. Although there is a strong preference to implement, the vocabulary is not a requirement unless the binding strength is explicitly made required in an implementable profile	
Representative	The value set has been used in at least one normative implementation in the past, and is available as a reusable component if desired	
Example	The value set contains only a few codes to explain the intent of the value set	

independently (e.g., HL7 V3). Some standards do not support the concept at all. A detailed explanation is given as part of the HL7 V3 discussion in "Additional Healthcare Data Exchange Standards". As indicated earlier, some standards provide a means of conveying this information in the basic information model structures (such as the datatypes), whereas other standards intend it to be included in a bound value set, e.g., including a code "U" for unknown.

5.6.3 *Fixed Value (Constant)*

A standard may provide a fixed value conformance construct to allow for denoting a constant value. The use of fixed values only makes sense in the context of applying constraints to the base standard for a given use case (a process called profiling). Analysis of a use case may result in the determination that only one value is valid out of a set of possible values for an element.

In principle, a fixed value may or may not be present in the specified element. In practical terms, a fixed value only makes sense when combined with usage that requires a value. When combined with a usage of "must support", it must be assumed that the standing of the constant is binding; therefore, depending on how the construct is specified in the standard, an actual value may or may not be included. Of course, best practice and common expectation are that the fixed value for this element will be included. Additionally, a well-defined standard would ensure that Required usage is applied to any element having a fixed-value conformance construct. Regardless, the use of the fixed-value conformance construct requires that only this single constant value shall be used in the message or document instance.

In HL7 v2.x, constraint of a message structure to a specific event code is an example of how a fixed-value conformance construct may be used. When a patient transfer message needs to be transmitted, the event code is set to the literal "A02" (which is selected from a set of possibilities). It is important to note that the event code must be sent in order to identify the message instance as a patient transfer. In another use case example, if only female patients are to be included, the code for administrative gender is constrained to the single code "F" for female, a fixed value.

5.6.4 *Default Values*

A default value is a pre-determined value that is assigned to an element. If a dynamic value is not provided for the element in the message or document, the recipient performs the processing of the element populated using the pre-determined value. Unlike with a fixed value (constant) element, the actual value populating an element that is assigned a default value can be different from the default value (i.e., the default is overridden if a value is present in the message or document). The use of a default value is a common means of saving space by omitting data. This approach requires the recipient to know which value should be used by default when a value is omitted. Default values require either an additional negotiation in advance between sender and receiver in order to define those values, or stipulation of the default in a specification. During runtime, default values cause additional computational effort on the sender side to determine whether the data for the element can be omitted, and on the receiver side to determine the default value. The use of default values is not recommended.

Taking the use case example from the previous section in which only female patients are to be included and modifying the use case slightly to allow for inclusion of male patients as well, a value set constraint to a single value would not be permitted, because the elements may need to support a value representing either female or male. The assumption in this example is that male patients would be an exception, so missing gender information can be assigned a default value of "female". Consequently, the gender information for male patients must be conveyed specifically.

Use of a default value only made sense in an era when keeping the size of the message as small as possible was critical due to capacity limitations on the wire, and leaving out such information was a way of reducing the size of the message. Now, the size of the message is of little concern. The use of default values does not make sense today (although inexplicably they are still specified in some implementation guides), and it represents bad practice, because neither the size of the transmitted message nor computation time is really reduced. Another argument against use of a default value is the uncertainty about the value itself, as there is no distinction between an element that is left out of the message intentionally or left out erroneously.

5.6.5 *Placeholder Values*

Another, related concept is the transmission of placeholder values in cases where an element is Required but no valid data are available. A very good example of such a case is the sending of "John Doe" in the patient name elements when the name of the patient is unknown. A null flavor can be sent in HL7 V3, and in HL7 v2.x an empty name element should be sent with a tag (type code) denoting "temporarily unavailable", a method introduced in HL7 v2.7. In some standards, however, no mechanism exists for conveying the non-availability of data for an element (e.g., earlier versions of HL7 v2.x). Placeholder values are used in lieu of a null flavor or an element with the type code, which points to a deficiency of the standard.

5.7 Conformance Statements

Conformance statements[19] are normative statements of requirements explicitly expressed in a natural language or formal language. In a sense, conformance statements are a catch-all mechanism for specifying requirements that aren't conveniently defined using the conformance constructs. Some specifications, such as CDA templates, use explicit conformance statement extensively. Basically, CDA templates are expressed as a collection of conformance statements. An example of a CDA conformance statement is [6]:

SHALL contain [1..1] component/structuredBody (CONF:4082).

(a) This component/structuredBody SHOULD contain [0..1] component (CONF:4130) such that it a. SHALL contain [1..1] Reporting Parameters section (templateId: 2.16.840.1.113883.10.20.17.2.1) (CONF:4131).
(b) This component/structuredBody SHALL contain [1..1] component (CONF:4132) such that it a. SHALL contain [1..1] Patient data section—NCR (templateId: 2.16.840.1.113883.10.20.17.2.5) (CONF:4133)

Certain conformance constructs, such as cardinality and vocabulary requirements, are embedded in the CDA conformance statements. HL7 v2.x, on the other hand, uses conformance constructs extensively to specify requirements and uses explicit conformance statements sparingly.

[19]Conformance statement is an overloaded term. At a low-level it is used for expressing requirements in a specification. At a high-level it is used to express a capability of a system or product; the low-level use is described in this section.

5.8 Data Semantics

Data semantics defines a concept (logical meaning) binding to a data element. That is, data semantics conveys the sort of data an element is carrying and how those data should be interpreted. Data semantics can be highly subjective. The "Patient Identifier" element provides information for identifying a patient; the definition of this element provides the meaning of the data. A model can be developed to define the semantics and to relate them to concepts (data elements). HL7 V3 has sophisticated models and element definitions. HL7 v2.x describes the semantics as part of the data element definition. HL7 FHIR lands somewhere between these two approaches. In all cases, the semantics of an element can be refined through profiling that addresses a specific use case.

5.8.1 Models

Correct behavior of systems and associated interfaces requires the use of proper models, otherwise achieving interoperability becomes very difficult. For example, if a one-to-many relationship exists between persons and patients, then this ratio should be implemented the same way for all of the interfaces involved, or specific meanings based on this structure will not be supported correctly. Both, the example presented with the introduction of optionality in Sect. 5.3.1 and the example data repository schema developed in Chap. 2 certainly help explain the associated requirements.

As introduced in Chap. 2, even if a straight forward approach to developing and implementing specific structures exists, full compatibility can only be achieved if the underlying models are the same. A thorough analysis of this subject would exceed the limits of this book and, therefore, is not covered.

5.9 Encoding

Correct encoding of data is essential to the operation of interfaces and, in many cases, is underestimated or even not covered at all. An application typically provides a graphical user interface (GUI) that provides the capability for the user to enter data. This feature hides the internal representation of the data from the user. As an example, if the user has to enter a date, a calendar can be presented that shows a month of the year and that allows the user to select the day. Such a presentation can provide additional features to allow for marking a set of days, a date range, or a point in time, use of which can be explained by tool tips that display when the cursor is moved over the calendar. The manner in which the data are stored internally is unseen by the user. Normally, the ability to recover the exact data that are entered is the only aspect of interest. In the case of a data exchange, the

Fig. 5.12 Encoding

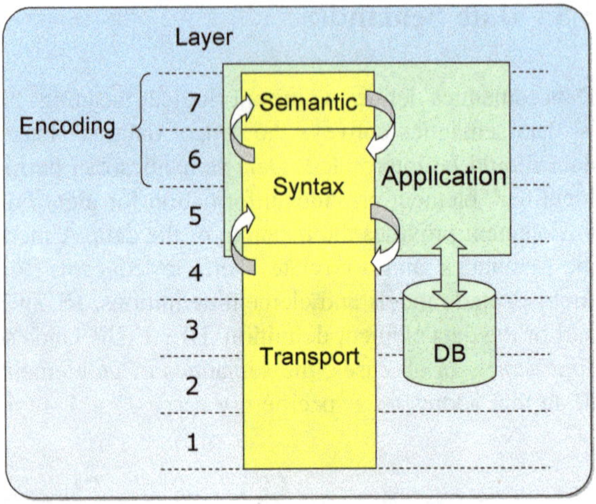

differences among the various representations are important. Entities wishing to exchange data must agree upon a common representation. A conversion of the data into a serialized representation must be performed before sending. On the other end of the exchange, the serialization is unraveled into the data representation used by the receiving system.

The encoding occurs between the ISO levels six and seven, which is marked in Fig. 5.12. The information presented to the user is handled on level 7, but for data exchange the information must be transformed to a correct syntactic representation on level 6. This process, including some examples, is explained below.

5.9.1 Display-Oriented Encoding Concepts

As mentioned in the introduction of this section, data are normally only handled inside an application. What counts as far as the user is concerned are how the data are entered and correct retrieval and display of the data after they have been stored. When data must be exchanged, the characters representing the data must undergo a special treatment so they do not conflict with the characters needed for managing the data representation. This treatment is called escaping. For certain use cases, like reporting, textual data should embed formatting commands to allow for user friendly display. And finally, the character sets are important for presenting the data correctly to the user.

5.9.1.1 Escaping

The characters needed to handle and manage the encoding are, of course, excluded from direct use. Nevertheless, one has to find an alternative way to express them if

Table 5.22 Example encodings in XML

Representation (as data)		Encoding in XML
5 < 10	⇔	<text>5 **<** 10</text>
Walter **&** Sons	⇔	<text>Walter **&** Sons</text>

Table 5.23 HL7 v2.x ER7 escape characters

Code	Description	Resulting escape sequence		
		Pos[a]	“\”[b]	“x”[c]
F	Field separator		\F\	xFx
S	Component separator	1	\S\	xSx
R	Repetition separator	2	\R\	xRx
E	Escape character	3	\E\	xEx
T	Subcomponent separator	4	\T\	xTx

[a]MSH-2 position. Field separator is MSH-1
[b]Using the escape delimiter “\”
[c]Using the escape delimiter “x”

they occur within the data. The method used is typically called *escaping* and is part of all programming languages

Table 5.22 provides some examples showing the encoding of text in XML. Other encodings have similar requirements, which we will demonstrate and explain later. Special characters that are needed to support the encoding are excluded from direct use. In other words, if the characters that have a special meaning occur within the data, special handling in the form of a certain replacement is required. For comma-separated files the replacement is a “comma”, and for XML it is the angle bracket (“<“, “>“) and ampersand (“&”). Consequently, the “less than” character and the ampersand in the two examples in Table 5.22 must be *escaped* by the correct representation as defined for XML, which is “<” and “&”.

For HL7 v2.x the replacement is the set of characters defined in the message header, which—according to their definition—may vary. An explanation can be found in Chap. 4 in Section HL7 Version 2 ⇒ Encoding.

The way escaping is done varies as well. For most programming languages it is done by pre-pending the corresponding character with another special character like the backslash (“\”) in “C”. In HL7 v2.x escaping is done by replacing the corresponding character with a sequence of special characters.

As a consequence, all characters used as a delimiter[20] (which is defined in the message header) must be replaced using the appropriate sequence. For HL7 v2.x, the escape sequence itself varies in the end, as can be seen in Table 5.23. A correct

[20]For HL7 v2.x, the carriage return character also belongs in this category, requiring a proper escaping. Errors for wrong handling are, in most cases, visible for text fields, allowing the user to enter multiple lines of text.

Table 5.24 Example encodings in HL7 v2.x ER7

MSH-2	Representation (as data)		Encoding in ER7
^~\&	Walter **&** Sons	⇔	Walter **\T** Sons
0123	5 < **10**	⇔	5 < **2R22S2**

implementation has to account for escaping delimiters that appear in data, otherwise an application is non-conformant[21] to the underlying HL7 v2.x ER7 encoding rules.

Two different examples are given in Table 5.24 using the standard encoding (first row) and an alternative encoding (second row). The strings displayed to the user are shown in the 2nd column from the left. The leftmost column provides the characters to be used for the encoding in HL7 v2.x and conveyed in the message header (MSH-2), i.e., those characters must be escaped in a transmitted message when used in the data. The characters that are replaced and their encoding replacements in the message are marked in bold.

The two examples demonstrate how encoding is accomplished depending on the delimiters. In the first example, the ampersand must be escaped, while in the second the digits are used as delimiters so they enforce an escaping. As explained with Table 5.23, those characters are replaced by a sequence of characters.

Consequently, in HL7 v2.x the escaping is definitely not limited to certain data types but applies to all. A correct implementation takes care of all data elements and checks for their correct encoding in a certain environment. The implementation should consider the current set of encoding characters and allow for individual (bilateral) use among trading partners.

Switching to an alternative set of encoding characters immediately reveals whether problems during encoding and decoding will occur or not. If a sending interface is, for example, appending a second component to a field that normally should be composed of a single component only, and if the receiver does not manage the encoding correctly, i.e., without considering a delimiter on component level, the whole set of data—both components together including the delimiter—is taken as the data being sent. Of course, the wrong data are erroneously stored then, or—in case of coded information—the codes are not correctly identified, leading to unexpected results.

A very good way to confirm proper encoding is to enter data containing the characters that are used for encoding during testing. For XML these data are “<” and “>”, while for HL7 v2.x the pipe symbol (“|”) and caret (“^”) are good candidates.

[21]It must be noted that most applications do not account for escaping delimiters, which is the reason for many compatibility issues and the request to constrain the set of delimiters to fixed values.

5.9.1.2 Text Formatting

Text also can be formatted similarly to the manner in which characters are escaped. Some data exchange standards allow for special sequences to highlight (most often interpreted as **bold**) specific fragments within *normal* text. In contrast to escape sequences, text formatting is typically restricted to elements of certain data types. For HL7 v2.x, this kind of handling is defined for the data types "TX" (text) and "FT" (formatted text). The appropriate formatting commands are listed in Table 5.25.

Text formatting is, of course, restricted to those data exchange standards allowing for a higher level of encoding. Most of them are based on XML, including the text formatting ("markups") known from HTML.

HL7 v2.x has taken the liberty of using escape characters to allow for formatting commands stemming from the UNIX world. They are taken from the "old" text formatting language "roff" (Table 5.26) and include the appropriate escape sequences. Table 5.27 provides an example of how a short text with a headline in bold and a paragraph break would be represented in HL7 v2.x. The codes denoting this are surrounded by the "standard" escape sequences:

Table 5.25 HL7 v2.x ER7 text formatting commands (for data types FT, TX and CF)

Command	Description
H	Begin highlighting
N	End highlighting (i.e., return to *normal* text)

Table 5.26 HL7 v2.x ER7 formatting commands (for data type FT)

Command	Description
.sp <number>	End current output line and skip <number> vertical spaces
.br	Begin new output line
.fi	Begin word wrap or fill mode
.nf	Begin no-wrap mode
.in <number>	Indent <number> of spaces, where <number> is a positive or negative integer
.ti <number>	Temporarily indent <number> of spaces where number is a positive or negative integer
.sk <number>	Skip <number> spaces to the right
.ce	End current output line and center the next line

Table 5.27 Example for HL7 v2 text formatting

Example	Encoded representation
Anamnesis The patient has diabetes	\H\Anamnesis\N\\.br\The patient has diabetes

5.9.1.3 Character Sets

A very different kind of problem, which only occurs under certain conditions, is the character set itself (Table 5.28). Uninformed implementers erroneously insert data directly into the message instance. This usually results in:

- no character set specification,
- lack of proper encoding (in this case escaping), and
- no mention of changes[22] in the character set.

If the communication partners are using the same character set, and the transmitted data are processed directly, thus, the associated problems would not be noticed.

A point to note is the escape sequences: to switch between the various character sets, escape sequences are necessary, but these sequences are not defined for all character sets. In principle, according to the HL7 v2.x Table 0211, an appropriate escape sequence must be present for each allowed character set, which often is not the case.

The Japanese use for their preferred character set (ISO IR87) the escape sequences that are implicitly internally-defined so no special treatment is necessary. The current implementations show that this works well even if they do not manage it explicitly.

Note that delimiter definitions can be represented in 7-bit to ensure interoperability.

Table 5.29 provides the appropriate character codes for some characters that are used quite often. As can be seen, the problem with character sets has a higher incidence in non-English speaking countries:

Care must be taken when communicating with data-delivering devices, because they are mostly bound to ASCII.

Example: To explain the impact on different encodings, Table 5.30 provides a simple example from the German language. The hexadecimal encoding of the word "Grüße" (Engl.: regards/greetings) is shown:

The extraction of data on the sending side, as well as transmission and simple storage of the received byte string without any special treatment will lead to problems. The prevalence of this problem, however, primarily depends the countries and the domain. For example, in the administrative domain in English speaking countries the occurrence is unlikely, because only standard characters are used. In the medication domain the probability is much higher if the single character representation for "½" or "¾" is used to denote the administration of drugs. Another good example is the device communication in Germany with different character sets used in the computer and the device itself, so the German "Umlaut (encoding)" ("ä", "ö", "ü" and "ß[2]") is highly problematic.

[22]Some databases like mySQL/Maria allow for individual character sets for table columns.

Table 5.28 Text encodings (explanation) [7]

Encoding	Usage
ASCII[a] = US-ASCII = ANSI X3.4-1986	8-Bit character set, but only 7 bits are used, so only 128 characters are contained (33 control codes and 95 printable characters)
Codepage 437 = CP437 = DOS-US = OEM-US	8-bit character set used in USA in a Windows command line (=DOS-Box)
Codepage 850 = CP850 = DOS-Latin-1	8-bit character set used in Western European countries in a Windows command line (=DOS-Box)
Codepage 1252 = Windows-1252 (sometimes also called ANSI)	Windows standards character set for Western European countries (8 bit) Cp1252 contains all characters from ISO 8859-1 and ISO 8859-15, but partially with a different encoding
ISO 8859-1 = Latin-1	8-bit character set for HTML web pages, includes "äöüß", but no "€" (compare with 8859-1, 8859-15, 1252 and Unicode)
ISO 8859-15 = Latin-9	Comparable to ISO 8859-1, but it contains "€" and some specific characters for French
UTF-8[b]	This is the most common encoding for Unicode. It is used with some operating systems (GNU/Linux, Unix) and partially in web services (e-mail, web). The characters are encoded with different lengths, ranging from 1 to 4 bytes
UTF-16	It is used in some operating systems (Windows, OS X) and programming languages (Java, .NET) for their internal character encoding. The characters are encoded using 2 or 4 bytes
UTF-32	This is the four byte encoding for Unicode
EBCDIC[c] 273	8-bit character set, which is primarily used with IBM legacy systems (AS/400, iSeries)
HTML-Entities	"named entities" are used in HTML source code (but not XHTML and XML) for specific non-ASCII characters

[a]ASCII = American Standard Code for Information Interchange
[b]UTF = Universal Multiple-Octet Coded Character Set (UCS) Transformation Format
[c]EBCDIC = Extended Binary Coded Decimal Interchange Code

Unicode: In the family of character sets, Unicode is superior. It is in principle a collection of characters from a lot of different countries. Currently it covers more 65,000 different characters. The set of characters for a specific country are organized into pages, so that each character is assigned a unique number in combination with the page. The encoding is then defined algorithmically allowing use of the

Table 5.29 Text encodings (example characters) [7]

Encoding	Ä	ö	Ü	ß	§	€	½	²	√	Σ
ASCII	–	–	–	–	–	–	–	–	–	–
Codepage 437	84	94	81	E1	–	–	AB	FD	FB	–
Codepage 850	84	94	81	E1	F5	–	AB	FD	–	–
Codepage 1252	E4	F6	FC	DF	A7	80	BD	B2	–	–
ISO 8859-1	E4	F6	FC	DF	A7	–	BD	B2	–	–
ISO 8859-15	E4	F6	FC	DF	A7	A4	–	B2	–	–
UTF-8	C3 A4	C3 B6	C3 BC	C3 9F	C2 A7	E2 82 AC	C2 BD	C2 B2	E2 88 9A	E2 88 91
UTF-16	00E4	00F6	00FC	00DF	00A7	20AC	00BD	00B2	221A	2211
EBCDIC 273	C0	6A	D0	A1	7C	–	B8	EA	–	–
HTML-entities	& auml ;	& ouml ;	& uuml ;	& szlig ;	& sect ;	& euro ;	& frac12 ;	& sup2 ;	& radic ;	& sum ;

Table 5.30 Example encoding for the German word “Grüße”

Example	G	r	ü	ß	e
ANSI	47	72	FC	DF	65
UTF-8	47	72	C3 BC	C3 9F	65
Codepage 437	47	72	81	E1	65

necessary number of bytes (from one to four with UTF-8), pairs (one or two) of two bytes (UTF-16), or a fixed length with four bytes (UTF-32). Based on the contents, conversions between the different encodings can be made. However, without special treatment the different encodings are incompatible with each other.

The HL7 InM (Infrastructure and Messaging) WG decided on 16.3.2010 to disallow the character sets UTF-16 and UTF-32 for HL7 v2.x messaging. These two sets are basically only alternative forms of representation for UNICODE and can thus certainly be represented by UTF-8 alone, meaning a fundamental incompatibility between the different applications can be avoided. UTF-8, however, is designed so no fundamental problems are caused in the overlap with ASCII.

Byte Order Mark (BOM): When using Unicode it is possible to use different orders on the bytes in the stream, especially with UTF-16 and UTF-32 (Table 5.31).

UTF-8 really does not make use of the byte order; nevertheless, an “invalid” character sequence is defined, which helps in deciding the order that is used.

Table 5.31 Byte order mark (BOM)

Encoding	UTF-8	UTF-16	UTF-32
Big endian notation	EF BB BF	FE FF	FE FF 00 00 00 00 FE FF
Little endian notation	EF BB BF	FF FE	FF FE 00 00 00 00 FF FE

5.9.1.4 HL7 v2.x XML Encoding

The XML encoding for Version 2.x ("HL7v2.xml") uses XML structures and elements, which are based on the abstract message syntax (AMS) and represent an alternative to the standard encoding (ER7). The structures are implemented compatible to ER7, however, there are some differences:

- Segment groups are clearly identified, which puts the structural elements at a level deeper and makes them addressable directly. Enhancing the message structure definitions by introducing new groups will result in structural incompatibilities, because the affected segments are moved one level deeper.
- Fields are expressed based on the type of data if it is a composite data type. This approach becomes problematic when developing and refining the data type by adding further components to newer versions of the standard, which can lead to incompatibilities. The same effect will occur when specific implementations introduce additional components. Here, complete documentation, including the data type definition for the changed elements in form of implementable profiles, becomes necessary.

On the one hand (apart from the available XML tools), implementations based on the XML encoding have a certain advantage, because the structures are clearly identifiable. On the other hand, enhancements lead to incompatibilities by introducing new substructures.

ER7 Versus XML: Both of these encodings require appropriate handling of special characters. Although this requirement is understood and performed correctly for XML, it is called into question for ER7. The intent of previous discussion in this section is to convey that each encoding requires a special handling of those characters that are necessary to manage the appropriate encoding. Of course, the way the handling is accomplished and the number of affected characters varies between those two encodings.

5.9.2 Presence/Absence of an Element

Within a message or document[23] instance an element can be either present or absent. Additionally, the presence or absence of an element can have different flavors. Figure 5.13 provides the set of possibilities that a standard might support in specific encoding.

[23]In this book, concepts are typically explained in the context of messages, but the concepts apply equally to documents.

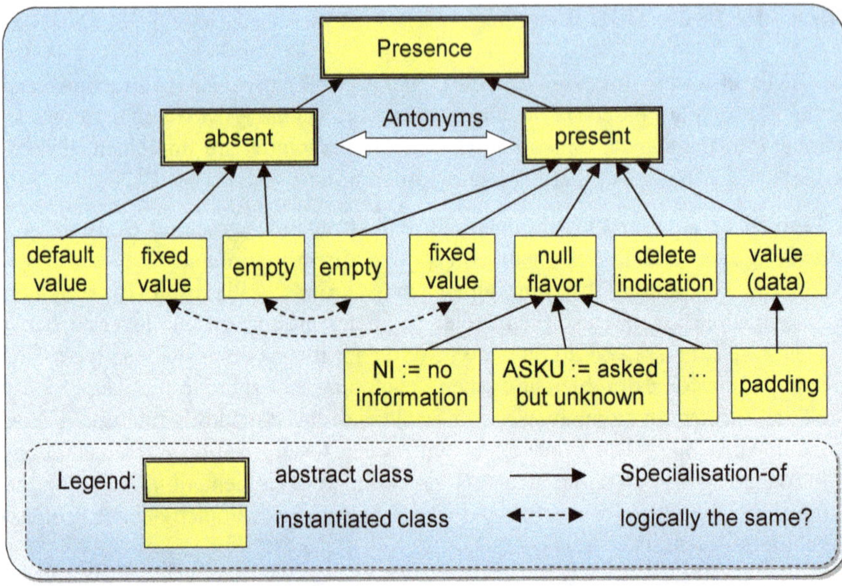

Fig. 5.13 Possible states for the presence of an element

A message (or document) instance is a serialization of a set of data according to an abstract specification. The serialization is managed by an encoding specification. Early standards (during the beginning of the 1990s) used a fixed format, such that the position in the exchanged character sequence was clearly defined and delimiters were not necessary. Consequently, each record had the same length and did not allow for variations. Modern standards are based on hierarchical representations with optional and repeating elements. This capability requires the use of delimiters or at least some means to divide the conveyed string into its constitute parts.

The representation of available data is easy. (Encoding specialties of specific characters are explained in a subsequent section.) If a fixed length is given for an element and the data to be conveyed in this element have a length that is less than the specified length, then the data are filled with special characters; this function is called padding. Typically, for alphanumeric characters trailing blanks are added, while for numeric data leading zeros are used. Fortunately, no HL7 standards make use of padding. DICOM, however, requires an even number of characters for text elements. If no clear definition is provided for how to identify padded values, different applications may treat padding differently, maybe by overwriting valid values or interpreting the padded characters as real values. Most application developers are not aware of their specific responsibilities for handling these values.

The option to convey information about missing data (null-flavors) is explained later on and is bound to the possibility of an adequate representation. The Implementation Technology Specification (ITS) for HL7 v3 has built in this feature, while HL7 v2 has almost no means of finding an appropriate backward-compatible

Table 5.32 Example encoding for HL7 v2.x

<table>
<tr><th>ER7 encoding</th><th>XML encoding</th></tr>
<tr><td>…
PID|||||Smith^Jane|
…</td><td>…
<PID>
<PID.3>
</PID.3>
<PID.5>
<XPN.1><FN.1>Smith</FN.1></XPN.1>
<XPN.2>Jane</XPN.2>
</PID.5>
</PID>
…</td></tr>
</table>

representation. Most of the other data exchange standards are not mature enough to support this notion.

In the case where no data are available, the encodings have two different options for representing the situation. In the standards that are used currently, different kinds of encoding may be applied:

- ER7 (HL7 standard Encoding Rules for Version 2.x)
- XML (HL7 XML encoding)
- DICOM

As indicated in Fig. 5.13, for specific implementation technologies like ER7 and XML, an empty element can be present or absent (shown in the dashed box in the middle). Table 5.32 provides examples for ER7 and XML, demonstrating the difference between present and absent elements:

As HL7 encoding rules (ER7) at least treat an element as present,[24] whether a field is absent or empty cannot be determined. Table 5.32 shows that ER7 does not distinguish between an empty present element (PID-3) and an empty absent element (PID-7). In HL7 v2.xml encoding, the elements are clearly distinguished as can be seen with the missing “PID-7” element in the right column of Table 5.32. In other words, in XML the representation for the missing element PID-3 is present, while the representation for PID-7 is absent. This approach leads to the phenomenon that, depending on the way the encoding is specified for missing values, one can or cannot determine between those two representation forms.

Another aspect is the handling of default and fixed values. They are used if no information is available from a message directly and are dependent on the

[24]If the implementation of HL7 v2 ER7 is performed correctly, one can access any field, component or sub-component in a segment—even if it is not defined! As an example, the access to PID-255.3.1 should not fail, but return an empty string. Of course, an interface program will only access the elements it is aware of. A common solution to these problems, however, is to append new elements to existing standard segments, although this behavior is improper; and access to such an element in a message from a trading partner not supporting these additions should not return an error.

Table 5.33 Summary of presence/absence capabilities in standards

Standard	HL7					
Version	v2.x	v2.x	V3	FHIR	3.0	
Encoding / Element	ER7	XML	XML	XML		xDT
Absent elements	Not possible, i.e. no distinction from a present information	Yes	Yes	Yes	Yes	Yes
Present elements	Always	Yes	Yes	Yes	Yes	Yes
Empty elements	Yes	Yes	Yes	Yes	Yes	Yes
Null flavor[a]	No: currently not possible[b]	No: currently not defined[c]	Yes	No	No	No
Delete indication	Yes	Yes	No	No	No	No
Value (i.e. populated)	Yes	Yes	Yes	Yes	Yes	Yes

[a]In most standards null flavors are realized by special values

[b]For HL7 v2.8 a proposal has been discussed to introduce null flavors through a generic approach, but this proposal has been tabled as of this writing due to uncertainty about its backward compatibility, and, therefore, it is not introduced in HL7 v2.x yet

[c]HL7 v2.xml provides a richer syntactic representation then HL7 ER7. Therefore, it would allow for null flavor representations

availability of pre-negotiated data. These two classes are treated as specializations of "absent" because of this property, and their use has been explained earlier in this chapter. An absent element is treated as empty if no default or fixed value can be assumed.

5.9.2.1 Summary of Presence/Absence Capabilities

Table 5.33 provides an overview of how the presence and absence capabilities are handled in various standards. As indicated, different capabilities exist.

5.9.3 Parsing

An important consideration in a data exchange standard is the ease in which the underlying message structure definition can be parsed. Message and document instances are usually comprised of tree structures. A parser needs some help in analyzing these structures to recreate this tree, i.e., at every point in this structure the parser needs to know exactly where it is—or what comes next. XML encapsulates the substructures by placing parenthesis around them. Other encodings like HL7 v2 ER7 and the German xDT do not provide any details. In other words, the parser must be made aware of the structure he has to parse, including repetitions and substructures.

5.9.3.1 Message Substructures

An essential capability of a standard is to support elements (including sub-elements) that can repeat in the message structures. A marker of some kind is required to denote the beginning and end of this substructure. If this marker is unique within a sequence of characters, detecting multiple occurrences of an element is straight-forward.

XML maintains the hierarchical nature of structures in its serialization. Other representation forms convert hierarchical structures into flat (linear) representations. HL7 v2.x and the German xDT are examples of the latter. The German xDT standard uses "fields" (named by their number) that are listed sequentially. These fields control the encoding so they may occur on different repetition levels ("nesting"). Because those fields are used uniquely within a message, the structure can be identified quite easily. An implementation developer must be aware of all the fields being used as a starting point for a repetition. With xDT, each repetition must be implemented individually based on the number used for the field. HL7 v2, as another example, uses segments in the message structure specifications; but, in contrast to xDT, the segments are neither unique in a message (e.g., OBX) nor mandatory in the first position of a repeating group[25] (e.g., the ORC segment in the ORU_R01 message structure is optional). As a consequence, the correct parsing of the appropriate message structure becomes a challenge, because a guess must be made and, in case of an error, the parsing process must track back to a previous reliable point.

For HL7 v2.x, a message structure identifier (e.g., ADT_A01) was introduced in v2.3.1 to support and enhance the parsing process. The message structure provided a "map" of the segments that could be expected. As of this writing, the authors are uncertain how many vendors make use of this feature.

5.9.3.2 HL7 v2.x: Implicit Segment Structures

A problem discussed in this book already is the many implicit information contents. An implementation of the standards is simplified considerably if this information is

[25]In newer versions of HL7 v2.x, two new segments (SGH and SGT) are defined that should support marking the beginning and end of a group, implicitly helping in parsing the message structure. Starting with v2.8.1 these segments are used in OMQ_O42 only and not added to older messages for backward compatibility reasons.

Table 5.34 Message structure "ADT^A24: Patient Link" with explicit information (marked in bold)

ADT^A24^ADT_A24	ADT message	Chapter
MSH	Message Header	2
[{SFT}]	Software Segment	2
[UAC]	User Authentication Credential	2
EVN	Event Type	3
<	**PATIENT_1**	
PID	Patient (1) Identification	3
[PD1]	Patient (1) Additional Demographics	3
[PV1]	Patient (1) Visit	3
[{DB1}]	Patient (1) Disability Information	3
>	**PATIENT_1**	
<	**PATIENT_2**	
PID	Patient (2) Identification	3
[PD1]	Patient (2) Additional Demographics	3
[PV1]	Patient (2) Visit	3
[{DB1}]	Patient (2) Disability Information	3
>	**PATIENT_2**	

also shown explicitly in message instances. In the following message structure, the explicit information content is inserted as "single-choice" elements (in red). (The current specification does not include those details.) This means of expressivity was definitely available in the standard since the first HL7 Version 2, but only since v2.3.1 has it been mentioned explicitly. Fortunately, some HL7 working groups recognized the issue and began to include these options with HL7 v2.8 in 2014. The message structure in the following example still has no additional explicit information, unfortunately, but it is an ideal candidate to use for an explanation.

In the above example from the Table 5.34, the two segment sequences for the identification of the two patients are identical in the original specification. A correct assignment of semantics, however, can only be determined by the order respectively position of the segments in the message. Accessing "PV1" alone does not allow for any conclusion about its assignment to the first or the second patient. To determine its assignment, one must know whether the PV1 segment occurs before or after the second PID segment. This problem results in additional difficulties for the XML encoding, because simple XPath expressions are identical. In the example shown above, PV1 may be fixed by the position information, but not in other examples.

An explicit name is indicated by the text in red. In the XML encoding, this solution would mean placing the segments in their own (named) sub-group, thus simplifying access to the content. (This change, introducing the substructures, would then be incompatible with existing implementations using the XML encoding.) Thus, weighing optimal encoding against backward compatibility is necessary.

5.9.3.3 HL7 v2.x: Explicit Message Structures/BNF

A problem equivalent to the segment structures is the reusability of complete messages. For example, the approximately 60 ADT messages consist of three basic structures—when ignoring the few query messages:

- ADT basic message
- Merge message
- Link message

The basic message varies for most of the ADT messages, by optional structures being omitted (minor in scope), or by the order of the segments (which is not always one hundred percent equal). This fact exposes a disadvantage of not using the meta-model approach when defining the standards: in principle, similar messages vary and must be developed dedicatedly. Apart from the additional development costs for the manufacturer, the voting and maintenance requirements for the standard itself are unnecessarily increased.

The introduction of "Message Structure Identifiers" helps as a first step in identifying exactly the same message structures as such. Note: unfortunately, this identifier will not be taken into account when advancing the standards, so messages that previously had the same structure will be "enhanced" to a new but different message structure, thus starting new discussions. In a second step, these message structure identifiers (MsgStructID) should be used to eliminate duplicate definitions for the same message structures in the standard and, thus, reduce the size of the standard, since each structure is then specified only once. In a third step, one could also harmonize the varying structures and substructures in total. This proposal leads to compatibility issues in general, but it would solve the problem of varying structures permanently, as it then provides each structure only once.

This proposal is not accepted by the community precisely because of the compatibility issues! Conversely, the discussions triggered by these "inconsistencies" and the associated additional expenses are not being discussed. According to the author's opinion, the resulting expenditures add up to an amount that justifies such a drastic step.

5.9.3.4 HL7 v3 Message Structures

HL7 Version 3 overcomes some of the problems discussed above by using a dedicated methodology that introduces the derivation of message structures by adding constraints from one model to the next.

5.10 Summary

Essential to any well-defined standard are the mechanisms it provides to specify requirements. The better standards provide a rich set of conformance constructs to promote the specification of requirements in a consistent, unambiguous, and easily interpretable manner. This chapter provides in-depth descriptions, analysis, and recommendations for use of the common conformance constructs found in standards, including Usage, Cardinality, Vocabulary, and Length.

Conformance constructs can be viewed as a shorthand notation for expressing explicit statements of requirements. Use of conformance constructs provides a more powerful approach than an explicit list of (narrative) conformance statements. Conformance constructs, which lend themselves to a better and more concise presentation of requirements, are much better suited for automated processing and validation and are easier for developers to consume and understand.

The use and sophistication of the conformance constructs vary significantly among the standards. This chapter presented the concepts at a generic level. Understanding the basic principles of the constructs and their impact will allow the reader to interpret the standards they use more accurately.

Other important aspects that are presented are the encoding, representation and formatting of data, and the use of character sets. The permanently and repeatedly occurring problems for encoding and decoding messages and documents originate with these factors. The possible divergent uses of character sets are a general problem that is identified in this chapter and requires an independent treatment in interface development. Finally, this chapter elaborates on the pre-conditions needed for correctly parsing the information transmitted in a message or document.

Generally speaking, SDOs should make an effort to improve requirement specifications. One recommended approach is to define a rich set of conformance constructs.

References

1. Adapted from HL7 Version 2.8 Chapter 2B Conformance, Section 2.B.7.4, http://www.hl7.org.
2. HL7 Version 2 Implementation Guide: Laboratory Value Set Companion Guide. Release 1 – US Realm DSTU – March 2016 http://www.hl7.org.
3. HL7 Tables Project Wiki. HL7 Vocabulary and Conformance Working Groups. http://wiki.hl7.org/index.php?title=V2_Code_Table_Project
4. HL7 Value Set Binding Project Wiki. HL7 Vocabulary and Conformance Working Groups. http://wiki.hl7.org/index.php?title=Binding_Syntax
5. HL7 Specification: Characteristics of a Formal Value Set Definition, Release 1. http://www.hl7.org/implement/standards/product_brief.cfm?product_id=437
6. HL7 Implementation Guide for CDA® Release 2: Early Hearing Care Plan (Universal Realm) Draft Standard For Trial Use February 2013.
7. Horn T. Encoding, http://www.torsten-horn.de/techdocs/encoding.htm

8. DICOM. Digital Images and Communication in Medicine, http://www.rsna.org/Technology/DICOM/index.cfm
9. Fast Healthcare Interoperability Resources, http://www.hl7.org/fhir
10. Health Level 7 (HL7). HL7 Standard Version 2.5, ANSI/HL7 V2.5-2003, June 26, 2003, http://www.hl7.org.
11. HL7 Version 2: XML Encoding Syntax, Release 1. ANSI/HL7 V2 XML-2003; June 4, 2003; Release 2. ANSI/HL7 V2 XML-2012; 2012.
12. Health Level 7 (HL7): HL7 Standard Version 3, http://www.hl7.org.
13. Snelick R: HL7 v2 Value Set Specification Proposal. Profiling Vocabulary in HL7 v2 Implementation Guides. Original September 2013; last update June 2015. http://hl7v2tools.nist.gov (Publications/Presentations and Technical Documents).

Chapter 6
Principles of Specifying Conformance

6.1 Introduction

The focus of this chapter is to provide a review of and general guidance for specifying conformance in data exchange standards. The guidance is grouped into three notions:

- Definition of conformance keywords
- Conformance clauses
- Specification of conformance requirements

These three notions should be included, or at least referenced, in all standards documents. Consistent and unambiguous specification of requirements is vital to the development of implementations and test suites. Well-defined standards and the accompanying conformance test tools lead to better implementations.

Standards, regardless of the quality, are just artifacts. They are a means to an end. The goal of any standard is the eventual *binding* of the specified requirements into correct, reliable software. To accomplish this goal, the standard must be a clear, precise, unambiguous, complete, and testable enumeration of detailed requirements. Using a natural language (e.g., English) to provide this detailed specification is a challenge in itself because natural languages are not precise and lend themselves to ambiguities; however, as stated in [1] and expanded upon here, there are principles that one can implement to help ensure a precise, implementable, and testable standard. A good standard should (1) define what/who needs to implement the standard, (2) distinguish between normative (mandatory) and informative sections of the standard, (3) use universally accepted key words to specify requirements, (4) provide unambiguous definition of requirements, (5) be modular, with minimal or, if possible, no redundancy, (6) be adaptable to accommodate needed changes,

F. Oemig and R. Snelick, *Healthcare Interoperability Standards Compliance Handbook*, DOI 10.1007/978-3-319-44839-8_6

(7) adhere to a compliance hierarchy (profiles), and (8) be technology- and design-independent from a software development perspective. If a standard embodies these principles, it stands a good chance of being implemented correctly. In order to substantially increase the likelihood of producing correct implementations, however, tests must be developed that determine whether a specific implementation is conformant to the referenced standard.

Recommendations (1), (2), (3), and (4) are addressed in this chapter. Chapter 7 addresses recommendations (5), (6), and (7). Recommendation (8) is straight-forward and needs no further explanation.

Conformance requirements (normative statements) are the expressions that convey the criteria to be fulfilled in an implementation of a specification [2]. A well-defined specification should follow all of the recommendations presented in this chapter. As stated previously, these recommendations fall into the following categories:

- Definition of Conformance Keywords
- Conformance Clauses
- Definition of the Conformance Requirements
  - Conformance constructs used to specify implicit requirements
  - Normative statements[1] used to specify explicit requirements

The conformance keywords define how requirements are specified and interpreted. There must be a common understanding of the terms used when writing the requirements, otherwise readers can interpret and implement the requirements differently, which will lead directly to interoperability issues. The conformance clause[2] provides a high-level list of requirements. The clause may provide options or levels of requirements to which implementers can claim conformance. The conformance claim gives an indication as to what components of the specification an implementer has implemented. The definition of conformance requirements provides a detailed, unambiguous description of what the software must be capable of supporting. The manner in which the requirements are expressed can be implicit or explicit. The focus of this chapter is to provide conformance specification principles and guidance on how to apply those principles to the development of a specification. Consistent and unambiguous specification of requirements is vital to any good standard.

---

[1]We use the generic term "normative statement" to describe explicitly written requirements. Forthcoming is a discussion on synonymous terms.

[2]A Conformance Clause is sometimes referred to as a Conformance Statement in various standards.

6.2 Overloaded Terms

6.2.1 Declaring Requirements and Conformance

The terms used to describe individual requirements in a specification, as opposed to the collective set of requirements in a specification, are often overloaded. Additionally, multiple terms are used to describe both notions. Terms used to describe individual requirements (e.g., on a data element) include *predicate constraint*, *conformance statement*, *conformance requirement*, and *invariant* (we have used the generic term "normative statement" to refer to these concepts in this chapter). Often the requirements are defined by the conformance constructs of the standard (implicit). In cases where these constructs are not defined, or where the conformance constructs are not suitable (capable) to document all requirements, the terms listed above are used to refer to documentation of requirements that have to be stated explicitly (i.e., without the use of the conformance constructs). Terms used to describe a set of requirements in a specification or how an implementation fulfills those requirements include *conformance statement* and *conformance clause* (often paired with a conformance claim). Table 6.1 provides a summary of the notions and the terms used.

In this book, we will refer to these terms in the context in which they are used. For example, when discussing CDA and referring to a requirement within a template, we will refer to that requirement as a conformance statement. Likewise, when referring to a set of requirements in FHIR, conformance statement will be used. In addition, we will provide synonymous terms to communicate clearly to the reader

Table 6.1 Common terms for declaring requirements and conformance

Notion	Term	Known uses	Definition(s)
Individual requirement	Predicate constraint	HL7 V3	Provides an explicit normative statement (requirement) expressed in text or a testable expression that defines a constraint. Conformance constructs provide an efficient mechanism to state and categorize requirements; these are implicit statements that can replace explicit statements
	Conformance statement	HL7 CDA HL7 v2.x	
	Invariant	FHIR	
	Conformance requirement	Many; generic term	
Set of requirements	Conformance statement	DICOM FHIR HL7 v2.x (for query)	"*…is a set of requirements for a desired implementation or a description of how a target application fulfills those requirements in a particular implementation*" [3]
	Conformance clause	Many W3C	"*The conformance clause of a specification is a high-level description of what is required of implementations. It, in turn, refers to other parts of the specification for details*" [4]

the intended notion. In general, we will use the term "normative statement" or just "requirement" to refer to an individual requirement within the standard and will use "conformance clause" to refer to a set of requirements. Hopefully, this approach will reduce the ambiguity of the overloaded term "conformance statement". As with other concepts expressed in this book, the most important aspect is to understand the meaning of the terms and how to apply them. A secondary aspect is to recognize what they are referred to, because it is important to understand where and when the terms are used (the same or differently) such that a common understanding exists, especially when discussing issues across various standards.

6.2.2 Requirement Documents

"Specification", "standard", and "implementation guide" are some of the terms used to describe documents that define implementation requirements for a specific purpose. Depending on the context, one term may be used instead of another. Most often the differences are subtle, but there are ways to distinguish between these terms. The terms are not universally accepted nor are they used consistently in SDO deliberations or documents. The general distinction made in this book is as follows:

- Specification—the most generic term to describe a requirements document
- Standard—used when referring to a particular instance of a base (SDO) requirements document (e.g., the HL7 V3 Standard)
- Implementation Guide—used when referring to a targeted use case requirements document (e.g., an Immunization Messaging Implementation Guide)

As one reads down this list, the definition for each term becomes more specific. Thus, referring to an implementation guide as a specification is acceptable but not all that informative.

6.3 Conformance Keywords

An essential component of any specification is the identification of conformance keywords (also referred to as conformance verbs). The first step for defining requirements is to have a clear understanding of the language for expressing those requirements, which is accomplished by first defining the conformance keywords. The conformance keywords must be used to describe all requirements and must be applied consistently. The conformance keywords help identify the requirements and testable criteria.

It is recommended that specifications adopt, in principle, the *Key words for use in RFCs to Indicate Requirement Levels* (commonly known as RFC 2119) [5]. Depending on the type of specification and its purpose, a subset of the keywords may be appropriate.[3] Below is an example of a subset of the keyword definitions extracted from RFC 2119 and adopted by an HL7 v2 implementation guide [8]:

KEYWORDS:

The key words "**MUST**", "**MUST NOT**", "**REQUIRED**", "**SHALL**", "**SHALL NOT**", "**SHOULD**", "**SHOULD NOT**", "**RECOMMENDED**", "**MAY**", and "**OPTIONAL**" in this document are to be interpreted as described in RFC 2119. The following definitions are excerpted from the RFC:

MUST or the terms "**REQUIRED**" or "**SHALL**", mean that the definition is an absolute requirement of the specification.

MUST NOT or the phrase "**SHALL NOT**", mean that the definition is an absolute prohibition of the specification.

SHOULD or the adjective "**RECOMMENDED**", mean that there may exist valid reasons in particular circumstances to ignore a particular item, but the full implications must be understood and carefully weighed before choosing a different course.

SHOULD NOT or the phrase "**NOT RECOMMENDED**", mean that there may exist valid reasons in particular circumstances when the particular behavior is acceptable or even useful, but the full implications should be understood and the case carefully weighed before implementing any behavior described with this label.

MAY or the adjective "**OPTIONAL**", mean that an item is truly optional. One software supplier may choose to include the item to enable certain capabilities while another software supplier may omit the same item. In either case, the communication partner cannot be expected to either provide it (sender) or process it (receiver) without clear and voluntary agreement between the partners.[4]

An implementation which does not include a particular segment/field/component marked as optional **MUST** be prepared to interoperate with another implementation which does include the optional segment/field/component, though perhaps with reduced functionality. In the same vein an implementation which includes a particular segment/field/component marked as optional **MUST** be prepared to interoperate with another implementation which does not include the optional segment/field/component.

It is good practice for a specification to select a given set of keywords. A common set is **SHALL**, **SHALL NOT**, **SHOULD**, **SHOULD NOT** and **MAY**. Another convention is that the keywords are capitalized and perhaps also in bold text. It is important to use these conventions consistently throughout the document, allowing the reader to identify conformance requirements quickly. Additionally, these terms should not be used in lower case as part of the general text to avoid confusion. The keywords and conventions listed in this paragraph are the ones used in the examples to follow in this chapter.

---

[3]This is not to say that the definitions are to be altered, only that all parts of RFC 2119 need not be included. For example, a specification may choose to use only the verbs SHALL, SHALL NOT, SHOULD, SHOULD NOT, and MAY.

[4]Chapter 7 presents a methodology for specifying and documenting these agreements.

ISO/IEC Directives Part 2 uses a similar set of keywords but restricts the concept to a single term. That is, it uses only the keyword listed to represent the concept. The ISO/IEC list of keywords includes [6]:

- SHALL
- SHALL NOT
- SHOULD
- SHOULD NOT
- MAY
- NEED NOT
- CAN
- CANNOT

Regardless of the set of keywords chosen, it is important that the keywords are indicated as part of the specification, are well-defined, and are used consistently in the specification. In addition, the same keywords with the same meaning should be used in all specifications derived from a *base* standard.

Requirements specified using the keywords are expressing *explicit* conformance requirements. Many more requirements may be specified *implicitly* through the use of the conformance constructs (as described in Chap. 5). It is important that the conformance definition of the conformance constructs define keywords and apply them when specifying the requirements of the conformance constructs. This topic will be expanded upon in this chapter.

6.3.1 Impact of Keywords on Requirements

What impact do the keywords have on a specification? What does it really mean when the keywords **SHALL**, **SHOULD**, or **MAY** are used? If these keywords are not used as defined, the authors of the specification may have a particular intent for a certain requirement, but the keyword may be interpreted with a different meaning by an implementer. Below are three statements using the various keywords, each expressing a similar but a different *obligation*. We describe the meaning of each statement and the impact on the implementation.

(1) EI.3[5] (Universal ID) **SHALL** be valued with an ISO-compliant OID.[6]
(2) EI.3 (Universal ID) **SHOULD** be valued with an ISO-compliant OID.
(3) EI.3 (Universal ID) **MAY** be valued with an ISO-compliant OID.

[5]This example is taken from HL7 v2.x; EI is the *Entity Identifier* data type and in this instance is a reference to the 3rd component (Universal ID) is made.

[6]Although not indicated here, a precise definition (or reference to) of what constitutes "an ISO-compliant OID" is necessary.

For (1), the statement is an absolute requirement, and the implementation must follow this criterion. When tested for conformance the implementation is in error if the data element EI.3 is not valued with an *ISO compliant OID*.

For (2), the statement is a recommendation, and it is considered best practice for implementations to value EI.3 with an *ISO compliant OID*. Often, specification authors will introduce such statements as best practices with the intent of making the statement a requirement in a future version of the specification. The indication of **SHOULD** has no standing with the assessment of conformance. That is, the implementation is conformant (with regards to this specific statement) whether it adheres to the statement or not. A conformance test tool may be designed to issue a warning for recommended *requirements* and often is designed to do so. The conformance assessment must not interpret this as an error if the statement is not implemented.

For (3), the statement is optional and an implementation may decide to value EI.3 with an *ISO compliant OID*. The relevance with regards to conformance assessment is the same as that of **SHOULD**; the implementation is conformant whether it adheres to the statement or not; however, conformance assessment should not express a warning if the statement is not implemented, since the statement is optional. The distinction between SHOULD and MAY is that SHOULD is considered best practice and implementers should make an attempt to support such features. MAY is optional, and whether it is supported or not is at the discretion of the implementer.

6.3.2 Nested Requirements

Requirements can be nested, forming a hierarchy, and specified with the use of conformance keywords. Under certain circumstances, provisional specification of recommended and optional components is desirable. The provisional specification affords a mechanism for indicating that, when a component is supported, it must be supported according to the definition provided. For example, a *high-level* component that is optional is provided with a fully specified declaration of what it contains. That is, the high-level component may be specified with a **MAY**, but it may have many decedent components in which some or all are specified with a **SHALL**. If an optional or recommended component is implemented, then it must be implemented in accordance to the decedent requirements, i.e., the **SHALL** statements now becomes binding.

It is important to note that the definition of the provisional requirements does not place any conformance requirements on implementations that claim conformance to the given (base) specification in which the optional component is defined; however, in a derived specification (or implementation) where there is a claim of conformance to the provisional requirements, those provisional requirements become mandatory (i.e., if you choose to implement the optional component, all decedent requirements are now binding). For example, if a segment in HL7 v2.x is defined as optional (O) and has four fields that are required (R), then those fours fields must be implemented if the optional segment is implemented (i.e., made required in a derived specification).

6.3.3 Normative and Informative Statements

The keywords NORMATIVE and INFORMATIVE also describe important concepts in the authoring and interpretation of specifications. As a component of the conformance clause, part of the specification can be NORMATIVE or INFORMATIVE. The NORMATIVE section or part of the specification indicates the required aspects and must be included when claiming conformance. The INFORMATIVE section or part of the specification is provided for informational purposes and is intended to assist with the understanding or use of the specification. The INFORMATIVE sections do not contain any provisions that are required for conformance.

6.4 Conformance Clause

Another essential conformance principle of a specification is the conformance clause. As defined in [4], "*The conformance clause of a specification is a high-level description of what is required of implementations. It, in turn, refers to other parts of the specification for details. Ideally, readers can find any conformance-related information from its conformance clause which serves as a root source*".

The conformance clause defines the requirements, criteria, or conditions that must be satisfied by the implementation to claim conformance. The conformance clause identifies *what* must conform and *how* conformance can be met [7]. A conformance claim[7] is a declaration by an implementer of the requirements in the conformance clause that their implementation satisfies.

The conformance clause typically indicates only the high-level conformance requirements. The requirements may be stated in terms of a profile, a set of profile components, or identifiable parts of a specification. Profile and profile components are mechanisms that provide a structured approach to specifying requirements. Chapter 7 explores this subject further. The detailed requirements are contained and delineated in the other parts of the specification. For example, a conformance clause in an HL7 v2 implementation guide could indicate a number of profiles available to

[7]As mentioned earlier, different terms are used in various standards. Sometimes (at a high-level) conformance statement is used by an implementer to "make a statement" or "claim" about their implementation.

the implementer and describe the components that pertain to the profiles. This is the level of detail the conformance clause would contain. The detailed requirements in support of a profile or profile component are specified in other parts of the specification.

The conformance clause also can describe options in the form of profiles and levels. Profiles can be used to define a set of requirements within the specification. The profiles may use modular components[8] (See Chap. 7). The conformance clause may state which profile must be implemented or provide a choice (or options) of profiles that could be implemented. For instance, some profiles may be required whereas others are optional.

The conformance clause can contain levels that indicate the various degrees in which conformance requirements can be specified. For example, the lowest level could indicate the minimum set of requirements necessary. Another level could indicate additional requirements. The highest level would indicate full conformance. Example specifications that employ this design strategy include the HL7 Version 2.5.1 Implementation Guide: S&I Framework Lab Results Interface (LRI) [8] (See Chap. 7, for a detailed example) and the *ELGA Interoperabilitäts-Stufen*—ELGA interoperability levels (EIS) of ELGA, the Austrian ehealth program [9]. The profile mechanism can be used to describe the conformance levels.

As described in [7], the rationale for a conformance clause is as follows:

- promotes a common understanding of conformance and what is required to claim conformance to a specification,
- facilitates consistent application of conformance within a specification,
- facilitates consistent application of conformance across related specifications,
- promotes interoperability and open interchange,
- encourages the use of applicable conformance test suites,
- promotes uniformity in the development of conformance test suites.

6.4.1 Conformance Claim

A ***conformance claim*** is a declaration made by an implementer indicating the requirements in the conformance clause that their implementation satisfies. A conformance claim is a self-declaration made by the implementers stating the capabilities of their application. Conformance testing is a process by which the conformance claim can be verified. The level of rigor in which claims are verified will vary among testing programs (See Chap. 15).

[8]This is good practice.

The W3C [10] provides an example set of requirements for declaring a conformance claim. Key components of a conformance claim are the date of the claim, what is being claimed (e.g., a profile or a level), application components, and versioning information.

6.5 Specifying Conformance Requirements

The most critical aspect of a standard is the precise specification of the requirements. Requirements must be stated in a clear and concise manner if there is to be any chance of a consistent interpretation and implementation. Such specification of requirements is articulated in the form of a normative statement. A normative statement is a formal method of expressing a requirement and can be expressed in a natural written language or a formal definition language. A formal definition language is preferred, but not always obtainable, and can be cryptic at times. Often the normative statement is expressed in the natural written language for the reading of the specification and codified as machine process-able for use in associated tooling [11–13] (see Chap. 9).

The principles for specifying conformance must be followed for creating the conformance requirements whether using *implicit* normative statements or *explicit* normative statements. The distinction between implicit and explicit normative statements is determined by the manner in which they are specified in the standard. Both forms express a requirement. Implicit statements are described in terms of a conformance construct (e.g., usage) and are sometimes organized in a table (or another form) that provides a convenient, compact representation of requirements. Explicit statements express the requirement narratively (often verbosely). Implicit statements unravel into explicit statements based on the explicit definition of the conformance construct used to define them. The sections to follow describe both forms and the best practices for specifying requirements. Whenever possible, implicit statements are preferred due to readability, compactness, and amenability to automated processing.

6.5.1 Implicit Definitions with Conformance Constructs

Chapter 5 describes common conformance constructs typically available to authors of data exchange standards. These constructs can be considered the tools of the author for defining conformance requirements. This chapter provides the principles for applying these concepts in practice. A primary goal is to improve the quality and consistency of standards documents and the resulting implementations.

The conformance constructs are essential components for defining requirements in a specification. Chapter 5 describes the concept of the constructs; however, it does not explicitly define the requirements on implementations. The same technical term may have different meanings in different standards and two different terms may have the same meaning. Therefore, every standard must define a detailed description of the conformance construct requirement so the reader understands the requirements. In order to specify requirements, a clear and concise understanding of the conformance constructs is necessary. Conformance keywords are employed to describe the constructs. Another important tool that provides additional understanding of the constructs is conformity assessment. Chapter 12, provides a set of truth tables that gives outcomes of observed instances for each conformance construct. The assessment may differ slightly from standard to standard,[9] but it must be described such that the reader knows exactly what the author is trying to convey. Otherwise, misunderstanding will lead to incorrect implementations and hinder interoperability.

A definition is provided for each of the conformance constructs in terms of the conformance requirements it imposes. These definitions can't be used universally, as is indicated for a set of healthcare data exchange (communication) standards in Chap. 4 and pointed out in Chap. 5, because the same representation of a conformance construct is used to represent different (although similar) concepts (e.g., "R" usage in HL7 v2 and HL7 V3). The most important aspect to recognize is that within a given standard[10] the concepts must be clearly defined so they can be interpreted correctly and consistently. It does not necessarily matter if they are universally accepted as long as they are well understood with regard to the concepts they are conveying; however, as pointed out previously, harmonization across standards would be beneficial to all stakeholders. Certainly within a family of standards one would expect that consistency would be mandatory, but, unfortunately, this is not the case. For example, the IHE HL7 v2 Integration Profiles define different conformance constructs than those in the HL7 standards ("R2" as opposed to "RE") with a similar[11] meaning [14]. In addition, various HL7 v2 implementation guides provide their own interpretation of the conformance constructs provided in Chap. 2B *Conformance in the HL7 v2 Standard.* Implementation guides need to follow exactly the conformance rules provided by the base standard, otherwise there is a disconnect among the specifications using the same underlying standard, which unnecessarily complicates common application architecture and, therefore, a vendor's product line.

---

[9]Most of the standards do not provide such an assessment. Sometimes it can be extracted from explanations given in the standard (but, if not given explicitly, it is difficult to enforce the same interpretation of requirements among implementers).

[10]As can be seen with the introduction of the various standards in Chap. 4, they are on a different maturity level of how deep the conformance constructs are explicitly defined.

[11]Analysis of the background of these two conformance concepts reveals that they are similar and in some views identical; there is disagreement among authors and implementers, which results in unnecessary confusion.

When providing a definition for the conformance constructs, we use the SHALL, SHALL NOT, SHOULD, SHOULD NOT, and MAY keywords described earlier in this chapter.

We will consider a few of the conformance constructs and provide a definition of each. We then will specify the requirements for a message element based on this definition in a table format. An explanation of the meaning of the requirement is then translated into explicit normative statements. This is a common method for expressing conformance requirements in data exchange standards. The table format contains implicitly expressed requirements that are expandable to explicitly expressed requirements. As mentioned, it is preferred to capture most requirements implicitly and write explicit requirements only when necessary. Note, the term implicit as used here is meant to describe shorthand notations as a convenient method to express verbose explicit requirement.

Data exchange standards have the generic concept of *usage* that determines the *presence* or *non-presence of an element* for a sending application (and processing requirements of this element for the receiving application). For the analysis to follow, however, only the sender side is considered. A standard might employ the concept of *required* and define it as follows:

1. A required element SHALL be implemented[12]
2. A required element SHALL be valued and sent

For a given element *x* the requirements can be translated to:

1. Element *x* SHALL be implemented (implementation requirement)
2. A value for Element *x* SHALL be sent (operational requirement)

This expression of normative statements is a convenience mechanism to convey requirements. The definitions of the conformance constructs impose requirements when applied to aspects of a specification. This method of specification lends itself to common requirements that apply in general to data elements. Chapter 5 went into detail about the conformance constructs that fit this mode. This section concentrates on expressing the explicit normative statements derived from the common constructs. For every conformance construct that is defined in a standard, explicit normative statements (requirements) need to be expressed such that implementers can understand unambiguously the meaning of the requirement. Conformance assessment of such constructs also improves the understanding of the construct but is rarely done in any of the data exchange standards; this topic is addressed in Chap. 12.

Table 6.2 illustrates an example from an HL7 v2 PID segment definition. A row in the table describes a number of requirements placed on an element. For the "Administrative Sex" element (Sequence 8 in the PID segment) the specification indicates requirements for the data type, usage, cardinality, and value set. Assuming the implementation guide that contains the PID segment specification expresses or

[12]In other words, supported by the application.

Table 6.2 Excerpt of an HL7 v2.5.1 PID segment definition

SEQ	Element name	Data type	Usage	Cardinality	Value set	Comments
...						
8	Administrative Sex	IS	R	[1..1]	HL70001	Patient's gender
9	Patient Alias		X			Excluded for this implementation guide, see Sect. 1.3.1
10	Race	CWE	RE	[0..*]	HL70005	Note that state and/or national regulations may dictate other behaviors
...						

references the interpretation of the conformance constructs (e.g., what does R mean), the following inferences can be made for PID-8:

(1) PID-8 (Administrative Sex) SHALL be used to communicate information about the administrative gender of the patient.[13]
(2) PID-8 (Administrative Sex) SHALL use the data type IS.
(3) PID-8 (Administrative Sex) SHALL be implemented (supported).
(4) A value for PID-8 (Administrative Sex) SHALL be sent.
(5) One and only one instance of PID-8 (Administrative Sex) SHALL be supported.
(6) One and only one instance of PID-8 (Administrative Sex) SHALL be sent.
(7) The implementation SHALL support all codes (concepts) in the HL70001 value set specification.[14]
(8) The implementation SHALL support only the codes (concepts) in the HL70001 value set specification.
(9) PID-8 (Administrative Sex) SHALL be valued with a code in the HL70001 value set.

For the sake of this example, it is assumed the implementation guide indicates that the value set binding is a requirement and that the only allowed values for this element are specified in the value set (for this message profile and any derived message profiles). This is an important point in this case, since the data type associated with element PID-8 is "IS". The "IS" data type indicates that this is an

[13]Additional text is provided in the standard that describes the concept being conveyed by the element. Moreover, the implied requirement for the application is to support the concept of Administrative Gender (as a pre-condition), which is typically agnostic to the interface specification.

[14]We assume that the value set specification indicates these requirements. Unfortunately, too often seen in practice value set specifications in implementation guides are underspecified and/or ambiguous.

HL7 User table. Per the HL7 v2.x base standard, requirements for "IS" elements are suggested values and can be redefined. Therefore, it is important for the implementation guide to indicate that the value set has been defined and is now a binding requirement. For details on how to *correctly* specify value sets and their implications, see Vocabulary topics in Chaps. 5 and 7.

Another point to be made is that some of the requirements expressed are compound requirements and need to be further unraveled. For instance, PID-10 (Race) specifies the complex data type as "CWE—Coded with Exceptions". This data type is made up of components, each of which may have requirements for usage, cardinality, length, value set, and so on.

As mentioned, other requirements that need to be specified, but can't be expressed using the convenience form provided by the conformance constructs, can be conveyed with explicit normative statements. The focus of the remainder of this section of the chapter is on principles for writing these requirements.

6.5.2 Explicit Definition with Normative Statements

Explicit statements of conformance express the requirement narratively (often verbosely). An example (as is the list given in the previous section) of an explicit requirement is the normative statement "The EI.3 (Universal ID) data element SHALL be valued with an ISO-compliant OID". Below we provide a set of recommendations for writing normative statements. The guidelines apply at multiple levels for conveying conformance requirements; that is, the guidelines apply to stating the requirements for the conformance constructs at the standard level and for the targeted requirements in an implementation guide.

6.5.3 Principles for Writing Conformance Requirements

The list that follows provides a set of principles and guidelines for writing conformance requirements in the form of explicit normative statements.[15] Requirements should be expressed using conformance constructs when possible and practical. Requirements that can't be expressed in terms of the available conformance constructs should be described in the manner given below. The goal for using this approach is to provide implementers with requirements that are more understandable. It is especially important for requirements to be understood and implemented correctly in data exchange standards. Incorrect interpretation or

[15]As described earlier, normative statements are referred to as predicate constraints, conformance statements, and by other terms.

instantiation of requirements is a common reason for interoperability issues. This list includes and extends the list of recommendations provided by the NIST [15].

1. Do restrict each conformance requirement to one atomic (simple) statement (i.e., do not comingle requirements).

   a. Address a single requirement in a normative statement.
   b. Keep each requirement as simple as possible. Multiple one-facet requirements are more understandable and manageable to test (and to audit in the event a test fails) than one multi-part requirement.

   For example, consider the methods for expressing the same set of requirements. *Method 1*:

   (1) **CS-001**: MSH-9 (Message Type) **SHALL** contain the constant value 'ORU^R01^ORU_R01'.[16]

   Method 2:

   (2) **CS-002**: MSH-9.1 (Message Code) **SHALL** contain the constant value 'ORU'.
   (3) **CS-003**: MSH-9.2 (Trigger Event) **SHALL** contain the constant value 'R01'.
   (4) **CS-004**: MSH-9.3 (Message Structure) **SHALL** contain the constant value 'ORU_R01'.

   The normative statement[17] of Method (1) describes a compound requirement. Although this statement is certainly clear and unambiguous, it combines three separate requirements into one normative statement. When an error is reported, potentially one, two, or all three aspects may be the source of the error. The source of an error may not be readily clear, especially if the compound normative statement is complex. Three separate assertions can be made to assess conformance to this requirement and relay precise non-conformity information to the implementer. Furthermore, Method (1) of specifying a requirement may also impact other requirements which in this example fixes the delimiters and does not allow for further testing of alternatives in encoding.
   The set of normative statements given in (2), (3), and (4) is generally the preferred method. Each statement addresses a singular requirement, and errors are easily and precisely identified to trace back to the requirement that caused the failure (e.g., Method (1) is not granular to the component level). This is especially true for a set of less related requirements.
2. Do label each normative statement with an identifier that has a numeric component. Identification provides traceability and enables machine processing and rendering.

[16]This example assumes the component delimiter is fixed to the constant value '^' which in HL7 v2 standards may be changed by implementers at run time to a different character.

[17]Referred to as a conformance statement in HL7 V2.x.

a. Once assigned, do not change the identifier of a normative statement (i.e., don't renumber/refactor), e.g., in subsequent versions of a published specification.
b. If a normative statement is removed do not reuse the identifier.
c. Do not be concerned that normative statement identifiers are not ordered sequentially in the document.

3. Do use consistent language for specifying normative statements.

   a. Establish and use a set of conformance keywords.
   b. Use the conformance keywords to indicate the conformance level of the statement. For example, use "SHALL" to signify a requirement; "SHOULD" to signify a recommendation; and "MAY" to signify optional.
   c. Be consistent in the use of the conformance keywords. For example, always use "SHALL" (i.e., don't use "SHALL" and "MUST" interchangeably).
   d. Be consistent in the use of action verbs. For example, in HL7 v2 the terms *"is populated", "contains", and "is valued"* often are used to indicate the presence of a value. Establish one term and adhere to it.

4. Do establish a pattern (grammar) for each type of normative statement. This allows the reader to quickly identify the type of normative statement.

   a. For example, establish patterns for elements with constant values, element equality, etc.
   b. If possible, provide the exact grammar how these patterns are created. (A good example is the vocabulary binding syntax for HL7 V3 (CDA) implementation guides [16].)

   The examples provided in Principle 1, Method 2 above illustrates establishing a pattern for a type of normative statement. In this case a clear pattern is established for defining elements with constant values.

5. Do specify "what" the requirements are; do not specify "how" requirements are to be satisfied (implemented) or tested.
   For example, a normative statement such as:

   The receiving application SHALL persist the LOINC code associated with the laboratory result.

   The normative statement describes what must be done but not how. One vendor may choose to store explicitly the LOINC code in their database where as another could store a local code and use a mapping service to derive the LOINC code. In either case the LOINC code associated with the laboratory result can be retrieved upon request and thus satisfies the requirement conveyed in the normative statement.

6. Do make requirements technology neutral.
7. Do make normative statements self-contained (i.e., avoid footnotes and external references).

8. Do indicate explicit dependencies when based on a condition not already implied.[18] For example, consider the following normative statement.

   If RXA-5.1 (Vaccine Administered) contains the value "998" (No Vaccine Administered) and RXA-5.3 (Code System) contains the value "CVX" then RXA-20 (Completion Status) ***SHALL*** *contain the constant value "NA".*

   In this case, it is evident that the requirement to populate RXA-20 with the literal value of "NA" is dependent on the value of RXA-5.1 and RXA-5.3. This dependency could also be documented in the implicit requirements in the tabular specification (see Table 6.2 as an example) in form of a condition ("C").

9. Do not indicate dependencies if known from another implicit or explicit requirement. For example, consider the following two normative statements.

   (1) *MSH-2 (Encoding Characters) SHALL contain the literal value "^~\&".*
   (2) *If MSH-2 (Encoding Characters) is valued it SHALL contain the literal value "^~\&".*

   MSH-2 is a required element and therefore normative statement (1) is sufficient. Normative statement (2) has the extraneous qualifier "*If MSH-2 (Encoding Characters) is valued*" since this requirement is captured in the implicit usage normative statement for the MSH-2 element.

10. Try to use positive wording, especially when defining conditions. For example, consider to turn the condition around:

    If not [field xxx equals yyy] then do aaa else do bbb.
    but
    If field [xxx equals yyy] then do bbb else do aaa.

6.6 Scope of Conformance Specifications

The purpose of an implementation guide is to describe the requirements for an implementation based on a given use case or use cases. All requirements need to be directly tied back to (and supported by) the use case. This includes all aspects of the specification. The conformance constructs provide the tools for the authors in expressing requirements. Extraneous requirements that do not cover an aspect described in the use case must not be specified in the implementation guide, which includes codes in a value set, since they may imply support for certain functionality.

Implementers are not obligated to claim conformance to an implementation guide. The reason a certain standard or implementation guide is implemented is out of the scope for this book. Once implementers do make a claim of conformance,

[18] An example of a condition that is implied is "RE" usage in HL7 v2.x.

however, they are indicating that they are capable of supporting all requirements. Implementers claiming conformance to an implementation guide (or aspects of the guide as allowed) are obligated to implement all requirements as stated regardless if it meets their business practices or not. Purchasers of such systems are provided, in essence, a contract of what they have bought. In practice, a certain client may not want or use all capabilities provided. On a per instance basis, a vendor may work with customers that only need support for a given subset of capabilities. This approach is acceptable; the implementation can be configured as needed. It is good practice for the vendor/purchaser to document those requirements. The system capabilities may also be extended as allowed by the standard (implementation guide), and the resulting implementation should be documented. Such documentation provides the vehicle by which the appropriate conformance claim can be made.

If the use case needed by the vendor is slightly different than the use case described in the implementation guide, site agreements can be made. This constitutes another profile or profile component. Such components may or may not be compliant with the source implementation guide (in all cases, this delta should be documented). Extensions to the implementation guide are expected to be made to meet site specific requirements. Extensions should be in compliance with the implementation guide, otherwise, interoperability is at risk. The scope of testing (to be discussed in chapters that follow) is to ensure a certain level of capabilities. This provides purchasers with a degree of confidence in the capabilities of the product. The implementation guide provides one source of that documentation.

Local requirements (or lack for need of requirements) should not be considered in the creation of the standard development organization's (SDO) implementation guides. What needs to be considered in the development of an implementation guide are the requirements for an implementation in general and not any particular site installation implementation. The purpose is to define the requirements of capabilities of the implementation based on the stated use cases (this is the scope), but still allow for extensions to facilitate re-use of the specification.

Therefore, good practice for implementation guides (and additionally software instances) is to allow for options (for documented extended use cases)[19] from which a vendor can select so the application can realize enhanced functions that may be used in various use cases and/or sold to different customers. Implementation guides should also seek to leverage or reuse components of other guides, thus forming a hierarchy of profiles (requirements). This topic is further explored in the next chapter (Chapt. 7).

[19]Such extensions (options) can be documented as profile components as described in Chap. 7.

6.7 Summary

A characteristic of a well-defined standard is the way in which the requirements are expressed. Implementers must have a clear and concise understanding of the requirements so they can be interpreted consistently. This common understanding is a pre-requisite for interoperability. Each standard must employ certain principles, including definitions of conformance keywords (the foundation to express requirements); stating the conformance clause (a statement of what is required to be implemented); and the specification of requirements (based on the conformance constructs and principles for specifying requirements). Detailed specification of requirements allows for common interpretation and provides the foundation for subsequent testing of implementations.

References

1. Gebase L, Snelick R, Skall M: Conformance Testing and Interoperability: A Case Study in Healthcare Data Exchange. 2008 Software Engineering Research and Practice (SERP08), WORLDCOMP'08 July 14–17, 2008, Las Vegas, NV.
2. ISO Reference - ISO/IEC *17000.* Conformity assessment - Vocabulary and general principles. first edition 2004-11-02
3. Fast Healthcare Interoperability Resources (FHIR); Definition of Conformance Statement. https://www.hl7.org/fhir/conformance-definitions.html
4. QA Framework: Specification Guidelines W3C Recommendation 17 August 2005; http://www.w3.org/TR/qaframe-spec/
5. Keywords used for use in RFC's to indicate Requirement Levels. http://www.ietf.org/rfc/rfc2119.txt, http://tools.ietf.org/html/rfc2119
6. ISO/IEC Directives, Part 2. Rules for the structure and drafting of International Standards, Annex H: Verbal forms for the expression of provisions. Edition 6.0, 2011-04 http://www.iec.ch/members_experts/refdocs/iec/isoiec-dir2%7Bed6.0%7Den.pdf
7. Conformance Requirements for Specifications – OASIS, v1.0. March 15th, 2002. Editors: Rosenthal L, Skall M. National Institute of Standards and Technology (NIST), http://www.oasis-open.org/committees/download.php/305/conformance_requirements-v1.pdf.
8. HL7 Version 2.5.1 Implementation Guide: S&I Framework Lab Results Interface interoperability standards (DSTU) July 2012; http://www.hl7.org
9. ELGA. Vernetzte Gesundheit. http://www.elga.gv.at/
10. Understanding WCAG 2.0, Understanding Conformance; http://www.w3.org/TR/2007/WD-UNDERSTANDING-WCAG20-20071211/conformance.html
11. Messaging Workbench (MWB). Developed by Peter Rontey at the U.S. Veterans Administration (VA) in conjunction with the HL7 Conformance Special Interest Group; http://www.hl7.org.
12. NIST Implementation Guide Authoring and Management Tool (IGAMT). http://healthcare.nist.gov/NIST-TOOLS/index.html
13. *Open Health Tools Model-Driven Health Tools* (MDHT) Project https://www.projects.openhealthtools.org/sf/projects/mdht/
14. Oemig F. IHE Internal Technical Terminology, v0.6, http://www.ihe.net, http://groups.google.com/group/iheterminology/attach/7804505ee72e6ed9/IHE+Terminology+v07.zip?hl=en&part=2, last accessed Feb. 11 2016, http://www.hl7.org/documentcenter/public/wg/ictc/IHE%20Terminology%20v06.zip, last accessed Feb.11 2016

15. PRINCIPLES for Writing Conformance Requirements. http://www.itl.nist.gov/div897/ctg/conformance/Principles4Requirements.pdf
16. HL7 Vocabulary Binding Syntax. http://wiki.hl7.org/index.php?title=Binding_Syntax
17. HL7 Version 2 Implementation Guide: Laboratory Value Set Companion Guide. Release 1 – US Realm DSTU – March 2016 http://www.hl7.org.
18. Snelick R. HL7 v2 Value Set Specification Proposal. Profiling Vocabulary in HL7 v2 Implementation Guides. Original September 2013; last update June 2015. http://hl7v2tools.nist.gov (Publications/Presentations and Technical Documents).

Chapter 7
Principles of Effective Profiling

7.1 Introduction

A major challenge for the healthcare industry is achieving interoperability among proprietary applications provided by different vendors. For example, each hospital department may use one or more applications that need to share clinical and administrative information with other applications. Each application may require multiple communication interfaces that must be modified and maintained. This approach is a difficult way to achieve interoperability. Alternatively, interoperability can be achieved through the use of standardized interfaces, which can reduce the cost of building and managing unique interfaces for each associated application. Developers can build applications that conform to the standardized interface definition, increasing the likelihood of interoperability and reducing cost. Maintenance cost is also reduced, since there are fewer unique interfaces to maintain. One obstacle to achieving usable standardized interfaces is that the base standards are often not defined at a granular enough level to support a specific use case or local requirements; therefore, the base standard must be further defined or "constrained". The mechanism for constraining standards is called profiling (Fig. 7.1).

The standards described in Chap. 4 and Appendix provide only a foundation (framework) to be used as a starting point and were designed to accommodate the many diverse business processes that exist in the healthcare industry. This universal design was necessary to gain broad industry support; however, attempting to accommodate such wide-ranging requirements resulted in standards that include numerous optional elements as well as other aspects[1] that are not completely defined, making alignment of interface implementations overly difficult.

---

[1]For example, a constrained value set definition specific to a particular data element (is generally not provided at the base standard level).

F. Oemig and R. Snelick, *Healthcare Interoperability Standards Compliance Handbook*, DOI 10.1007/978-3-319-44839-8_7

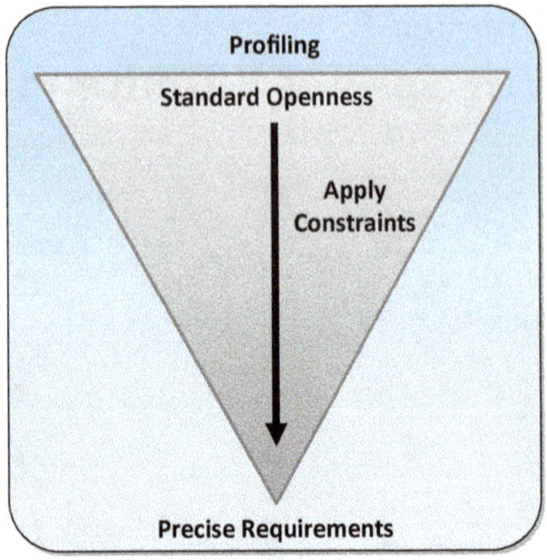

Fig. 7.1 Profiling standards

For these reasons, further definition of the base standard (through constraining or extending) is necessary to support a particular use case. Profiles are created to provide precisely defined requirements. Profiles reduce or eliminate the optionality (or openness) of a base standard. Profiling can be applied to messages, documents, and other objects, such as FHIR resources. They also are used to manage and document requirements that are necessary and sufficient for implementation. The precepts of profiling are general and they apply universally, although the mechanics of how profiles are realized vary from standard to standard. The concepts, hierarchy framework, and use of profiles are the subjects of this chapter.

7.2 Profiling: Definition of Terms

The terms implementation guide, profile, integration profile, conformance profile, message profile, and conformance message profile, etc., do not have clear (nor consistent) definitions in practice and are often used interchangeably (and inappropriately). This reality is a source of confusion for many authors, readers, and implementers alike. In addition, depending on the context in which they are used, the meanings of the terms have different implications. To help clarify, we provide definitions (See Table 7.1) for these terms and will use these definitions for discussion of *profiling* concepts.

Broadly speaking, implementation guides and integration profiles are *containers* for conformance profiles. In short, implementation guides and integration profiles describe the use case(s), the applications (actors) involved, and the workflows (including the transactions and interactions); and they also can specify functional requirements. A conformance profile in the context of a messaging standard describes the requirements for a single interaction (e.g., Send Immunization History —VXU V04 message in HL7 v2.x). An implementation guide or integration profile

Table 7.1 Definition of profile related terms

Term	Description
Profile	Profile is a generic term often used to refer to a conformance profile or integration profile. Knowing the context in which it is used is important for determining what it means. In general, a profile is a refinement of a standard artifact (at any level) or artifacts through constraint and extension
Conformance profile	A conformance profile is a refinement to either the underlying standard or another conformance profile; it normally specifies constraints on messages or documents, but is also used to specify extensions as an integrated part for further refinements[a]
Message profile	Message profile is a synonym for conformance profile that explicitly refers to a messaging standard such as HL7 v2.x
Conformance message profile	Conformance message profile is another synonym for conformance profile that explicitly refers to a messaging standard such as HL7 v2.x
Template	A template is used in CDA on different levels (document, header, section, entry) and denotes a conformance profile
Data type flavor	In HL7 Version 3 conformance profiles on data types are called data type flavors[b]
Implementation guide	An implementation guide is created to organize a collection of conformance profiles for specifying a set of related interactions described in a use case or use cases. Implementation guides typically describe broader conformance requirements such as application functionality. Such requirements may include how a set of messages are to be used to enact certain application functionality among applications (actors)
Integration profile	An integration profile is an implementation guide and is the term used in the IHE Technical Frameworks. It describes the workflow for a specific use case. It combines actors, interactions (e.g., messaging requirements), and functional requirements. Conformance profiles can be and often are a key component of an integration profile. An integration profile can bind conformance profiles derived from multiple standards, such as HL7 v2.x and CDA, to address a particular use case/workflow. Note: Integration Profile and Implementation Guide can be used interchangeably

[a]It can be applied to FHIR resources and (Web) Services as well
[b]The German Message Profiles for HL7 v2.5 contain data type flavors since 2003, although they do not provide a unique identification. HL7 v2.x as of early 2016 is beginning the process of formalizing data type flavors as well.

often describes numerous conformance profile definitions. For instance, the IHE Patient Identification Cross-Referencing (PIX) integration profile [1] defines a conformance profile for each of the HL7 v2 administration interactions (A01: Inpatient Admission, A04: Outpatient Registration, A05: Inpatient Pre-admission, A08: Patient Update, and A40: Merge Patient), the associated acknowledgement interactions (ACK: Acknowledgement), and the query/response interactions (Q23: Query and K23: Response).

Another example of a guide that describes a set of relevant conformance profiles for a specific domain is the CDC HL7 v2.5.1 Release 1.5 implementation guide for

Table 7.2 Immunization implementation guide list of message profiles

Profile identifier[a]	Message definition	Profile	Related profiles
Z22[b]	VXU V04	Send Immunization History	Z23
Z23	ACK V04	Acknowledgement	Z22
Z34	QBP Q11	Request Immunization History	Z31 Z32 Z33
Z44	QBP Q11	Request Evaluated History and Forecast	Z42 Z33
Z31	RSP K11	Return a List of Candidates Profile	Z34
Z32	RSP K11	Return an Immunization History Profile	Z34
Z42	RSP K11	Return Evaluated History and Forecast	Z44
Z33	RSP K11	Acknowledgement with No Person Records	Z34 Z44

[a]The identifier is the HL7 v2.x conformance profile identifier. The CDC implementation guide uses a text identifier. Best practice is to create an accompanying OID
[b]The letter "Z" in the profile identifier does not imply a "Z" event

immunization messaging [2]. Table 7.2 lists the base message definitions and derived profiles included in that guide. The left column of this table indicates the identifier of the profile and the column on the right side lists the valid profile transaction pair(s) for each profile. For example, the profile Z22—Send Immunization History defines (refines) the requirements for a VXU V04 message **interaction**. When it is paired with the Acknowledgment profile (Z23), a **transaction** is defined. The implementation guide provides use cases, actor definitions, transactions, and limited functional requirements. Each refinement of a message definition (e.g., VXU V04) specifies a **conformance profile** (e.g., Z22) and corresponds to an interaction. The collection of conformance profiles and associated use case information defines the **integration profile (implementation guide)**. This explanation should help the reader understand the subtleties of the overloaded term "profile". Conformance profiles are building block components and can be used (and reused) in integration profiles (implementation guides). A collection of profile identifiers can be declared in a conformance clause for an application's or product's claim of conformance (e.g., a claim of conformance to an integration profile).

Figure 7.2 illustrates a generic logical organization of an Integration Profile. There is no universally accepted rule for what constitutes an implementation guide or integration profile. For example, HL7 v2.x implementation guides usually focus on interoperability definitions and include limited application functional requirements (mostly implied); whereas IHE integration profiles usually include functional requirements to a greater degree. HL7 typically has not defined functional requirements, but has left this task to implementers or profiling development organizations such as IHE. More recently though, HL7, through the ONC S&I Framework, has created functional requirement guides to support the ONC Health IT Certification Program associated with EHR Meaningful Use (See [3], for an example).

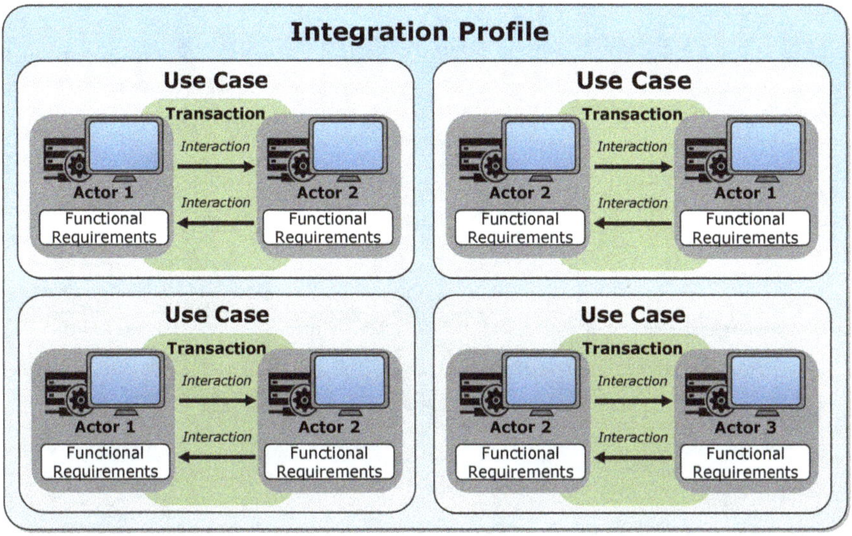

Fig. 7.2 Generic integration profile organization. Note the *left-hand side of the diagram* indicates the case where the Actors are the same but for a different Transaction

Figure 7.3 illustrates how a representative integration profile might work for a set of related immunization use cases. This diagram illustrates a use case (e.g., Send Immunization), the actors involved (i.e., EHR-S and IIS-Immunization Information System), and a set of relevant transactions (e.g., Z22/Z23) and interactions (e.g., Z22-VXU).

Figure 7.4 depicts the logical organization of the immunization messaging interoperability solution. The solution is predicated on four specifications (three of which are shown in the white folded-corner boxes in the diagram):

1. EHR Functional Requirements (in progress)
2. Interoperability Specification (HL7 v2.5.1 Messaging Implementation Guide)
3. IIS Functional Requirements (in progress)
4. Transport Specification (not shown)

The HL7 v2.5.1 implementation guide specifies the eight conformance profiles listed in Table 7.2. Separate implementation guides have been written for the transport and functional requirements.[2] Although not formally assembled as an integration profile, the collection of specifications defines an interoperability solution. The 2015 Edition ONC immunization messaging certification criterion requires that a subset of the solution be supported by certified EHR technologies.

[2]The Functional Requirements specifications are not yet published, so the diagram indicates a desired state. The 2015 Edition ONC Health IT Certification Program Final Rule does include display requirements for EHRs.

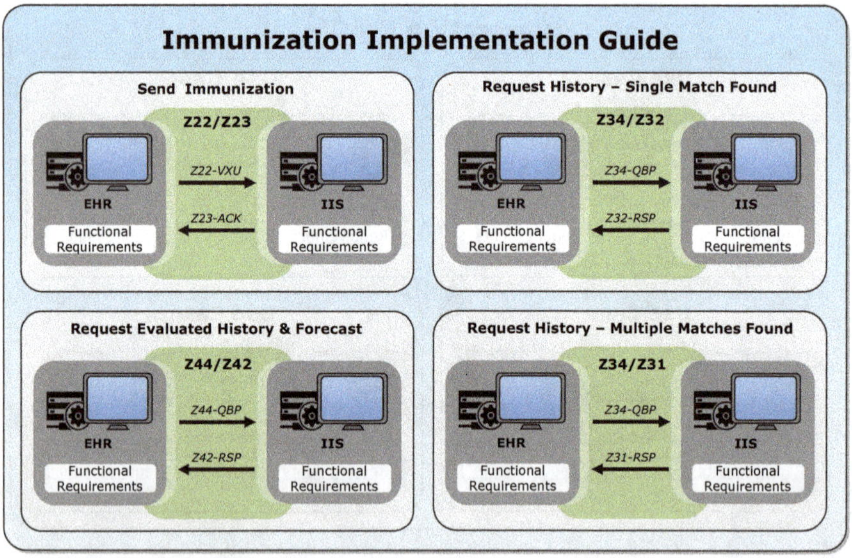

Fig. 7.3 Representative immunization implementation guide (this diagram does not indicate all possible use cases and transactions described in the implementation guide. A sample of the most relevant use cases is provided to illustrate the organization of the guide. Here the term implementation guide is used instead of integration profile, because the specification is HL7-based, and HL7 typically uses implementation guide)

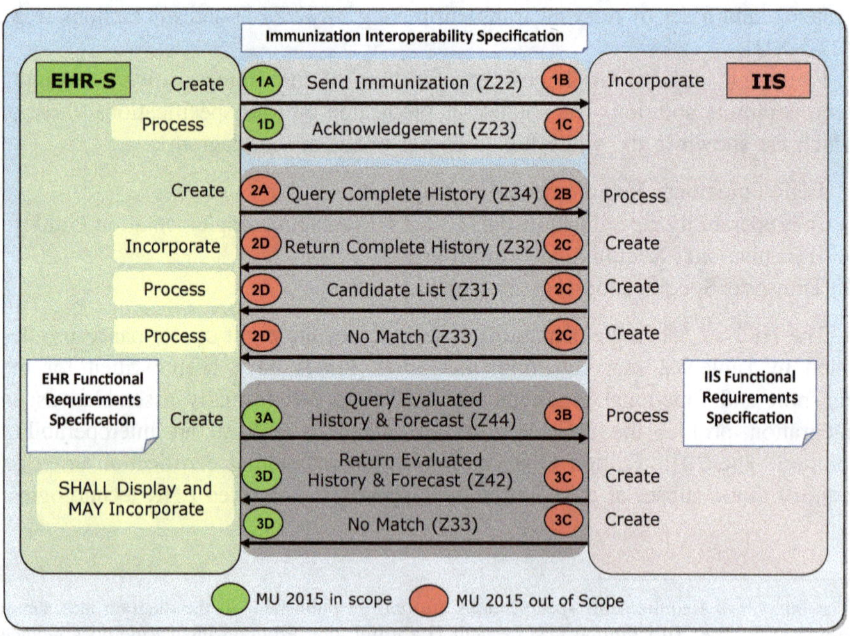

Fig. 7.4 Immunization interoperability solution organization

More details on how each of these base message definitions are *profiled*, managed, and organized are described as the principles of effective profiling and are explored in this chapter.

7.2.1 Profile Components

A profile component defines a part or a certain aspect of a profile and is used to aggregate correlated requirements and/or to differentiate requirements from another profile or profile component. It provides a mechanism to support a set of reusable requirements. A profile component can be applied to any construct or section of a profile. Profiles and profile components can be combined to develop and manage other profiles. A profile component in a family of profiles can be used to identify different levels of requirements for the same use case or to identify the differences in requirements for different, but closely related, use cases. An example of the former is for the suite of HL7 v2.5.1 Lab Implementation Guides where profile components are used to specify an option of using globally unique ("GU") identifiers or non-globally unique ("NG") identifiers. Although this may not be "best practice" for an interoperability specification, profile components do provide alternate approaches to solve a single problem (See [4]).

Examples of profile components include the patient photo, patient weight and height (as observations), and diagnoses, each of which can be re-used in different ADT message profiles. Defining them individually and separately eliminates redundancies. The use of profile identifiers in the message header helps to identify what "features" a message instance supports. Profile components and their use are elaborated on later in this chapter.

The data type flavors and Common Message Element Types (CMETs) in HL7 Version 3 represent profile components on a very granular level. They are reused in refined message information models (RMIMs).

The templates introduced with HL7 CDA represent profile components that are applied to different parts of a document. The details are explained in Appendix (Additional Healthcare Data Exchange Standards).

In HL7 FHIR, profile components are defined as extensions to resources or as specializations of resources themselves.

7.2.2 Annotations

An annotation is descriptive text that accompanies a standard element definition or concept and provides additional information pertaining to the use of the element (i.e., it is an elaboration of the concept as it relates to the use case to which it is being applied). Annotations do not introduce new requirements in the form of constraints or extensions; they are informative and are often part of profile definitions. Annotations are sometimes referred to as implementation notes or usage notes.

7.3 Refinement of a Standard

When we talk about profiling, we are declaring a refinement to the base standard in the form of constraints and extensions. Profiling in this context is at the conformance profile level (e.g., on a single message or document). Chapter 5 defines and describes the common conformance constructs that are used to specify requirements in a standard. These constructs are used to specify constraints on data elements and to provide a "toolbox" for authors to specify requirements. Each conformance construct (e.g., usage) has different levels of constraint specification. Profiling is the process of refining the constraint according to the rules of the conformance construct. For example, in HL7 v2.x an element that is declared as optional (O) in the base standard can be constrained ("profiled") to required (R). The conformance constructs and allowable constraint models are defined by each standard. The constraint rules provide the mechanism to make a requirement more specific (i.e., "to tighten" a requirement). A more specific specification produces a shorter path to interoperability.

Figure 7.5 illustrates the basic principle of constraint profiling. The base standard defines a segment, "EXP", which is used for a specific purpose and typically could be used in many conformance profiles. Examples of a segment definition include patient identification or a generic observation. The example in Fig. 7.5 shows that the segment is being "profiled" for use in a conformance profile for an admission message and also in a conformance profile for a discharge message. The base standard specifies the segment definition, which defines a number of elements,

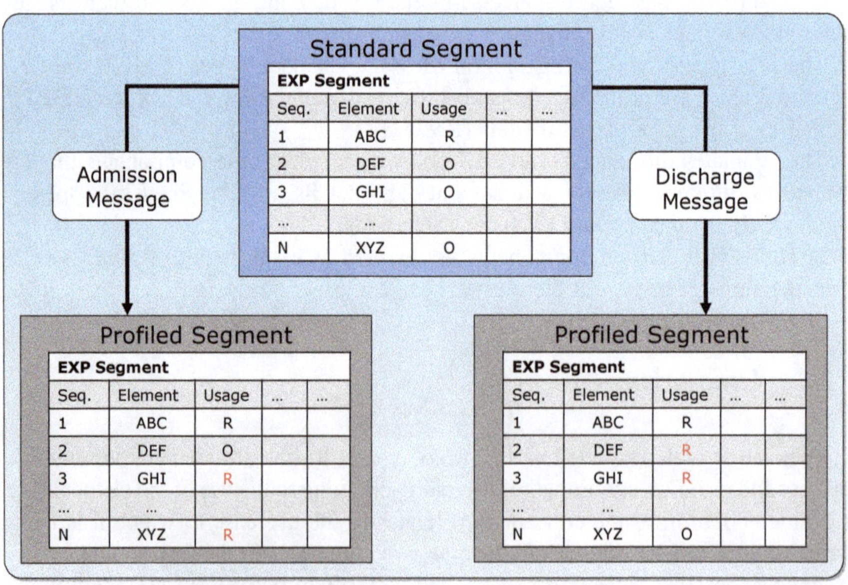

Fig. 7.5 General constraint profiling example (usage)

and these elements have certain attributes (conformance constructs). One attribute is optionality (or usage), and the initial requirement is set by the base standard (ABC = R (required), DEF = O (optional), GHI = O, and XYZ = O). The profile for the admission message constrains the segment definition based on the use case. Elements GHI and XYZ have been constrained from O to R. Similarly, the discharge profile also provides constraints to the base standard to satisfy the discharge use case, and the discharge profile constrains the segment definition differently. In the sub-sections that follow, the general concept of profiling is presented for the common conformance constructs.

7.3.1 Profiling Methodology Summary

Figure 7.6 summarizes the concepts of profiling [5]. A profile is a refinement of the base standard and such refinements can be articulated as annotations (informative), constraints (normative), and extensions (normative). The constraint model presented in Fig. 7.6 is for a single interaction (i.e., a single static conformance profile). The dynamic (transactional) aspects would be considered within the scope of an integration profile (and be constrained and extended according to the same principles).

7.3.2 Constraints

Chapter 5 listed the mechanisms for defining and subsequently refining the requirements through constraining. Table 7.3 provides a summary of the various constraint types. The balance of this sub-section expands on these notions and provides examples for each. Note: the term “element” refers to a generic object describing data and can be interpreted as, for example, a “message element” in HL7 v2.x, a “model element” in HL7 V3, or a “resource attribute” in FHIR.

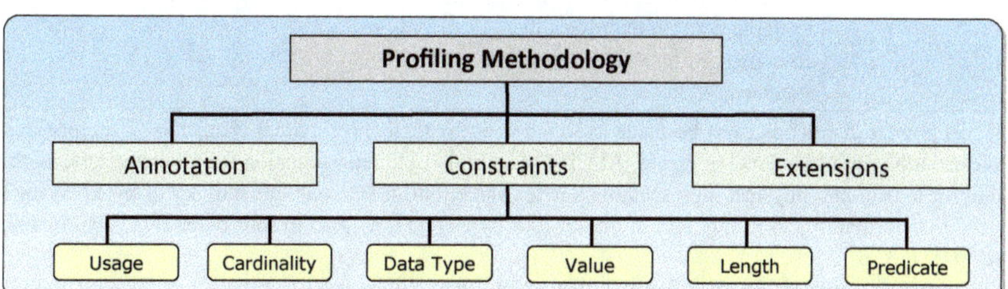

Fig. 7.6 Profiling methodology summary

Table 7.3 Constraint types

Constraint type	Description	Examples
Usage	Indicates requirements for the presence (appearance) of an element. Also referred to as Appearance or Optionality indicator	M—Mandatory (V3) R—Required (v2) Element must be supported and must be present
Cardinality	Indicates the number of occurrences for an element by specifying the minimum and maximum bounds. Also referred to as repetition	[0..1] Element may be omitted and it can have at most one occurrence
Data type	Defines the data element structure and, at the primitive level, the type of data it may contain. Constraints include type substitution and specialization (when combined with other constraint types)	String, Date, Time, Address, Numeric, Coded Element, etc.
Content (value set)	Defines the allowable values for a coded element (i.e., a list of values)	M, F, U, O
Length	Defines a constraint on the number of characters[a] that may be present in one occurrence of an element. Can specify a maximum or the minimum and maximum bounds	80 Element must have at most 80 characters
		[2..4] Element must have at minimum 2 and at most 4 characters
Conformance statement (predicate constraint)	Provides an explicit normative statement expressed in text or a testable expression that defines a constraint. A conformance statement is used when a conformance construct is insufficient to specify a requirement. Patterns can be established to categorized predicate constraints such as a simple constant[b] (e.g., element ABC = "15")	OBR-8 (Observation End Date/Time) SHALL be equal to or later than OBR-7 (Observation Date/Time)
Co-constraint	The co-constraint is a related concept that is used to express dependencies among a set of data values. Such constraints are normally expressed in a table format. The example in the example column expresses the co-constraint in a conformance statement style	If the code in OBX-3 is 30956-7 (Vaccine Type) then OBX-2 shall be "CE" and OBX-5 shall be a value drawn from the CVX value set

[a]At this point a distinction must be made as to whether the logical (printable) characters or the physical representation on a byte level is meant. ASCII has a single byte representation for all characters, so the value for logical and physical representations is the same; but in Unicode, the number of bytes depends on the transformation, so it may end in one to four bytes (UTF-8), two to four bytes (UTF-16) or four bytes (UTF-32).
Data exchange standards do not make this distinction; they merely refer to "characters" when counting the length. For data exchange and on the application level, the amount of "logical" data (characters) counts. However, a specification should clearly state what "type of length" is used

[b]Some standards include constant (or fixed value) as a common conformance constraint

7.3.2.1 Usage (Optionality) Constraint

Usage (also referred to as optionality or appearance) determines, from an *implementation* perspective, whether an element in the message or document instance needs to be *supported.* Additionally, from an *operational* perspective usage determines whether the element has to be *present* in the message or document instance. A usage is assigned for each element in the base standard. In addition, the base standard has rules that define the allowable set of constraints that can be applied for profiling an element (for example, an element that is required in the base standard cannot be profiled to an optional element). Figure 7.5 above and its accompanying explanation describe the application of a Usage constraint.

7.3.2.2 Cardinality Constraint

Cardinality defines the allowable occurrences for an element. It is expressed as an interval or range. For example, "[0..5]" would indicate that the element need not occur in the instance at all or it may occur up to five times; an implementation must support up to five occurrences of an element that has this cardinality definition. A cardinality definition of "[1..5]" is a valid constraint of the "[0..5]" cardinality definition; in this case, the element must appear at least once and may appear up to five times.

7.3.2.3 Data Type Constraint

A data type is a container of data and in a data exchange standard can be complex or primitive. A complex data type contains more than one complex or primitive data type. Essentially, a complex data type is a grouping mechanism for related concepts on a very low level. For example, a data type for "address" may contain data elements for street name, city, state, and zip code. A primitive data type is a container of data that indicates the type of data it may contain (e.g., a String or a Numeric value). Complex data types eventually resolve to primitive data types in the end. Data types can be thought of as buckets that hold data. In programming languages, a complex data type is referred to as a data structure (e.g., C) and a class (e.g., Java) whereas a primitive data type equates to *normal* data types in programming languages (e.g. integer or string in Java).

A constraint applied to a data type is a specialization of the data type (i.e., a more specific definition of the data type's constituent elements). The primitive elements are further constrained by applying constraints of the conformance constructs. For example, the base standard may define a data type as shown in Table 7.4 and a specialization of this data type can be defined as Table 7.5.

DT_2 is a specialization (also referred to a data type flavor) of DT_1. Once defined, instances of DT_1 can be constrained to DT_2. Other variations of this

Table 7.4 Example data type specification

DT_1	Usage	Cardinality
Element 1	R	1..1
Element 2	O	0..*
Element 3	O	0..1
Element 4	O	0..*

Table 7.5 Constrained example data type specification

DT_2	Usage	Cardinality
Element 1	R	1..1
Element 2	**R**	**1..5**
Element 3	**X**	0..**0**
Element 4	O	0..**10**

concept exist; this example provides one way in which a data type can be constrained. It is common for a profile to define multiple flavors of the same base data type for different use cases or purposes. An example could be the specialization of addresses to national (not country, but federal states) or international (country) addresses.

7.3.2.4 Content (Value Set) Constraint

A value set is the set of codes that may be used to populate an element in a message or document instance. The value set is associated with a specific element (which is known as "binding"), and the bound value set should only contain codes that are meaningful for that element in a given context (use). Base standards often do not or cannot provide the necessary granularity or depth of specification because they are designed to have broad utility. Therefore, the base standard provides a starting point, and it may specify a code system (or, in HL7 v2.x, a table), may provide normative or informative (e.g., example) value sets, or may merely provide a placeholder (i.e., define a concept domain). The process of profiling elements that are bound to code values includes providing the value set definition, the binding to the element, and the strength of that binding.

For example, an element may be defined in a base standard for specifying the "unit of measure" of an observation, and the vocabulary binding of that element is to the UCUM (Unified Code for Units of Measure) code system. A given use case may restrict an element that conveys observation data to (only) a patient's height, and thus profiling would entail creating a value set containing desired codes related to units of measure appropriate for height that are provided in the UCUM code system. Table 7.6 illustrates an example of a value set constrained for height observations; four codes are selected from the hundreds of available UCUM codes. This set, along with a normative binding to an element defines the requirements for an implementation (i.e., the implementation shall support this set and only this set for this element for the defined use case).

Table 7.6 Constrained value set for height observations

Code (value)	Description	Code system
[in_i]	inch—length	UCUM
[ft_i]	foot—length	UCUM
cm	centimeter—length	UCUM
m	meter—length	UCUM

A similar use case may be found in Europe. Here the specification author may choose to profile the value set differently, e.g., include only cm (centimeter) and m (meter). In this instance, the set shown in Table 7.6 could be constrained to only those two values.

Appropriate value set constraints should define and bind a value set containing only the values suitable for a particular data element; however, often this rule is not followed. A common issue found in specifications is a single value set being applied to multiple elements for the sake of convenience, even though not all values in the value set are meaningful (suitable) for every element. The implementer is left to figure out which values in the given value set are appropriate for the data element in their particular use case. (See [6] for a detailed description of the issue and a proposed solution for defining value sets in v2.x specifications).

7.3.2.5 Length Constraint

Length is defined as a constraint on the number of characters that may be present in the data value of one occurrence of a data element (object). The definition is system-independent; the number of character is what is important at the application level. The application must be designed to ensure that storage space is adequate to suit the defined length, even if more bytes are necessary to physically store the data.

Length is interpreted as a restriction on an element's data value, not on the presence or absence of the element. The Length Constraint is generally expressed in the form of a minimum and a maximum indicating the number of characters an element may have. A constraint on length restricts the range and thus reduces the capabilities, e.g., [1..2048] to [1..1024]. In some sense the length constraint is a bit counterintuitive when compared to usage. Usage requires that an application add capabilities, whereas a constraint on length may mean reducing an application's current capability (as configured). The specific needs of a use case will dictate whether length constraints must be applied. For example, if the length is derived from a specific (closed) value set that enumerates all possible values, the constraint may be introduced by removing codes from the value set, thereby possibility constraining the length). This action may lead to increasing the minimum length (if the shortest values are eliminated) or to decreasing the maximum length (if the longest values are eliminated), so a narrower range for length could be specified.

7.3.2.6 Conformance Statement (Predicate Constraint)

A conformance statement[3] (also referred to as a predicate constraint) is in its more granular form a normative statement that specifies a requirement. An example is OBR-8 (Observation End Date/Time) SHALL be equal to or later than OBR-7 (Observation Date/Time). It provides a *catch-all* mechanism for expressing a constraint that can't be defined by the other constraint types (conformance constructs). Specific business rules can be captured with conformance statements.

The forms in which a conformance statement can be expressed vary from standard to standard and can appear as a text description or a computable expression. In both forms a specific syntax should be used to ensure that the requirement details are complete and to improve readability for the developer/implementer.

7.3.2.7 Co-constraints

The co-constraint is a related constraint concept that is used to express dependencies among a set of data values. An HL7 v2 message in which healthcare observations are conveyed is one example of how co-constraints are used. Such constraints typically follow the form of "if OBX-3.1 = LOINC code *XXXXX-X* then OBX-2 SHALL BE "CE" and OBX-5.1 SHALL contain a value from the value set *YYY*" or a similar form. A co-constraint is not limited to use with observations, but appears most frequently with observations. A convenient way to illustrate a set of co-constraints is to present them in a table format (Table 7.7 illustrates an example for Immunizations [2].

Usually the OBX-3 (Observation Identifier) is the key upon which data dependencies are based. For example, when OBX-3 contains the LOINC code 30980-7 (for Vaccine Type), the data type in OBX-2 must be "CE" (for coded element), and OBX-5 (the Observation Value) must contain a code from the CVX value set (specifically from the Vaccine Group). This example shows how co-constraints are typically expressed in HL7 v2. Other mechanisms can also be used, and they are used in different standards.

Co-constraints are defined in HL7 FHIR for resources and in HL7 CDA in the form of templates in the same way. HL7 Version 3 uses the Object Constraint Language (OCL) to phrase co-constraints on the model level.

---

[3]The term conformance statement is also used to indicate, from a high level, the capabilities of an implementation or system (i.e., a set of things that the implementation or system is claiming it can do). In the context of this section, conformance statement simply refers to a statement of a requirement. See Chap. 6 for a discussion on the use of overloaded terms for specifying requirements at various levels.

Table 7.7 Excerpt of co-constraints of immunization observations

LOINC (OBX-3)	Description	Data type (OBX-2)	Value set (OBX-5)	Units (OBX-6)
30973-2	Dose number in series	NM	Not applicable	"NA" from HL70353
59782-3	Number of doses in series	NM	Not applicable	"NA" from HL70353
59783-1	Status in immunization series	CE	Local value set	
30956-7	Vaccine type	CE	CVX—Vaccine Group	
30980-7	Date next dose is due	DT_D	Not applicable	
59779-9	Immunization schedule	CE	ScheduleIdentifier	
30963-3	Vaccine funding source	CE	FundingSource	

7.3.3 Allowable Constraints

For each of the conformance constructs described above, the standard defines a set of "allowable constraints" (i.e., the rules for profile compliance) that can be applied. Allowable constraints are a means of restricting requirements in the base standard (or another profile) to make those requirements more specific. As such, elements that are "Required" cannot be relaxed, e.g., changed to "Optional". Chapter 8 provides a detailed examination of constraint rules for each of the conformance constructs.

7.3.4 Extensions

Extensions provide a mechanism for specifying a concept (e.g., a data element) that is not expressed in the base standard but is needed for a particular use case. This mechanism allows for new concepts to be specified in an "as needed" manner to support particular implementations. When using extensions, the data elements should be described and documented sufficiently in a profile such that trading partners can reach a common understanding. Extensions should not be used in cases where a concept already exists in the base standard. The base standard provides a common method for defining extensions, thus ensuring consistent application of the mechanism. One weakness of extensions is that the same concept can be extended in many different forms. If a given concept is found to be specified frequently as an extension, such common extensions should "bubble-up" to the base standard (or at the very least be a candidate to be included in the base). A good way to enable interoperability when extensions are being used is to provide a registry (or registries) where existing solutions for a certain problem/requirement can be posted, queried, and reused if applicable.

Each base standard has a different strategy for handling extensions. Some standards prohibit their use, because the use case is narrow and fixed (e.g. the German xDT family). This type of standard is called a "closed" specification. Other standards, e.g., HL7 v2, H.PR.I.M. and DICOM, seek to provide almost all data elements such that extensions are less likely to be needed. These types of standards are called an "open" specification, because extensions are allowed. HL7 v2 allows extensions via the Z-Segment mechanism. A third type of standards, e.g., FHIR, provide a core set of data elements with the expectation that extensions will be used frequently by design. This type of standard also is called an "open" specification.

7.3.5 Conformance Approaches: Constraints Versus Extensions

When designing base standards, authors must be aware of the trade-off between including a concept in the base standard or allowing the concept to be addressed with an extension. If the concept is introduced in the base standard, then constraints that fit the requirements of the use case are applied during the process of profiling. Extensions likely will need to be defined later if the concept is not included as part of the base standard. Both approaches are valid for determining how to address a concept, but the advantages and disadvantages of each one must be weighed. The time invested in developing a more detailed standard up-front pays off through providing better guidance for implementers; and the time saved when a simpler specification is developed up-front means a significant amount of effort is required to be invested later on for defining customized extensions.

7.4 Profile Hierarchy

As described in [7], a profile is distinguished from a base standard in that, through the application of the conformance rules to the base standard, the openness permitted by the base standard is ultimately restricted. Applying this restriction enables implementation of an interface that is based on the profile without needing to make further modifications to the specification. A base standard allows for numerous ways to define a message (or document) for data exchange; profiles reduce the number of possible definitions to a manageable set, and their use helps to ensure that systems attempting to communicate with each other implement compatible definitions. It is important to recognize that profiles do not eliminate other possible definitions permitted by the standard; rather, profiles select a specific group from the total set of definitions allowed. In this regard, a profile imposes a constraint on

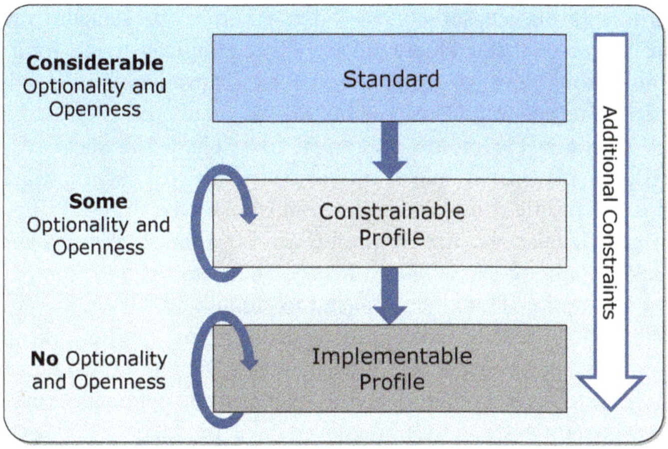

Fig. 7.7 General profile hierarchy

the base standard such that the resultant constrained specification may be used to implement the interface more efficiently. The profile also introduces discipline into the relationship between the interface partners in order to promote harmony in the actual implementation and to facilitate support for a certain use case. Interface partners that faithfully implement the requirements defined in the profile likely will have a shorter path to interoperability.

Profiles innately form a logical hierarchy as layers of constraints are applied to a base standard. Although the various standards have different conventions for naming the profile levels, the principles are the same. The three general profile levels are:

- Standard Profile
- Constrainable Profile
- Implementable Profile

Figure 7.7 illustrates the basic profile hierarchy and the degree of constraints applied at each level. The standard-level profile (hereafter called "standard profile") represents the base standard definitions and constraints,[4] and establishes the framework for a specific type of event (e.g., an unsolicited vaccination record update—VXU V04 message type in HL7 v2.x). Treating the standard as a profile aids in related discussions and management. At this level, the overall structure ("pattern"), including the data type definitions, are established; however, the full declaration of requirements has yet to be specified, and therefore considerable openness still exists. For example, the allowable structure of segments is defined in the HL7 v2.x base standard, but which segments are to be included for a particular use will not have been determined.

[4]Some standards, such as HL7 FHIR®, do not include constraints at the base level; this refinement is performed at subsequent levels.

Other profile levels are subsequently derived from the standard profile. The standard profile can be defined more precisely by adding constraints for a particular use (e.g., the national level of requirements for the unsolicited vaccination record update message) to create a Constrainable Profile (hereafter called "constrainable profile"). A constrainable profile is derived from either the standard profile or another constrainable profile, and it further constrains the definition attributes in accordance to the profile compliance rules stipulated by the standard (Fig. 7.7). For example, a state-level constrainable profile can be derived from a national-level profile by adding more constraints for this specific state. At this point, an element with a usage of "optional" may be changed to "required".

In a constrainable profile, analogous to the standard profile, not all element attributes are fully constrained. An Implementable Profile (hereafter called "implementable profile") defines all elements such that all optionality and openness have been removed. All interfaces deployed in a production setting are implementable profiles whether they are documented (explicitly stated) or not documented (implicitly stated). It is highly recommended that interfaces be completely documented to the implementable profile level using the profiling mechanisms described in this book and provided in the various standards. See the "Uses of Conformance Profiles" section in this chapter for the benefits of this approach.

An implementable profile may also be derived by further constraining another implementable profile. In this case all openness has been removed, however, additional constraints on attributes are applied; for example, in HL7 v2.x, the usage "required, but may be empty" can be *strengthened* to "required" if the particular use case needs it to be.

As described previously, constraints can be added iteratively, thereby forming a hierarchy of profiles; but a certain set of rules must be followed. A profile can only further constrain, not relax, the requirements defined in its *parent* profile. For example, if an element (e.g. field) is "*required*" in the parent profile, the element can't be profiled to "*optional*" in a (compliant) *child* profile, because "*optional*" would be relaxed relative to "*required*".

The allowable derivations for profiling are described for each interoperability standard (e.g., HL7 v2.x [8]). (Non-compliant profiles are discussed later in this chapter.)

Whenever a standard provides choices for implementers, this kind of profile hierarchy is applicable; hence, it is valid for HL7, IHE, DICOM and other standards.

7.4.1 Profile Hierarchy in Use

Two typical real-world scenarios demonstrating the use of the profile hierarchy model are presented in Fig. 7.8. In the first case a national-level constrainable profile is developed. A hospital (group) adopts and refines the national-level guidance provided in the realm-specific constrainable profile. The hospital procures a vendor's product that can be configured to satisfy the requirements. The hospital

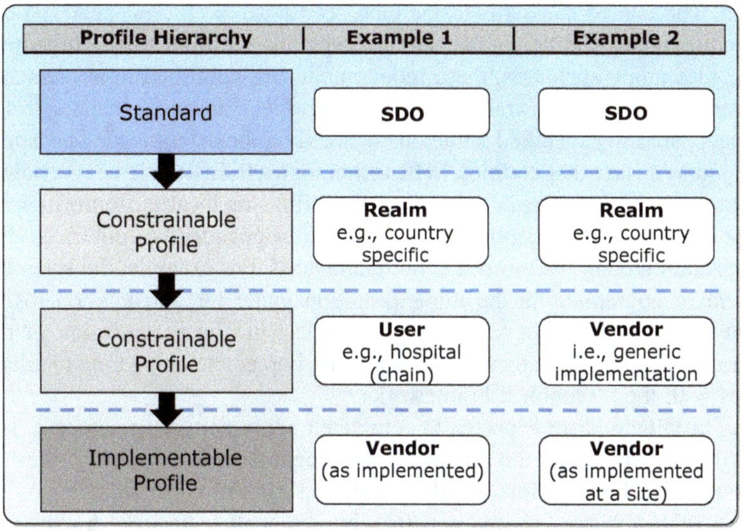

Fig. 7.8 Example profile hierarchy

and the vendor finalize the requirements and the software is installed. The resultant interface is documented as an implementable profile. Alternatively, the hospital could have provided their desired implementable profile directly to the vendor.

In the second case, a vendor refines the national-level guidance profile and provides a generic implementation based on this constrainable profile. When working with clients for whom this profile closely satisfies their requirements, a final refinement is made at the specific sites. The vendor often will (or should) provide the documentation for the installed interface in the form of an implementable profile. The examples shown in Fig. 7.8 can be nested and refined to any depth as appropriate.

7.4.2 Profile Hierarchies for Standard Specifications

The concept and use of constrainable profiles is important in practice, as this level is often (and should be) what standards organizations (e.g., the HL7 affiliates [9]) specify. These profiles can be thought of as a set of harmonized requirements, and they are useful at a national level or at any intermediate level down to the local site implementation. Employing implementable profiles at a high-level, such as nationally, often precludes widespread adoption because of their restrictiveness; therefore, this practice is not recommended and should be avoided (a profile hierarchy should be used instead as is explained with Fig. 7.8).

Use of the message profile hierarchy is the strategy employed in the United States by the Office of the National Coordinator's (ONC) HIT Certification

Program. The named standards in the ONC certification criteria specify "*national level*" requirements—although they are not explicitly named as such. Regarding the HL7 v2 messaging standards, these requirements are published in implementation guides and realized as constrainable message profiles—meaning that a selected set of elements are fully specified while others are yet to be determined. This approach is intended to ensure that certified EHR technologies (CEHRT) have a certain level of common capabilities while providing flexibility for local customization; however, these implementation guides are developed independently from each other, so harmonization among the profiles is not guaranteed. For example, the specification of patient demographics in the implementation guide for transmission to immunization registries does not necessarily coincide with the specification of patient demographics in the laboratory results reporting implementation guide or what IHE specifies with their Technical Frameworks.

Local installations are expected to complete trading-partner agreements. That is, they will further refine the national-level requirements to satisfy their local requirements within the framework established by the constrainable profile for exchange of healthcare information. It is important that the local trading-partner agreements do not relax or conflict with the national-level requirements. The certification of the EHR products seeks to ensure a minimum level of capability that often will not meet all local requirements. Once local trading-partner agreements are put in place, the certified EHR technology and partner systems will need to be implemented and configured accordingly. For example, a provider and their state immunization registry will coordinate data exchange requirements. The referenced EHR certification criterion interoperability standard (i.e., the constrainable profile) provides the foundation, but additional requirements may be necessary for the particular jurisdiction (specified in a more restricted profile derived from the constrainable profile). In that case, the system receiving the HL7 v2 messages (i.e., the immunization registry) must be able to consume and understand the state-level information according to CEHRT in order to achieve the desired interoperability, because the original requirements are still in place and valid. To ensure accuracy and integrity for this exchange of information, local site testing must be performed. At present, this aspect of testing is not part of the ONC Health IT Certification Program; however, starting with CEHRT that meets the constrainable profile requirements provides a shorter pathway to achieving site-specific interoperability. Discussion on the topic of testing is provided in detail in Chap. 11.

Figure 7.9 shows a simple use of a profile hierarchy for the unsolicited vaccination record update message described previously. A constrainable profile for national-level requirements is created from the HL7 v2.5.1 base standard. This standard is referenced in the ONC 2014 and 2015 Editions of the transmission to immunization registries certification criterion. Vendors' products are certified to this standard. Various states can further constrain the national-level profile to meet their local requirements. The states could create a constrainable profile (more likely) or an implementable profile. Ultimately, what a vendor implements is defined in an implementable profile. Tools such as the NIST Implementation Guide Authoring

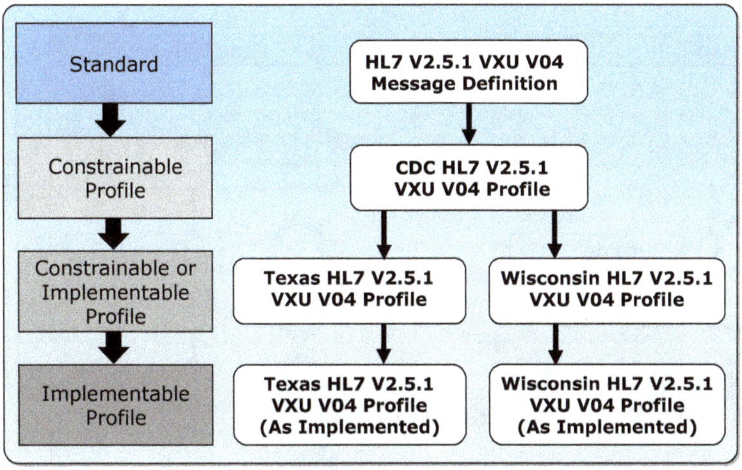

Fig. 7.9 Example profile hierarchy for send immunization history

and Management Tool (IGAMT) [10] and the Messaging Workbench (MWB) [11] can be used to author and manage HL7 v2 profiles (see Chap. 9).

7.4.3 Non-compliant Profiles

In practice, sometimes profiles are not used as prescribed in this book and in the standards. Deviation from a particular standard may be warranted in certain cases if the standard doesn't accommodate a specific need or if it is too restrictive for the use case. Such matters should be brought to the attention of the appropriate SDO. In the meantime, non-compliant profiles can be used as an effective tool to handle these (non-optimal) circumstances. Although the non-compliant profile may not follow some base-level standard rules, the fact that the deviations are documented allows trading partners to manage the non-compliance in a proprietary way.

In an ideal situation, every specification is based on a standard or a profile and provides additional constraints according to the defined constraint rules. If a profile relaxes (weakens) a constraint, the resulting profile is deemed a non-compliant (conflicting) profile.[5] Non-compliant profiles should be avoided if possible.

---

[5]The intent of the IHE Technical Frameworks is to specify only compatible message profiles in the different integration profiles. However, a thorough examination (as of 2013) reveals that different IHE integration profiles have specified message profiles that are incompatible with each other. Therefore, a single implementation cannot be compliant with both specifications, and configuration is necessary

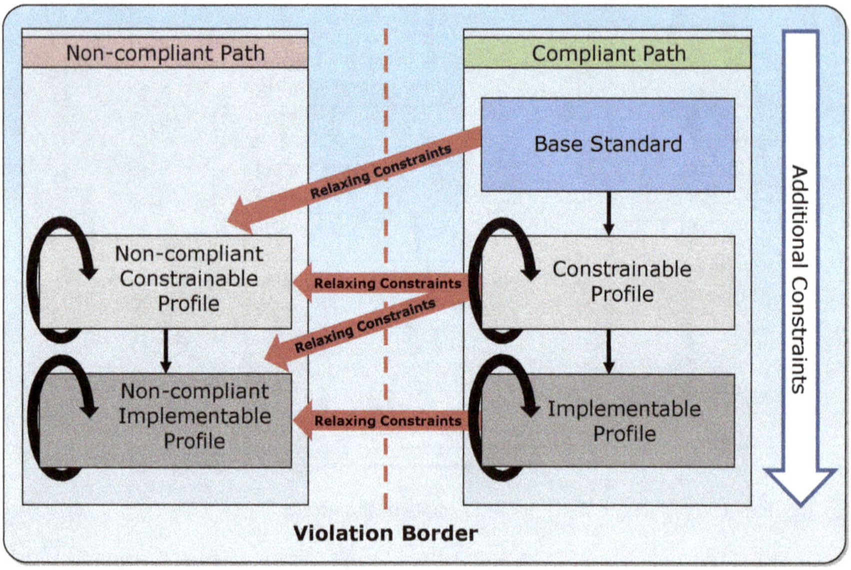

Fig. 7.10 Profile hierarchy with non-compliant profiles

Figure 7.10 depicts the profile hierarchy that accounts for non-compliant profiles. The right side of the diagram indicates the preferred path of profiling as was described earlier. The left side of the diagram indicates the non-compliant profile path. As shown, non-compliance can be introduced at any level in the hierarchy.

7.5 Profiling Case Study: HL7 v2

To provide a detailed explanation of profiles and their use, we describe the profiling mechanisms as defined for HL7 v2.x and draw from a case study described in [12]. Understanding this use case will give the reader a knowledge base that can be quickly applied to other standards. Along the way, specific profiling approaches in other standards are pointed out to help the reader compare and contrast profiling methods. As mentioned previously, even though the mechanics for each of the standards may differ, the profiling concepts are universal.

7.5.1 HL7 v2.x Profiles: Background and Motivation

There are numerous healthcare data exchange standards in the US and internationally for communicating administrative and clinical data. The most widely used standard is the Health Level Seven (HL7) Version 2.x *Application Protocol for Electronic Data Exchange* (hereafter HL7) [8]. This standard is designed to support application-to-application message exchange. An HL7 *message* contains data for real-world events, such as admitting a patient or sending a laboratory result (e.g., a CBC—complete blood count). For each event, HL7 defines an *abstract message definition* that is composed of a collection of segments (data units, e.g., Patient Demographics) in a predetermined sequence. Rules for building an abstract message definition are specified in the HL7 message framework, which is hierarchical in nature and consists of building blocks generically called *elements* [8]. These elements are *segment groups*, *segments*, *fields*, *components*, and *sub-components*. The requirements for a message are defined by the message definition and the constraints placed on each message element. The constraint mechanisms are defined by the HL7 conformance constructs which include usage, cardinality, value set, length, and data type. Additionally, explicit conformance statements (predicate constraints) are used to specify other requirements that can't be addressed by the conformance constructs.

Applications using HL7 v2.x are generally connected in two ways: via point-to-point or via middleware such as communication server (integration engine) products. Point-to-point entails connecting each pair of applications directly to each other independently of other applications. In the communication server approach, all applications are connected to a centrally located message broker instead of directly to each other. A set of HL7 v2.x message definitions specifies the requirements between the communicating applications. Although the message definitions are specific, there are many ways to specify a particular HL7 interaction (i.e., the definitions may not be compatible). In practice, two vendors' interface specifications may not quite match, and the differences between them must be addressed when developing the data exchange connection. With the point-to-point approach, each new set of messaging interfaces requires a separate implementation. If a communication server is used, a new mapping transformation definition needs to be defined whenever a new application is added to the existing group of connected applications. In both cases, the breadth of the specification leads to cumbersome and ad hoc interface implementations. System implementations such as these are prone to error, are difficult to maintain, and do not scale easily.

To help alleviate these shortcomings, the HL7 v2 standard[6] introduced the concept of *conformance message profiles*. Message profiles provide an unambiguous description of HL7 messages by defining processing rules and by specifying specific requirements for each element in order to support a particular use case.

[6]Via work performed in the HL7 Conformance and Guidance for Implementation and Testing (CGIT) Working Group.

7.5.2 HL7 v2 Conformance Profile Defined

Message profiles[7] constrain HL7 messages by adding requirements for a particular interaction. A message profile provides a mechanism for specifying a single message definition. An implementation guide often is created to organize a collection of message profiles for specifying a set of related HL7 v2.x interactions described by a use case or use cases. Implementation guides typically describe broader conformance requirements, such as a use case model, a dynamic definition, a static definition, and application functional requirements. IHE integration profiles can be characterized as high-level or generic implementation guides [1].

The *use case model* provides a description of the process being addressed, defines actor responsibilities, and describes a sequence of actions performed by the sending and receiving applications. The *dynamic definition* describes the interaction between the sender and receiver in terms of the expected acknowledgments (or other transactions such as query/response). The *static definition* provides a precise explanation of the message structure and constraints for a single message (this is the message profile). *Functional requirements* describe the application (or actor) level requirements. Such requirements may include how a set of messages are to be used to trigger certain application functions. The message profile's definition, use, and organization within an implementation guide are key issues addressed in this section.

A message profile can be represented as an XML document, and Fig. 7.11 shows an excerpt from an example XML profile. Each element in the message profile is listed along with its associated attributes. For a more detailed description of a message profile, refer to the HL7 standard, chapter 2B (Conformance) [8]. It is important to note that the attributes and constraints a profile places on a message provide a clear and unambiguous definition, thereby facilitating the design, implementation, and testing of interfaces (especially when represented in a computible form) [12, 13, 14].

The rules for constructing a message are described by the message framework. In addition, for targeted real-world events (for example, "Admitting a Patient") a specific abstract message structure (ADT_A01) is defined. The message structure defines a template or format that the message must follow; it defines explicitly the elements and the order in which the elements must appear in a message instance. For example, in Fig. 7.11, the "PID" segment contains the field "Set ID – PID" and so forth. The usage attribute refers to the circumstances under which an element appears in a message [8]. For example, the "Driver's License Number" component in the profile excerpt is required (Usage = "R") and must be present in a valid message instance. Cardinality refers to the minimum and maximum number of occurrences an element may have [8] in a message instance. An example of an

[7]Message profiles are not to be confused with the Integrating the Healthcare Enterprises (IHE) integration profiles. Often IHE integration profiles will use HL7 v2.x message profiles.

```
...
&lt;Segment Name="PID" LongName="Patient Identification" Usage="R"
        Min="1" Max="1"/>
 <Reference>3.4.2</Reference>
  <Field Name="Set ID - PID" Usage="R" Min="1" Max="1"
        Datatype="SI" MaxLength="4" MinLength="1">
  </Field>
...
  <Field Name="SSN Number - Patient" Usage="X" Min="0" Max="0"
        Datatype="ST" MaxLength="16" MinLength="1" />
  <Field Name="Driver's License Number - Patient" Usage="R" Min="1 Max="1"
        Datatype="DLN" MaxLength="66" MinLength="1">
    <Component Name="License Number" Usage="R"
              Datatype="ST" MaxLength="20" MinLength="1" />
    <Component Name="Issuing State, Province, Country" Usage="R"
              Datatype="IS" Table="0333" MaxLength="20" MinLength="1" />
    <Component Name="Expiration Date" Usage="O"
              Datatype="DT" MaxLength="24" MinLength="1" />
  </Field>
...
```

Fig. 7.11 Excerpt from an HL7 v2.x message profile (XML representation)

element cardinality is "[0..1]", which indicates that the element does not have to appear in the message instance and it can only have one occurrence if it does appear. A table[8] of allowable values can be defined and associated with a certain element. For example, see the "Issuing State, Province, Country" component in Fig. 7.11. This element must be populated with a data value that is defined in HL7 Table 0333. The length attribute defines the minimum and maximum allowable number of characters a value can include for a *particular element. The data type defines the kind* of data an element can contain.

7.5.3 Message Profile Components Defined

A message profile component (hereafter profile component) defines a part of or a certain aspect of a profile and is used to differentiate requirements from another profile or profile component. A profile component can be applied to any construct or section of a profile. A profile component in a family of profiles can be used to identify different levels of requirements for the same use case or to identify the differences in requirements for different, but closely related, use cases.

[8]Since the example is HL7 v2 the term *table* is used, but this can be thought of as a *value set*.

In one case, a specification may need to express different levels of conformance. For example, a profile in the specification may be written to require the use of Object Identifiers (OIDs) for all Universal ID data elements. Another profile may be written in which use of OIDs for these data elements is a not requirement (i.e., other identifier types are allowed to be used). An intermediate profile may be written that requires certain, but not all, of these data elements to support the use of OIDs. This specification is, in principle, describing three levels (as mutually exclusive sets) of conformance requirements. These three profile levels can be described using a base profile definition and three profile components. The profile components describe the differences in the requirements (this approach can be thought of as a substitution mechanism). A similar approach as the one described here is employed in the "HL7 v2 2.5.1 Laboratory Results Interface (LRI)" implementation guide's laboratory results message profiles (ORU_R01 message structure) [15] (the LRI guide is a named standard in the 2014 Edition criteria of the ONC Health IT Certification Program). Although profile components are currently used in this manner, it is debatable whether allowing multiple incompatible solutions for a regulatory certification program is a good idea. For more details, see the case study for the family of laboratory specifications in this chapter.

In another case, a profile component may need to be employed to express requirements for a different, but closely related, use case. Here the creators of the new profile component leverage the requirements in an existing profile, since that existing profile contains many common requirements. The "HL7 v2.5.1 Electronic Laboratory Reporting (ELR) to Public Health Release 2" implementation guide uses the concept of a profile component in this manner [16] (i.e., it further builds on the LRI implementation guide). Section 7.11.3 of this chapter provide detailed descriptions of the use of profile components in the LRI and ELR implementation guides.

In the first case above, the use case is the same, but the requirements in which it can be achieved are different. The profile component is expressing a different level of conformance. In the second case above, the use case is similar, but there are several important differences, and, therefore, the requirements are different. The profile component concept is used to leverage the in-common requirements defined by the profile while allowing any different requirements to be defined in a profile component.

Profile components can be used as "*building blocks*" to specify a complete profile (set of requirements) as identifiable sub-units. As such, they can express common requirements, additional requirements, or substitute requirements. Profile components are an efficient utility to manage and define a family (a related set) of profiles.

The descriptions of the different conformance levels, profiles, and profile components are found in the conformance clause section of a specification. Based on the information provided in these descriptions, an implementer is able to make a conformance claim as to which level of conformance they support.

7.6 Vocabulary Profiling

Vocabulary profiling was introduced at a high level earlier in this chapter. Chap. 5 provided the foundation for vocabulary specification. This Sect. 7.6 and the next Sect. 7.7) discusses in detail the techniques for specifying, constraining, and managing vocabulary. The topic of vocabulary is explored further in Chap. 12 in the sections entitled Vocabulary Conformance and Vocabulary Conformity Assessment.

Vocabulary is a complicated and convoluted subject. An attempt will be made here to provide the basic concepts (in a generic fashion) and insight into the key factors that should be considered when working with vocabularies. Every standard approaches the specification and profiling of vocabulary in a different way; there is no common methodology or glossary of terms to use. The approach presented here is representative of one school of thought and by no means expresses a consensus viewpoint.

Figure 7.12 indicates the types of vocabulary bindings that are typical for each profiling level. The base standard level supports broad use cases, so it follows that the vocabulary bindings are more at the concept and code system level. As use cases are developed and refinement of a specification occurs at the constrainable profile level, more information becomes known, and, therefore, relevant value sets begin to emerge. At the implementation level, all coded elements must be linked to a specific value set. In some implementation level specifications, an element is bound to a code system, which is then deemed implicitly to be the value set (although explicit designation is recommended).

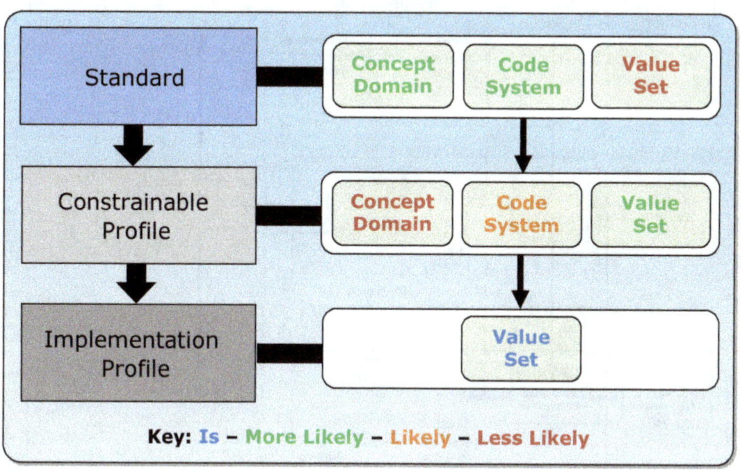

Fig. 7.12 Typical vocabulary bindings

7.6.1 Vocabulary Binding and Profiling

Specification of vocabulary conformance is a multidimensional process. It involves successive refinement of both the informational model and vocabulary in parallel. The figure (Summary of Vocabulary Mechanics) in Chap. 5 provides an overview of these vocabulary conformance mechanics. The ultimate goal of the specification is to bind coded data elements to a specific set of codes to facilitate a precise implementation.

As described previously, specifications are refined via the process of profiling. The labels in the boxes that are lined up along the left-most side of Fig. 7.13 illustrate a profile hierarchy progressing from a general (abstract) specification to a completely constrained and precise implementation. Each of the three rows, demarcated in the diagram by the horizontal dashed lines, shows the successive operations performed on both the specification of the data elements and the vocabulary objects with which they are associated. This successive constraint is shown in the diagram starting with the top row, then continuing with the next row down, and, finally, ending with the bottom row. To reduce the clutter in the diagram, this process is shown using only a single example data element that is associated with a "simple" value set consisting only of codes from one code system; but all of the indicated items exist for each and every one of the coded data elements in any profile. The binding of a coded data element is either to an internal value set or an external value set (indicated by "XOR" in the diagram).

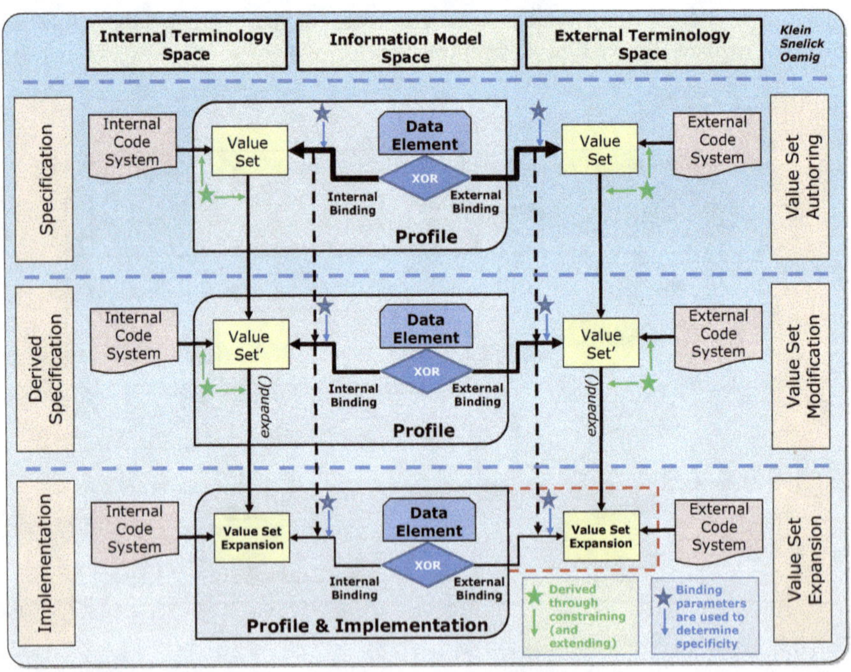

Fig. 7.13 Vocabulary binding and profiling: a high-level perspective

The labels in the three boxes across the top of the diagram indicate the three parallel constraint processes by which specification of vocabulary conformance occurs. The steps related to the process of defining, refining, and maintaining the sets of coded concepts are illustrated in the portion of the diagram that is below the box labelled "Internal Terminology Space". This information applies to those vocabulary objects that are handled by the same organizational processes used for constraining a profile and/or the base specification. These internal value sets may come from the base specification or may be created as entirely new sets for the profile being developed. The central portion of the diagram below the box labeled "Information Model Space" illustrates the processes wherein the profile definitions are created. These definitions include data elements and their bindings to value sets, as well as various parameters controlling use and extensibility (described in detail in the sections to follow). The portion of the diagram below the box labeled "External Terminology Space" shows that the governance processes for these vocabulary objects are handled by an organizational entity that is outside of, and separate from, the entity developing the profile (although some communication may exist between these entities).

One goal of the profile constraining process is to define a binding to vocabulary that ultimately is implementable for each data element that is assigned a coded element data type. This binding is necessary for all coded data elements for an operational implementation, and the binding can be to a value set that is created and maintained within the confines of the profile definition (internal) or to a value set that is created and maintained externally. An *internal binding* refers to a value set binding in which the code system is defined within the specification (typically the base standard, but the values may also be defined within any of the profiles being derived from the base standard). This value set is created or copied from another internal source and subsequently bound to a data element. For an external binding, the code system is always maintained by external stewards. Those stewards (or in some cases another third party) may create a value set, or they may copy an external value set expansion into the profile during the final implementation constraining process (as shown within the red dotted line in the diagram).

Examples of external steward organizations include ISO and WHO (which define many international code systems), IHTSDO (SNOMED CT), Regenstrief (LOINC), and VSAC (the Value Set Authority Center of the US National Library of Medicine, which develops and publishes value sets for use in implementing the US "Meaningful Use" regulations). In many (but not all) of these cases, the value sets also are developed externally to the profile constraining activity, but they may have some modifications originating from "inside" the profiling activity. Finally, the labels in the boxes positioned along the rightmost side of the diagram describe the sequential activities that are performed on the code systems and value sets as constraint of the profile moves towards Implementation level refinement.

It is important to note that these three profiling activities shown in parallel may be performed independently and do not have any timing-based relationships between them that can be considered during the iterations of the profiling cycles.

A value set is derived from one or more code systems or another pre-existing value set through the process of constraining and extending (this action is represented in the Fig. 7.13 diagram by the green stars and green arrows). The constraint and extension mechanism applies to both internally and externally defined value sets, and is part of defining and using the binding parameters.

The binding of a data element to a value set is annotated in Fig. 7.13 by the blue stars. The specification (i.e., the profile) makes this association explicit. The binding includes parameters that are used to define specificity. This required specificity includes details related to the code system (such as its release version), the requirement to use the codes in the value sets (as opposed to custom codes or free text), and the limits of or guidance on further constraint of the value set for a subsequent profile. These specificity parameters are explained in detail in the sections to follow.

Value set authoring is the initial phase of specification in either of the Terminology Spaces. As a profile is constrained for a specific use case, the value sets are refined to match the needs of that use case. This phase is labeled as "Derived Specification" in the second row of the diagram. The operations on vocabulary during this phase can be described as a "Value Set Modification", where the value sets that were established in the specification to which the constraints are being applied are further constrained (and/or extended); this notion is indicated in Fig. 7.13 with the green stars and arrows. Note that extending may involve adding codes from a code system to the value set. The thickness of the binding (black) arrows that point from a data element to a value set box in the diagram decreases in each of the sequential three rows to indicate a more precise (and often smaller) set of values. Note that more than one derived specification may be produced for a set of related or similar use cases during each iteration (i.e., profiling cycle) of the operations shown in the portion of the diagram below the Information Model Space label.

The bottom "Implementation" row represents the implementation profile and its realization (the actual configured system that is in production). In the transition from the "Derived Specification" to the "Implementation", further constraints (and extensions) may be specified. Additionally, once the value set definition has been finalized, its set of specific values can be realized (e.g., enumerated) through the process of value set expansion. This action, indicated in the diagram by the label "*expand()*" on the vertical arrow in the second row, is an operation that may be performed manually at the local installation site or by a terminology service that is available to the profile authors, developers, and system implementers. The value set expansion is the code set instance in a form directly suitable for implementation. Note that under some circumstances, a data element in an Implementation Profile may still be bound to a Value Set Definition that has not yet been expanded to an explicit list of values ("Value Set Expansion"). In these cases, the development of the final Implementation Profile involves further constraint and parameterization of the Value Set Definition, so the final expansion may be completed at the time of implementation of the system, and will be deterministic at that time.

7.6.2 *Use of Extensibility and Stability*

Figure 7.14 shows value set attributes of Extensibility and Stability (See Chap. 5 for definitions) along with the allowable settings these attributes may take on related to the specification space and their impact in post specification and runtime environment. The requirements for value sets are determined when specifications are created initially in the base standard, and then these requirements are subsequently refined through the mechanism of profiling. The specification (and the impact of that specification) of the extensibility and stability for a value set can be considered in three distinct spaces: the specification space, post specification space, and operational space. In the specification space, the extensibility of a value set can be designated as "open" or "closed". Constrainable profiles (which include the base standard) can specify value set extensibility as either "open" or "closed". For implementation profiles, the value set extensibility is closed. At this point in the creation of the specification, the use case is definitive; therefore, the universe of allowable values for the element is known and is documented as such. Any desired change would have to occur in another version of the specification with a new value set. Extensibility is a construct in the context of the specification space; modification of a value set outside the specification space is controlled by Stability and is discussed next.

There are circumstances when, although the completed state is known, it is anticipated that additional updates to a value set will be necessary. In some cases, the updates can be managed, published, and communicated in an orderly manner.

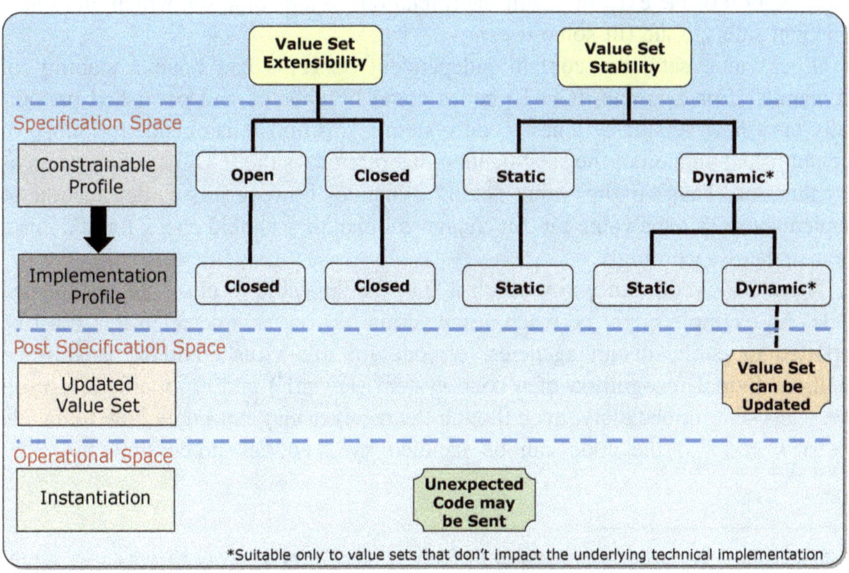

Fig. 7.14 Extensibility and stability use in specifications

This situation occurs in the post specification space, and it is indicated by the value set having a stability of "dynamic". In other cases, the real-world circumstances necessitate communication of an unknown code. There is no pre-coordinated agreement about this code, but there can be a pre-coordinated agreement that an unknown code is possible. Standards do not provide an explicit and distinct mechanism to support this notion; however, the notion is sometimes conflated in other mechanisms which dilutes the specification.

For most internal value set bindings (at least for HL7 v2.x), the settings predominantly are "closed" and "static" (and for implementation profiles, extensibility has to be "closed"). A stability of "static" is appropriate for value sets where all concepts needed for the use case are known at the time of specification. These value sets may also have dependent concepts or those in which the value set is tightly-coupled to the underlying technical infrastructure; that is, the concepts have certain dependencies within the use case, and any change that is made has a significant and consequential impact on implementations. For example, if a value set for laboratory results defined a *state machine* using various status codes (preliminary, final, corrected, etc.), it would be unacceptable to allow another *state* to be defined outside the bounds of the specification. This example is one in which the value set codes are tightly-coupled to the technical infrastructure. A more subtle example is the definition of the abnormal flags (HL7 v2 Table 0078) that indicate the result interpretation. The code "H" indicates "above high normal" and "HH" indicates "above upper panic limits". If an intermediate setting is needed, for example, "HU" for "very high", then this concept should be defined as part of a new version of the interoperability specification and value set (and not as part of a local value set or a dynamic value set). Adding an intermediate value changes the interpretation of the existing result interpretations in the value set, which, in turn, is a patient safety issue (in some uses).

Other value sets that contain independent concepts can have a stability of "dynamic". For example, ICD-10 codes could be updated and published periodically (as a new version or a new code system). This update is outside the scope of the published version of the specification that references the ICD-10 code system as a value set. Tagging the value set as dynamic, however, is a notification to implementers that the value set can change and that they should check for and make their updates accordingly.

There are circumstances in which it may be desirable to allow an unexpected code. An example might be when a new strain of a virus is detected that must be reported to public health agencies. A code for this virus could be established (without formal recognition of a code system steward[9]) and reportable lab result messages sent immediately, even though the receiver may not know how to handle the new code. If the code can be handled by "generic" processing, however,

[9]Although the code would be expected to be forthcoming. The necessity of having a code for the concept immediately prevents an orderly deliberation and document process (which will happen later).

a complete understanding of it by the receiver may not be necessary. Also, when the code and the associated concept are published officially, receivers that update to this new value set can then process this information in a meaningful way (if so desired). This circumstance is indicated in the "Operational Space" as an "Unexpected Code may be Sent". As of this publication, none of the SDOs have a mechanism in their vocabulary machinery that supports this notion independently.

Vocabulary specification should provide a way to indicate whether a data element definition allows or disallows unexpected (unpublished) codes. The mechanism should not be conflated with existing mechanisms (i.e., Extensibility and Stability). Implementers must be able to distinguish concepts of extensibility and stability from the case of unexpected codes in operational environments. Such information would enable precise specifications and robust implementations. Systems could handle the "expected" unexpected code for data elements specified with this attribute and report a violation for data elements in which unexpected codes are not allowed. For most data elements, unanticipated and unexpected codes would not be expected (in well-defined specifications).

7.6.3 Profiling at the Code Level

Similar to, but not equivalent to, usage for data elements is the concept of usage for the codes in a value set. Vocabulary usage is a mechanism for defining and setting the scope of the concepts to be included, considered for inclusion (or exclusion), or excluded in a value set definition.

Table 7.8 defines usage indicators for profiling vocabulary. Required (R) usage indicates that the code must be supported (and thus can be used); Permitted (P) indicates that the code can be *profiled* to R, P, or E in a derived profile; and Excluded (E) indicates that the code must not be supported (and thus cannot be used) for the given element. The Permitted usage indicator is only applicable to constrainable profiles, i.e., it cannot appear in an implementation profile (it must become an R or an E). Permitted usage can be included in a closed value set (at the constrainable profile level). In this situation, the set of all known concepts are defined, but some concepts are left to be profiled at the implementation level based on local requirements/needs.

The assignment of the usage codes to define a value set presented here is similar to (***but not quite equivalent***) to the concept of *min* (=Required), *max* (=Required ∪ Permitted ∪ Excluded), and *ignore* (=Excluded) in HL7 V3.

Figure 7.15 indicates the relationship of vocabulary usage to the profiling hierarchy. The value set is deemed to be "scoped" (at the constrainable profile level). At the base standard level, all codes have an implied usage of Permitted.[10] The base standard defines a set of concepts and the representative codes. The

[10]Although this is not explicitly stated but can be inferred.

Table 7.8 Vocabulary profiling usage

Usage	Name	Conformance	Allowable usage[a]
R	Required	The code SHALL be supported	R
P	Permitted (applicable to constrainable profiles only)	None; to be specified	R, P[b], E
E	Excluded	The code SHALL NOT be supported	E

[a]Allowable usage in a derived profile
[b]Not allowed in an implementation profile

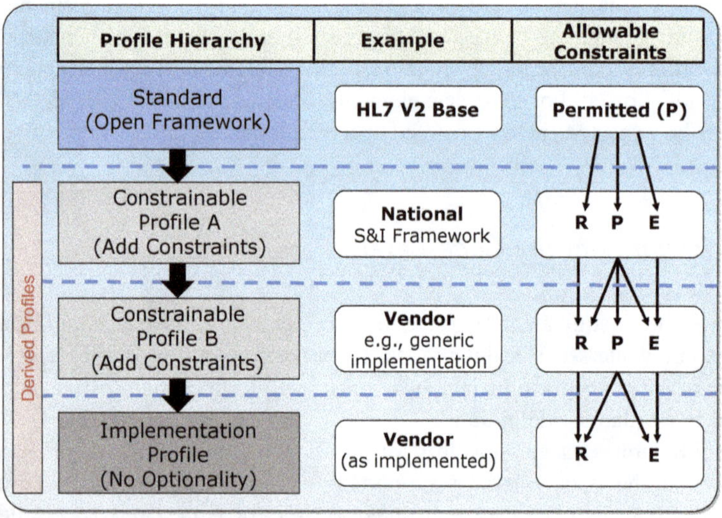

Fig. 7.15 Vocabulary profiling usage and allowable transitions

binding strength determines how the value set can be used in derived specifications. If the binding strength is "Required", and if the concept that needs to be conveyed is available in the code set, then the code must be used. The use case analysis determines which codes are applicable for the element to which the value set is bound. An important point to make here is that the base standard would have defined a set of codes with associated concepts. A binding strength of Required means that the value set must be used; however, only the codes that are appropriate to use for the element to which the value set is bound should be specified in derived profiles. This analysis should be completed for every element to which the base vocabulary is bound. In practice, specification at this granular level rarely occurs in implementation guides.

Figure 7.16 presents a typical vocabulary specification for administrative gender at the base standard level. The table indicates the value (or code), a description,

Value	Description	Usage	Code System
A	Ambiguous	P	HL70001_v2.5.1
F	Female	P	HL70001_v2.5.1
M	Male	P	HL70001_v2.5.1
N	Not Applicable	P	HL70001_v2.5.1
O	Other	P	HL70001_v2.5.1
U	Unknown	P	HL70001_v2.5.1

Fig. 7.16 Base standard sample vocabulary definition

usage, and the code system to which each value belongs. Typically, usage is not designated at the base standard level; Permitted is the implied usage for each code.

Also, unless explicitly stated otherwise, a vocabulary specification at the base standard level has open extensibility. Extensibility is rarely restricted in a base standard.

Figure 7.17 shows a vocabulary profiling example using an abbreviated value set definition. Starting with the base standard definition, a set of concepts and associated codes are defined. The Usage for all of the codes is Permitted, and the value set definition has "open" extensibility. This value set definition is equivalent to the sample vocabulary definition in Fig. 7.16 (but the description and code

Additional Constraints →

Base		Constrainable		Implementable	
Value	Usage	Value	Usage	Value	Usage
A	P	A	E	A	E
F	P	F	R	F	R
M	P	M	R	M	R
N	P	N	E	N	E
O	P	O	E	O	E
U	P	U	P	U	E
E = Open		E = Closed		E = Closed	
S = ?		S = Static		S = Static	

Fig. 7.17 Example vocabulary profiling 1

system columns are omitted for brevity in Fig. 7.17). The usage of each code in the value set is determined based on the use case analysis conducted during the development of a derived specification. In the Constrainable profile in Fig. 7.17, the usage for codes "F" and "M" is profiled to Required; for "A", "N", and "O" the usage is profiled to Excluded; and usage for "U" is left to be decided in another derived specification (e.g., a local implementation). Furthermore, the specification authors decided that no additional codes can be added in derived profiles (Extensibility = "closed"), and that this value set is not suitable for revisions post publication of the specification (Stability = "static"). Next, Fig. 7.17 shows that, at the implementable profile level, the local use case dictated that the concept represented by the code "U" was not needed, therefore, it is profiled with a usage of "E". A different local use case could specify that the concept is needed, in which case the usage for the code "U" would be set to "R".

In the next example (Fig. 7.18), the use case for the implementable profile warranted an additional concept represented by the code "X". This extension is valid since the value set has Extensibility set to "open" in the constrainable profile. If the Extensibility had been "closed" in the constrainable profile, the code "X" could not have been added to the implementable profile (to be considered compliant with its *parent* profile).

The example in Fig. 7.19 shows that a new concept (represented by "Y") was added in the constrainable profile, and another concept (represented by "Z") was added in the implementable profile. The Base standard is "open", which allows for the addition of code "Y" in the Constrainable Profile; likewise, the Constrainable

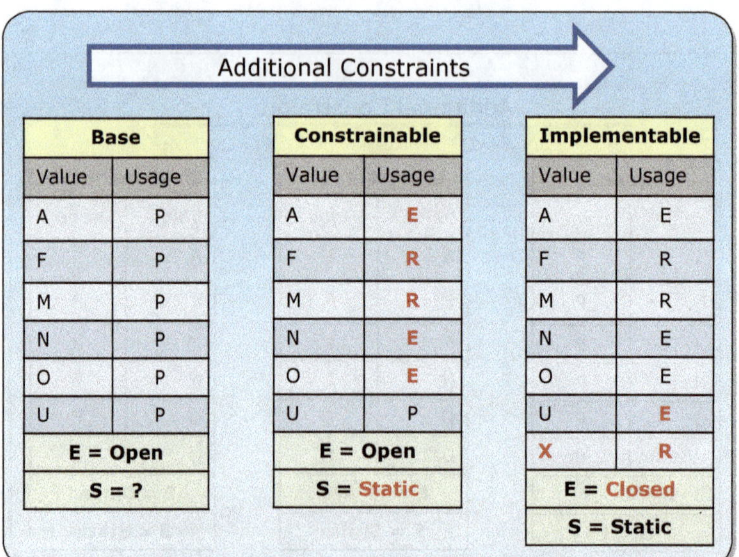

Fig. 7.18 Example vocabulary profiling 2

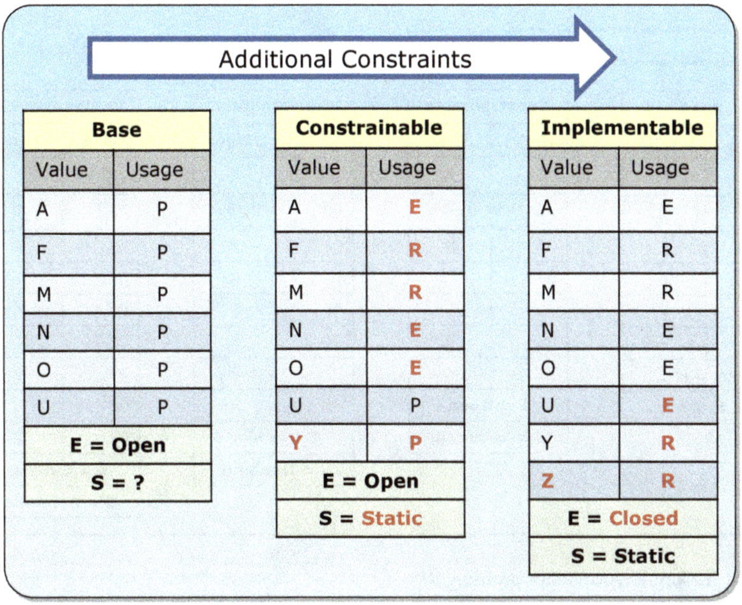

Fig. 7.19 Example vocabulary profiling 3

Profile is "open", which allows for the addition of the code "Z". It is important to note that the *extensibility* is a construct that is in the specification space, so as long as the specification authors indicate that it is "open", additional codes can be added as the use case is refined. This is the case even when the Stability is "static", because this describes another dimension of specification; that is, whether the value set can be modified post specification by an external steward. In this example, the authors deemed this value set not to be modifiable post specification.

Figure 7.20 demonstrates how the use of a dynamic value set might be defined in practice. Initially at the base standard level, not only is the concept domain known, but a particular code system is specified. An example might be the set of CVX codes for reporting immunizations. When published, the base standard specified codes "01" through "06". It might be assumed that the binding strength and all code usages are defined as Required; however, generally no indication of this explicit requirement is given in the standards. It may also be assumed for this vocabulary definition that Extensibility would be "open", and, for Stability either "dynamic" or "static" might be assumed (but again, typically no indication is given in the standards). Therefore, in Fig. 7.20 all usages are initially shown as Permitted, Extensibility is set to 'open', and Stability is set to '?' (unknown, but to be defined). In a constrainable profile (e.g., at the national level), it is likely that a newer version of the CVX code system exists, as years may have passed since the publication of the base standard and the development of an implementation guide, so the constrainable profile would reference the latest CVX code system. Figure 7.20

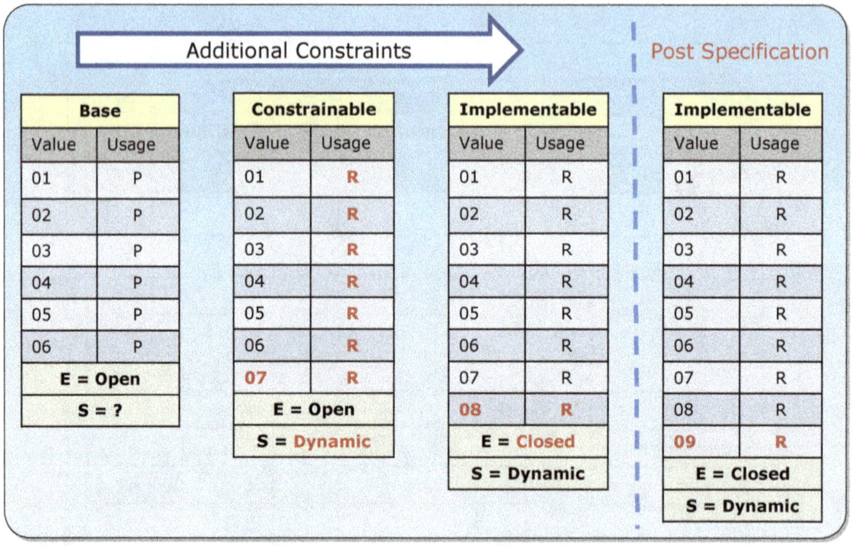

Fig. 7.20 Example vocabulary profiling 4

illustrates this possible change; the immunization represented by the code "07" has been added to the code system. Stability for the constrainable profile is defined explicitly to be "dynamic", which is an indication that post specification the implementer can expect this code system (implicitly a value set) to change. At the implementable profile level, another update has been made to the CVX code system: code "08" has been added. This change may have occurred by the time a particular implementation was installed, as the CVX code had been updated since the publication of the national level specification. Implementers should use the latest version of the code system available. Additionally, the implementers should be aware that subsequent revisions will be made and should plan accordingly. This situation is depicted in Fig. 7.20 as a post specification revision; code "09" has been added. When the immunization message is transmitted, the version of the CVX code system used should be indicated (but it rarely is). Some data exchange standards support this capability (e.g., in later versions of HL7 v2.x with the message profile identifier), while others do not. In HL7 v2.x, the dynamic value set can be considered a profile component, and the sender can indicate support of a specific version of the value set.

Another situation to be aware of is the deprecation or status (e.g., made inactive) of codes in an external code system. In such a case, the usage of the code needs to be clearly indicated in the specification. In the previous example, what if code '03' is made inactive by the external steward of the code system in the post specification space? Is it valid to continue to send the code? The answer depends on the value set specification tied to the anticipated use. If the value set is deemed to support newly administered vaccines, then the specification would indicate that inactive codes are now "excluded" and a new value set is created. However, if the use is for the messaging of historical vaccines, then the inactive codes are still valid (and therefore "required"). Separate value sets and bindings should be included in the specification to articulate the requirements precisely.

These examples illustrate the various ways in which a value set can be specified. The vocabulary profiling mechanism provides a flexibility utility such that a broad set of value sets can be specified.

An analysis should be performed for each coded element in the specification to determine which codes from a source code system are applicable for that particular element. Unfortunately, this level of definition usually does not occur in practice. Developers, therefore, must decide for themselves which codes apply to a particular element. For example, in many HL7 v2.x implementation guides, HL7 Table 0203 (identifier type) is universally applied to every element that includes an identifier type with no profiling (i.e., HL70203 is simply referred to or is copied as is from the base standard). There are over one hundred identifier types, and in most cases only a few of the codes are pertinent to any given data element. Figure 7.21 presents one possible solution for specifying the appropriate level of detail.

		Binding ID	1	2	3	4
Concept Domain = Identifier Type		**Strength**	R	R	R	R
		Extensibility	Closed	Open	Open	Open
Value Set Root Name = HL70203_USL		**Stability**	Static	Static	Static	Static
		Profile ID	LRI	LRI	LRI	LRI
		Binding	PID-3.5	PID-18.5	ORC-12.13	OBX-23.7
Value	**Description**		**Usage**	**Usage**	**Usage**	**Usage**
AN	Account Number		E	R	E	E
BA	Bank Account Number		E	E	E	E
DL	Drivers License Number		P	E	E	E
FI	Facility Identifier		E	E	E	R
MR	Medical Record Number		R	E	E	E
NPI	National Provider Identifier		P	E	R	P
PT	Patient External Identifier		R	E	E	E
SS	Social Security Number		P	E	E	E
XX	Organization Identifier		E	E	E	R

Location	Element Name (Identifier Type)	Value Set	Strength
PID-3.5	Patient Identifier List	HL70203_USL.1	R
PID-18-5	Patient Account Number	HL70203_USL.2	R
ORC-12.13	Ordering Provider	HL70203_USL.3	R
OBX-23.7	Performing Organization Name	HL70203_USL.4	R

Fig. 7.21 Creating a collection of value sets and binding to a data elements

The Identifier Type in HL7 v2.x is bound to a number of data types and is used in higher-level elements. In a given specification, many data elements will use the Identifier Type for many different purposes. The base standard provides a set of codes for common identifier types that apply to a broad spectrum of identifiers. This set can range from a medical record number to a bank account number. For a particular element, however, only a few of the codes might be applicable.

At the base standard level all codes in a code system can be implicitly considered Permitted, thus giving the most flexibility for specification in derived profiles. An analysis must be performed for each element that uses the code system in order to ascertain which codes actually do apply. Figure 7.21 shows a sample list of codes for HL7 Table 0203. It also indicates four elements to which this code system is bound in the base standard. For each binding, a value set is created that is shown in the form of a separate column. For the Patient Identifier List-Identifier Type (PID-3.5) element, analysis of the particular use case is necessary (e.g., analysis related to the Lab Results Interface (LRI) determined that support for the Medical Record Number (MR) and Patient External Identifier (PT) codes are required). The Driver's License Number (DL), National Provider Identifier (NPI), and Social Security Number (SS) codes are Permitted, while the rest of the codes are Excluded.[11] For the Patient Account Number-Identifier Type (PID-18.5) only the Account Number code is applicable. Value sets for Ordering Provider-Identifier Type (ORC-12.13) and Performing Organization Name-Identifier Type (OBX-23.7) are defined as well. In addition to specifying the usage for each code, other attributes for each element-specific value set are determined, such as the Binding Strength, Extensibility, and Stability. Essentially, the collection of value sets in Fig. 7.21 are domains for the concept of identifier type, and elements can be constrained by indicating the domain.

The table in the lower part of Fig. 7.21 shows examples of value set bindings that might appear in a specification (each row in the table would be in the associated element location in the specification). The upper part of the diagram shows the value set collection. Each column represents a value set and lists the associated attributes and vocabulary constraint usage for each code in the value set. Some of the attributes appear both in the specification and the value set collection, which allows for easy cross referencing (since they can be specified in separate documents).

The Binding ID is a qualifier to the Value Set Root Name (HL70203_USL) and, when combined, they provide the binding in the specification (e.g., HL70203_USL.3 is used to bind to the Identifier Type of the Ordering Provider element). The binding qualifier may be included as part of the binding definition in the specification (as shown in Fig. 7.21) or it may not be included. If the qualifier is

[11]For the complete HL70203 table many more codes would be listed, most of which would be "Excluded" with a handful set to "Permitted" for these four data elements.

not included in the specification (profile), then the profile and the value set collection are separated, which means the value sets could be changed without requiring changes to the specification. The approach promotes effective management of updates, however, versioning must be accounted for and stakeholders need to be notified.

Although these value sets are shown to be bound to particular elements for a particular profile, value sets are defined independently in order to promote reuse of the value set. As an example, perhaps several value sets could be created from the administrative gender code system, and then the different value sets could be referenced in many specifications (not only HL7 v2.x, but any other specification based on other standards such as CDA and FHIR). This approach to value set reuse requires broader vocabulary management.

7.6.4 Summary

As should be evident from the information presented in this section, the specification, profiling, and use of vocabulary is a complicated and convoluted subject. An attempt was made here to provide the basic concepts (in a generic fashion) and to provide insight as to the factors that should be considered. Every standard approaches the specification and profiling of vocabulary in a different way; there is no common methodology or glossary of terms. The approach presented here is representative of one school of thought and by no means expresses a consensus viewpoint. For each implementation project, the vocabulary model and approach of the given standard have to be examined and applied. The level of granularity presented here illustrates leading practice for the definition of element-specific value sets; however, many of the standards don't provide a rich enough vocabulary mechanism to enable achievement of this granularity. This issue should be addressed by all SDOs. The methods provided here are similar to a methodology that was proposed for HL7 v2.x and applied to the set of laboratory specifications developed as a Standards & Interoperability Framework project.

7.7 Vocabulary Management

The need for code systems and value sets to be updated creates issues for specifications and implementations. These updates have a very direct impact on implementations especially. This section provides some insight into the issues to help inform solutions for vocabulary management related to implementations.

7.7.1 Managing Code Systems

Figure 7.22 illustrates typical changes in code systems over time as new releases are published. Some codes are added, while others are made inactive. Note that it is a violation of good vocabulary practices to remove codes completely from a code system when a new version is released, as it makes interpretation of historical records difficult. Good practices recommend that if a code is removed from a code system, a new code system must be created. In Fig. 7.22 this is indicated with Code System "y" since code 'X" was removed.

In case that only codes are added without changing the semantics of the other codes, or codes are merely changed to inactive (or deprecated), then a new version is created. This is typically the case with terminologies like LOINC and SNOMED CT. Figure 7.23 depicts this situation.

A challenging issue arises when a code system contains the concept of "Other" or "Not otherwise Specified". This is a very common occurrence especially for classifications like the WHO code systems (the families of ICD), but also in many of the HL7 Version 2.x code systems (tables). When a code system has such a concept, then the meaning of this concept is dependent upon the other codes in the code system. If this group of other codes is changed in a new version, either by adding codes or removing codes, then the "Other" code has a changed meaning. The implication of this is that when historical records are accessed for analysis, the meaning of any records containing "Other" must be analyzed with all of the codes

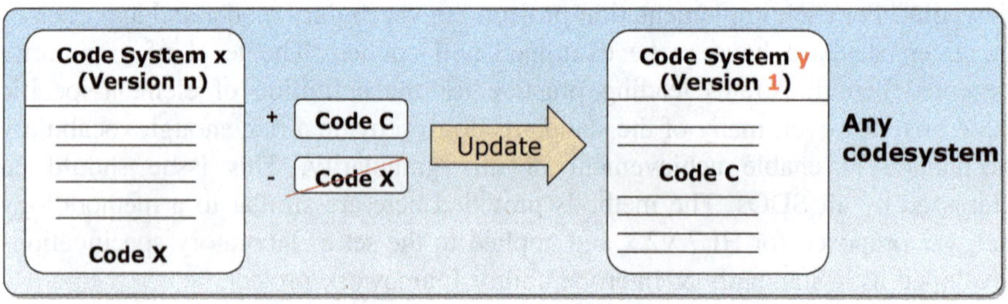

Fig. 7.22 Typical versioning of any code system

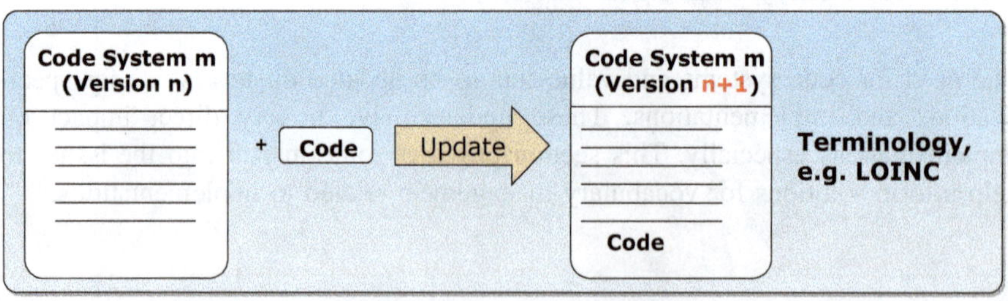

Fig. 7.23 Versioning of terminologies

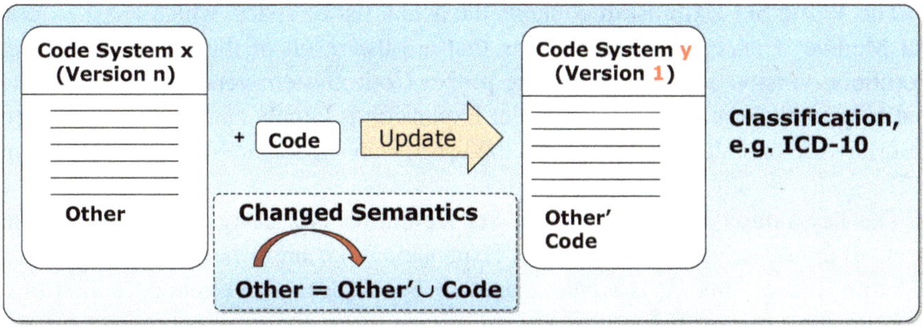

Fig. 7.24 Versioning of classifications

in that record being drawn from the version of the code system (and value set) in use at the time the record was created. If this is not done, then an incorrect assumption of the meaning of the record labeled with code "Other" may be made which can lead to invalid statistical analysis results or even patient safety issues. For this reason, it is very strongly recommended that when any records are stored using code systems that may contain the concept "Other", the code system version for each and every code value stored with the record also be stored. Figure 7.24 illustrates the update process for such classifications.

7.7.2 *Value Set Definition and Expansion*

A Value Set describes a collection of concepts drawn from one or more code systems grouped together for a specific purpose (e.g., orderable laboratory tests from LOINC). Note that the phrase "Value Set" usually is taken to mean both the *Value Set Definition* and the *Value Set Expansion*.

A **Value Set Definition** is a set of metadata that describes the scope of the intended member Concept Representations, provenance of the included information and, most importantly, a set of instructions that describe (always in a computable manner) which code system Concept Representations should be in the Value Set Expansion Code Set. As such, the Value Set Definition is then applied to one or more Code System instances to determine the Value Set Expansion Code Set Member Concept Representations. In essence, the Value Set Definition (specifically the Content Logical Definition described below) functions like a query into the Code System(s) to retrieve the concepts as described in the definition. This is true for every Value Set Definition. It is not restricted to only definitions that use a logical or "intentional" definition; it is also true for simple explicit lists of individually selected concepts. As long as the Value Set Definition is not locked to a single Code System version, even simple code lists can result in changing Value Set Expansion Code Sets if the codes in the original definition are retired in later Code System versions [17].

The **Value Set Expansion** contains the actual list of codes, which are the Code Set Member Concept Representations that are the result of the proper Value Set Definition version applied against the proper Code System version. The metadata that may be associated with a Value Set Expansion is largely confined to that which describes the operation that produced the list of codes from the Value Set Definition [17].

The key notion is that the Value Set Definition is a design and specification oriented construct, and the Value Set Expansion is an implementation construct.

From time to time, it is advantageous to NOT specify an explicit version of a code system in the Value Set Definition, in order to essentially delegate the updating of the code list in the value set to the publishers of the code system. Such Value Set Definitions are known as '*Dynamic Value Sets*'.

7.7.3 Managing Dynamic Value Sets

The concept of stability was discussed earlier. A value set can be specified as either static or dynamic. The term "dynamic" implies possible "automatic" changes without editing the definition. These changes occur in a controlled, managed, and documented fashion. At a given point in time, a dynamic vocabulary has the characteristics of a static vocabulary because the expansion can be enumerated explicitly. A stability of *dynamic* is only an indication that the vocabulary can change outside the space of a version of an interoperability specification or profile. Figure 7.25 illustrates this point.

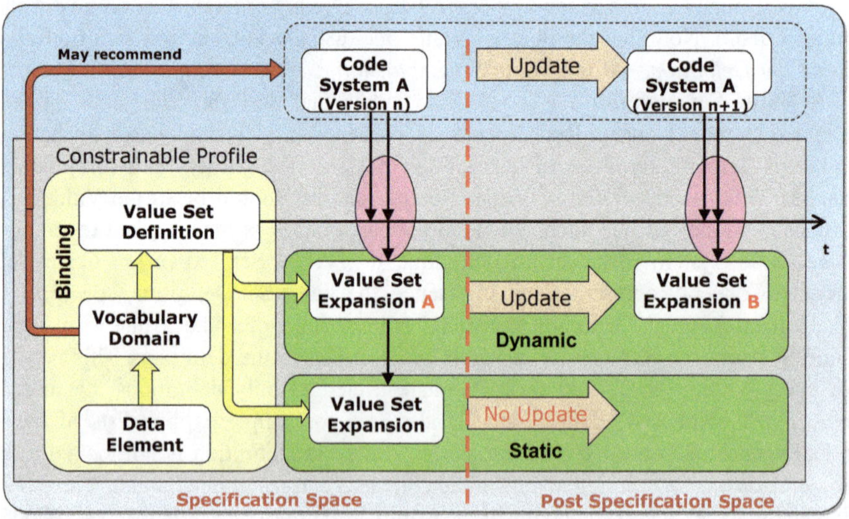

Fig. 7.25 Updating a code system to a new expansion

Figure 7.25 presents the various factors that have to be considered in the design and management of vocabulary specifications. The left side of the diagram indicates concepts and actions that are made during the development of the specification. For a particular data element, a vocabulary binding is made. Eventually, the binding is made to a specific value set definition. For a static binding, the value set expansion is fixed and remains fixed in the specification and post specification space (lower green box). The source of the value set expansion can be a specific version of a code system that will not be updated.

If the stability of the vocabulary binding is dynamic (upper green box in Fig. 7.25), then an updated version of the code system may be specified in the post specification space. The value set definition remains the same but the value set expansion changes (i.e., the codes in the value set are different). The pink circles in Fig. 7.25 indicate this expansion process.

Note that a value set itself may have the characteristic of 'static' or 'dynamic', but this characteristic may also be applied by the binding. Specifically, a value set that has been published by an external terminology authority as having dynamic stability may have a binding which 'locks it down' for a particular profile to be static. Note however, that a value set whose definition is 'static' cannot be made dynamic in the profile; the property of 'static' cannot be overruled.

Another common situation is the replacement of a code system that may especially occur with classifications like ICD10. WHO as the responsible terminology authority provides updates on a regular basis formally leading to a new code system. The intent of the value set definition is to use the newest code system. In such a case, the value set expansion is updated with the codes from the new code system which is shown with Fig. 7.26. Note however that this operation does not

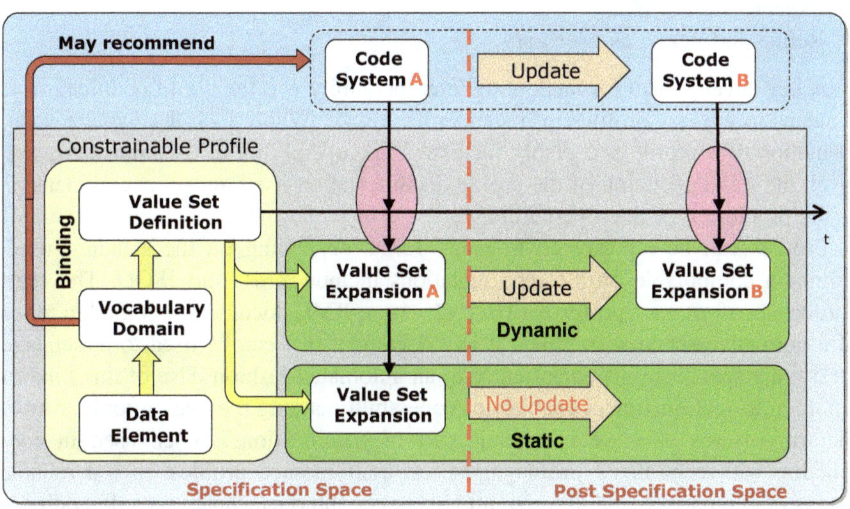

Fig. 7.26 Replacing code systems in a value set definition

happen 'automatically' as in the case when a new code system version is made available; it must be an explicit change to the Value Set Definition (updating it to a new version).

7.8 Uses of Conformance Profiles

A message profile applies use case specific constraints to the base standard in order to eliminate the potential ambiguities and implementation alternatives that the standard permits. Whether the underlying interface architecture is point-to-point or brokered through middleware, profiles give organizations a better way to manage system integration. Profiles can be used to implement an interface directly. All partners who have agreed to use the interface view the message profile as a contract specifying the exact behavior expected of each participating application. The basic steps that an analyst performs to design and implement an interface are summarized below. Message profiles can help with every step.

- Analyze the needs of the interface to determine requirements, including the use case, the dynamic interactions, the static definition (content), and the vocabulary.
- Document the interface in a standard way, e.g., using a message profile.
- Implement the interface. Profiles support automated code generation [e.g., HAPI] and mapping of internal data to interfaces.
- Develop a test plan; include creation of the test cases, generation of test messages, and building of test tools; the test plan should account for syntactic, semantic, and use case scenario testing, and the handling of error conditions.
- Execute the test plan.
- Refine and iterate as necessary.

A key development for facilitating interoperability was the use of codification as a means to express profiles in a standardized way. While natural language documentation of a profile acceptably facilitates interoperability at the implementation level, the standardization of the profile documentation itself adds a new dimension to the promotion of interoperability.

Profiles can be represented in many forms depending on the standard used. Common computable profile representations include XML and JSON. The standardized conformance profile for HL7 v2.x is an XML document specified in terms of a normative schema. In effect, it is a document that can be used to understand messaging specifications consistently in an automated fashion. Use of this kind of common format document enables interoperability among messaging tools, which, in turn, ensures effective communication of specifications. When used in conjunction with centralized profile registries, conformance profiles offer a reliable means of comparison and differentiation between interface capabilities. In addition, the profile may be used as a common basis for highlighting vendors' value-added product features, such as profile-directed code generation and profile-directed message automation. Another important outcome from the development of the standard message profile is the ability to use the profile directly in message instance validation, as employed by the NIST EHR certification conformance test tools [14, 18, 19, 20] and IHE Gazelle [21]. Machine computable profiles are also leveraged in HL7 CDA, FHIR, and other standards.

Although the practice is not recommended, the standards allow for creation of localizations (e.g., "Z" elements in HL7 v2.x) that give users the ability to extend the standard in a way that satisfies site-specific needs. Prior to the existence of profiles, documentation of localizations was ad hoc. Through the use of profiles, localizations can be clearly documented and, therefore, tested.

7.9 Profile Design and Management

This section presents an approach for designing and managing profiles such that profiles and profile components can be leveraged. When writing a set of related profiles (or a family of profiles, such as those in IHE or for a particular domain such as laboratory orders and results) it is important to reuse the profile and profile components in order to harmonize the requirements and to gain efficiency. The concepts of the profile hierarchy and profile components provide an effective approach for managing and documenting extensions.

Figures 7.27, 7.28, 7.29 and 7.30 illustrate possible configurations for composing a family of related profiles. The design principle is to develop a common or base profile component that applies across a family of profiles with the intention of using the profile component concept to specify *complete* profiles.

In the first depiction (Fig. 7.27), a base profile component is developed that expresses all of the common requirements for a related set of profiles. Profile component 1 and profile component 2 are also created for aspects that are not defined in the base profile component. Combined, the three profile components are used to describe a complete specification, Profile 1.

For the second depiction (Fig. 7.28), the base profile component and profile component 1 are reused and combined with profile component 3 to specify Profile

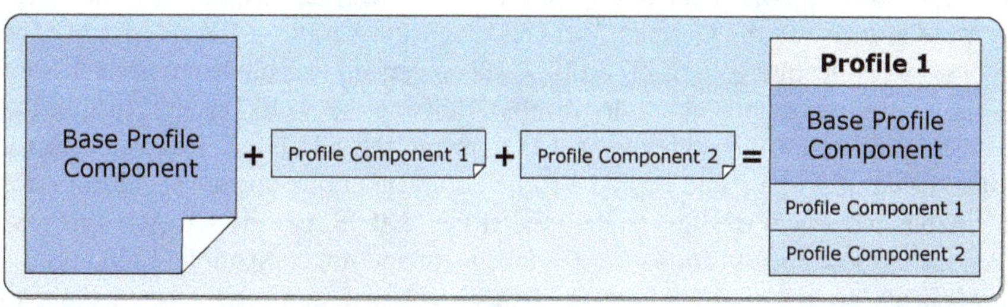

Fig. 7.27 Profile design principles—Example 1

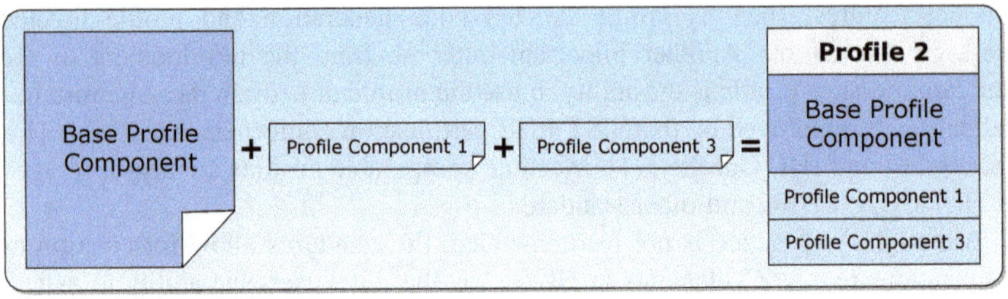

Fig. 7.28 Profile design principles—Example 2

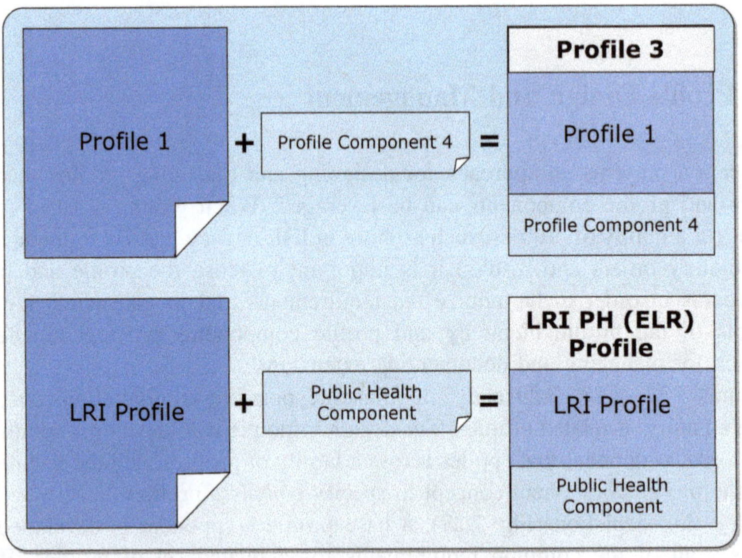

Fig. 7.29 Profile design principles—Example 3

2. In the third depiction (Fig. 7.29), Profile 1 is combined with profile component 4 to create Profile 3. Example 3 demonstrates how use case expansions can be managed. Using this approach, the ONC S&I Framework working groups developed a set of HL7 v2.5.1 laboratory profiles, and HL7 v2.5 message profiles were built in Germany as the German National Extension based on IHE ITI PAM. The laboratory results interface (LRI) profiles were extended to include requirements for public health (reportable laboratory results). Relating this to Example 3, Profile 1 is the LRI profile, profile component 4 documents the additional requirements for public health reporting, and Profile 3 is the complete public health specification for reportable laboratory results (called Electronic Lab Reporting—ELR). Previous versions of these specifications were independent and not compatible. Using profile components provides an efficient mechanism to reuse and repurpose in order to

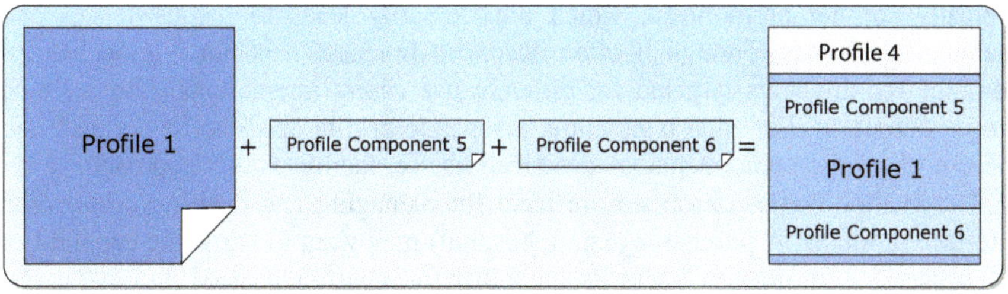

Fig. 7.30 Profile design principles—Example 4

accommodate a different, but closely related, use case. Profile components also help reduce implementation efforts by clearly indicating the essential differences.

Profile components can also express new requirements that replace requirements established in a base profile component or profile. This approach often is used when different levels of profiles are developed, or when the profile provides utility outside the original intent of the profile. The forth depiction (Fig. 7.30) illustrates a case where a subset of requirements for an existing profile are overridden. Here, Profile 1 is used; however, certain aspects are redefined according to the constraint rules and are documented in profile components 5 and 6, which results in Profile 4. It is important to note that if the new profile is intended to be a refinement in the existing profile hierarchy, then the requirement replacement is limited to further constraints (in essence, this is a level). However, if the intent is to establish a new specification to address a similar (but different) use case, then there is no restriction on the requirement replacement since it is a new profile (i.e., it is not intended to be a specialization of the original). Here, the use of profile components is a mechanism to leverage an existing specification.

For each of the complete specifications illustrated in Figs. 7.27, 7.28, 7.29, and 7.30, the resulting profile can be a constrainable or an implementable profile.

The key design principle involved is that when related specifications are being developed, the authors should leverage as much information as possible from existing profiles, or they should design/create base profiles that are a harmonization of requirements for a related set of use cases. The profile components can be developed at any level of granularity; however, caution should be exercised when creating profile components at a fine-grained level or when specifying numerous details. Often, having to manage many building block artifacts can outweigh the benefits these artifacts are supposed to provide. If management tooling is available, then fine granularity of profile components is attainable. A good practice is to introduce an orthogonal structure of the individual requirements (e.g., data type constraints) in one case, message fragments (e.g., for insurance or diagnosis data) in a second case, and value set definitions in another instance, which would allow for easy integration and combinations (i.e., a data type specialization should not include a specific value set binding, as it significantly reduces the ability to reuse).

Frequently, standards developers fully specify each of a related set of profiles, entailing duplication of sizeable sections of the standards document. These profiles typically are not harmonized, which unnecessarily leads to inconsistences and maintenance issues. Though it often occurs in practice, it is not a good idea to combine requirements targeted for different use cases (interactions) into a single profile definition. For each interaction, a separate profile needs to be defined, and the use of profile components, as described above, facilitates this approach.

The methodologies described are ideal for managing and creating customized interface products. A purchaser (e.g., a hospital) may want to know the capabilities of an interface in order to assess its suitability for a particular need. In most cases, the vendor provides an interface that supports many features, most of which typically are driven by market demand. The system is designed to be configurable so as to support a variety of specific interface needs. The use and documentation of profiles is a powerful mechanism to manage system configurations. In essence, each installation of an interface is an implementable profile whether it is documented explicitly or not. All of these aspects can be described exactly in the form of profiles as well. The vendor might publish what could be called a "configurable implementable profile", which declares the implementation capabilities and allows a prospective purchaser to compare the profile to their needs. Once an interface has been installed, the capabilities are clearly defined and configured as the implementable profile, and, ideally, this profile is documented.

7.9.1 Profile Identification Management

To simplify profile management and claims of conformance, an identification mechanism for the base profile, profile components, and the coordinated profile is important. In principle, all of these items can be managed the same way. In HL7 v2.x, this management typically is achieved by using OIDs. In message instances, the claim of conformance is indicated by a profile identifier or a series of profile component identifiers. Using the ELR example above, a pre-coordinated identifier could be created and messaged; or the LRI profile and ELR profile component identifiers could be messaged. In either case, each claim refers to the same set of requirements. Any receiving system or validation tool then knows exactly what to expect and process accordingly.

7.9.2 Publishing the Specification

An important design principle for publishing the specifications is to avoid creating numerous new specifications when each one expresses only small variances in requirements from an original specification. Producing essentially duplicate specifications in this manner causes management and maintenance issues later on when modifications are made in the base profile component. If possible, the profile should be part of the original specification and should be distinguished as a profile variance through the profile component mechanism (and assigned a profile component identifier). If, however, the new profile is created after the profile from which it is derived is published, then only the variations from that original profile should be published in the new specification. Often this new specification document will consist of only a few short pages, allowing the implementers to be alerted quickly and efficiently to the modifications from the original (base) profile.

If the specification is developed via an authoring tool, then the user is afforded various options for publishing since the tool is handling the rendering and maintenance. NIST is developing such a tool to enable this manipulation of profiles for HL7 v2 (See Chap. 9, ref. [10]). IGAMT builds upon the concepts developed in the Messaging Workbench (MWB) [11, 12]. The tool will allow for the development of the profile components; and, since all artifacts related to the profile are machine processable within the tool, the user will have the option to publish a specification that just expresses the variances of a profile, that expresses the complete profile, or that is composed of other artifacts, such as the XML representation of the profile.

Another tool is ART-DECOR [22], which supports the development, maintenance, and testing of templates for CDA. This toolkit follows the same basic principles although the profile hierarchy paradigm is not developed to the degree described above.

7.10 Pairing Sender and Receiver Profiles for Use

Profiles document a set of requirements (or capabilities) for systems. A profile is applicable to a sender, a receiver, or to both if a common expectation is sought. An interaction profile pair associates a sending profile and a receiving profile, e.g., for an ADT message. A profile pair at the transaction level is for the initiator and the responder, e.g., an ADT message and an ACK message. The focus of this section is on the interaction profile pair.

Sender and receiver profiles can be paired in various ways to satisfy a targeted use. The profile pair binding can have various patterns including:

- One-to-one
- One-to-many
- Many-to-one

Regardless of the profile pairing pattern, a set of expectations is specified in a *higher-level* constrainable profile for each sender and receiver in the use case. In practice, the expectations can vary substantially. For example, in one case the sender and receiver may have mutual expectations about how the data are processed, and in another case the sender may be agnostic about how the data are processed. Any combination of the profile pairing patterns and processing expectations is valid.

It is important to note again that the use case defines these expectations, because it describes how the sender and receiver are interpreting requirements for the same message. In the subsections that follow, a representative set of profile pairings are presented along with general expectations of the sender and receiver in the context of a given use case, however, the details about a specific use case are not considered.

7.10.1 One-to-One Profile Pairing

A common profile pairing is an exchange between a sender and receiver in which there are mutual expectations. In this case, the sender and the receiver share the same (or nearly the same) profile and, therefore, implement a common set of requirements. An example is the US Realm Laboratory Results Interface (LRI), where the sender has an expectation that the receiver will process and use the data in a prescribed way. From a regulatory perspective in the US, the Clinical Laboratory Improvement Amendments (CLIA) places the responsibility on the sender (i.e., the Laboratory) for ensuring that the laboratory results are correctly consumed, processed, and displayed by the receiving system (e.g., an EHR). As such, nearly identical constrainable profiles are specified to meet the requirements of the use case.

Figure 7.31 illustrates that a common profile is used, which signifies mutual expectations for the data exchange. The use case documents how the profile pair is to be utilized.

In another example, the profile pairing may exhibit the one-to-one pattern, but it may not have strongly-correlated expectations about how the exchanged data are handled. Again, these expectations are described in the *higher-level* use case.

Note that in this example, and the examples to follow, an examination of the requirements and their compatibility is limited to the usage conformance construct in order to simplify the explanation of the concept. Analogous analysis applies to the other constraints. In Fig. 7.31, the common expectation for the sender and receiver is indicated by the same usage settings.

7.10.2 One-to-Many Profile Pairing

The one-to-many profile pairing pattern typically is used for broadcast applications in which there is loose correlation of sender and receiver expectations. The sender has no or limited expectations about how the receiver processes and uses the data. The sender is providing a *service* for the receivers. It is the responsibility of a receiver to ensure that the sender is providing the information necessary to complete the particular use case. An example is the ADT (Admissions, Discharge, and Transfers) use case. Typically, ADT systems will broadcast a patient's information

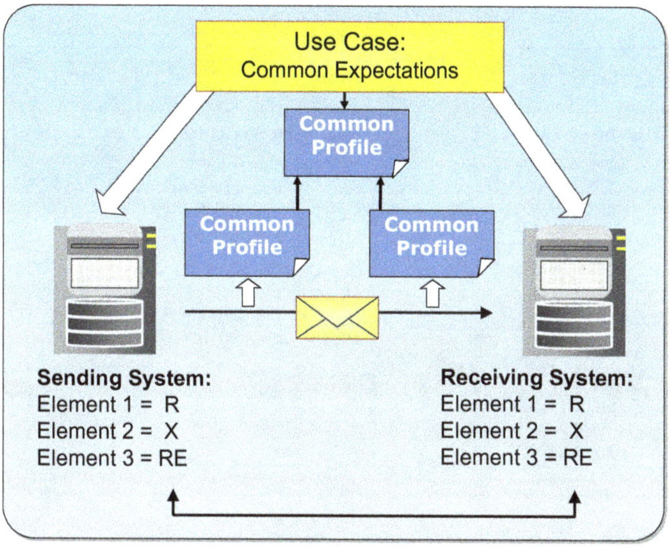

Fig. 7.31 One-to-one profile pairing pattern (mutual expectations)

to a number of other systems (which may be internal or external to the sending entity). In such a case, the sender will provide as much information as possible about the patient. This information can be documented in a profile and implemented by the sender. The sender is providing an indication of what it is able to give. The requirements for the sender often are derived from the collective set of receiver requirements, which is typically fluid, as receiver requirements can change and/or other receivers can be added to the network. Each receiver can provide a profile to indicate what it needs. In essence, the sender profile is a *superset* of the receiver requirements.

Figure 7.32 illustrates a single sending system along with three receiving systems and excerpts from their profiles. As shown, the sending system profile provides support for all the elements needed by all of the receiving systems. For example, for Receiver 1, the sending system sends Elements 1 and 2, and if known, Element 3. This set of elements satisfies the needs of Receiver 1, because this receiver requires Element 1 (which is supported by the Sender), does not need Element 2 (and will discard it), and does support and will process Element 3 if it is provided by the sender. The *higher-level* use case indicates the expectations of the sender and receiver. Each receiver has its own use case that informs what data are to be received from sender (and, hence, defines the sender profile). The sender has no expectation about how the data are processed by the receiver—this processing requirement is specified in the *higher-level* use case. The profiles in this pair are compatible with each other, since the receivers are provided the data they are requesting.

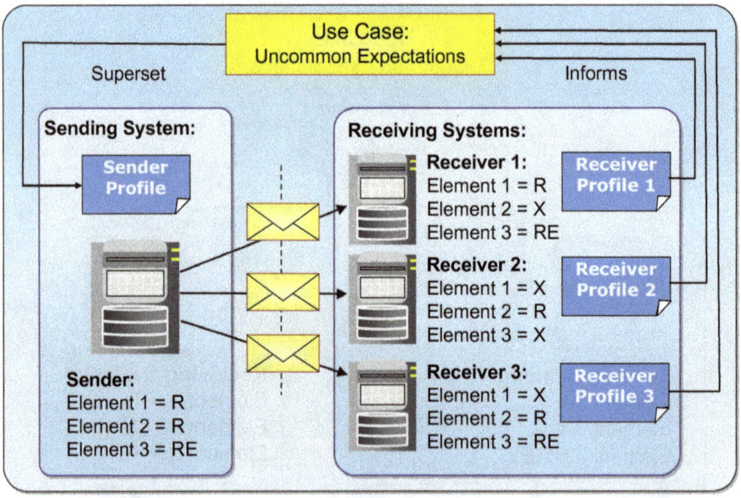

Fig. 7.32 One-to-many profile pairing pattern (receiver-side expectations)

Profile compatibility is covered in more detail in Chap. 8. However, a brief discussion is warranted here to explain why Fig. 7.32 shows that the pairing of a sender usage of R (or RE) and a receiver usage of X is allowed (and is compatible). Compatibility is a concept that is considered from the receiver's perspective. A simple question used to assess compatibility is: will the receiver be provided the information it needs? In this example, and unlike the example of mutual expectations, the sender has limited expectations or responsibility for the treatment of the data that are sent. The need for the data is driven by the business requirements of the receiver. The receiver takes the information it needs to fulfill its use case and ignores (processes and discards) unwanted data. If the sender had expectations about the processing of one or more data elements, then these expectations are documented in the *higher-level* constrainable profile, and both sending and receiving profiles would specify a usage of *required* for each element for which there is a common expectation.

7.10.3 Many-to-One Profile Pairing

The many-to-one profile pairing pattern is typically for use cases in which there is a single collection point for data. Figure 7.33 illustrates a case where multiple senders exchange information with a single receiver. This situation is common in the public health arena where, for example, multiple providers send data to an Immunization Information System (IIS).

For this example, the use case defines a common set of messaging requirements (as indicated by the common usage settings in Fig. 7.33). As with the previous

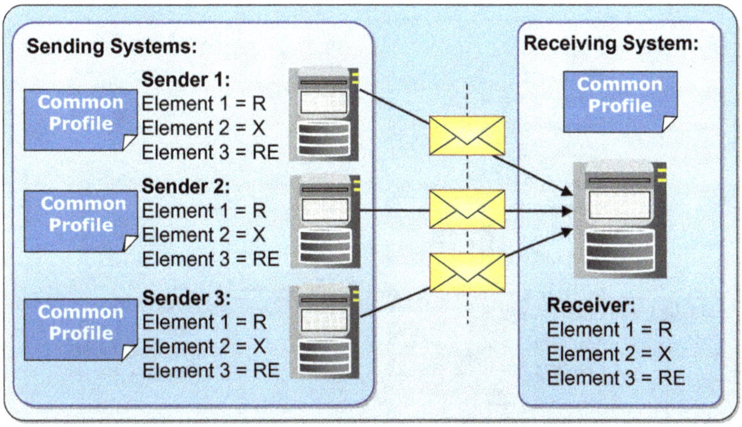

Fig. 7.33 Many-to-one profile pairing pattern (Example 1)

examples, these requirements, along with the processing expectation, are defined in the common *higher-level* constrainable profile (not shown in this diagram). The processing expectations can be mutual (more or less), sender side oriented, or receiver side oriented. In the case of the US national guidance for immunization, the processing expectations are mutual (more or less) for the sender and the receiver. This use case is explored below and is related to the many-to-one profile paring pattern.

In immunization systems, two basic types of information are collected: patient identifying information and vaccination events. The IIS is not the source of truth for the patient identifying information, so the patient identifying information is generally loosely correlated in the exchange. The submitter provides patient identifying information to allow patient matching and consolidation of immunization histories, but the submitter is agnostic about how the IIS processes or records patient identifying information. However, the IIS is tasked with storing and creating a complete vaccination history, so the sender expects the IIS to accept and store all submitted vaccinations,[12] which must be available for retrieval later. In this regard, the vaccination requirements between the sender and receiver are mutual (strongly-correlated).

As shown in Fig. 7.33, the data collected by the receiver are provided by many sources, and, therefore, the information about a particular patient may not match the information of any individual sender (provider). For example, an IIS may have information about a patient from both a doctor's office and a pharmacy. Some data

[12]In this case, the sender's expectation is in a "collective" sense. For a particular instance, data may be processed and discarded because the receiver recognizes that the data are duplicate and the existing data are of better *quality*. A typical case is where the receiver has data from the provider who administered the vaccine and the duplicate data newly received are a historical recollection provided by the patient.

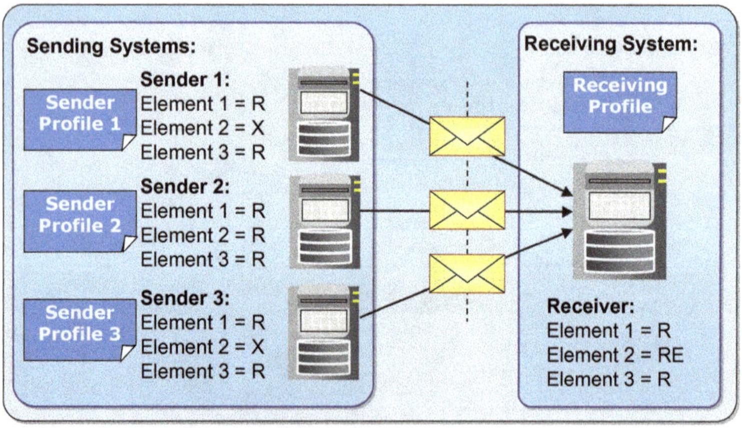

Fig. 7.34 Many-to-one profile pairing pattern (Example 2)

may be submitted by both sources (such as patient demographics) while other data may be unique to one system or the other (such as childhood immunization information from the doctor's office and a recent influenza immunization from a pharmacy). The *high-level* use case would address this situation. An individual sender would expect the IIS to handle the information they submitted, but also would expect it to handle additional and modified data.

It is important to note that expectations set for particular data elements will vary according to each use case. In some cases, the expectation may be to process and store received data, and in other cases it may be to make the data available to perform a function and then discard them. For example, patient demographic data are sent within the immunization scenario, but there is limited or no expectation that these data will replace the data that exist in the IIS. An individual provider usually is not the source of these data. In this case, the data are needed by the receiver to seek a match to an existing patient. Once the function is performed the data may be discarded.

A similar case is where not all senders have the capabilities desired by the receiver. As shown in Fig. 7.34, Sender 1 and Sender 3 are not capable of supporting a certain requirement. For example, a particular EHR-S may not be capable of reporting refused vaccines, however, other systems in the network support this capability, and the information is useful to the IIS. In this case, the receiver publishes a profile that includes the *superset* of sender capabilities (or, more appropriately, the receiver's *wish list*), but does not require support of all capabilities desired. In the example presented in Fig. 7.34, this situation is indicated by the designation of "RE" usage for Element 2. If the data are provided, the receiver can process the information, but the receiver is not dependent on the data to operate. To reiterate, it is the use case that sets the expectations and describes the relationship between the sending and receiving profiles.

7.10.4 Design Considerations: Profiling Pairing

A design question to consider is: should all profile pairings adhere to the one-to-one pattern? In this paradigm, the sender and receiver share the same (or nearly the same) profile and, thus, expectation about the handling of the data from the sender and receiver perspective is documented in the profile. Take, for example, the use case where the sender is broadcasting to a set of receivers. The sending system documents, in the form of a profile, the superset of requirements that accommodates all receivers. The sending system extracts information from its data model, maps the data to the superset profile, and sends a superset message. When additional requirements are needed in the receiver set, additional provisions are made. The sender unilaterally updates its profile and then broadcasts updated messages.[13] The receivers, based on an original agreement, are prepared to accept unexpected data and deal with them appropriately. Such fluid expectations have advantages in terms of efficiency, operational tolerance, and expansion of capabilities with little or no negotiations in operating interfaces. Alternatively, the sender could tailor messages based on each receiver's profile. Upon data extraction from the data model, the sender maps the data and creates a message specific to a particular receiver based on the negotiated profile. This tight association binds the sending and receiving set of requirements together. There is no ambiguity between what the sender is providing and what the receiver is expecting. The receiver always gets what it expects and nothing more. The robustness of the interface sets a clear expectation and reduces the chance of misconceptions and, therefore, error in interpreting and using the data. The downside of this approach is the increased effort involved in each sender/receiver negotiation and interface implementation. The practicality of this approach also must be considered: is it feasible or optimal to implement it in today's environments? In some circumstances there are clear benefits, in others, maybe not; but achieving the goal of tight associations may reduce gaps in the interoperability bridge. Implementers need to examine the use case and weigh the trade-offs relative to cost and effectiveness.

7.11 Case Studies

7.11.1 Localization Using Profile Components

Applying the combination of the profile hierarchy, profiles, and profile components provides an effective way to manage local specifications. A typical domain for which localization is needed is public health, where a national-level profile is created and additional requirements (constraints) are specified at the state- or jurisdictional-level. A constrainable profile for the national level is created for a

[13]This is an underlying basic principle of many data exchange standards such as HL7 v2.

particular interaction (e.g., send immunization record). State level requirements could be expressed in a profile component. When combined with the national-level profile, the result expresses the complete requirements for the state.

This method naturally forms a hierarchy that indicates one profile is a "proper" constraint of the other. The national-level profile is a constrainable profile and the state profile is an implementable profile (assuming all optionality has been constrained) or a further constrained constrainable profile. Conformance claim is made to the most constrained profile (e.g., the state-level profile).

Figure 7.35 illustrates how states can leverage the national-level profile and refine it for their local requirements. Given that vendors may implement their products to support the national-level requirements, the state could provide them with the additional requirements documented in a profile component. It is anticipated that the states will have minimal additional data requirements, therefore, most variations probably will be in different value set definitions and bindings. In this case, the efforts for the vendors are reduced to a minimum, since value set adjustments are everyday business when installing new interfaces. This mechanism provides an effective approach for both the vendors and states to manage the variations.

Tooling can aid in the management of these variations. NIST's IGAMT tool is specifically designed and streamlined to support the localization requirements presented here. In this tool, the national-level profile is pre-loaded, and then modifications are made to that profile based on the local requirements. The delta between the two versions, along with explanatory text, can be published for each local profile. In addition, the end user obtains the benefits derived from the machine computable profile, including a customized conformance validation tool. More information is provided on this topic in Chaps. 9 and 11.

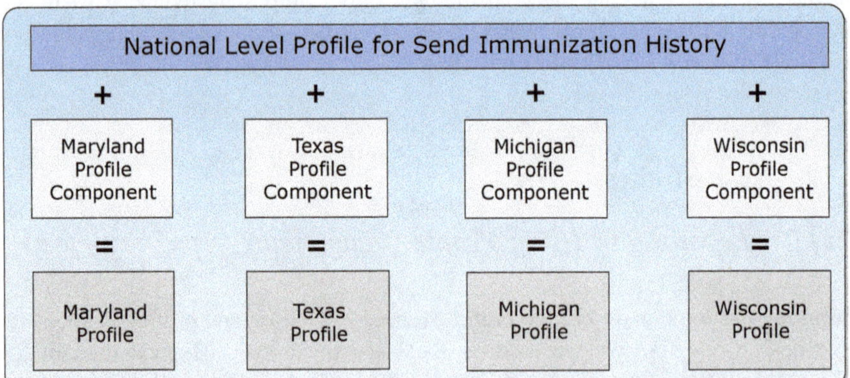

Fig. 7.35 Managing localizations using profile components

7.11.2 IHE Integration Profile

The different IHE Technical Frameworks for the various domains also provide some good examples of how profiles can be leveraged. The primary purpose of each framework is to define workflows by specializing appropriate messages or documents. IHE allows for further localizations, which have been accomplished, for example, with the French and German National Extensions to IHE ITI Patient Administration Management (PAM). Both of these localizations specify further requirements on the national level in the form of constrainable profiles. Users have the latitude to define additional requirements for their individual use cases in the form of profile components or derived profiles.

7.11.3 Laboratory Orders, Results, and Public Health

Combining the concepts of profiling and profiling components in the form of a profile hierarchy provides an effective and flexible manner in which to organize variations in related specifications. Figure 7.36 illustrates another example of how profiling is used to organize and manage a set of related profiles for specifying laboratory orders, laboratory results, and reportable laboratory results to public health. This example is taken from the S&I Framework family of laboratory HL7 v2.5.1 implementations guides. For the purpose of illustration, a simplified profile organization is shown (i.e., only a subset of the profiles and profile components are presented versus all that are contained in the family of implementation guides). See [15, 23] for details.

To provide context for this discussion, Fig. 7.37 shows the laboratory interoperability solution and each interaction as it relates to the in-scope ONC Health IT certification criteria.[14] Since it is critical that all of the specifications in the solution are compatible, a concerted effort was made to ensure that concepts and object instantiations were in alignment. Profile components, and reuse of those components, facilitated this design goal.

The workflow starts with the LIS sending the laboratory order compendium to the EHR-S, indicating the orderable laboratory tests that the specified clinical laboratory supports. The EHR-S incorporates this order list and associates it with the particular laboratory. When a lab test needs to be performed for a patient, a provider uses the EHR-S capabilities to select from this list (and possibly other lists as well) to order the lab test. This action triggers the LOI event. The LOI message is sent to the appropriate LIS system being used by the clinical laboratory. The lab order message is received by the LIS, the laboratory performs the test that was

[14]To simplify the diagram, the acknowledgement interactions are omitted, which is not to diminish their importance. When errors occur, correct recognition and response by the receiving system is a critical aspect of this workflow.

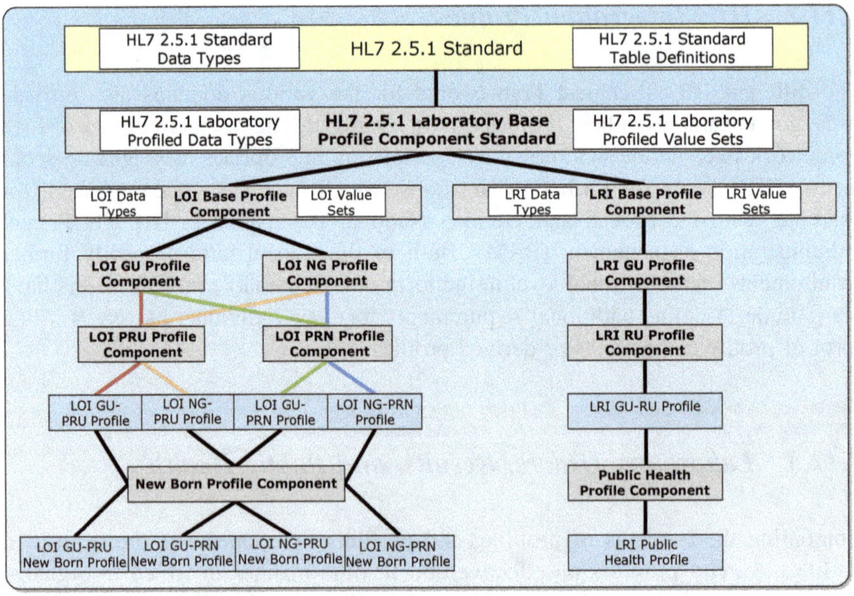

Fig. 7.36 Lab orders and results profile organization [this diagram shows a representative profile subset and possible profile organization for the laboratory interoperability solution (not the actual realization defined in the LOI and LRI implementation guides)]

ordered, and the LIS responds back to the EHR-S with one or more LRI messages (containing lab results). The EHR-S subsequently associates the lab results with the appropriate patient record in the EHR-S, and incorporates the results. If the results are for a "reportable" lab, then the EHR-S creates and sends an electronic laboratory results public health message (listed in the diagram as ELR, since this acronym was the original name used for this interface) to a public health agency.[15] The ELR interaction is based on the LRI profile with the addition of the public health component. The EHR-S typically takes the LRI results received from the LIS and adds other patient information to this interaction to create the public health message (as prescribed by the profile component).

The workflow described represents one path through this landscape; many others exist. The diagram indicates some of the more prevalent workflows, including workflows where the LISs are being used in commercial laboratories, which are where most lab reports to public health originate.

Figure 7.36 illustrates a subset of profiles for the interoperability solution shown in Fig. 7.37. All derived profiles originate from the standard profile. The goal is to manage a number of related profiles that are specified in multiple interface solutions.

[15]This workflow coincides with the ONC 2014 Edition Certification criteria. The more likely scenario is that the LIS sends the reportable results directly to Public Health. Both scenarios are valid and in both cases the ELR specification is applicable.

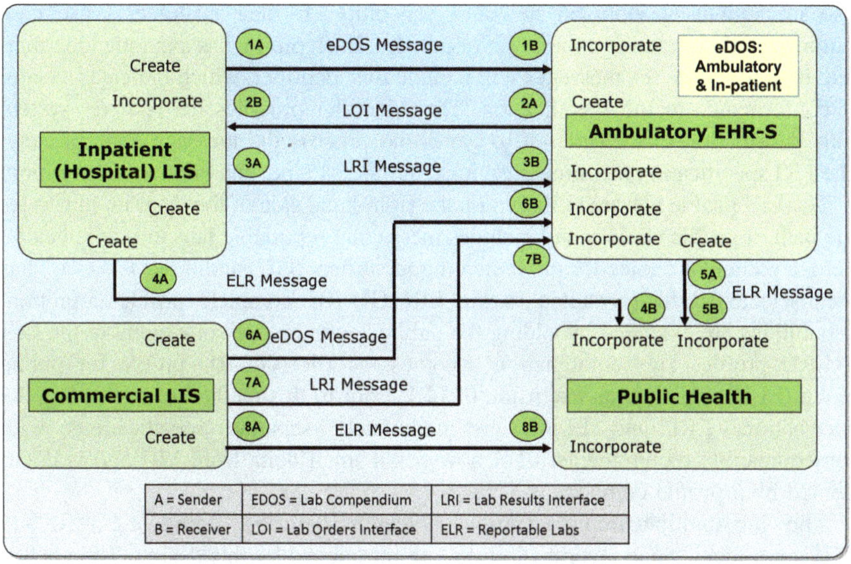

Fig. 7.37 Laboratory interoperability solution

The fact that there are multiple implementation guides is irrelevant; however, these guides do provide a logical separation of the use cases. When grouped together and supplemented with functional requirements, the laboratory interoperability solution is comparable to the IHE's integration profiles.

The first level of profiling involves creating a common set of requirements that can be applied across the spectrum of the set of laboratory specifications. Data type specializations are the most prevalent profiling activity at this level. Here, a common set of data type variations can be established and used in each of the profiles. This is an important step, since the set of transactions will need to have a harmonized set of data elements in many cases. A further refinement is made at the LOI and LRI profiling levels. Here, further specializations of data types are realized and specific value sets are defined. For example, at the standard-level, a particular table may have been established that is all-encompassing for the lab workflow in general; however, some codes are unnecessary or illogical for a given use case and interface definition. This level of specification is appropriate at this stage.

The lab specifications support various options for unique identifiers and for unique order and filler requisition numbers. These implementation choices are documented as profile components and are designated as GU (Globally Unique Identifiers), NG (Non-globally Unique Identifiers), PRU (Unique Placer Order Number), PRN (Non-Unique Placer Order Number), etc., for LOI. The GU and NG components are also used in the LRI specification. The left side of the Lab Orders and Results Profile Organization diagram (Fig. 7.36) shows the various LOI implementation choices and how they produce four combinations. Vendors may also implement an optional newborn capability (if their customer's use case requires it), thus creating another set of profiles. Each profile has a unique identifier, and, in production, the messages will include this identifier, which indicates a claim of conformance to the specification. This identifier provides the receiver system with information that enables it to parse and process the message appropriately. The LRI specification has similar options, but they are not shown in the illustration.

The LRI profile hierarchy shown on the right-hand side of the diagram illustrates one path of profile choices and includes messaging reportable labs to public health. Here, a particular choice for implementing identifiers (GU) and order IDs (RU) has been selected, which resulted in the LRI GU-RU complete profile definition. Capabilities are extended by adding the public health profile component to the LRI GU-RU profile. This combination becomes the LRI GU-RU profile for public health (ELR), which is an extension of LRI. Prior to this method of organizing the information, LRI and ELR were completely separate specifications with non-compatible requirements. ELR now has a small delta from LRI and is documented by a profile component.

Allowing multiple implementation choices as described above, e.g., GU and NG, is not ideal, since incompatibilities are introduced by this design. The goal of the standards community is the use of globally unique identifiers; however, given the current state of vendors' systems, a bridge that allows both GU and NG identifiers was deemed necessary for the near term. The profiling mechanisms provide a straight-forward way to accommodate this need. As demonstrated, the profiling mechanism can be used to manage a series of related specifications in an efficient manner.

7.11.4 HL7 v2.x Message Profiles (in Germany)

Figure 7.38 depicts the profile hierarchy used in Germany. Based on the original standards, a translation (i.e., interpretation) was created from 1993 to 2003. This version is widely accepted in Germany and is used as the basis for many implementations, although it has never passed an official balloting process. In Fig. 7.38, this fact is represented by the hatched background. This version also is used as the basis for the message profiles that were created and balloted by HL7 Germany and are, thus, regarded as normative for use in Germany. On this basis, vendors can then define and implement any additional constraints following the profiling rules, as is shown in the lower part of Fig. 7.38.

The constrainable profiles were built in the form of a hierarchy consisting of a foundation specifying basic profile components and specific message profiles by combining the profile components. For example, three different profiles for Admission were defined. The message header in the message instance should specify which variation (profile) is intended (i.e., to be transmitted):

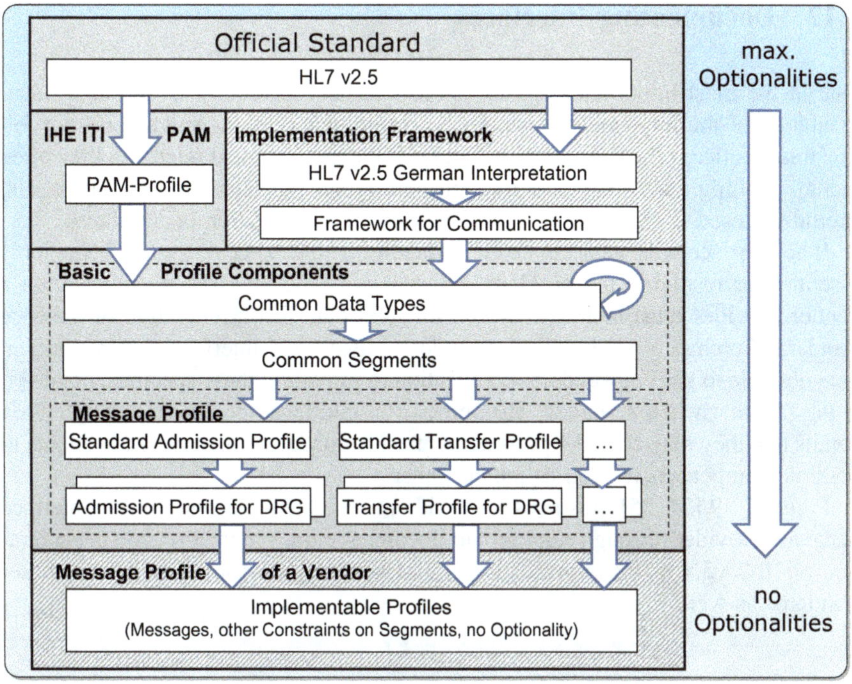

Fig. 7.38 Profile hierarchy (in Germany)

- Standard admission message,
- Admission message for DRG,[16] or
- Admission message with insurance data for billing purposes (not shown)

After the latest harmonization work, the current message profiles are compliant to the IHE ITI Patient Administration Management (PAM) integration profile and the German message profiles originally defined in 2003. They currently represent the official German National Extension to IHE ITI PAM.

An important aspect is the documentation for the profiles. As described previously, each refinement of the basic specification is a profile (component), but it is not typically recognized as such and, therefore, is not documented accordingly.

As shown in Fig. 7.38, the profile definitions are derived from other profile definitions and are clearly identified by corresponding (profile) OIDs.

In most (other) cases, however, such OIDs are neither defined nor stored (with their specification) in a (central) register, therefore, one can neither uniquely identify individual variations of messages nor verify them. HL7 International provides such a registry.

[16]Diagnosis Related Group.

7.12 Documenting Interfaces

One of the most important steps for successful interoperability is thorough documentation of the implemented interfaces. Unfortunately, most vendors do not follow this practice. When vendors do document the implemented interface, they often include nothing more than an extract of the original standard. Profiles can be, and should be, used to facilitate the comprehensive documentation of interfaces.

If an interface fails, an accurate understanding of the expected system behavior is essential for resolving the problem, which is why the interface documentation a vendor provides must include more information than just a reiteration of the base standard. Purchasers should seek complete and correct interface documentation. One obstacle to gaining vendors' cooperation in providing these specifics, however, is the fact that when a vendor "customizes" an interface, the hidden configuration details that they may consider proprietary must be made transparent and available to possible competitors as well as the customer.

Figure 7.39 [24, 25] illustrates that, with an accurate description of the interface behavior provided through appropriate documentation, preparation for the migration of HL7 v2.x to V3 is made easier. The same applies for a migration to other standards as well.

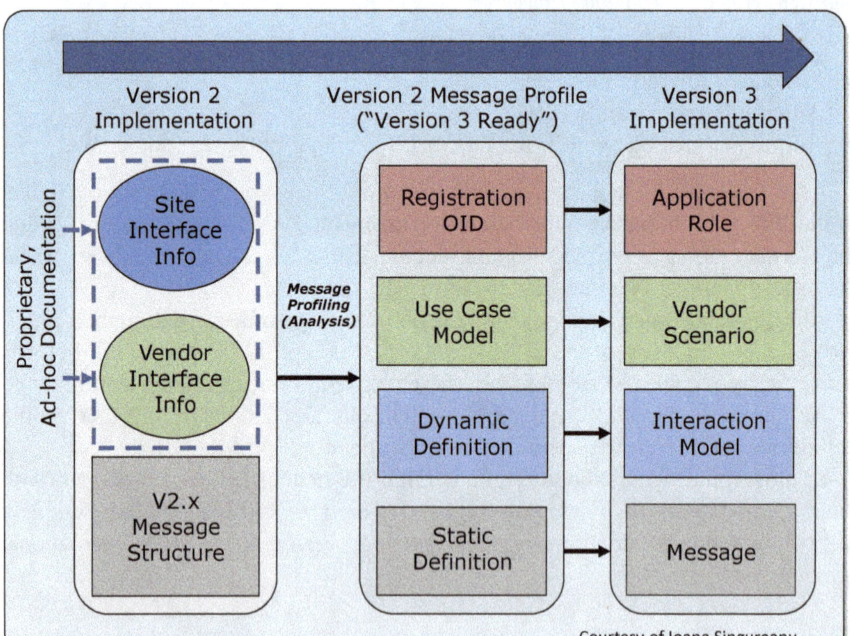

Fig. 7.39 Migration of HL7 v2.x to V3

The HL7 version 2 messages require additional information that will be implemented in a relatively "static" manner. This information includes constraints, such as an element's usage and number of occurrences, the interpretation of segment contents, or the presence of pre- and post-conditions for a message. In cases where an interface is used, there are further constraints, such as the binding to specific catalogs (vocabularies), which should not be fully specified but only referenced. The information needed for the HL7 v2.x messages also covers the static and dynamic definitions and the various scenarios in the V3 standard.

7.12.1 Profile and Implementation Relationships

Figure 7.40 shows the relationships between profiles and implementations and the associations that can be drawn among them. Profiles at the various levels provide a source of the documentation about what is to be implemented or what has been implemented. Purchasers can use profiles to express their requirements. Likewise, vendors can use profiles to convey system capabilities. Such documentation can be used to assess needs and capabilities. If the documentation is provided in a standardized computable format then efficiencies can be gained in assessing compatibilities. Comparisons also can be made between vendor interface implementations for a given use. In Fig. 7.40, Implementable Profile (E) and Implementable Profile (F) can be assessed for profile compatibility (shown as point 6). Profile E and F are

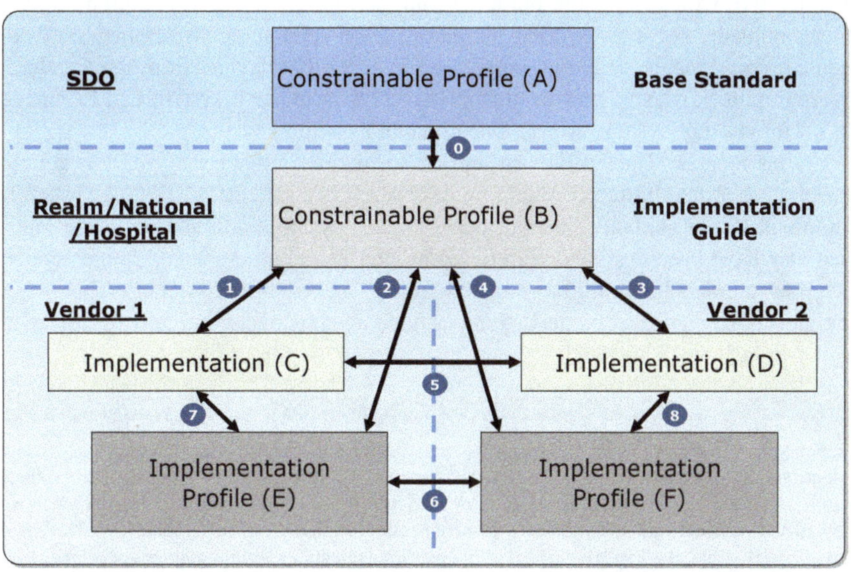

Fig. 7.40 Profile and implementation relationships

documentation of requirements for what is to be implemented or what has been implemented.

These profiles are derived from the constrainable profile (B), shown as points 2 and 4. These implementable profiles constrain the national (or realm/hospital) profile that is typically specified in an implementation guide. Profiles (E) and (F) are said to be compliant with Profile (B) if the rules for adding constraints are faithfully followed. Likewise, Profile (B) is said to be compliant with Profile (A) if the rules for adding constraints are faithfully followed. In this case Profile (B) is constraining the base standard (A). The base standard can be considered a constrainable profile.

Implementations (C) and (D) are conformant to Profiles (E), (F), and (B) if the software implements the requirements as stated in the specification (shown as points 1, 3, 7, and 8 in Fig. 7.40).[17]

Finally, Implementations (C) and (D) are said to be interoperable if they can exchange information and use the exchanged information as intended (shown as point 5).

Compliance and compatibility are terms that are used to indicate relationships between profiles (that is, its documentation). Conformance is a term that is used to indicate the relationship between a profile and an implementation. Interoperability is a term that is used when discussing the relationship between implementations. Table 7.9 summarizes these relationships and the various assessments that can be made.

The ultimate goal in development of an interface is to ensure that two implementations of that interface are interoperable with each other. The final step before deployment of an interface is to test the interface. In the simplest case, this test is performed “live”; i.e., two systems are directly tested with each other, for example, as in the IHE Connect-a-thon. For a hospital, performing a live test is often difficult to accomplish, because of their implementation-specific requirements, undocumented requirements, or documented requirements that deviate from the standard. At minimum, however, one would like to know whether a system can exchange data with another system or not. Documentation is the key.

Claims such as “The system can support/speaks HL7” that are by vendors are not informative or helpful to potential purchasers, nor is a statement like “the system is compliant to the guidance” useful, because each system participating in the interface may have been designed with different interface requirements. As an example, usage for an element could be set to “Required” in one of the systems. This usage setting is not a significant issue as long as this system is not acting as the receiver of

[17]A constrainable profile is not typically an artifact that is considered to be implementable (points 1 and 3). It is included in this diagram to show that, in some cases, implementations are developed only to the requirements specified in a constrainable profile and not to optional (or undefined) aspects. In essence, the constrainable profile is an implementable profile, although not explicitly documented as such; and therefore, in this regard, the implementation can be said to be conformant to the constrainable profile.

Table 7.9 Assessment of profile and implementation relationships

Test type	Dimension	Artifact	Description
Profile compliance (Points 0, 2, 4)	Hierarchical	Profile	Profiles are tested against each other to determine whether one is a constraint of (i.e., consistent with) the other. Profile compliance testing is appropriate when additional constraints are specified to successive profiles in the hierarchy (e.g., standard to a constrainable profile to an implementable profile)
Implementation conformance (Points 1, 3, 7, 8)	Hierarchical	Implementation	Provides an assessment of how well the application fulfills the requirements specified in a profile. This is conformance testing. ONC Health IT Certification is an example of conformance testing
Profile compatibility (Point 6)	Peer	Profile	Profiles are tested against each other to determine whether the pair can be used by applications to successfully exchange information (interoperate). If a profile pair that constrains the same underlying profile conflict with each other, chances of interoperability for applications that implement these profiles are diminished
Implementation interoperability (Point 5)	Peer	Implementation	Applications are tested with each other to determine whether they can successfully exchange information (interoperate). Applications that implement the same profile or compatible profiles and have successfully passed conformance tests have increased likelihood of interoperating. IHE connect-a-thons are an example of interoperability testing

information and the partner sending systems are not transmitting this information; however, this scenario could result in a problematic mismatch between a sender and receiver if the sender transmits a message without required information and the receiver subsequently cannot process the message.

To mitigate the downside of not being able to perform live testing of two systems (Point 5), an alternative must be sought (Point 6). Table 7.9 gives possible avenues for making this assessment as long as sufficient documentation is provided.

7.12.2 Documentation Quality

A standard provides the foundation for implementers and includes many options, which can lead to multiple interpretations and implementations that exhibit different behaviors depending on the options chosen by the implementers. Given the possible variations in implementation behavior, it is essential that vendors' claims for conformance to the standard are backed by documentation that clearly describes the capabilities supported. This documentation can be articulated in varying degrees of completeness and quality. To emphasize the importance of documentation, we describe characteristics of documentation quality. Some aspects are hierarchical in nature, forming levels of quality. Other aspects are necessary to ensure completeness. Table 7.10 presents documentation quality levels.

It is important to note that this quality hierarchy is designed for assessment of documentation and not for systems. The primary goal is to support assessment of the compatibility capabilities of proposed interface implementations. This determination of the quality of the associated documentation provides a first-level review prior to interoperability testing with implementations.

Table 7.10 represents a tiered structure of the steps for determining the quality of documentation related to vendors' conformance claims. Substantiating a claim is most meaningful when applied to an implementable profile.

7.13 Summary

This chapter explains a methodology for specifying and managing local interpretations of a data exchange. The ability to share relevant information among diverse healthcare systems and provide consistent data across applications will help improve the quality of care. It will also improve patient safety and reduce the cost of healthcare. Healthcare SDOs define the specifications for interfaces that allow centrally-located and distributed information systems to communicate. The standards establish rules for building interfaces and provide many optional features to accommodate the diverse needs of the healthcare industry. For interfaces to be implemented reliably, however, a precise and unambiguous specification must be defined. Healthcare data exchange standards introduced the concept of profiles that state precisely the structure and constraints of a message or document. The use of profiles promotes interoperability by providing a common format to trading partners for documenting interface specifications.

There are three levels of profiles that form a hierarchy, including the standard level, the constrainable level, and implementable level. A profile component defines a part or a certain aspect of a profile and is used to differentiate requirements from another profile or profile component. A profile component can be applied to any construct or section of a profile. Combining the concepts of profile levels and profile components provides authors of implementation guides the tools they need

Table 7.10 Documentation quality hierarchy

Documentation claim	Description
Undocumented unsubstantiated claim	A developer of an implementation claims conformance to a given standard; however, the claim is unsubstantiated
Documented unsubstantiated claim	A developer of an implementation provides evidence of a claim with documentation of the interface. The documentation can be in any format (e.g., a text document) and the contents of the claim are not substantiated Note: For example, the provider of the documentation (e.g., a vendor) may copy paragraphs from the original standard; this approach represents the type of documentation at this level
Documented standard unsubstantiated claim	The documentation fulfills the requirements of the conformance profiling mechanism provided by the underlying standard. A text document of a state-level (e.g., guide for Immunization for Texas) profile is an example
Documented standard machine processable unsubstantiated claim	The documentation is machine processable, such as HL7 v2.x XML conformance profiles or a HL7 CDA template. Tools can aid in the development of machine processable documentation. The MWB and IGAMT are examples for HL7 v2.x, MDHT and ART-DECOR for CDA. Documentation at this level enables automated comparison of specifications and implementations
Documented standard (implementable profile level) machine processable unsubstantiated claim	The documentation is a conformance profile fulfilling the criteria for implementable profiles in a machine processable format. Such documentation defines precisely the capabilities of the implementation. Tooling, as mentioned previously, can provide the machine processable documentation and also allows for verification that this claim is an implementable profile
Substantiated claim	The implementation is verified to a claim (i.e., a claim in this list) made in the documentation. The verification is performed in a testing or certification program. Different levels and types of programs exist (see Chap. 15)

to effectively create and manage a set of related profiles. A profile can be represented in a standardized form that enables automatic processing of many facets of the supporting operation, including publishing and validation. System developers can take advantage of profiles to simplify implementations that support both similar and disparate interface requirements.

To ensure interoperability among healthcare systems, installations must be implemented correctly—and conformance testing is essential [13]. Employing a comprehensive testing program at the onset of an implementation leads to more reliable systems, and ultimately, reduced costs. Profiles provide the mechanisms that promote better testing of implementations. Employing an implementation and testing strategy (See Chap. 11), based on profiles and tools to support them, will improve interoperability among healthcare systems.

References

1. Integrating the Healthcare Enterprises (IHE) Technical Framework. http://www.ihe.net/technical_framework/
2. HL7 Version 2.5.1 Implementation Guide for Immunization Messaging; Release 1.5, October 1, 2014. http://www.cdc.gov/vaccines/programs/iis/technical-guidance/downloads/hl7guide-1-5-2014-11.pdf
3. HL7 EHR-S Functional Requirements: S&I Framework Laboratory Results Messages, Release 1, US Realm Draft Standard for Trial Use March 2016; http://hl7.org
4. HL7 Version 2.5.1 Laboratory Results Interface (LRI) Implementation Guide, Release 1. DSTU Release 2. September 2015. http://www.hl7.org.
5. Singureau I (Editor). Adapted from Standard Profiling Process (SPP): Constraints, Extensions, and Annotations. Draft for Review (excerpt from HL7 HDF 1.5).
6. Snelick R: HL7 v2 Value Set Specification Proposal. PowerPoint Presentation for Profiling Vocabulary to HL7 v2 Implementation Guides. Original September 2013; last update June 2015. http://hl7v2tools.nist.gov (Publications/Presentations).
7. Snelick S, Oemig F: Principles for Profiling Healthcare Data Communication Standards 2013 Software Engineering Research and Practice (SERP13), WORLDCOMP'13 July 22-25, 2013, Las Vegas, NV.
8. Health Level 7 (HL7) Standard Version 2.7, ANSI/HL7, January, 2011, http://www.hl7.org.
9. German Message Profile Architecture. 2004-2007. http://www.hl7.de/download/documents/Profile_2.1.zip.
10. NIST Implementation Guide Authoring Management Tool (IGAMT). https://hl7v2.igamt.nist.gov/igamt.
11. Messaging Workbench (MWB). Developed by Peter Rontey at the U.S. Veterans Administration (VA) in conjunction with the HL7 Conformance Special Interest Group; http://www.hl7.org.
12. Snelick R, Rontey P, Gebase L, Carnahan L: Towards Interoperable Healthcare Information Systems: The HL7 Conformance Profile Approach. Enterprise Interoperability II: New Challenges and Approaches. Springer-Verlag, London Limited 2007 pp. 659-670.
13 Snelick R, Gebase L, O'Brien G: A Framework for testing Distributed Healthcare Applications. 2009 Software Engineering Research and Practice (SERP09). WORLDCOMP'09 July 13-16, 2009, Las Vegas, NV.
14. NIST Laboratory Results Interface (LRI) EHR Conformance Testing Tool. Supports 2014 ONC Health IT Certification. http://hl7v2-lab-testing.nist.gov.

15. HL7 Version 2.5.1 Laboratory Results Interface (LRI) Implementation Guide, Release 1. DSTU Release 1. July 2012. http://www.hl7.org.
16. HL7 Version 2.5.1 Electronic Laboratory Reporting (ELR) to Public Health Implementation Guide, Release 2. Work in Progress. http://www.hl7.org.
17. HL7 Specification: Characteristics of a Formal Value Set Definition, Release 1. http://www.hl7.org/implement/standards/product_brief.cfm?product_id=437
18. NIST Immunization Conformance Testing Tool. Supports 2014 ONC Health IT Certification. http://hl7v2-iz-testing.nist.gov/.
19. NIST Syndromic Surveillance Conformance Testing Tool. Supports 2014 ONC Health IT Certification. http://hl7v2-ss-testing.nist.gov/.
20. NIST Electronic Lab Reporting (ELR) Conformance Testing Tool. Supports 2014 and 2015 ONC Health IT Certification. http://hl7v2-elr-testing.nist.gov/.
21. Gazelle eHealth Test Framework for Interoperability. http://gazelle.ihe.net/.
22. ART-DECOR Expert Group. https://art-decor.org
23. HL7 Version 2.5.1 Laboratory Orders Interface (LOI) Implementation Guide, Release 1. DSTU Release 1. http://www.hl7.org.
24. Singureanu I: Making Version 3 Implementations 'Version 3 Ready' Paves the Way to Successful Migration, 20.10.2003. http://www.hl7.org/Library/Committees/Conf/V2-V3-Migration.pdf, last accessed November 2016
25. Singureanu I, Juurlink MA: Conformance Tutorial Jan, 2001. http://www.hl7.org/Library/Committees/Conf/ConformanceTutorial.ppt, last accessed November 2016
26. Conformance Documentation Hierarchy, v07. http://www.hl7.org/documentcenter/public/wg/ictc/605%20conformance%20documentation%20v07.doc
27. HL7 Version 2.x Proposal #605: http://www.hl7.org/memonly/dbtracker/attach/605.doc.
28. HL7 International: Refinement, Constraint and Localizations, www.hl7.org
29. HL7 International: Services Aware Enterprise Architecture Framework: Enterprise Conformance and Compliance Framework, http://gforge.hl7.org/gf/project/eccf/, http://gforge.hl7.org/gf/project/saeaf/

Chapter 8
Profile Relationships

8.1 Introduction

The use of profiles is central to documenting detailed specifications. When created, profiles can be expressed in numerous combinations and derivations. Chapter 7 discussed the various types of profiles; the focus of this chapter is how the profiles are related to each other and what constraints must be met in order to use the profiles correctly to achieve interoperability. Topics include profile compliance, compatibility, and versioning. Compliance is an indication of how faithfully a derived specification adheres to the requirements defined in the foundational specification (standard). Compatibility indicates whether two specifications define sets of requirements that are harmonized with each other, allowing systems that implement them to work together, i.e., interoperate. Versioning refers to identifying subsequent releases of a specification (profile). When specifying and maintaining profiles, these three dimensions interrelate, and all three must be taken into consideration. Figure 8.1 provides an overview of the profile relationships.

The use of interoperability and data exchange standards leads to evolution of the standards, including the enhancement of the base standard and releases of new versions. Derived profiles are developed and adapted from the underlying base standard. Furthermore, implementations of interfaces are developed and adapted according to the required profiles. And finally, the implementations behave as a sender or receiver of data. How do these different aspects interrelate, and what are their impacts on achieving interoperability? Taking all of these issues, as well as additional details, into account, Fig. 8.1 expands to what is shown in Fig. 8.2.

Figure 8.2 presents a view of the complex relationships between the various interoperability components. Table 8.1 lists descriptions of (and questions about) the components and their relationships that will help the reader navigate through this diagram.

F. Oemig and R. Snelick, *Healthcare Interoperability Standards Compliance Handbook*, DOI 10.1007/978-3-319-44839-8_8

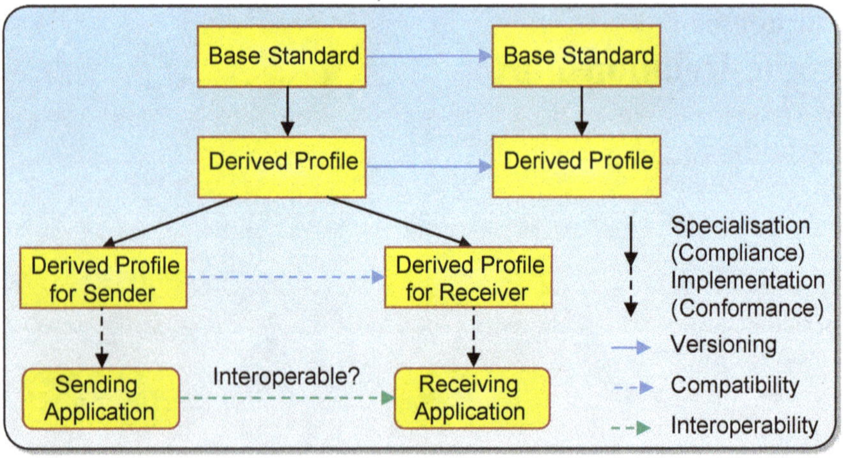

Fig. 8.1 Overview profile relationships

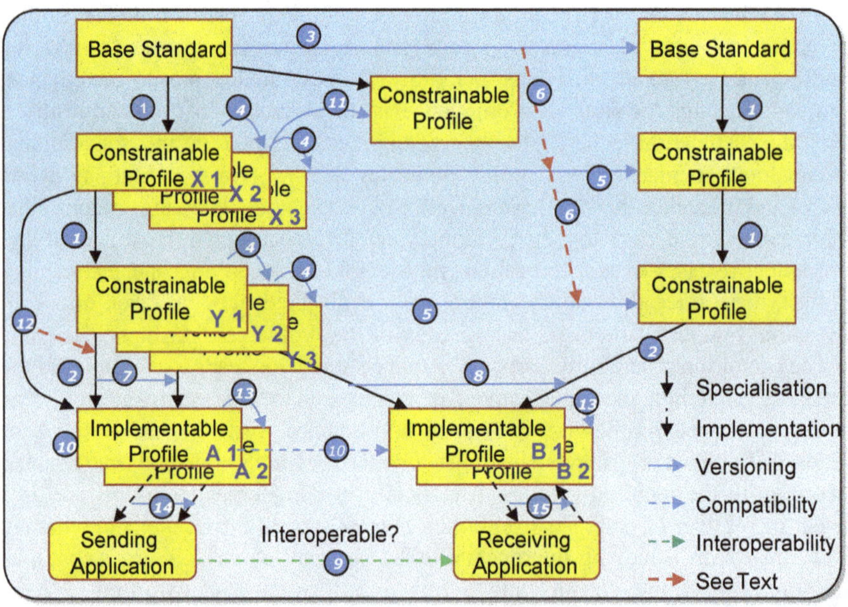

Fig. 8.2 Profiles and their relationships (detailed)

Table 8.1 Explanation of the points in Fig. 8.2

Point	Description	Questions to consider
1	Taking a base standard or another constrainable profile, one can introduce further constraints, so the resulting profile will have fewer available options	What are the rules that must be met in order to say the derived profile is compliant to the underlying profile? Does it make a difference whether the base standard or a constrainable profile is constrained?
2	No additional options are available for an implementable profile. However, there are still some ways to constrain it further, e.g., using value sets	Do the same rules apply for implementable profiles when they are derived from a constrainable profile (or directly from the base standard)?
3	Base standards are improved and released as new versions, but not all of these versions consider the notion of backward compatibility	Are changes in the standard backward compatible with regard to derived profiles and implementations? What changes are allowed in order to maintain this compatibility? Does a new version of the standard have a different impact on sending and receiving applications?
4	Constrainable profiles are updated and adjusted (possibly to address technical corrections, enhanced business requirements, or other needs)	When creating a new version of a constrainable profile, what are the rules to be met?
5	Constrainable profiles are migrated to a new release of the base standard	What must be considered or examined with regard to the base standard? What is the impact on derived profiles?
6	Updating a base standard implies specific changes on the updating derived profiles	Is there any impact on the changes to the next version of the underlying standard or base profile for a derived specification that requires ("triggers") a new (version of the) profile?
7	Migrating the implementation to a new version of a profile	What happens if an implementable profile is migrated to another version of the underlying profile? Are the changes the same as when versioning the underlying profile itself? Is there any need to update the implementation, or do the changes have no impact on active interfaces?
8	Migrating an implementation to a constrainable profile belonging to another version of the base standard	What is the impact of this migration?
9	Interoperability is determined from the perspective of implementations	What is necessary to say that implementations for sender and receiver are interoperable
10	Compatibility is determined from a receiver's perspective	What is necessary to say that implementable profiles for sender and receiver are compatible?

(continued)

Table 8.1 (continued)

Point	Description	Questions to consider
11	Releasing a new profile instead of a new version of an existing profile	Are there any rules that specify that some changes to a profile require the release of a new profile instead of a new version of this profile (4)?
12	Migrating an implementable profile to a more specialized constrainable profile (red arrow)	Under which circumstances does an implementation support the specialization of a specific profile (1), which typically adds new constraints, and is this implementable profile compliant to both?
13	Updating an implementable profile	Is there an effect on the trading partner when an implementable profile is updated?
14	Updating an interface on the sending side	When updating an implementation on the sending side, is there something to be considered with regard to (1) or (2)?
15	Updating an interface on the receiving side	When updating an implementation on the receiving side, is there something to be considered with regard to (13)?

All of the questions listed in Table 8.1 must be answered for the different conformance constructs covered in previous chapters, including:

- usage (optionality)
- cardinality
- length
- vocabulary
- data structures (as aggregations like address)
- data types (as representations like integer)
- conformance statements

For example, when considering usage, what are the compliance rules for creating a derived profile? What are the allowable transitions for a usage code? Likewise, when considering compatibility, what usage code pairs work between a sender and receiver? These questions are addressed later on in this chapter. Data structures are aggregations of primitive components, and, as such, the same compliance and compatibility rules can be applied individually to all primitive components. The rules for vocabulary are complex and have already been addressed in Chaps. 5 and 7.

Certain conformance constructs will have an influence on another conformance construct, as shown in Fig. 8.3.

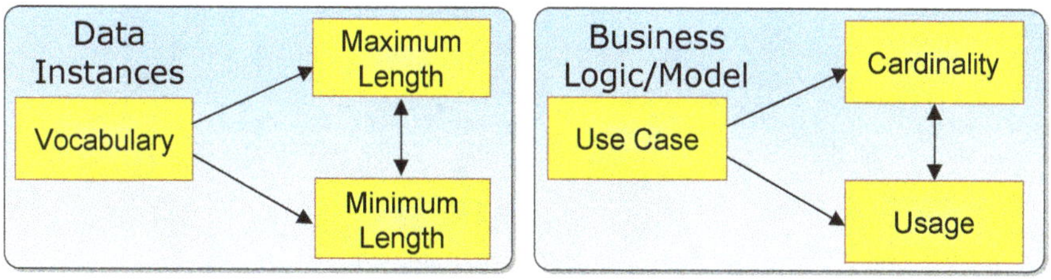

Fig. 8.3 Impact of profile specialization

The left side of the figure shows that minimum and maximum lengths influence each other, because the minimum length must always be smaller than the maximum length. Providing normative guidance for the length of data elements only makes sense in combination with specific vocabulary or in closed realms with very specific and detailed requirements. For example, an acceptable maximum length for the family name of the patient may be highly variable, so that a specific maximum length in Australia may be in conflict with the one in France. The vocabulary, minimum length, and maximum length constructs deal with actual data instances.

The right side of Fig. 8.3 addresses the business logic with respect to the underlying data model that controls whether an element must be present at all, and, if present, how often it has to occur. Usage and cardinality may be influenced by specific use case requirements, such as the Date of Death element must be populated with a value when a patient dies.

8.2 Specialization of Profiles

A consensus standard is, in essence, the amalgamation of all the requirements provided by the stakeholders (e.g., vendors, providers, payers, public health agencies, and government entities) involved in the development of this standard. Because such requirements cannot always be declared required/mandatory (for every implementer or use case), many elements are optional (i.e., they need not be provided), they allow for unlimited cardinality or lengths, or they are not bound to a specific vocabulary. This approach enables a broad acceptance of a standard, but it also leads to different manufacturers providing different implementations based on their interpretation of the standard, meaning interoperability is limited despite adherence to the same standard.

To address this shortcoming, profiles are employed to identify specific requirements for a particular use case. Profiles innately form a logical hierarchy, as layers of constraints are applied to a base standard. Recall the figure in Chap. 7 and repeated here (Fig. 8.4). Profiles have three general levels: Standard, Constrainable, and Implementable.

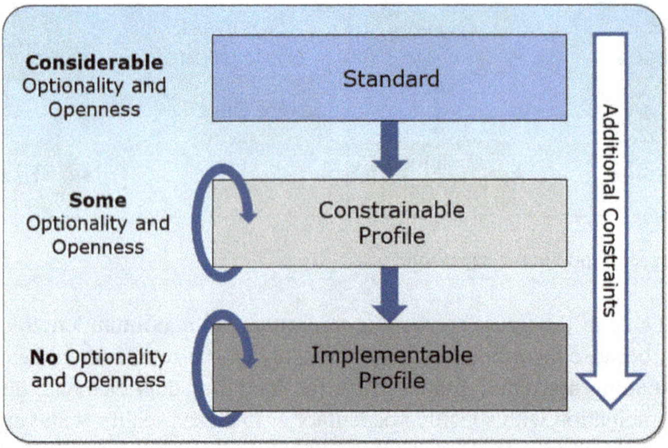

Fig. 8.4 General profile hierarchy

The specialization hierarchy for profiles (i.e., the compliance rules) is examined in this subsection. The profile compliance rules are indicated by points (1) and (2) in Fig. 8.2. For the most part, more constraints are added in derived profiles. For a compliant profile definition, the specialized (derived) profile will contain, at a minimum, the same constraints as the profile from which it was derived. In other words, the only available option for making changes to the profile definitions is to introduce additional constraints or make current constraints stronger.

The workflow for addition of further requirements is illustrated by the three vertically aligned boxes in Fig. 8.4. Adding requirements is achieved by strengthening or reducing the remaining flexibility present in the underlying profile.

The top level profile represents the standard and has the most flexibility—or in other words, it has the least number of constraints. A constrainable profile limits this flexibility by adding constraints, however, some choices still exist that ultimately are removed in implementable profiles. For an implementable profile, a declaration must be provided for each data element as to whether it is supported or not (along with other requirements defined by the conformance constructs). In the following subsections, an analysis is provided for constraining the different conformance concepts.

8.2.1 *Usage (Optionality) Compliance Rules*

A well-written standard will define unambiguously the allowable paths by which optionality is removed to create an implementable profile. As an example, Table 8.2 provides the Usage (or Optionality) indicators for HL7 version 2.8.1 [1], and Fig. 8.5

provides a graphical representation of the allowable transitions when profiling the base standard or constrainable profile to an implementable profile. Table 8.3 provides an expanded view of the compliance transition rules.

If the same usage indicator that is in the constrainable profile is used in an implementable profile provided by a vendor, the requirement becomes a self-declaration that is read as "has implemented" and "populates/consumes" or "does not populate/consume" for that data element.

Conditional usage for elements is not considered in Table 8.2, because it resolves to R, RE, O, or X usage based on the outcome of the condition. Conditions are used when referring to operational requirements or specific use cases.

In an implementable profile, ultimately only two possibilities are allowed: either a specific element is supported ("R or RE") or it is not ("X") [2].

Figure 8.5 uses the terminology that is used in HL7 version 2.x. As of version 2.7, "RE" will also be allowed, i.e., used in the standard. The solid arrows describe the allowed transition when constraining the base standard to a constrainable profile, or a constrainable profile to an implementable profile. The dashed arrows indicate the transitions when introducing more requirements in the profile type.

With version 2.7.1, the notation "C(a/b)" has been added to the profile mechanism to allow for a better formulation of conditions. The set of optionality concepts being used within the standard is a clear superset of the concepts used with

Table 8.2 Usage (optionality)

Usage	Implementation requirement	Operational requirement
R	The application shall implement "R" elements	The application shall populate/consume "R" elements with a non-empty value
RE	The application shall implement "RE" elements	The application shall populate/consume "RE" elements with a non-empty value if there is relevant data
O	None. The usage requirement for this element has not yet been defined. The requirement is to be determined	Is contingent on how the element is profiled
X	The application (or as configured) shall not implement "X" elements	The application shall not populate/consume "X" elements

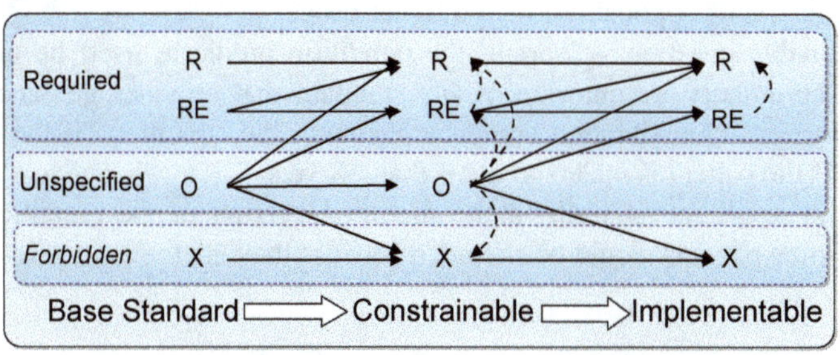

Fig. 8.5 Allowable usage constraints

Table 8.3 Compliance assessment for constraining usage

Base profile	Derived profile	Compliance assessment
R	R	Yes
R	RE	No
R	O	No
R	X	No
RE	R	Yes
RE	RE	Yes
RE	O	No
RE	X	No
O	R	Yes
O	RE	Yes
O	O	Yes
O	X	Yes
X	R	No
X	RE	No
X	O	No
X	X	Yes

profiles. Elements with a conditional usage indicator require a separate examination, because a specialization allows for different combinations depending on the characteristics of the constraint. This situation is explained in the next subsection.

8.2.1.1 Conditional Usage

Compliance assessment for elements with conditional usage [i.e., C(a/b)] is dependent on the respective true and false usage code specification. For example, if conditional usage for an element is specified as C(RE/O), the true usage code “RE” can be profiled to “RE” or “R” in a derived profile. The false usage code of “O” can be profiled to “R”, “RE”, “O”,[1] or “X”. The conditional usage codes may collapse to a single non-conditional code if the usage codes are profiled to the same code. For example, if the “RE” and “O” usage are both profiled to “R”, then the usage code can be specified simply as “R” and not C(R/R). Table 8.4 summarizes the possible constraints applicable to conditional usage.

A reasonable question is: should the condition predicate itself be allowed to change? The authors are unaware of any standard that provides guidance on this question. An example situation could be changing the condition “if the patient is male” to “if the patient is male and older than 18 years”. Any change to a condition changes the result set as well. In the modified version of the condition in this example, some patients would be excluded because they are too young. In principle,

[1]In a constrainable profile.

Table 8.4 Summary of compliance rules for constraining conditional usage

Base profile	Derived profile	Comment
C(a/b)	C(a/b)	The derivation remains unchanged
C(a/b)	C(a′/b′)	a' is a valid specialization (constraint) of a, and b' is a valid specialization of b; a and b can be constrained individually, the condition remains unchanged
	a	If b' is a valid specialization of b and this is equal to a. For example, C(R/O) and because of the specific use case being profiled it is desired to further constrain the false outcome to R. Therefore, the conditional is C(R/R), which resolves to R
	b	If a' is a valid specialization of a and this is equal to b. For example, C(O/X) and because of the specific use case being profiled it is desired to constrain the true outcome to never allow that element. Therefore, the conditional is C(X/X), which resolves to X
C(a/b)	a	If the condition is always met in a specific use case
C(a/b)	b	If the condition is never met in a specific use case

such a change causes the application to evaluate the data in a different way, but it does not change the related usage of this element and, therefore, does not change the handling of this element. It is unclear whether this kind of change should be an allowable "constraint". When changing a condition, careful consideration should be given to the potential impact on implementations.

8.2.1.2 Withdrawn Usage

Evolution of a standard may result in developing approaches for organizing data elements differently, perhaps using a better, more sophisticated representation. Due to such enhancements, it may become necessary to disable old existing data elements in the newer versions of the standard. The process of phasing out those data elements often occurs over several versions of the standard. If the standard makes use of positions to denote the semantics of a field (this is the case for ER7 with HL7 version 2.x or Hprim), an element cannot simply be deleted from the standard, because a shift in fields would alter the syntactic representation. The recommended approach, therefore, is to not permit its further use. Elements deemed eligible for deprecation are first marked as "B" for *backward compatible use only*. This usage indicates to profile developers and implementers that they are to abstain from using such elements. At a predetermined version of the standard, these elements are marked *withdrawn* ("W").

The usage code "B" in a constrainable profile can be profiled to another usage indicator; however, this approach is not recommended (unless it is being profiled to "X"), since the intent of the authors of the standard is that this element not be used in the future. The usage code "W" can only be profiled to "X", and use of "X" is recommended in the derived profiles (since "X" is implied by the authors).

8.2.2 Cardinality Compliance Rules

Table 8.5 lists the rules for constraining cardinality. The left most column indicates the cardinality for an element as defined in the base standard. The combination of the "Derived Profile" column (always m..n) and the "Valid Compliance Rule" indicates possible modifications of the cardinality constraint. The associated "Example(s)" column provides valid instances. Likewise, the "Derived Profile" column (always m..n) and the "Invalid Compliance Rule" indicate possible modifications (invalid in this case) of the cardinality constraint. The associated "Example (s)" column provides non-valid instances.

For instance, a cardinality defined in the base standard as [0..0] and then *constrained*[2] to [0..0] ($m = 0$ and $n = 0$) is a valid constraint (row 1—valid column), however, if *constrained* to [1..4] it is invalid (row 1—invalid column). In Table 8.5 it is assumed that "*m*" is always less than or equal to "*n*". Generally speaking, the cardinality range must be constrained by increasing the lower boundary and decreasing the upper boundary. The minimum cardinality has to be less than or equal to the maximum cardinality. Additionally, for some of the examples listed in Table 8.5 a specific value for a variable is used to facilitate the explanation.

Table 8.5 Compliance assessment for constraining cardinality

Parent profile	Derived profile	Valid compliance		Invalid compliance	
		Rule[a]	Example(s)	Rule	Example(s)
[0..0]	[m..n]	$m = 0$ and $n = 0$	[0..0]	$m \neq 0$ or $n \neq 0$	[0..1], [1..4]
[0..1]	[m..n]	$m \leq 1$ and $n \leq 1$	[0..0], [1..1]	$m > 1$ or $n > 1$	[0..3], [1..2]
[0..x]	[m..n]	$n \leq x$	$x = 3$, [0..0], [0..3]	$m > x$ or $n > x$	$x = 3$, [4..6], [0..4]
[0..*]	[m..n]	$m \leq n$	[0..200], [2..40]	$m > n$	[1..0], [5..1]
[1..1]	[m..n]	$m = 1$ and $n = 1$	[1..1]	$m \neq 1$ or $n \neq 1$	[0..1], [1..2]
[1..x]	[m..n]	$m \geq 1$ and $n \leq x$	$x = 3$, [1..3], [2..2]	$m < 1$ or $n > x$	$x = 3$, [0..3], [1..5]
[1..*]	[m..n]	$m \geq 1$ and $n \geq 1$	[1..1], [2..200]	$m < 1$ or $n < 1$	[0..0], [0..200]
[x..x]	[m..n]	$m = x$ and $n = x$	$x = 3$, [3..3]	$m \neq x$ or $n \neq x$	$x = 3$, [0..3], [3..4]
[x..y]	[m..n]	$m \geq x$ and $n \leq y$	$x = 3$, $y = 5$, [4..5]	$m < x$ or $y < n$	$x = 3$, $y = 5$, [3..6]
[x..*]	[m..n]	$m \geq x$ and $n \geq x$	$x = 3$, [3..3], [4…5]	$m < x$ or $n < x$	$x = 3$, [2..2], [2..6]

[a]In addition, "*m*" has to be less than or equal "*n*". As mentioned, this assumption applies to all cases in this analysis

[2]Or not modified in this case.

It is important to note that this analysis does not account for the dependencies that an associated usage (optionality) constraint places on cardinality constraints. For this table, the usage reference point is O-optional. For a cardinality of [0..1], a valid constraint is [0..0] as indicated in row 2—Valid Compliance column; additionally, [1..1] is also a valid constraint. In the context of a related usage, such constraints may not be valid. For example, for a cardinality of [0..1] and an associated usage of "RE-required, but may be empty", the maximum cardinality must be 1 (allowing for appearance of the element). Likewise, if the usage is "X-not-supported", then a cardinality setting of [0..0] is the only valid constraint of [0..1]. See chapter 2B in HL7 v2.7 (and later versions) for additional information on the dependencies between usage and cardinality.

Note that the set of constraints given in Table 8.5 can be applied to any profile level in the hierarchy (i.e., the constraint table can be applied *recursively*). Additionally, once a constraint has been applied, only further (or the same) constraint can be specified in the (another) derived profile. For example, if the base profile "A" has a cardinality of [0..1] that is constrained to [1..1] in a derived profile "B", then in derived profile "C" the cardinality constraint must remain as [1..1] (as indicated in row 5). Another example is if the base profile "A" cardinality of [0..*] is constrained to [1..5] in a derived profile "B", then in a derived profile "C" the cardinality can be further constrained to [2..4]. In this example, the constraint transitions went from [0..*] (row 4) to [1..x] (row 6), and finally to [x..y] (row 9).

8.2.3 Length Compliance Rules

The length conformance construct has three separate components for determining compliance: maximum length, minimum length, and conformance length.

8.2.3.1 Maximum Length

The maximum length is an indication of the largest number of characters that can be supported for a given element. When constraining the maximum length, the addition of constraints decreases the maximum length so that systems supporting the base profile are still capable of fulfilling the derived profile. This constraint seems to be counterintuitive relative to other requirements where capabilities are added; but here, increasing the maximum length of a data element would lead to adding more storage capacity in a database, which is not always possible. Allowing for less length is always possible without a change to storage capacity, while requiring more length could result in additional adaptations or development for implementations. Table 8.6 shows the assessment for constraining the maximum length.

Table 8.6 Compliance assessment for constraining maximum length

Base profile	Derived profile	Compliance assessment
n	n	OK
0	n	Error, if n > 0
m	n	Error, if n > m
m	n	OK, if m > n

Table 8.7 Compliance assessment for constraining minimum length

Base profile	Derived profile	Compliance assessment
n	n	OK
0	n	OK
m	n	Error, if n < m
m	n	OK, if m < n

8.2.3.2 Minimum Length

The minimum length is a construct that does not influence database requirements, i.e., storage capabilities. It is always combined with formatting guidance for certain values or the assignment of a set of specific values. An example of the former is numeric values that should have leading zeros. An example for the latter is a set of specific codes.

A value for the minimum length, therefore, is not arbitrarily defined, but is introduced by the above mentioned constraints on other conformance constructs. Once the list of values for an element is known, the minimum length can be calculated. Reducing the list of allowed values might eliminate the shortest value, meaning the minimum length would increase.

Furthermore, the increased minimum length should not exceed the maximum length, but this requirement is not shown in Table 8.7.

8.2.3.3 Conformance Length

For quite a significant number of data elements, length cannot be specified as normative because of highly diverging requirements within the different realms. Enforcing normative lengths across realms is not reasonable. Nevertheless, specifications should provide some guidance to implementers with respect to length requirements. Conformance length establishes the minimum number of characters that the application must support for a given element. For example, if the conformance length of the "Patient Last Name" element is 20, then the application can be expected to handle at least 20 characters. A derived profile can only decrease this "minimal maximum" length so that the interfaces are still able to handle messages according to the base profile, as is shown in Fig. 8.6.

Conformance length is a concept that is only applicable to base standards and constrainable profiles. When developing a standard or derived profile, the set of expected use cases are analyzed, and from that analysis a conformance length is

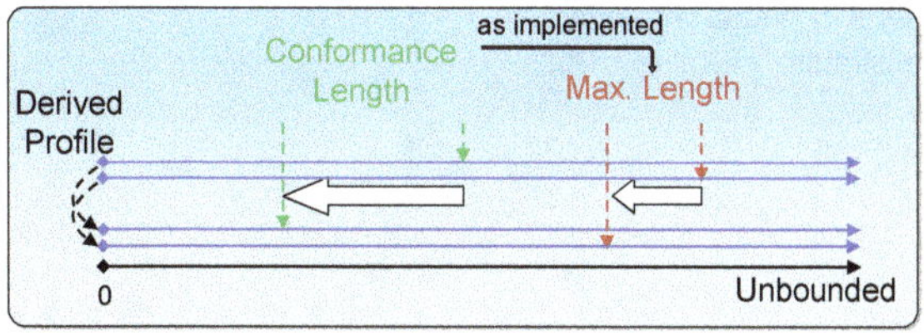

Fig. 8.6 Implementing conformance length

Table 8.8 Compliance assessment for constraining conformance length

Base profile	Derived profile	Compliance assessment
n	n	OK
0	n	OK
m	n	OK, if n < m
m	n	Error, if m < n

established. This information gives implementers an initial expectation as to what their application needs to support. A developer should treat this information as the lower boundary for the maximum length that is sufficient for most use cases. In implementable profiles the exact length must be known. Table 8.8 provides an assessment for constraining conformance length in derived profiles.

In principle, any conformance length allows for an unlimited maximum length in derived profiles. Therefore, the "real" maximum length may deviate from the conformance length of the base profile. At this point it, can be stated that the fewest number of problems will occur if the maximum length is equal to the conformance length.

8.2.4 Vocabulary Compliance Rules

How to apply constraints on vocabulary is a complicated subject that is heavily dependent on the vocabulary constraint model defined by a particular standard. In many of the standards, clear and concise profiling compliance rules do not exist. Chapter 7 presented the vocabulary profiling concepts in a standard agnostic manner. In principle, these profiling mechanisms relate to the vocabulary constraint mechanisms in the various standards. For example, comparisons of the approach given in Chap. 7 can be made with the CWE and CNE concepts in CDA. In this chapter, an overview of the compliance constraints is given; for details, refer to Chap. 7 or to a particular standard of interest.

8.2.4.1 Constraining Vocabulary

In healthcare data exchange standards, a lot of data are transmitted in the form of codes. The specifications make the code requirement explicit by defining different value sets. When creating a value set, analysis begins with a known universe of coded

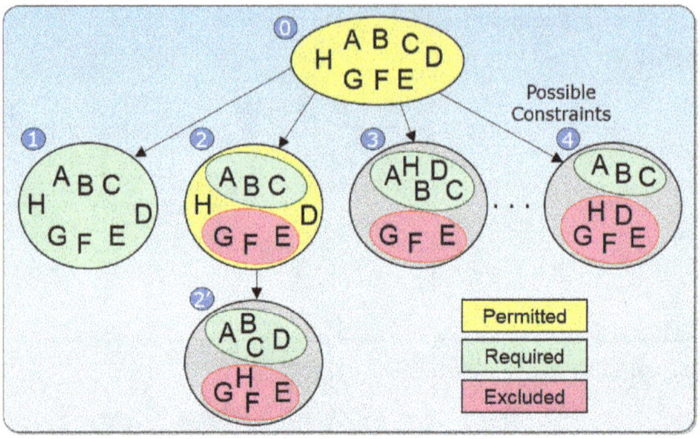

Fig. 8.7 Valid vocabulary constraints

concepts (codes) usually defined in a code system. This initial analysis is represented by assigning a usage code of "P-permitted" to all codes (this usage is implicit because the code is present in the code system). As the analysis of the use case progresses, usage codes will change from "P" to "R-Required" and "E-Excluded". These assignments are made in constrainable profiles. Eventually, in an implementation profile all "P" usage codes will be changed to "R" or "E" (either explicitly as documented in an implementable profile or implicitly in an implementation).

Figure 8.7 shows some possible workflows for generating valid vocabulary constraints for an initial value set[3] (Point 0—all codes permitted). A value set (Point 1) is created that includes the entire code system. Point 2 shows a value set in which codes A, B, and C are required, codes G, F, and E are excluded, and codes D and H are to be specified in a derived specification. Point 2′ shows a further constrained value set in a derived profile in which D is made to be required, and H is excluded. Points 3 and 4 show examples of other valid value set instances based on the initial code system shown in Point 0.

Note: Point 0 can be a set of codes from a single code system or from multiple code systems.

8.3 Versioning of Profiles

A version of a profile is a modification of a previous profile to which compliance is expected to be maintained in the creation of the updated version. That is, any change should not result in a negative impact on (break) existing implementations that are based on the previous profile. If significant changes are to be made based on a new scope or modified use case, then a whole new profile should be created. Publishing of a new implementation guide mostly means new profiles have been created. Applying leading practices for creation of new profiles, as described in

[3]In a real scenario, a code system typically will be the initial "starting" point.

Chap. 7, helps in writing the profiles and developing the associated interfaces more efficiently. Having said that, and given the effort involved in specializing profiles, creating a new version is, in most cases, not likely to occur unless it is needed in order to address technical errors.

A new version can be released under circumstances described in Table 8.9, which provides the assessment steps used for determining whether the creation of a new version is appropriate. This table is separated into two distinct perspectives called "Specialization (Profiling) Perspective" and "Implementation Perspective" that are presented as a pair of columns with an evaluation and a comment.

As can be seen with Table 8.9, the versioning of profiles may have a different impact on specialized (derived) profiles versus implementations. Therefore, it is recommended that new profiles be released instead of versioning existing ones.

Table 8.9 Assessment for versioning profiles

Change	Specialization (profiling) perspective		Implementation perspective	
	Evaluation	Comment	Evaluation	Comment
Extending a value set	Compliant	New value may be added to a value set if it is not directly added to the minimal set[a]. Otherwise, this value must also be supported by all derived profiles	Compliant	See comment on specialization (profiling) perspective
Limiting a value set	Non-compliant	May raise an error with derived profiles if the codes are marked as required	Depends	This depends on how the codes are dealt with: If they are not marked as required, this is fine
Increasing the maximum length	Compliant	This is automatically a constraint to specialized profiles	Non-compliant	The implemented length may be too small
Decreasing the maximum length	Non-compliant	May raise an issue on derived profiles when staying with the original length	Non-compliant	Decreasing the maximum length may introduce an error on the implementation if it supports the longer values
Increasing cardinality	Compliant	This is automatically a constraint to specialized profiles	Compliant	The implementation may not support the new maximum cardinality
Decreasing cardinality	Non-compliant	May raise an issue on derived profiles when staying with the original length	Non-compliant	See comment on specialization (profiling) perspective

[a]This is the set of codes out of this value set that must be supported at minimum

8.3.1 Example

Figure 8.8 provides an example scenario for a possible update (release of new versions) of constrainable profiles. (For consistency, the same identifiers that appear in Fig. 8.2 are used).

The "+", "o", and "−" character sequences in parentheses below the individual profiles indicate support, choice for support, and non-support of requirements[4] on elements (these could be a segment, field, or component). Furthermore, in order to keep the scenario simple, no specific hierarchies of constrainable profiles are introduced in the diagram. Figure 8.8 depicts one level for constrainable profiles and another level for implementable profiles. No apostrophe, one apostrophe, or two apostrophes indicate from which constrainable profile (C, C′ or C″) the implementable profile (A, A′, A″ respectively B, B′ and B″) is derived.

As can be seen with Fig. 8.8, the versioning of the constrainable profiles (4) clearly introduces new requirements. The resulting three constrainable profiles (C, C′, and C″) are valid specializations of the base profile (standard), which is marked with (1). The original implementable profile (A) on the sending side is a specialization of the first constrainable profile (C) that realizes exactly the requested constraints ("+") and nothing more ("o" ⇒ "−"). The updated interface for the sending application X (14) implements the updated profile (C′) by supporting implementable profile A′ (13) that is compliant to C′. The updated sending side interface (14) results in support

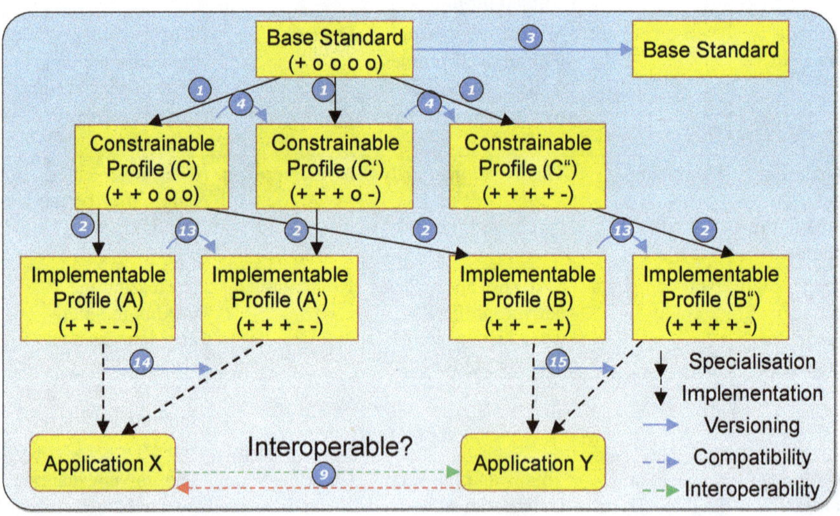

Fig. 8.8 Example update scenario

[4]This applies to any requirement defined by a conformance construct (e.g., usage, cardinality).

for an additional data element. From the sender perspective the updated interface is still compatible with the previous interface, so no problems should be expected despite the violation of backwards compatibility guidance.

The analysis for the receiving side (Application Y) reveals a different picture. The first implementable profile (B) is a valid constraint on profile C as well—with the difference that the fifth element is marked as required. Consequently, the interfaces for sending application X and receiving application Y are incompatible, because the interface on the sending side is not going to provide the requested data (9). When updating the receiving profile (B) to the latest release of the constrainable profile (C″, 13), the new profile (B″) is again a valid constraint (2); but this new profile breaks backward compatibility, because two new constraints (3rd and 4th) are introduced while an old constraint (5th) is removed. An update of the interface for the implementation according to this new implementable profile (B″) is not backward compatible. Furthermore, both interfaces for the two applications are neither compatible nor interoperable.

If the example update scenario depicted in Fig. 8.8 is modified by switching the direction of communication, thus changing sender (now Application Y) and receiver (now Application X) roles as indicated by the red dashed arrow, a completely different situation is established. The update of the interface for application Y as the sender (B ⇒ B″) still violates backward compatibility (15), but it is interoperable with the implementable profile (A) for application X (i.e., B″ and A). The updated interface for application X as the receiver (A ⇒ A′) is also interoperable with the updated interface for application Y as the sender (i.e., B″ and A′); but if the update for application X (14) is made before the update (i.e., A′ and B) for application Y (15), a brief period of incompatibility ensues, because the receiver requires an element (3rd in A′) that application Y does not provide (3rd in B).

Modifying this example by introducing another set of derivations made to the same set of constrainable profiles for sender and receiver results in another picture, as is shown in Fig. 8.9.

Updating the sending interface from A to A″ does not violate compatibility with the receiving interface (B). Also, an update from B to B′ is acceptable if this update (15) is made after (14) (A″ to B′); otherwise, a short period of incompatibility would occur.

Switching the sending (now Application Y) and receiving (now Application X) roles for both applications (red arrow) results in incompatibilities, because application Y as a sender does not deliver the data that application X needs as a receiver.

These brief examples demonstrate that a compatibility assessment, as a prerequisite for interoperability, must be performed very carefully.

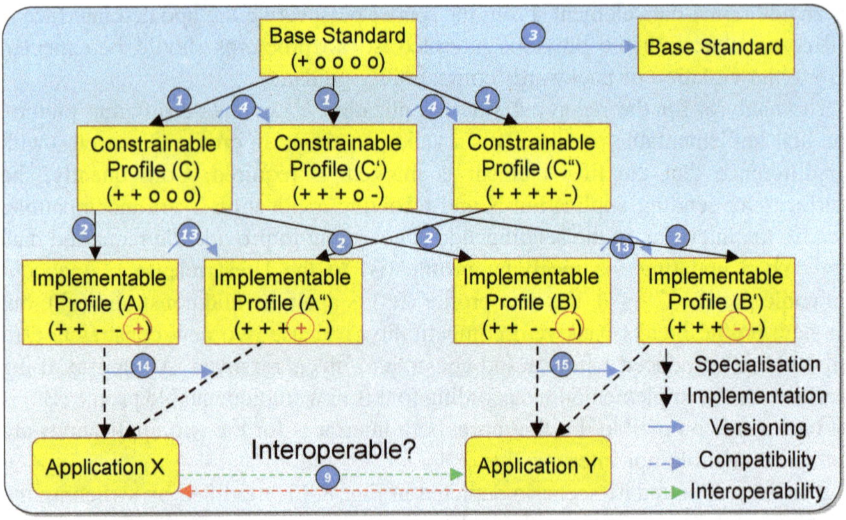

Fig. 8.9 Modified example update scenario

8.4 Creating New Profiles

Rather than publishing a new version of a profile (4, Table 8.9), an update to a profile must be published as an entirely new profile (1) if compatibility[5] issues cannot be resolved. In this situation, a new profile must be created because of fundamental requirement differences between the updated profile and the profile on which the updated profile is based.

8.5 Compatibility of (Sender and Receiver) Profiles

Table 8.10 indicates the allowable profile pairs for compatibility and addresses point (9) in Fig. 8.2. Note that the assessment in Table 8.10 is not an operational analysis; it provides a tool for evaluating whether the usage construct in a sender profile is compatible with that construct in a receiver profile. For a pair of profiles to be compatible, all element pairs in the profiles must adhere to the profile compatibility rules given in Table 8.10. For example, if the sender profile specifies an element as required and the receiver profile also specifies the corresponding element as required, then the profiles are compatible for that element. If, however, the sender profile specifies an element as not-supported and the receiver profile specifies the

[5]In this context, the term Compatibility is used to assess whether a profile is *compatible* to a new profile that is based on an original profile.

Table 8.10 HL7 v2.x sender/receiver pair profile compatibility rules

Sender	Receiver	Compatible	Comment
R	R	Yes	Sender and receiver have the same expectations
R	RE	Yes	Receiver supports this element but is not always expecting it
R	X	Yes	Receiver doesn't support this element
RE	R	No	Receiver is not guaranteed to get required data
RE	RE	Yes	Sender and receiver have the same expectations
RE	X	Yes	Receiver doesn't support this element
X	R	No	Receiver will not get required data
X	RE[a]	No	Receiver will not get the data it needs for certain use cases Note: there has to be at least one instance in which a data value is needed; otherwise, the element should not be profiled to RE. On the other hand, RE is the only construct to express the capability of the receiving system to handle data
		Yes	The element is not necessary for operation
X	X	Yes	Sender and receiver have the same expectations

[a]In this combination, compatibility depends on the use case. If the data are important in order to perform the use case, then this combination is not compatible. But if RE only declares the capability of the system, then this pair is compatible

corresponding element as required, then the profiles are not compatible for that element, since the receiver is expecting data that the sender will never provide. The same evaluation must be performed for all conformance constructs.

8.5.1 *Usage*

Having different alternatives for usage may result in a negative impact on message exchange. This section elaborates on the various allowable pairings. The following two tables do not take conditional usage into account; the implications of conditions are explained later.

Table 8.10 addresses implementable profiles where each element must be profiled; that is, no elements can be O or optional. Table 8.11 addresses additional optionality choices available for constrainable profiles.

Optional elements apply only to constrainable profiles. Often PDOs develop constrainable level profiles for national specifications (e.g., specifications used in the US for the Health IT Certification Program). Their goal is to specify elements that are needed to meet their use case requirements. Beyond that, they allow trading partners to negotiate among themselves regarding local customization of the remaining un-profiled (or optional) elements.

Defining compatibility among systems requires a comparison of the capabilities of the sending side to the requirements on the receiving side through the means of profiles. For assessing compatibility, use case requirements are defined in higher

Table 8.11 Compatibility analysis for optional elements

Sender	Receiver	Compatible	Comment
R	O	Yes	Receiver does not express any expectations or requirements on the data and may support this element in the future. Compatible receiver profiling in the implementable profile include R, RE, or X
RE	O	Only RE, X	Receiver does not expect data and may support this element in the future. Compatible receiver profiling includes RE, or X
X	O	Only X	Receiver does not expect data and may support this element in the future. However, it can only be compatible if it is constrained to X
O	R	Only R	Receiver requires the data. Compatible sender profiling option is R
O	RE	Only R, RE	Receiver expects data in certain instances. Compatible sender profiling options is R or RE
O	X	Yes	Compatibility sender profiling option is R, RE, or X
O	O	Possible	Compatibility can be achieved by following the rules for implementation profiles as given above

level constrainable profiles and are thus not considered. For example, the assignment of "R" usage for an element on the sending side expresses the fact (or the intent) that this element is always valued in every message instance that is sent. "RE" usage expresses the intent that data will be present in messages if the data are entered into the system or are made available in some other way. In other words, these usage requirements identify what a receiver can expect in messages being sent to them. Statements for a receiver are clear expressions of their requirements. Therefore, a required element ("R" usage) indicates that the receiver must get this information in order to be able to process the message or a specific part of the message. Having said this, the pairing "R ⇒ X" is deemed compatible, since the receiver can ignore a data element for which the sender always provides data, although this behavior may not fulfill a certain use case or meet external expectations. Use case requirements must, therefore, be introduced as higher level requirements ("R") in the form of a constrainable profile that must be fulfilled by both sender and receiver, i.e., the implementable profiles must be compliant to this higher level constrainable profile. Providing such a use case requirement would mean that the applications are compatible, although the receiver is not compliant (i.e., the receiver's implementable profile is not compliant with the constrainable profile). The receiver is conformant to its implementable profile, because this profile does not support the element; however, the fact that the receiver is not compliant prevents interoperability. In summary, specific aspects of compliance, compatibility, and conformance need to be met to enable interoperability.

The analysis of optional elements for profile compatibility provides guidance for pairing potential implementable profiles derived from constrainable profiles. A definitive assessment of profile compatibility can't be made until implementation profiles are developed; however, the guidance provided here will aid in the specification of constrainable profiles. As is to be expected, profile compatibility of constrainable profiles is directly linked to the requirements of the compatibility rules of implementable profiles.

8.5.2 *Cardinality*

Adding constraints to the cardinality of elements can be accomplished by narrowing the range of possible occurrences. Table 8.12 explains the possible restrictions.

8.5.3 *Length*

Most vendors do not provide details about the implemented length for data elements. In these cases, incompatibilities among senders and receivers can only be identified by a systematic testing of all data elements, which implies that each data element on the sending side must be populated to its maximum length. On the receiving side, all data in the messages must be evaluated to determine whether some values are being truncated, a manual and tedious process that can be automated by tooling if the implementable profiles specify the implemented length.

Table 8.12 Compatibility analysis for cardinality

Sender	Receiver	Compatible	Comment
[0..0]	[0..0]	Yes	Sender and receiver have the same expectations
[0..0]	[0..m]	Yes	Receiver can process data but can also handle absence of data
[0..0]	[n..m]	No	Receiver will not get required data, if n > 0
[0..1]	[0..0]	Yes	Receiver has no expectations[a]
[0..1]	[0..1]	Yes	Sender and receiver have the same expectations
[0..1]	[0..m]	Yes	Receiver supports more than the sender
[0..1]	[n..m]	No	Receiver will not get required data if n > 0
[1..1]	[0..0]	Yes	Receiver has no expectations[a]
[1..1]	[0..1]	Yes	Receiver processes the data
[1..1]	[1..1]	Yes	Sender and receiver have the same expectations
[1..1]	[1..m]	Yes	Receiver supports more than the sender
[1..1]	[n..m]	No	Receiver will not get required data if n > 1
[x..y]	[n..m]	Yes	If m < x
[x..y]	[n..m]	No	If n > y

[a]This case and similar cases are analogous to the sender usage of "R" and the receiver usage of "X". If the use case dictates that the sender expects the element to be handled, then the element must be profiled as "R" for both the sender and the receiver

Table 8.13 Testing possible combinations of implemented length

	Sender		Receiver	Compatible
Implemented minimum length	m	<	n	No
	m	=	n	Yes
	m	>	n	Yes
Implemented maximum length	m	<	n	Yes
	m	=	n	Yes
	m	>	n	No

At this point it can be noted that the receiver's capabilities must be greater than the sender's capabilities in order for them to be compatible (Table 8.13).

8.5.4 Vocabulary

Value sets can be created for senders and receivers independently. Since this is the case, under what circumstances are the value sets compatible? Figure 8.10 shows how a sender and receiver might profile a value set differently in a constrained profile. The sender excludes both D and H, while the receiver excludes D but includes H. In this case, the derived profiles (and therefore implementations) are compatible.

In general, if the sender is only sending a subset of the codes that are supported by the receiving application (Fig. 8.10), then the profiles are compatible. If the sender uses a code the receiver does not support, however (see element "D" in Fig. 8.11), a compatibility issue occurs.

According to the implementation guide, both derived profiles are compliant, because they specify valid constraints. The sender and receiver are not compatible, however, because the sender specifies code "D" as R-required while the receiver has specified code "H" as E-excluded. Thus, even if both sender and receiver implement their specified profiles correctly (that is, they are conformant), they are not interoperable. This example stresses the importance of trading partner agreements to address specific use case needs. In this case, the sender has an expectation about a code that is not supported by the receiver. Table 8.14 depicts the situation clearly in a row and column format.

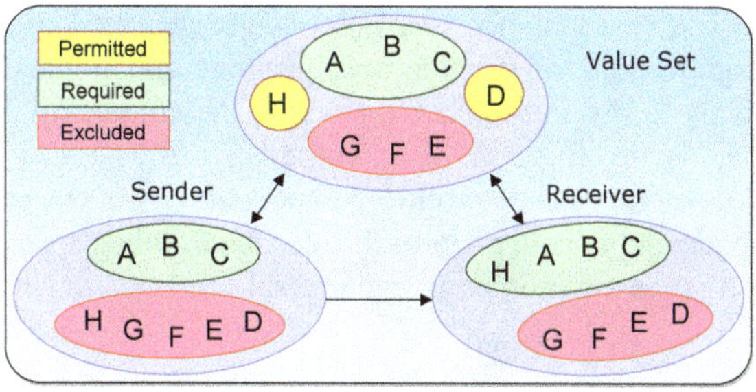

Fig. 8.10 Terminology assessment for sender/receiver implementations

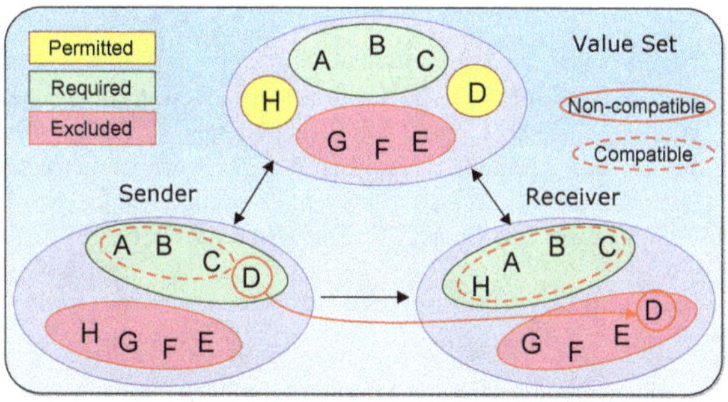

Fig. 8.11 Compatibility issues with supportive set of codes

Table 8.14 Compatibility analysis for vocabulary

Sender	Relationship	Receiver	Compatible	Comment
S := {c | c is supported by sender}	⊆	R := {c | c is supported by receiver}	Yes	The receiver has more supportive capabilities than the sender
	⊇		No	The sender can send a code that the receiver does not understand

8.6 Summary

Specifications—standards, profiles, and implementation guides—and implementations, with their accompanying documentation, are developed more or less independently from each other over time. New versions of base standards are released, profiles are adjusted or specialized, and applications—either in sender or receiver role—are enhanced with new features. This chapter examines compliance and compatibility related to the conformance constructs during versioning and specializing of profiles.

A practical example for updating interfaces of applications demonstrates how simple modifications of requirements, and the resulting changes in constrainable profiles, can lead to (temporarily) incompatible solutions. The scenario provided as an example is representative of what occurs every day.

The result of this analysis underscores the need for controlling the possible modifications of existing specifications and implementation such that interoperability is not impeded. Considering the complexity involved, the easiest solution may be to create a new profile and request that implementers migrate to it. Ultimately, using profile components as a means for modularization in a divide-and-conquer approach (see Chap. 7) helps vendors identify areas of concern and reuse the profiles in configurable and *intelligent* interfaces.

References

1. HL7 Version 2.8.1. http://www.hl7.org.
2. Oemig F, Blobel B. HL7 Conformance: How to do proper messaging? In: Bos L, Blobel B (Editors), Medical and Care Compunetics 4. Series "Studies in Health Technology and Informatics", pp. 298-307, Volume 127. Proceedings of the ICMCC 2007. Amsterdam, The Netherlands, IOS Press, http://www.icmcc2007.net, ISBN: 978-1-58603-71-2, ISSN: 0926-9630.
3. HL7 Version 2.x, Chapter 2B. http://www.hl7.org.

Chapter 9
Conformance Profiling Tools

9.1 Introduction

This chapter provides a survey of tools for creating and maintaining conformance profiles and implementation guides. The set of tools is a sample to give the reader an overview of their purpose and capabilities. Conformance profiling tools aid in the specification of requirements. As described, some data exchange standards also provides a framework that aids in constraining the standard for a specific use case. The standards provide "templates" (e.g., a base message) and conformance constructs. Profiling tools can take advantage of these elements to provide a structured and consistent approach for specifying and constraining requirements.

To realize the benefits of conformance profiles (whether they are for a message or a document), tools are needed to support their use. A collection of freely available tools is presented and includes:

- Messaging Workbench (MWB)—HL7 v2.x
- IGAMT—HL7 V2.x
- MDHT (Model Driven Health Tools)—HL7 V3 and CDA
- ART-DECOR—HL7 V3 and CDA
- Trifolia—HL7 CDA and HL7 FHIR
- Forge—HL7 FHIR

This list is not exhaustive. Furthermore, some of these tools are under continuous development, so their set of features may have changed since the publication of this book. Proprietary tools also are available. The goal of this chapter is to provide an overview of and insight into the most commonly used freely available conformance profiling tools.

In some instances the tools are designed for multiple purposes. For instance, the MWB includes capabilities not only for creating HL7 v2.x profiles but also for validating a message instance against a profile. Conformance testing tools are described in Chap. 14.

F. Oemig and R. Snelick, *Healthcare Interoperability Standards Compliance Handbook*, DOI 10.1007/978-3-319-44839-8_9

9.2 Messaging Workbench

The Messaging Workbench (MWB) [1] is a multifaceted productivity tool for HL7 messaging professionals. It was conceived at the Veterans Administration (VA) initially as a tool for developers of messaging specifications, and creation of these specifications is still the main focus of the tool. This capability has been enhanced over many years of development effort, driven to a large extent by association with the HL7 Conformance Working Group (WG). Currently, it supports the HL7 version 2 family of specifications. MWB incorporates all the version 2.x artifacts in the form of libraries that are readily available within the tool for use in specification composition, reporting, message instance decomposition, reverse engineering, validation, and test message generation.

The MWB is a Windows platform-based GUI tool. MWB profile building is facilitated by the incorporation of HL7 2.x version-specific artifact libraries (Fig. 9.1). Building a message profile from scratch is accomplished quickly by selecting a particular message from the message library list and compiling the message structure against the version specific segment library. Alternatively, the message structure can be entered manually independently from any predefined messages structure.

These steps result in the appearance of a hierarchical representation of all elements in the message in the form of a message tree, as can be seen in Fig. 9.2. Selection of individual message elements in the tree permits each one to be constrained and annotated as required by the particular implementation. The addition of

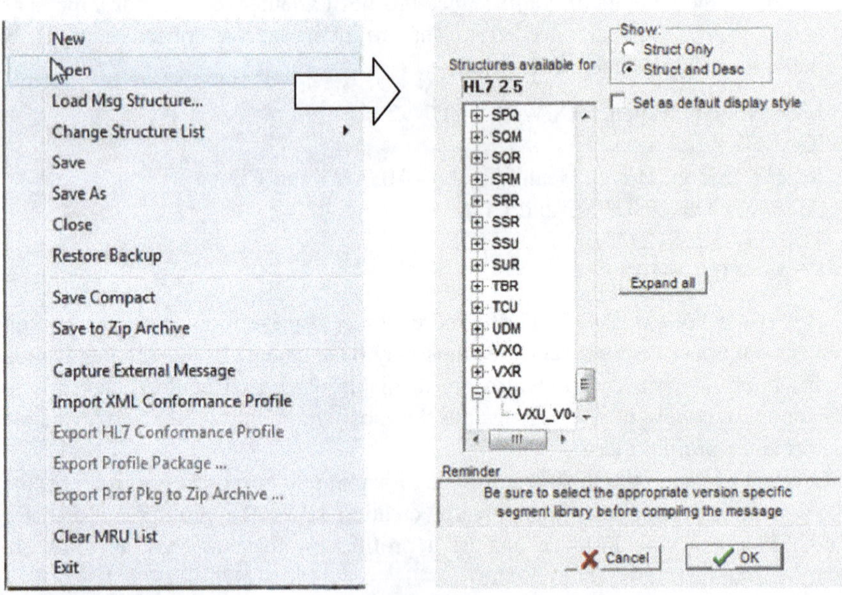

Fig. 9.1 MWB loading message structure

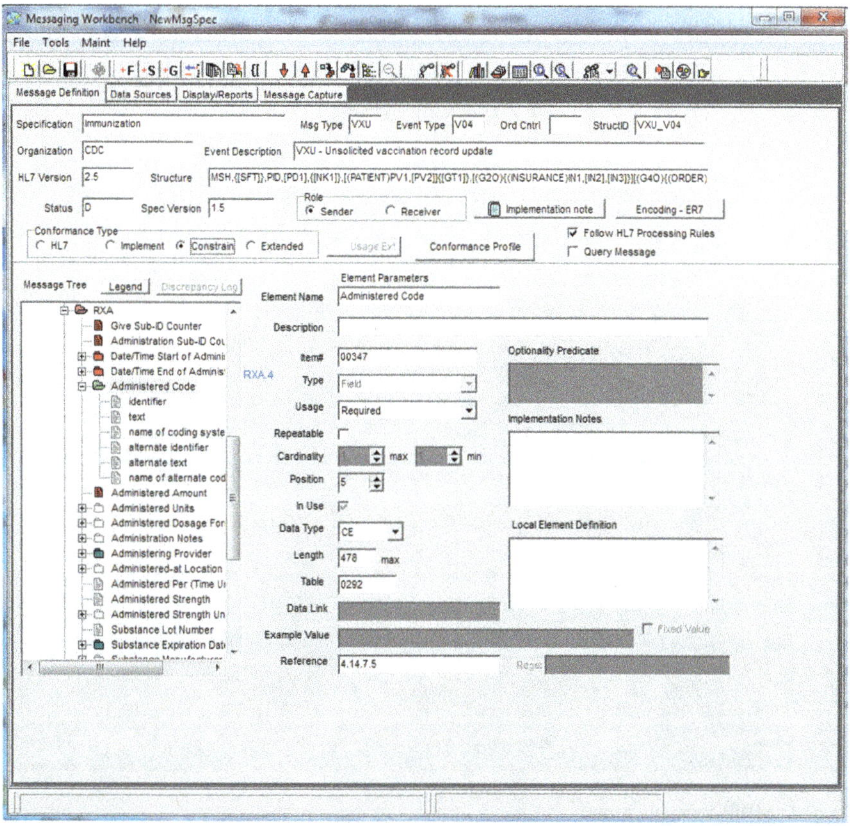

Fig. 9.2 MWB message profiling panel

use case information and diagrams, using the built-in diagram editor, typically supplements the constraint work. Additionally, the developer may constrain the profile vocabularies by selecting a subset of tables and table elements from the master table file library, which completes the constrained profile definition.

Another important part of the profile building process is the introduction of localized structures into the message. The HL7 standard promotes this aspect of messaging via the use of "Z" elements. The MWB supports the creation and incorporation of localized structures for all of the v2.x artifacts: message, segments, fields, data type, and tables.

The workbench also provides a set of reports that can be used for documentation purposes, and an example report can be seen in Fig. 9.3.

Once the profile is created it must be communicated to the interface partners. The MWB native profile format is a proprietary file structure that may be shared among the users of the MWB. In addition, the MWB provides a number of reports for alternate expression of the profile and message artifacts. The most important of

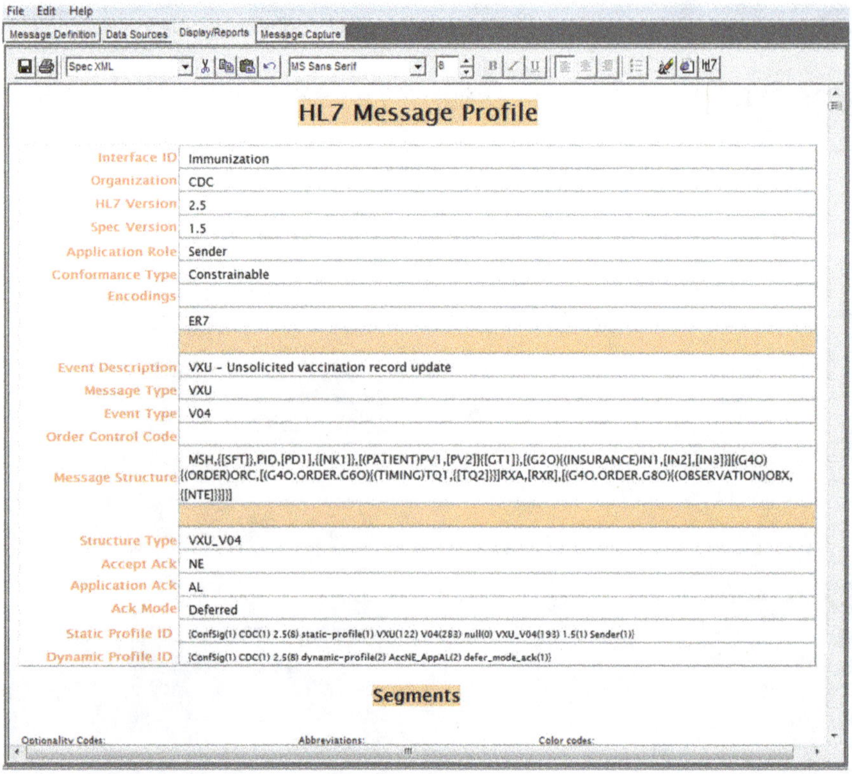

Fig. 9.3 MWB example report

these reports is the normative HL7 conformance profile, which is an XML document that validates against the HL7 DTD and schema. This format is especially important, because it imparts interoperability among tools that are capable of importing profiles that follow this normative representation.

While the MWB makes the initial profile construction a simple point-and-click operation, the effort required to adequately constrain and localize a profile is considerable. To ensure that these efforts may be conserved and, therefore, leveraged in future implementations, the MWB allows the developer to save the constrained artifacts in the form of libraries that may be reused and invoked in the same manner as the standard libraries.

The MWB may be used to receive and validate message instances, which is described in more detail in Chap. 14. It also has the capacity to decompose received message instances, making them available for individual analysis and for reverse engineering. The reverse engineering aspect is especially valuable for creating or updating the documentation of operating interfaces that may have little or no documentation. The MWB has the capability of generating syntactically correct test messages. It also has a mechanism to ensure data consistency among related message elements for generated messages, which facilitates development and implementation of rational test sets. Beyond this, the MWB has capabilities to verify, import, and export profiles; import new HL7 versions to create libraries; and to browse and register profiles. It also supports regular expression assessment of content.

The overall MWB goal, within the context of promoting interoperability among interface partners, continues to be to provide a light-weight, inexpensive means of interface development for applications and testing at the desktop level.

9.3 IGAMT

The NIST Implementation Guide Authoring and Management Tool (IGAMT) is a profiling tool used to build HL7 v2.x implementation guides (integration profiles in IHE terminology). Implementation guides are a collection of conformance profiles (a single interaction/message) bound together to describe a certain use case or work flow. IGAMT key capabilities include creating, editing, and browsing conformance profiles, value sets, and implementation guides. The general philosophy of IGAMT is similar to, and inspired by, the MWB. Key differences include the technology platform and expanded scope.

The MWB is a desktop application developed in Delphi and intended mostly for individual use. IGAMT is a Java web-based application intended for shared projects and individual use. A goal of IGAMT is to create and publish HL7 v2.x implementation guides using the tool.

The key capabilities of the MWB include the creation of conformance profiles, example messages, and message validation. IGAMT's main focus is on the creation of a collection of conformance profiles organized as an implementation guide (integration profile), and the tool includes complete publishing capabilities. Another focus of IGAMT is to support creation of local specifications based on the realm (national-level) implementation guides. A key feature is the capability to identify and publish only the delta between the national and local specifications if desired. A collection of defined implementation guides is maintained on IGAMT servers.

Unlike the MWB, IGAMT's focus is on the development of implementation guides and conformance profiles; as such, it does not support the creation of example messages nor message validation. IGAMT is one tool in an overall testing infrastructure. Separate NIST tools (and other tools) support other functionality independently. For example, the NIST Test Case Authoring and Management Tool (TCAMT) provides functionality for creating test cases and test messages (based on IGAMT conformance profiles). NIST also provides message validation tools, including those for IHE pre-connect-a-thons and connect-a-thons, the ONC Health IT Certification Program, and general HL7 v2.x testing. The validation tools include web-based applications and web services.

Figure 9.4 provides an overview of the NIST HL7 v2 testing infrastucture design and process. First, IGAMT is used to build implementation guides through

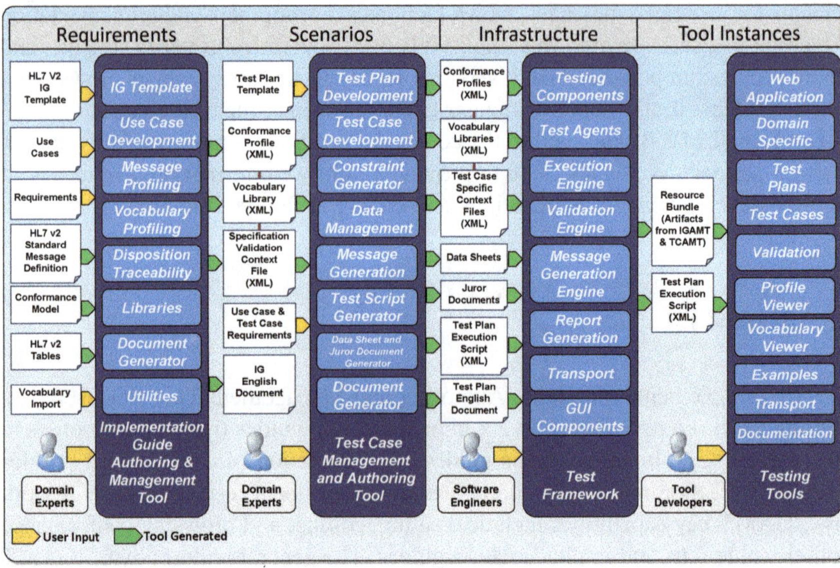

Fig. 9.4 NIST HL7 v2 testing infrastructure design and process

the entry of explanatory text and messaging requirements. Human readable documents and machine computable artifacts (e.g., an XML conformance profile) can then be exported. TCAMT imports conformance profiles and uses them as the basis from which test plans (a collection of test cases) can be developed. The test framework is a set of components that are used to build specific test tool instances. The test framework combines various components and artifacts created in IGAMT and TCAMT to build a specific tool. Additional information on testing infrastructures, frameworks, and tools can be found in Chaps. 13 and 14.

The left side of Fig. 9.4 illustrates the process and capabilities of IGAMT. The requirements for each use case need to be captured and documented when creating an implementation guide. Typically, this information is hand-crafted using a document editing tool such as Microsoft Word. IGAMT works the other way around; that is, the tool is used to capture and document requirements, and natural language artifacts are the outcome. Additionally, other machine processable artifacts (e.g., the normative XML conformance profiles) are produced that can be used as input for other purposes, such as message generation, test case development, message validation, and source code generation.

IGAMT's basic functionality allows the user to define a set of conformance profiles (which equates to a single message interaction in HL7 v2.x) organized as an implementation guide. Each conformance profile can be constrained according to the HL7 v2.x constraint model. IGAMT is pre-loaded with all of the HL7 v2.x message event types and tables. The tool design promotes the reuse of base components. For example, a data type library can be built and then used in various conformance profiles or implementation guides. Capabilities also include creation and

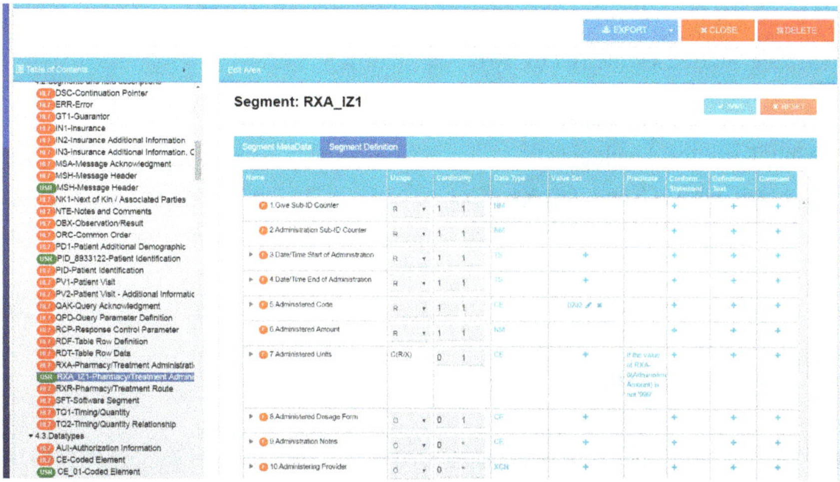

Fig. 9.5 IGAMT tables of contents and segment editing

management of value set definitions. Figure 9.5 shows a screenshot for profiling Field elements in a Segment. The left side shows the implementation guide table of contents, which is used for navigation in the tool.

IGAMT is designed to be a community tool, meaning it can be hosted as a central service in which there is single version of an implementation guide that is edited during development. Once requirements are determined through group discussion and deliberation, this information can be entered into IGAMT. Users can then immediately publish and have access to the current draft of the implementation guide.

Another important feature of IGAMT is the capability to support and manage creation of local implementation guides. For example, in the US immunization community, the national level implementation guide is pre-loaded into IGAMT. Following the conformance rules in the implementation guide, individual states can quickly add further constraints to meet their local requirements. Use of a common profile format helps provide consistency in the documentation and management of local variants. Such utilities help vendors manage their implementations and provide installations with validation tools when paired with testing frameworks (i.e., IGAMT artifacts are directly imported into validation tools).

9.4 MDHT

The Open Health Tools (OHT) initiative developed a Java based toolset to work with HL7 Version 3 and CDA: *Model Driven Health Tools (MDHT)*. This toolset is integrated into the Eclipse development environment and allows for an easy development.

It provides the following information and functionality:

- Getting Started Guide (CDA 101)
- Developers Guide
- Validation of CDA instances
- JUnit Tests for developers

The basis for MDHT is the MIF (Model Interchange Format) files that provide the necessary details to generate the corresponding Java classes. Figure 9.6 presents a few lines of Java source code to explain its use [2].

9.5 ART-DECOR

ART-DECOR is an open source tool suite used for creating and maintaining HL7 CDA templates, value sets, and data sets [3, 4]. ART-DECOR stands for **A**dvanced **R**equirement **T**ooling using **D**ata **E**lements, **C**odes, **OI**Ds and **R**ules, and its main objective is to allow stakeholders to work collaboratively together and collect their requirements in order to create profiles. This tool suite supports the collection and maintenance of requirements as profiles and other artifacts. These artifacts are made available through a repository of building blocks, primarily for HL7 Version 3 and CDA.

DECOR is a methodology used to model and document the information requirements of clinical users. This model is then used to link various "artifacts" like terminologies and templates together and generate documentation (implementation guides), XML, and test tools, etc. Supported by consistent version management, iterative improvement is fostered for all artifacts created during the working process .

DECOR is used to hold (among other things) data sets with a hierarchical list of concepts, data types, value sets, codes, identification schemes, business rules, and templates. The underlying data format is XML. Generation of HTML and PDF documents as well as XML materials is accomplished by transformation with stylesheets and other methods.

ART is the user interface of DECOR for creating and adapting DECOR files and artifacts. ART is based on the XML database eXist and uses XQuery and XForms.

The tool provides different views, allowing stakeholders from different domains to verify the specification. Figure 9.7 provides an overview of the metadata for a specific template including an XML example of the complete specification.

Primarily, ART-DECOR is used as a registry and repository for CDA templates. It supports the templates on document, header, section, entry, and data type levels. From an analysis perspective, the starting point of a specification is a data set that is designed to collect definitions in a hierarchical way from the clinician's viewpoint. Directly related to specification of data sets is the maintenance of vocabulary with codes from code systems and value sets. These codes are associated with the data set items and, subsequently, with the designed templates.

```
//create and initialize an instance of the ContinuityOfCareDocument
class

ContinuityOfCareDocument ccdDocument =
CCDFactory.eINSTANCE.createContinuityOfCareDocument().init();

//create a patient role object and add it to the document

PatientRole patientRole = CDAFactory.eINSTANCE.createPatientRole();

ccdDocument.addPatientRole(patientRole);

II id = DatatypesFactory.eINSTANCE.createII();

patientRole.getIds().add(id);

id.setRoot("996-756-495");

id.setExtension("2.16.840.1.113883.19.5");

//create an address object and add to patient role

AD addr = DatatypesFactory.eINSTANCE.createAD();

patientRole.getAddrs().add(addr);

addr.getUses().add(PostalAddressUse.H);

addr.addStreetAddressLine("1313 Mockingbird Lane");

addr.addCity("Janesville");

addr.addState("WI");

addr.addPostalCode("53545");

//create a patient object and add it to patient role

Patient patient = CDAFactory.eINSTANCE.createPatient();

patientRole.setPatient(patient);

PN name = DatatypesFactory.eINSTANCE.createPN();

patient.getNames().add(name);

name.addGiven("Henry");

name.addFamily("Levin");

CE administrativeGenderCode = DatatypesFactory.eINSTANCE.createCE();

patient.setAdministrativeGenderCode(administrativeGenderCode);

administrativeGenderCode.setCode("M");

administrativeGenderCode.setCodeSystem("2.16.840.1.113883.5.1");

TS birthTime = DatatypesFactory.eINSTANCE.createTS();

patient.setBirthTime(birthTime);

birthTime.setValue("19320924");

...

//write the document out to console

CDAUtil.save(ccdDocument, System.out);
```

Fig. 9.6 MDHT example Java source code

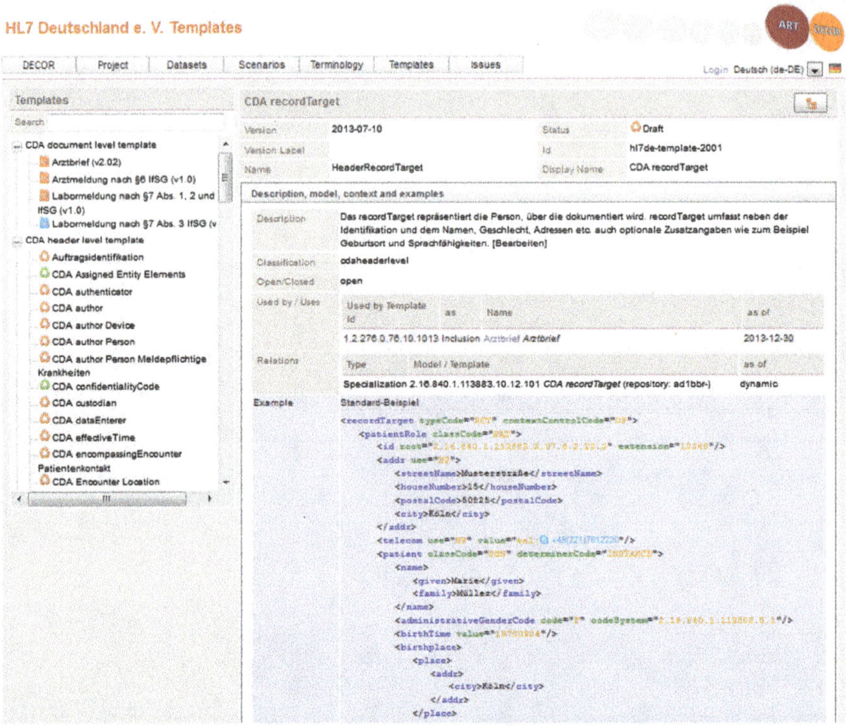

Fig. 9.7 ART-DECOR homepage of a specification project

The templates are essential building blocks of an implementation guide. All templates defined are shown in a list and can be compiled easily into an implementation guide. For maintenance purposes, such as editing or versioning, the individual templates are accessible individually.

To complete the analysis process, the elements from a template can be associated with the appropriate data set item. By this means a completed design process can be verified (Fig. 9.8).

ART-DECOR, therefore, supports the creation and maintenance of implementation guides. Figure 9.9 provides an overview of the way this information is presented to the user. The tool's display provides explanations, examples, vocabulary binding, and other attributes that allow users to specify and constrain templates.

As shown in Fig. 9.10, the clinician's view, reflected in the data set by concepts and lists with choices of terms, is completed by terminologists using terminology associations (right) and is completed by analysts, modelers, and template designers using templates and corresponding associations (left).

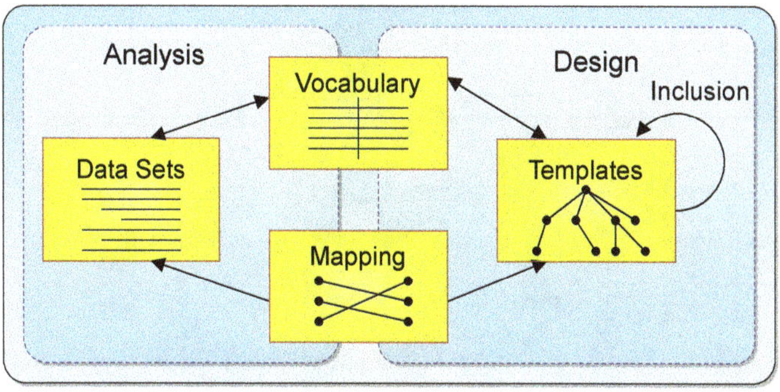

Fig. 9.8 ART-DECOR conceptual support

Item	DT	Card	Conf	Description	Label
h17:recordTarget					HeaderRecordTarget
	Example	<recordTarget typeCode="RCT" contextControlCode="OP"> <patientRole classCode="PAT"> <!-- ... --> </patientRole> </recordTarget>			
@typeCode		0..1	F	RCT	
@contextControlCode		0..1	F	OP	
h17:patientRole		1..1			HeaderRecordTarget
	Example	<patientRole classCode="PAT"> <id extension="186245" root="1.2.276.0.76.3.1.129.2.871"/> <patient classCode="PSN" determinerCode="INSTANCE"> <!-- ... --> </patient> </patientRole>			
@classCode		0..1	F	PAT	
h17:id	II	1..*			HeaderRecordTarget
	Example				
h17:addr	AD	0..*	O	Adresse des Patienten	HeaderRecordTarget
	Example	<addr use="HP"> <streetName>Dorfstraße</streetName> <houseNumber>54</houseNumber> <postalCode>51371</postalCode> <city>Leverkusen</city> </addr>			
h17:telecom	TEL	0..*	O	Kontaktdaten des Patienten	HeaderRecordTarget

Fig. 9.9 ART-DECOR template

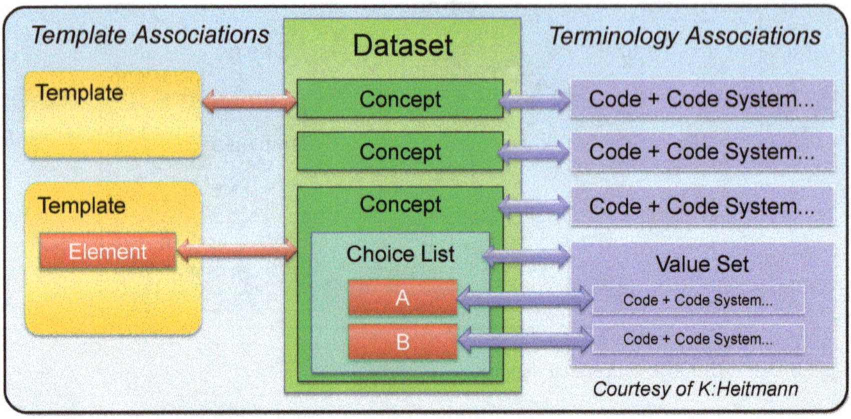

Fig. 9.10 ART-DECOR dataset

The ART-DECOR tool is project-oriented and supports the definition and management of clinical concepts and scenarios, allowing the definition of structure and semantics in terms of rules (templates, profiles), identification schemes, and terminologies (codes). It provides a forum for project-based problems, questions, and suggestions for changes (Fig. 9.11).

ART-DECOR has model-derived template prototypes that can be refined in the template editor to match the requirements collected and documented in the tool during the analysis phase (Fig. 9.12).

ART-DECOR provides the following features:

- Web-based collaboration platform
- Template Editor (HL7 V3, CDA, v2.xml)
- XML instance generation and validation
- Template import/export
- Documentation of templates and value sets (PDF, HTML)
- ISO-Schematron generator for open and closed templates
- Validation and testing engine, works collaboratively with IHE Gazelle Testing Tool Suite
- FHIR terminology services
- FHIR profile import/export (planned)

The ART-DECOR toolkit is used in a number of projects including IHE Europe, Austria (ELGA National eHealth program), The Netherlands (national screening program), and epSOS (European eHealth program).

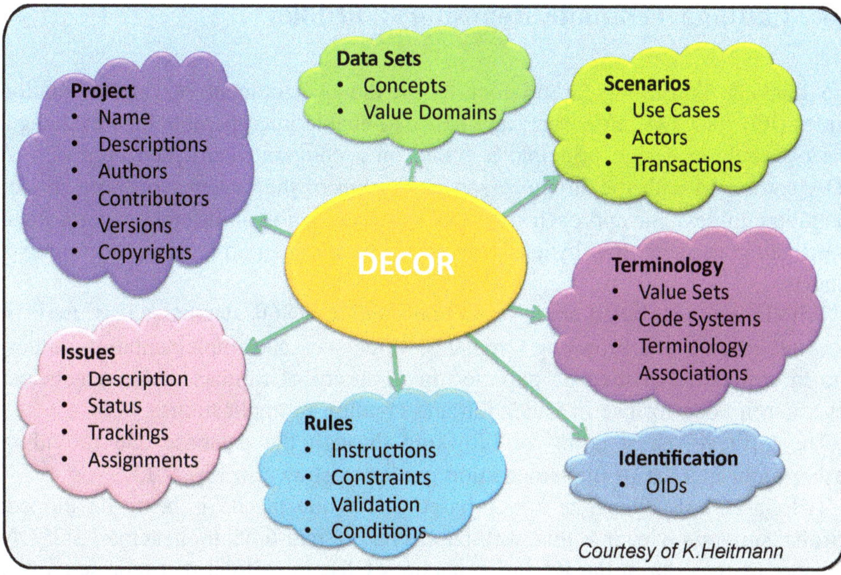

Fig. 9.11 ART-DECOR homepage of a specification project

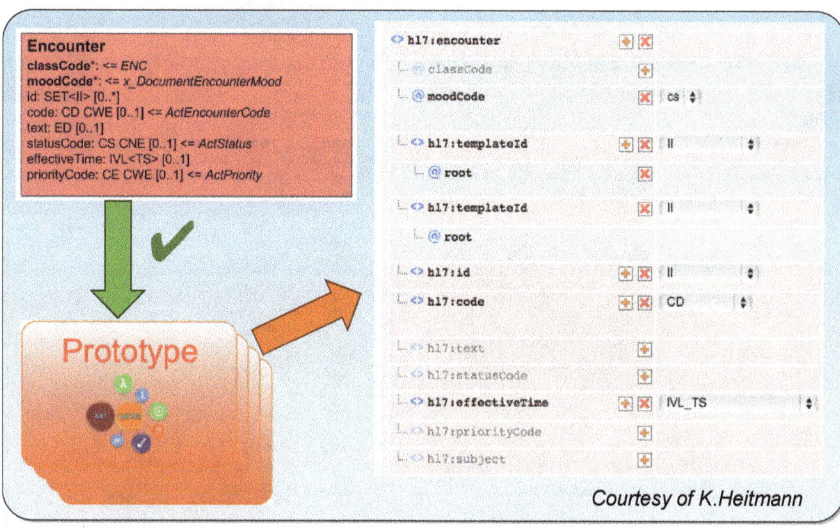

Fig. 9.12 ART-DECOR prototypes

9.6 Lantana Template Repository: Trifolia

The Lantana Consulting Group focuses on the development of implementation guides (IG) for CDA, eMeasure, and FHIR to enable interoperable data exchange. The overarching design principle is based on a component oriented approach of CDA combined with the structure and attribution of the contents of those implementation guides. The approach simplifies the cooperation of different experts when contributing to these IGs by entering all information in structured forms into a database.

Trifolia is a web-based application connected to a SQL database. It is used for creating, editing, and browsing templates, value sets, and implementation guides. The information can then be exported in a variety of formats and can generate Schematron code for use in validation and creation of applications.

The top-level entry point for browsing through the database and providing further input is a list of implementation guides as shown in Fig. 9.13.

Trifolia can also generate a web-based IG. While the IG is being developed, Trifolia supports viewing this web-based IG in real-time to generate a JSON snapshot of the data in the IG and generate a URL in Trifolia that represents that

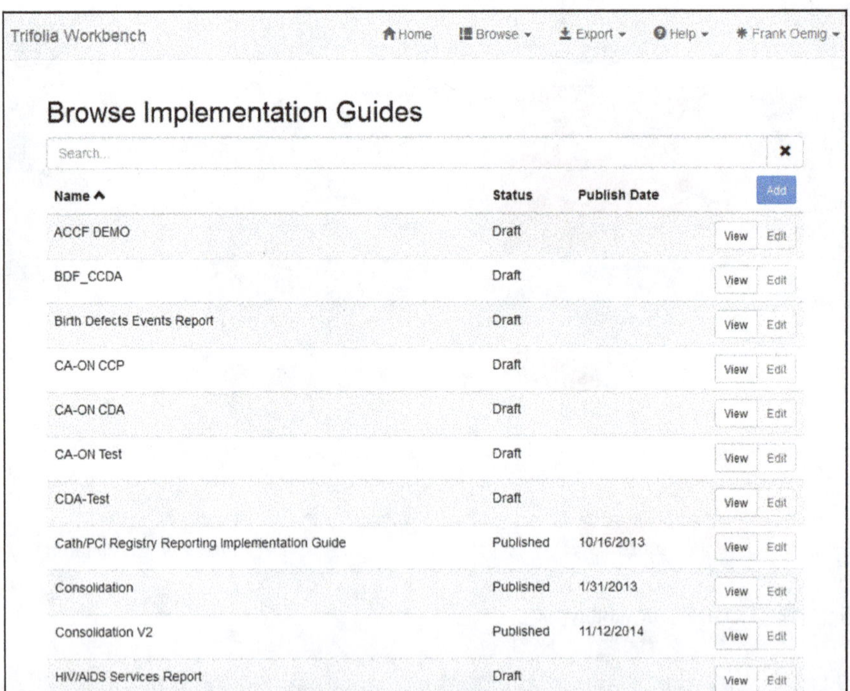

Fig. 9.13 Trifolia implementation guides

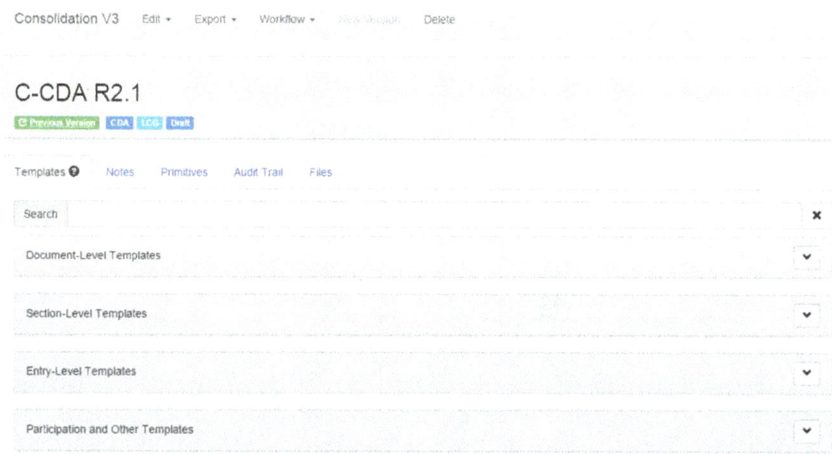

Fig. 9.14 Trifolia structure

specific point-in-time snapshot of the IG. The IG can be viewed directly within the Trifolia web application, or it can be downloaded for offline viewing.

After selecting an IG to view or edit, the internal structure, which is shown in Fig. 9.14, becomes visible. The most valuable aspect of the tool is the ability to edit implementation guides at the various template levels.

The Trifolia structured template editor tool allows users to design, review, manage, and document HL7 templates. Template Versioning capabilities identify and track version changes in templates (Fig. 9.15).

The Validation tab (Fig. 9.16) allows implementers to examine the validation messages for a specific template. Validation messages indicate structural recommendations or requirements on constraints.

The Constraints tab first shows only the element/attributes from the base standard/schema. Element/nodes (or nodes) that are associated with constraints are bold.

After selecting a node in the tree, the constraint editor window opens on the right side of the screen. The view that is displayed in the constraint editor depends on whether the node has been constrained. The constraints editor view also varies with the "Role" selected for the template editor as a whole (Analyst, Editor, and Engineer).

Computable constraints are constraints based on the element/attributes within the schema that can be represented using the fields supported by Trifolia (such as Conformance, Cardinality, Contained Template, Value Set, etc.). All computable constraints have a context, such as "@classCode".

Primitive constraints are free-text constraints that cannot be represented using the standard computable fields within Trifolia.

The next two screenshots shown in Figs. 9.17 and 9.18 provide the constraints defined at the section and entry level. Once the constraints are entered into Trifolia they are rendered into human readable natural language sentences.

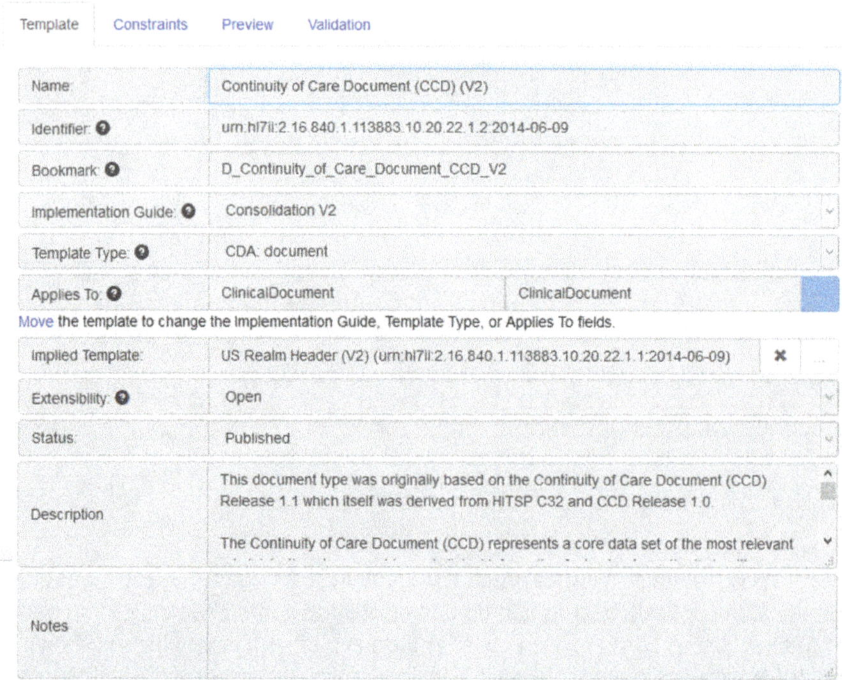

Fig. 9.15 Trifolia structured template editor

On the highest level, Trifolia manages the elements, e.g., @code, including their sub-elements, e.g., attributes, belonging to a template in the form of a hierarchy, as is shown in Fig. 9.19.

The Template Editor allows for managing the details of the constraint. In Fig. 9.20, the @code attribute is set to a fixed value as it appears in the Constraint Editor. In the lower part of the figure, a human readable expression is presented for this specific constraint. Figure 9.21 shows the @codeSystem attribute for a data element as it appears in the Constraint Editor.

A value set binding associates an element/attribute with a (pre-defined) value set. A value set specifies a set of codes drawn from one or more code systems. Specifying a value set allows the implementer of the template to choose a code within the value set that is appropriate for the scenario. Figure 9.22 shows the binding of an element to a value set in the Template Editor. The specification details entered into Trifolia are then rendered into a human readable implementation guide as is shown in Fig. 9.23.

Another export format for the same specification details is an XML Schematron file, as shown in Fig. 9.24, that can be used with a Schematron engine to validate CDA instances.

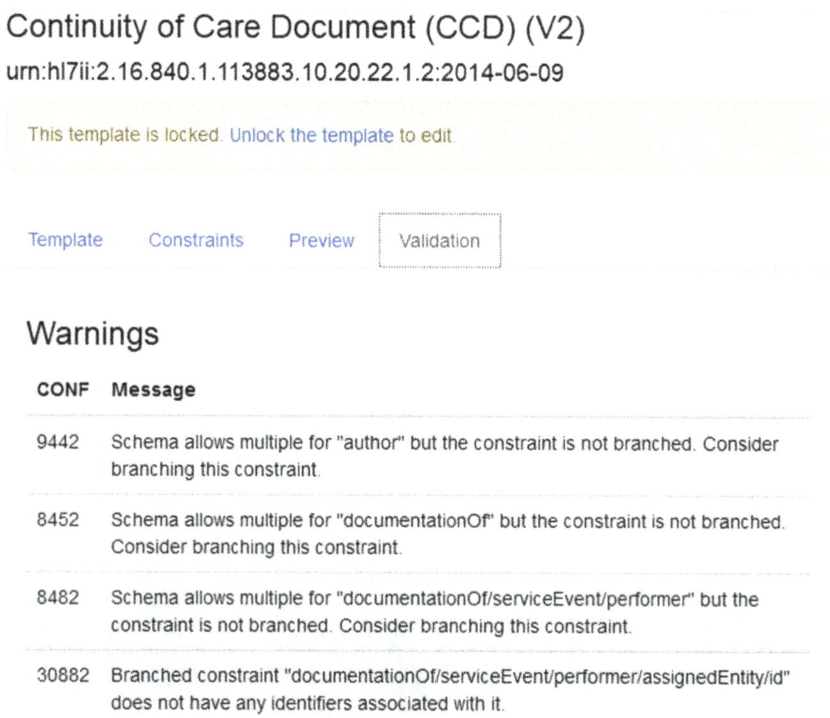

Fig. 9.16 Trifolia validation

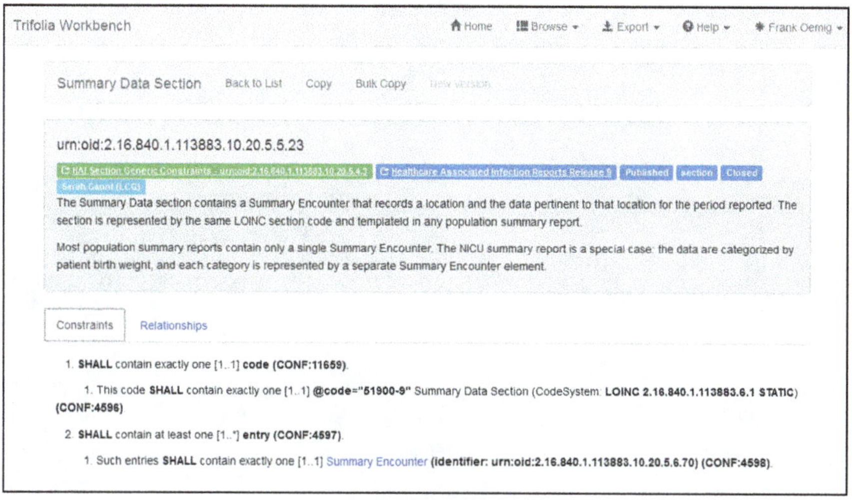

Fig. 9.17 Trifolia section level constraints

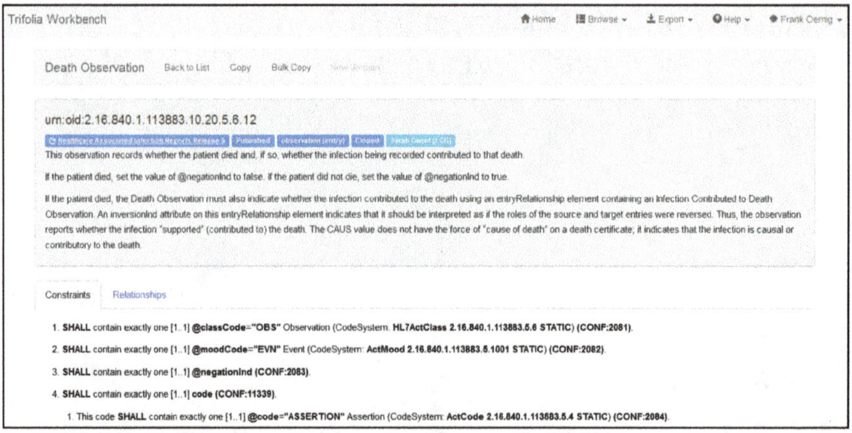

Fig. 9.18 Trifolia entry level constraints

⊟code	**19143**	**No**	**No**	**SHALL**	**1..1**	**CD**	
@nullFlavor				MAY	0..1	NullFlavor	
@code	**19144**	**No**	**No**	**SHALL**	**1..1**	**cs**	**11323-3, Health status**
@codeSystem	**32161**	**No**	**No**	**SHALL**	**1..1**	**uid**	**2.16.840.1.113883.6.1**
@codeSystemName				MAY	0..1	st	
@codeSystemVersion				MAY	0..1	st	
@displayName				MAY	0..1	st	
@sdtc:valueSet				MAY	0..1		
@sdtc:valueSetVersion				MAY	0..1		

Fig. 9.19 Trifolia structured list of template elements

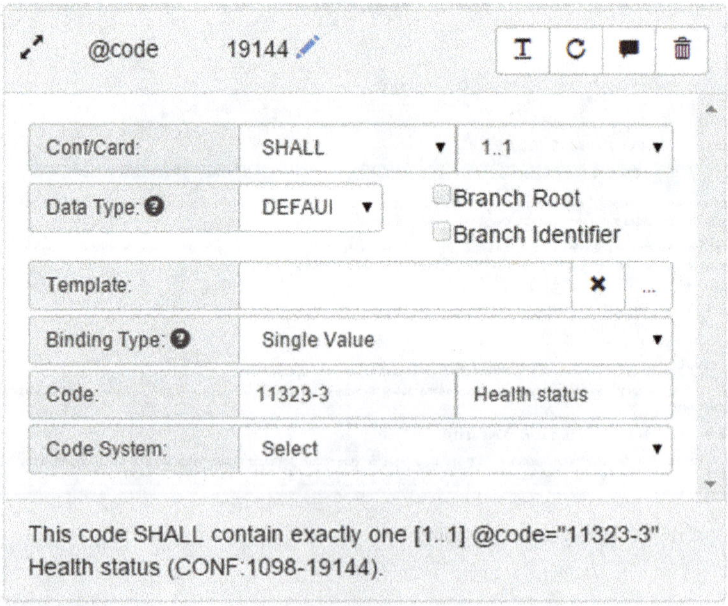

Fig. 9.20 Trifolia template editor (fixed value)

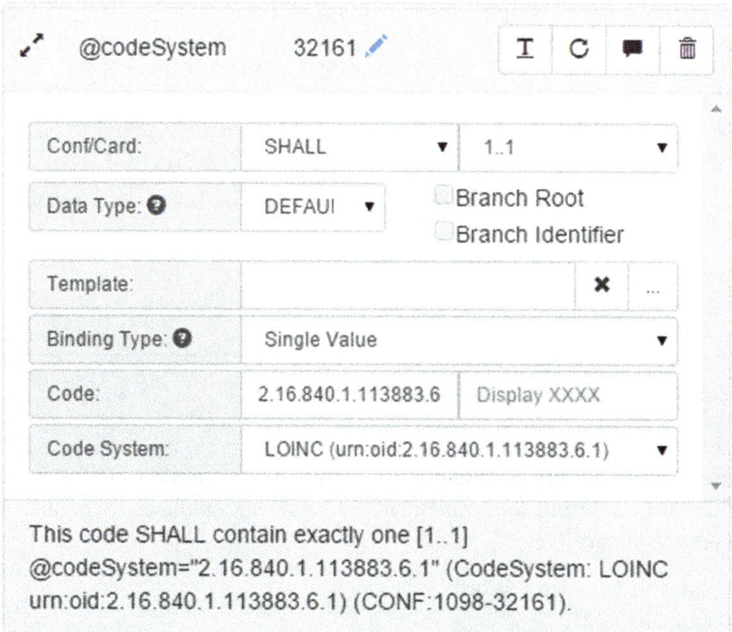

Fig. 9.21 Trifolia template editor (single code from code system)

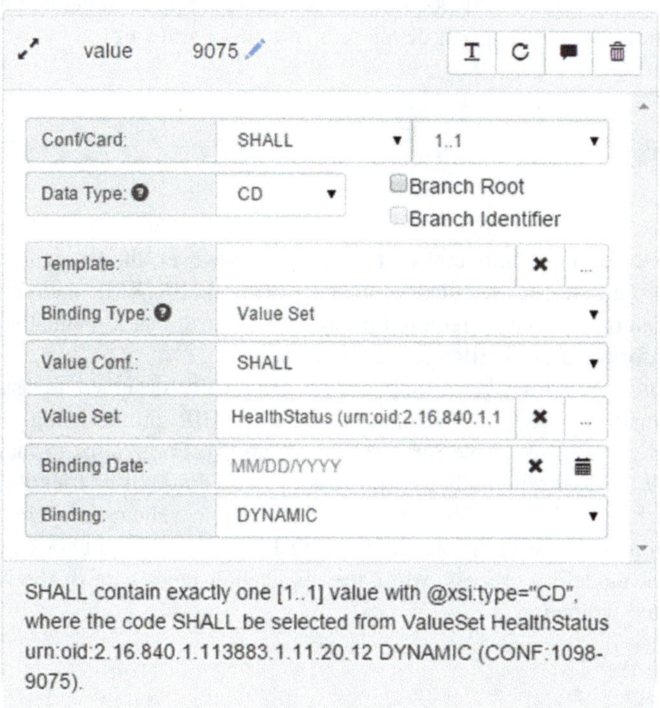

Fig. 9.22 Trifolia constraint editor (value sets)

7. SHALL contain exactly one [1..1] **value** with @xsi:type="CD", where the code **SHALL** be selected from ValueSet HealthStatus 2.16.840.1.113883.1.11.20.12 **DYNAMIC (CONF1098-9075)**.

Fig. 9.23 Trifolia implementation guide conformance statements

```
<sch:assert id="a-1098-9075" test="count(cda:value@xsi:type='CD'])=1">

    SHALL contain exactly one [1..1] value with @xsi:type="CD", where
    the code SHALL be selected from ValueSet HealthStatus
    2.16.840.1.113883.1.11.20.12 (CONF:1098-9075).

</sch:assert>
```

Fig. 9.24 Trifolia generated Schematron rule

As well as the editing functions to maintain the content, Trifolia provides capabilities for exporting the implementation guides, templates, Schematron, and associated vocabulary:

- Templates to Microsoft Word
- Templates to XML
- Standard IG Schematron
- Vocabulary

The export to a MS Word Document results in readable documentation, whereas the other three formats support developers in writing software.

9.7 Forge

It is possible to create and edit HL7 FHIR profiles manually, e.g., using a generic (XML) editor or a specially crafted Excel sheet. However, the manual approach is error-prone and requires detailed knowledge of the FHIR XML and/or JSON file formats. External tooling is required in order to confirm that a manually generated profile conforms to the FHIR specification.

Forge is a Windows-based application specifically designed to assist in the creation, maintenance, and publication of HL7 FHIR profiles (Fig. 9.25). The application is freely available for download from [5]. Forge aims to facilitate and support the FHIR profile authoring process by providing a user-friendly graphical editor interface in combination with automatic profile validation against the constraints defined by the FHIR standard. Using Forge, a profile author can focus on the medical modeling process, while the application takes care of the XML serialization and validation.

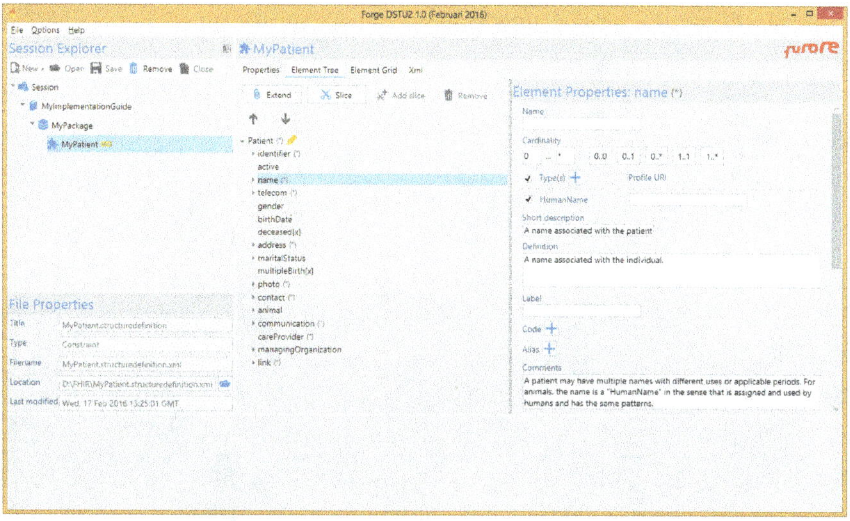

Fig. 9.25 Forge for DSTU 2

Forge supports the creation and maintenance of FHIR resource profiles and extension definitions. The application provides user-friendly access to the individual profile elements and element properties. Forge automatically handles and generates differential (constraints only) and snapshot (full) profile representations. Forge also supports the authoring of implementation guides and conformance packages. A conformance package represents a set of conceptually related conformance resources. An implementation guide combines one or more conformance packages together with the associated meta data and documentation (Fig. 9.26). Forge provides seamless integration of online FHIR servers (via import/export of conformance resources) and also supports the publication of profiles to online FHIR profile registries (e.g., simplifier.net [6]).

The FHIR team at Furore is developing Forge. FHIR .NET API, available on GitHub [7], is an associated project that is used extensively by Forge for profile (de-)serialization and validation.

Forge is under active development and strives to be compliant with the most recently published version of the FHIR specification. At the time of this writing, the most recent release supports the FHIR DSTU 2 (official version) specification published on October 24, 2015 [8]. An earlier application version that is compatible with the original FHIR DSTU 1 draft specification is also available for download, but it is no longer being actively developed. The application roadmap will closely follow the evolution of the FHIR specification.

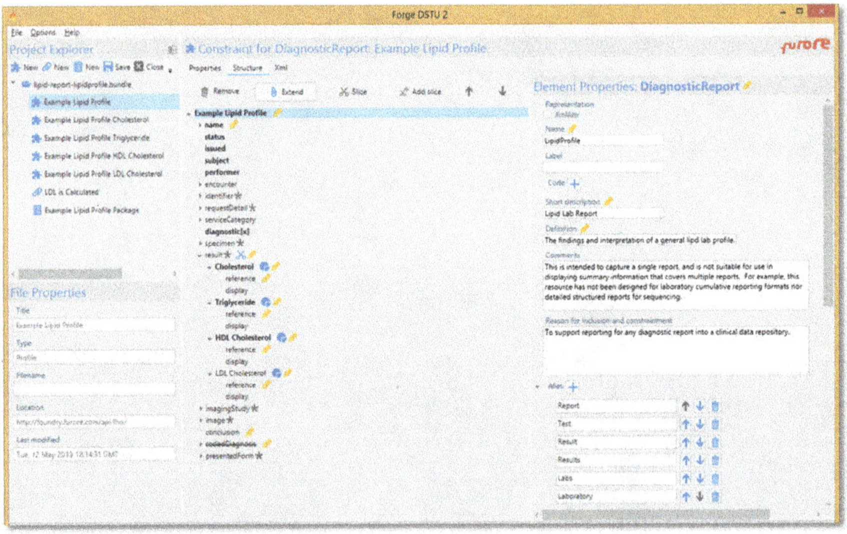

Fig. 9.26 Forge *lipid* example package

9.8 Summary

To realize the benefits of profiling, as explained in Chap. 7, appropriate tools must be available that help to create, maintain, and implement interface definitions. A brief survey of representative and freely available tools are presented to provide interested readers with an overview of the tool capabilities.

References

1. Messaging Workbench (MWB). Developed by Peter Rontey at the U.S. Veterans Administration (VA) in conjunction with the HL7 Conformance Working Group; http://www.hl7.org/
2. CDA Tools. Produce CDA Content using MDHT API. http://www.cdatools.com, last accessed June 6, 2016
3. Advanced Requirement Tooling - Data Elements, Codes, OIDs and Rules. http://www.art-decor.org, https://art-decor.org/art-decor/decor-templates–hl7de-
4. Heitmann K. ART-DECOR: Creating Templates with Prototypes and Building Block Repositories. https://www.hl7.org/documentcenter/public/wg/java/ART-DECOR-tooling-kheitmann-web.pdf, last accessed November 21st 2014
5. Forge: http://fhir.furore.com/forge
6. Simplifier. http://simplifier.net/
7. https://github.com/ewoutkramer/fhir-net-api
8. http://www.hl7.org/fhir

9. NIST. Implementation Guide Authoring and Management Tool (IGAMT). https://hl7v2igamt.nist.gov
10. Lantana Consulting Group. http://www.lantanagroup.com
11. Model-Driven Health Tools CDA Tools. http://cdatools.org
12. Trifolia Workbench HL7 Webedition. https://trifolia.lantanagroup.com/, https://trifolia.lantanagroup.com/IGManagement/List

Part III
Testing (and Tools)

Chapter 10
Testing Models

10.1 Introduction

Now that a clear understanding of what conformance means has been conveyed, let's explore why it is necessary, what are its benefits, and how appropriate application of the concepts by implementers and users can be assured. The third part of this book is devoted to the process, strategy, assessment, and instantiation of conformance and interoperability testing. This chapter presents a testing model classification framework that supports conformance and interoperability testing of distributed systems. This introduction provides the foundation and framework from which further discussions about testing can proceed. The various testing models are presented, along with their applicability and the requirements they impose for realization of a testing tool. Three distinct models are identified, and a description of the testing activities that can be performed within the model is provided for each one. The broad categories of testing activities include data instance validation, isolated systems testing, and peer-to-peer systems testing. The targeted systems are those that support data exchange standards.

A list and definition of the types of conformance and interoperability testing that can be conducted in a testing model are presented. A description and an illustration of a conceptual test tool design for each testing model is given. The details provided about the models and their testing capacity are intended to help promote a more structured approach to testing, in which the relationship between testing and test requirements is more clearly defined and the capabilities and limitations of testing tools are better understood. In broader terms, this approach should help the information technology industry and testing bodies identify and describe the depth and scope of their testing endeavors.

F. Oemig and R. Snelick, *Healthcare Interoperability Standards Compliance Handbook*, DOI 10.1007/978-3-319-44839-8_10

In Chap. 13, realizations of these testing models are described along with specific case studies. Chapter 14 presents examples of production tools that instantiate these design patterns.

10.2 Testing Objectives

Recognizing that testing is a complex, multidimensional, and often incremental problem leads to considering the use of multiple models for conducting testing. Each model can be used for conducting a—possibly overlapping—component of conformance or interoperability testing.

Conformance testing is a multi-faceted operation that can range from a simple assessment of whether a value in a message is valid to a nuanced appraisal of a system's reaction to a complex sequence of events. Testing the full range of conformance requirements is not always practical, but the evaluation of specific conformance requirements, such as the content of a data element, may be of interest. Ultimately, the goal of conformance testing is to enable interoperability among different implementations. Conducting interoperability testing adds another dimension to the requirements for the testing model.

A key aim of this chapter is to provide a clear explanation of the objectives for testing. The following questions are addressed:

- What are the testing objectives and scope?
- What testing models can be used to meet the testing objectives?
- What can be tested in each model?
- What requirements do testing models place on a test tool design and implementation?
- And, maybe most importantly, what does testing with a particular model reveal about the implementation that was tested?

In addition to addressing these issues, definitions are given for conformance and interoperability terms and concepts. Furthermore, a description of a typical scaled-down test organization hierarchy that can be used to guide and organize the testing plans and models is presented. In Chap. 11 the test organization hierarchy is expanded upon. A list of, and definitions for, the types of conformance and interoperability tests that can be performed to assess an application is presented. Next, for each of the three testing models, a description of the testing activities that can be performed within the model is given. Finally, each testing dimension and its inter-relationship with other testing dimensions is discussed. Testing dimensions include the test modes, such as automated versus inspection testing, and aspects of the test environment (e.g., the systems under test are on-site with the tester or the testing is conducted remotely over the Internet). These considerations are important when conducting testing.

10.3 Definition of Terms

This section defines (and, in some cases, elaborates on earlier definitions of) a set of terms used in this chapter and the chapters that follow. In some circles, these definitions may not be universally agreed upon, but establishing common definitions for use in this book will facilitate an understanding of the concepts presented.

Conformance: Conformance is defined as the fulfillment of a product, process, or service of specified requirements [1, 2]. The concept of conformance is essential to any standard for providing an objective measure of how closely implementations satisfy the requirements defined in the standard. Conformance is a term that describes a relationship between a standard and an implementation.

Syntactic Interoperability: If two or more systems are capable of communicating and exchanging data, they are exhibiting syntactic interoperability. Syntactic interoperability is required before any attempts of further interoperability can be achieved [3], i.e., syntactic interoperability is a prerequisite to semantic interoperability. Syntactic interoperability is domain-independent (e.g., base XML) and the meaning of what is exchanged is not important to its success [4]. In the literature, syntactic interoperability is sometimes referred to as Technical Interoperability.

Semantic Interoperability: Semantic interoperability goes beyond the ability of two or more computer systems to exchange information; it involves the ability for a sending system to communicate information automatically and have that information correctly interpreted by the receiving system (i.e., there is a shared *understanding*). To achieve semantic interoperability, both sides must defer to a common information exchange reference model [3]. Semantic interoperability is domain-specific and typically employs the use of codes (e.g., LOINC-Logical Observation Identifiers Names and Codes) and identifiers [4]. This level of communication is what the industry seeks to attain for healthcare interoperability.

Conformance Testing: Conformance testing entails the assessment of an implementation to determine if its behavior is consistent with the requirements for behavior as defined in a standard or other reference document. The term *behavior* is used here in a broad sense; for example, it could mean the action by which an implementation creates a message or document. The objective of conformance testing is to determine how completely and correctly the requirements of the standard have been met by the implementation. Note that conformance cannot be determined definitively; only a certain degree of confidence can be derived based on the quantity and quality of tests performed. Conformance testing is often referred to as *black box* testing, in which the details of the implementation are unknown, and only the inputs and outputs of the implementation are used for evaluation [1].

Syntactic Interoperability Testing: This kind of testing involves the assessment of an implementation to determine its ability to interoperate syntactically with one or more distinct systems. This testing might include assessing a system's capability for handling escape sequences or identifying the character set according to the rules defined in a standard.

Semantic Interoperability Testing: The focus of this kind of testing is on assessment of an implementation to evaluate its ability to interoperate semantically with one or more distinct systems. This testing might include extraction and interpretation of a coded data value and performing an agreed upon action based on a common understanding of that code.

System-under-Test (SUT): The software system that is being tested.

Testing Model: The testing models establish the method of operation in which a conformance or interoperability test is being conducted. Three such testing models have been identified: *Data Instance Test Model*, *Isolated System Test Model*, and *Peer-to-peer System Test Model*. The testing models are only defined here in terms of the necessary interactions to enable testing between the test system and the *system under test* (SUT) or test object. The hardware or software commonly associated with testing models is not addressed, because these elements are implementation dependent.

Test Object: The object that is being tested is called the test object; examples include a message, a document, or an application. The object may or may not have been created by the SUT (i.e., it may be created manually).

Test Artifact: Material used to test a test object are known as test artifacts. These artifacts are derived from the test requirements provided in the standards and are suitable for input or as props to perform an assessment. An example is an XML representation of an HL7 v2.x conformance profile as described in Chap. 7. The requirements are "codified" as assertions and can be processed by a validation mechanism.

Tester: A tester is the person or entity performing (administering) the testing. Typically, a first-party Tester is the creator of the product, e.g., a Vendor. A second party Tester is the user or purchaser of the product. A third-party Tester (often referred to as a third-party "neutral" tester) is an independent tester and is not affiliated with the product being tested. Certification testing is mostly (but not always) performed by third-party testers.

10.4 Test Organization Hierarchy

Important aspects of test planning are the organization and strategy, which are administered by the tester. It is advantageous to have a comprehensive and structured testing plan to ensure that testing objectives are met, that is, to ensure that the testing covers the evaluation of all aspects of the system that should be tested. Defining and applying an established organizational hierarchy at the outset of test suite development is important, as this hierarchy helps in the creation, management,

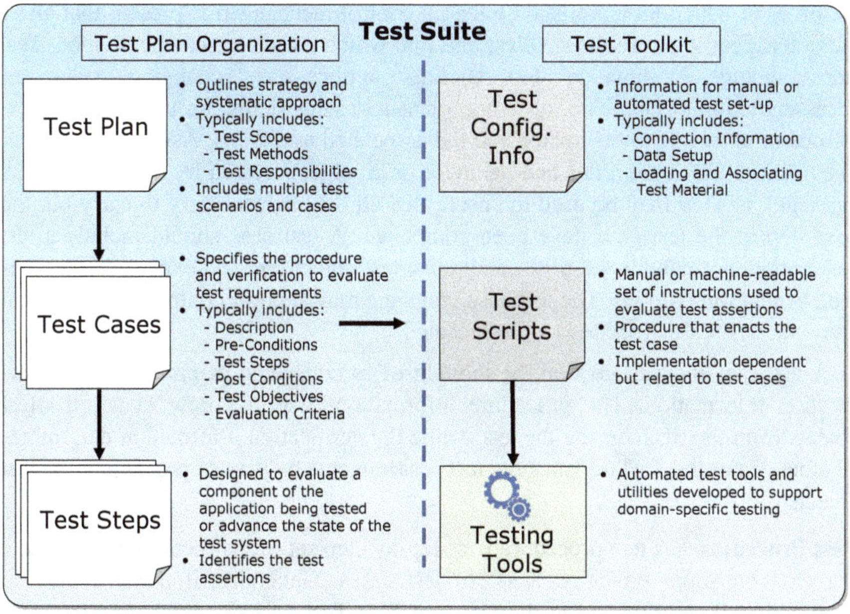

Fig. 10.1 Test organization hierarchy

and maintenance of test cases. In addition, an organizational hierarchy can provide the necessary documentation for demonstrating the purpose and tracing the results of using the test cases, which is especially important when the SUT fails a test. Figure 10.1 illustrates one such test organization hierarchy (this is a representative organization and is not necessarily universal). These concepts are expanded on in Chap. 11; the purpose of introducing them here is to aid in the explanation of the testing models. What follows is an definition of each component in the hierarchy. Additional related terms that do not appear in Fig. 10.1 are defined in Chap. 11.

Test Suite: A collection of test cases (usually organized in a test plan), along with the associated machinery and process to execute the test cases, is known as a test suite. A *test suite* should include documentation of the overall testing strategy, configuration requirements, and may control, via tooling, the invocation of test cases.

Test Plan: A test plan outlines the strategy and systematic approach to be used to evaluate an SUT. A *test plan* should minimally include test scope, test methods, test scenarios, test cases, test case coverage matrix, and test responsibilities.

Test Case: A test case is a specific executable test used to examine certain aspects of an object or system that is being tested and provides a detailed description of the steps that should be taken as well as the expected results. Test steps are executed in the order in which they are listed unless a control mechanism is present that alters the order. Test steps are the smallest unit into which a test case can be divided. Test steps include commands for starting applications, changing state, or accessing/loading data. The most important test steps define an action to be performed or an object to be created and the associated assertions. Assertions are used to evaluate SUT capabilities and behavior or an object created by the SUT (e.g., a message), or they may be used to ensure that all actions necessary to carry out the next step in the test case have been completed. A test case should include a test description, pre-conditions, post-conditions, test objectives, and expected outcomes (i.e., evaluation criteria). The test case language may support control structures that allow the test case workflow to be repeated.

A test case may, in general, be thought of as consisting of procedure and verification information. The procedure information describes how to get the test objects from the SUT during the test, while the verification information determines whether or not the SUT satisfies the test requirements by way of processing the test objects [5].

Test Procedure: A test procedure is a step-by-step set of instructions to execute a test case or, more typically, a set of test cases. Generally, it pertains only to instructions directly related to the test case (See Test Script).

Test Script: A script is closely tied to the test cases and the test procedure and provides a set of instructions for a particular test that will be carried out by a manual process or automated test tool. That is, it provides additional instruction on how to execute the test case, including test setup, the test environment (e.g., over the web), and other instructions needed by the Tester. It can be thought of as an *outer wrapper* to a set of test cases and the test procedure. Test scripts are typically created by organizations that execute the tests (e.g., the ONC Accredited Testing Laboratories).

Test Scenario: A scenario is also closely related to the test case, and it often is used to group test cases that involves a multistep business workflow. In some instances, a scenario may combine two or more test cases. A test scenario can be thought of as a particular use case instance (i.e., one path through the use case). Test scenario is a term often conflated with test case; for the purposes of the book, the term is used to describe a *higher-level* concept (i.e., a *grouping* of test cases).

Test Step: Conformance and interoperability testing can generally be conducted most effectively by dividing the testing into a number of steps. Each step in the testing process is designed to evaluate a component of the application being tested or advance the state of the test system. Test steps are components of a test case. Test steps typically equate to a single test action, e.g., creating a message or loading test data.

Test Assertion: A statement (preferably atomic) designed to evaluate an element or state of the SUT is called a test assertion. Assertions are derived from the test criteria (requirements). For example, for the requirement "the application shall populate the *administered code* element with a value identified in the vaccine administered code value set described in the CVX vocabulary", one or more test assertions are created to determine if the requirement is satisfied by the implementation. Typically, there is a many-to-one relationship between test assertions and a test step (because the test step can refer to a high level requirement that expands to many low level requirements). For example, validation of a CDA document will have many test assertions.

Test Criteria: Test Criteria specify requirements that are used to construct test cases and assertions that are designed to evaluate the SUT. The test criteria are derived from the test specification (e.g., a standard) that the system is being tested against. **Test Requirement** is synonymous with Test Criteria, which is a term that is used at various levels. For example, ONC, when issuing the Health IT certification rules, provides high-level criteria that reference a standard, e.g., incorporate laboratory results using the Laboratory Results Interface (LRI) standard. This standard fulfils the high-level criteria by providing an expansive set of requirements. Ultimately each criterion is addressed by assertions.

Test Configuration Information: Configuration data necessary for executing the test cases defined in the test plan are known as test configuration information. Configuration is necessary at two levels: the tool level and the test case level. At the tool level, connection information is necessary so that the tool can communicate with the SUT (if the test requires communication). At the test case level, various configuration information is typically necessary, including loading the system with data, setting the system to a particular state, and loading and associating the appropriate test material needed by the test tool.

Test Tool: An application that can be used in conducting conformance or interoperability testing is called a test tool. A test tool can interact with users, the SUT, or other test tools (e.g., Test Agents). The test tool executes the test cases and can be referenced in a test script.

Test Agent: A test agent is an implementation of functionality that—at a minimum—enables all interactions necessary for testing to be carried out with the SUT. Test agents (also referred to as simulators) are implementations of actors (or applications) that support the functionality of the underlying specification of the actor. The test agent does not have to be a complete reference implementation; it only needs to support the functionality of the actor to support testing of applications. Test agents are stand-in *applications* with which the SUT would normally interact.

It is important to note that the Test Suite container shown here is a typical framework and not universally adopted in practice. Variations of these components, use of different terminology, and commingling of concepts are commonplace. Although, a common approach is always desirable, the important point here is that a testing program identifies such terms and concepts, and develops a systematic approach to testing.

10.5 Test Evaluation Types

Conformance and interoperability testing can be conducted effectively by dividing the testing into a number of categories based on the evaluation specific criteria. The criteria address the evaluation of one or more components of the application being tested or one or more aspects of the application's behavior.

The system components and behavioral aspects to be tested include the following:

- Documents and messages (conformance)
- Transport protocol usage
- Application functional behavior
- Syntactic Interoperability
- Semantic interoperability

These testing types form layers and are interrelated to some degree. For example, messaging requirements directly influence the functional requirements of an application. In addition, when testing a complete system, one layer of testing is dependent on another layer.

One theme of this book is to focus on the data exchange standards; however, such standards can't be completely created in a vacuum. As mentioned previously, the data exchange standards influence functional requirements. In practice, functional requirement specifications often are not created by SDOs, which hinders the testing process for the latter three testing types. The IHE integration profiles do provide functional requirement specifications, but they are rarely specified at a level of depth and completeness to support *working* interoperability. For example, there is no mention of how receiving systems are to process data elements. If the data element is important enough to be sent, then an associated functional requirement must be bound to it. At some point the functional requirements (business rules, if you like) need to be expressed in such a manner that they are related to the data exchange specification and are testable. Otherwise, complete system testing for interoperability is not possible. An effort is being made to achieve this goal through the work of the ONC S&I Framework suite of HL7 v2 laboratory specifications [6].

The following information elaborates on the methods for evaluating each criterion introduced above.

Object Conformance Testing: Evaluates a test object for conformance to a specification. The specification contains the requirements for creating valid instances of the test object.

Object conformance testing has two modes of operation, context-free and context-based, as described in Chap. 11. Context-free testing does not have an associated test case. Context-based testing is tightly bound to a test case and test data.

Transport Protocol Usage Testing: To test the application's use of the transport protocol, an evaluation of how an application packages and extracts messages and documents is made. This type of testing assesses an application's use of an allowed communication protocol. That is, on sending, a check to ensure the application correctly packages messages before sending them is performed, and on receiving the application is checked to make sure it correctly extracts the message content from the package it was received in.

Testing Application Conformance to the Data Exchange Standard: One element of evaluating application behavior is assessment of an application's reaction to valid and invalid variations in data content. This type of testing examines application responses to received messages. For example, an application's reaction to variations in message structure and content are evaluated with this type of testing. Messages or documents are sent with variations in the encoding characters and with valid and invalid content. A valid response from the receiving application is an indication that it processed a valid message (document) or recognized an invalid message (document). This type of testing accommodates the acknowledgement protocols as defined by the specification.

Functional Requirements Testing: Evaluates a system's capabilities based on functional requirements—this is conformance testing of functional requirements. Functional requirements define a functional (system behavior) capability, e.g., update a patient record. To test functional capabilities, an evaluation of the application's interpretation of message content is made. The evaluation is made based on the actions taken by the application when new messages are received or by inspection testing. The application's response to the initiating system is also evaluated. Generally, this type of testing consists of sending the application valid messages and evaluating the responses returned by the application for correct semantic content (when the SUT is a server). Alternatively, inspection testing can be employed. When the SUT is a client application it will be instructed to create a message or document, usually via a user interface. In order to conduct Functional Requirements Testing, a test scenario is created in which a sequence of orchestrated transactions is composed to test adherence to specific functional requirements.

When there is no mechanism to automatically extract data from a system (i.e., a standardized query and response protocol), then various forms of inspection testing are necessary. Inspection testing may include an assessment of the application's display, log files, configuration files, direct data base queries, or whatever mechanism the systems provides for gaining insight into its operation. Depending on the system, all such mechanisms may not be available to the tester. More information on Functional Requirements Testing and approaches to testing sending and receiving applications is given in Chap. 11.

Syntactic Interoperability Testing: Interoperability testing is designed primarily to establish that two applications are able to exchange data successfully. No evaluation of the application's processing of the data is made with this type of testing.

Semantic Interoperability Testing: This type of testing is the second phase of interoperability testing. If two applications establish that they are capable of exchanging data, semantic interoperability testing attempts to determine if they correctly process the data exchanged as intended.

Functional testing (i.e., *application conformance testing of functional requirements*) can be performed irrespective of the data exchange standard. For example, the functional requirements for an application do not change based on how the data is obtained (e.g., HL7 v2.x, HL7 V3, FHIR, etc.). Semantic interoperability testing determines that two systems can function (process and use the data) as intended for the given data exchange standard (e.g., example HL7 v2.x). Therefore, semantic interoperability testing extends the scope of testing performed in functional testing. Semantic Interoperability Testing has to account for the information mapping to and from the information model employed by the systems. It seeks to determine if the systems employ a compatible information model and use the concepts in the same manner. In functional testing, the data exchange component is essentially detached from the testing; that is, the syntactic and information mapping aspect has already been performed.

10.6 Testing Models

In the previous sections, a set of distinct testing types were introduced that can be used to evaluate the components of an application that are essential to its overall functioning. Below, the conceptual models are described in which these testing types can be carried out.

Data Instance Test Model: This testing model is composed of one or more testing tools and the test object. The test tool uses the specification as the basis to evaluate the test object.

- *Object Conformance Testing*
  - Validates a test object against a specification.
  - E.g., the content of an XML document evaluated against a schema
  - Is context-free or context-based (has associated test data)

Isolated System Test Model: This testing model consists of a SUT and testing tools designed to interact with the system. The SUT may interact with test agents or validation testing tools.

- *Includes Data Instance Testing Capabilities*
- *Transport Protocol Usage Testing*
- *Testing Application Conformance to Data Exchange Standard*
  - Expanded test coverage of conformance requirements

  - Valid and invalid instances
  - Multiple test cases conducted

- *Functional Requirements Testing*

  - Test scenario is created to orchestrate a sequence of transactions

Peer-to-Peer System Test Model: This testing model consists of one or more vendor systems and a testing infrastructure designed to interact with and evaluate one or more of the vendor systems.

- *Includes Isolated System Testing Capabilities*
- *Syntactic Interoperability Testing*
- *Semantic Interoperability Testing*

To some degree, Syntactic and Semantic Interoperability Testing can be assessed in Isolated System Testing, albeit with a test tool. The degree to which semantic interoperability testing can be performed is dependent on the quality of the test cases and test agent (reference implementation). However, interoperability testing must ultimately be conducted with real systems in test environments.

10.6.1 Data Instance Testing Model

In the Data Instance Testing Model, a test is conducted with a test object and a testing tool. The goal is to perform evaluation of data content against a set of conformance rules. The tool may be a validation service. An example of data instance testing is validation of an HL7 v2.x message instance against an HL7 v2.x conformance profile [7].

The means of delivery is not important; any means by which the object can be delivered to the testing tool is satisfactory. That is, a file may be used to deliver the data or the test object may be delivered using the underlying transport protocol.

The objective of data instance testing is to assess the adherence of the test object to the conformance requirements defined by a specification. The specification typically will include requirements that define the structure or syntax of the data, along with semantic requirements for interpreting the data. The syntax may be defined by a formal grammar using a BNF (Backus-Naur Form) notation, an XML schema, or another notation. In these cases, precise evaluation of data items for conformance with the syntactic requirements will be possible. Generally, the specification also will include allowed values for instances of the data object, and these need to be evaluated for conformance with the requirements of the specification.

Figure 10.2 depicts the Data Instance Testing Model. In this illustration, the test object is delivered manually (i.e., the tester access point is via an uploaded file or cut-and-paste of the test object). Replacing the tester icon with a system is another instance of this test model in which the test object is delivered directly via the system that created the test object (still only the object is validated, not transport or

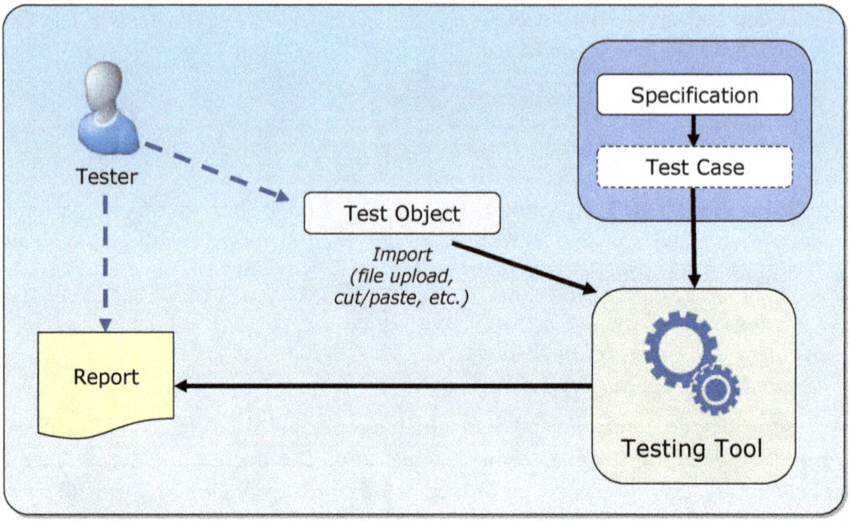

Fig. 10.2 Data instance testing model

the way it is created). As noted, the Data Instance Testing Model supports different testing types and, therefore, may or may not have an associated test case. The Data Instance Testing Model validation component is leveraged and is an integral part of the test models to follow.

10.6.2 Isolated System Testing Model

In the Isolated System Testing Model a test is conducted with the SUT and a test tool. The SUT may interact with test agents and validation testing tools. Since conformance testing is the main objective in using this model, Object Conformance Testing is a key capability. Additionally, the Isolated System Testing Model supports Transport Protocol Usage Testing, Testing Application Conformance to the Data Exchange Standard, and Functional Requirements Testing.

Transport Protocol Usage Conformance Testing asserts that an application correctly implements an allowed communications protocol. That is, on sending the application correctly packages messages before sending them, and on receiving the application correctly extracts the message content from the package in which it was received. SOAP[1] is an example of a transport protocol.

The Testing for Conformance to the Data Exchange Standard evaluation type tests that an application (SUT) correctly sends messages and that the application

[1]Simple Object Access Protocol.

(SUT) correctly responds to all messages, valid and invalid, that the application (SUT) receives. All responses are evaluated to ensure that they adhere to the requirements defined in the relevant specification. This type of testing evaluates an application's reaction to variations in message structure and content. Messages that the application is expected to support are sent to the application, changes are made in the encoding characters used, and valid and invalid variations in content are sent; often, boundary conditions are tested, and optional elements can be included. The goal is to "poke" the system in various ways in an attempt to provide *full* test coverage. The criterion for evaluation is receipt of an application response indicating that it processed a valid message or recognized an invalid message. At this level, little semantic evaluation of the response can be made. These tests expand the test coverage of conformance requirements and typically involve multiple test cases that can be executed in a batch mode.

The objective of Functional Requirements Testing is to evaluate the capabilities and behavior of an application. As with the previous testing method, it generally consists of sending the application valid messages and evaluating the returned responses. In this case, though, the response message is evaluated for their semantic content (when the SUT is a server). When the SUT is a client application, it will be instructed to create a message or document, usually via a user interface. In order to conduct Functional Requirements Testing, a test scenario is created in which a sequence of orchestrated transactions is composed to probe a certain functional requirement. In the analysis, certain data values are examined to assess support of the requirement. For example, a sequence of messages (stimulus) can be made for a new record and an update of the record. A query can be made to retrieve the record. The response is evaluated, and inferences can be made. In other cases, functional requirements are assessed by inspection testing.

Isolated system testing typically accounts for the majority of testing that is conducted. Once a system has successfully undergone conformance testing, interoperability testing usually proceeds more easily. This topic is expanded upon in the Chap. 11.

Figure 10.3 depicts the Isolated System Testing Model in which the testing methods described in this section are conducted. The SUT interacts with a test tool designed to assess conformance of the SUT. In this model there is direct communication between the test tool and the SUT via the communication protocol (not shown in the figure). The test tool may include functionality of an application with which an SUT would typically interact in an operational environment. Often, multistep tests are conducted in this model, involving numerous interactive communications between the test tool and the SUT. Chapter 13 provides a realization and example of the Isolated System Testing Model.

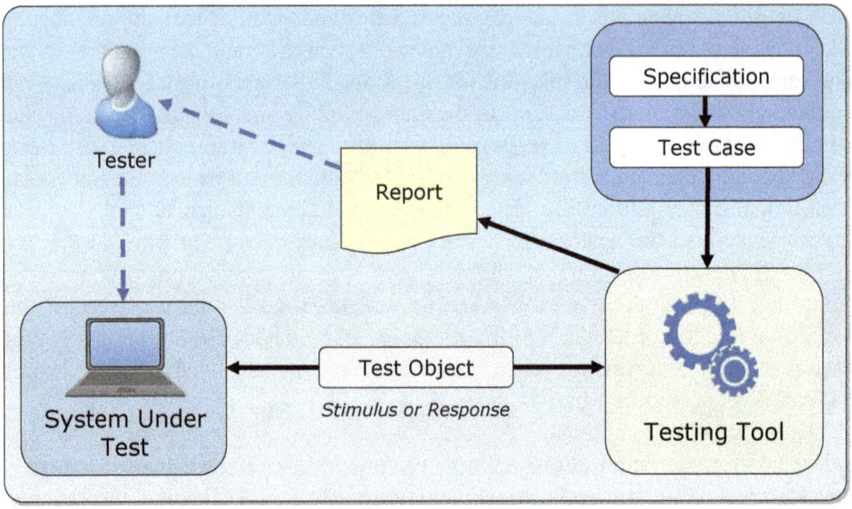

Fig. 10.3 Isolated system testing model

10.6.3 Peer-to-Peer System Testing Model

Testing is conducted among a group of vendor systems with this model. A vendor system may interact with a test tool or other vendor systems. Peer-to-peer system testing is designed to test interoperability among one[2] or more systems. Conducting conformance testing prior to interoperability testing can greatly facilitate the ease with which interoperability testing can be performed. Peer-to-peer system testing may include some or all of the conformance testing described for isolated system testing. When conformance testing is conducted in advance, peer-to-peer testing then specifically targets interoperability testing.

The objective of syntactic interoperability testing is to establish that two applications are able to exchange data successfully. No evaluation of the application's processing of the data is made with this type of testing. Semantic interoperability testing is the second phase of interoperability testing. If two applications establish that they are capable of exchanging data, this type of testing attempts to assess if they also correctly process the data exchanged. Semantic interoperability testing is the end step in which all layers of requirements are tested.

Figure 10.4 illustrates the Peer-to-peer System Testing Model. This model poses different and significant challenges in testing than the models examined previously. In this environment, data exchange is made among a group of systems. The test model no longer has direct interaction with the systems under test. Here an intermediary or a proxy can be employed to intercept, log, and route messages to their

[2] In a testing environment with one vendor implementation and one or more test agents, interoperability testing can be *simulated*.

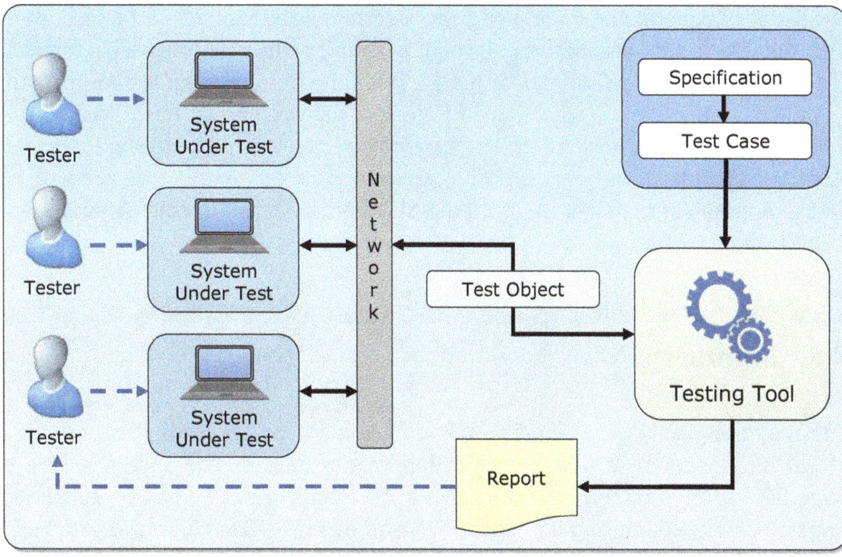

Fig. 10.4 Peer-to-peer system testing model

intended destination (in the diagram, this capability is shown generically as the test tool that is obtaining test objects from the network). The conformance test cases that were developed for Isolated System testing can be leveraged in Peer-to-peer testing. The abstract test cases could be identical, however, execution of the test steps, configuration requirements, and test management will differ. By ascertaining that the conformance requirements are now met in an environment where the SUTs are interacting, a declaration can be made about the interoperability capabilities of the systems. Chapter 13 explores an interoperability test bed design that instantiates the Peer-to-peer Testing Model.

10.7 Additional Testing Considerations

An important aspect to consider in testing is the testing mode. Automated testing, inspection testing, and hybrid testing are orthogonal (independent) to the testing model used. Automated testing mode implies that the evaluation of the SUT's behavior is automated. Inspection testing involves a human monitor. The hybrid mode is a combination of automated and inspection testing. The goal is to achieve automated testing whenever possible. However, in some circumstances it may not be possible, or the cost of automation is too high—for example, a test case stating "display the patient's medical record on your EHR screen for the patient with id

MR88408". Trying to automate such a test assertion is difficult; inspection testing is more suitable in this instance, as all requirements can be verified against a check list. The functional requirements of the SUT often will dictate the testing method.

Another important consideration in testing is the operational (testing) environment. Tests can be conducted on-site in a closed network or conducted over the Internet. Network access and firewalls are a few of the issues that need to be addressed in an environment in which the SUTs are expected to communicate over the Internet.

10.8 Summary

A testing approach for evaluating an application's adherence to requirements defined in a standard or other specification was examined. The approach was to divide the testing requirements into a number of categories that can be addressed separately. By decomposing the requirements in this way, a modular and structured approach to comprehensive testing of an application can be formulated. To accomplish this, a testing strategy has been defined that is based on this decomposition and the development of a testing plan and that can be realized through the implementation of a test suite built out of a number of test cases. With this approach, it is possible to evaluate systems effectively for both conformance and interoperability.

A number of tools for supporting testing in these models have been created in the community. The structured and modular approaches established in this work form the basis for building a testing infrastructure for evaluating implementations of healthcare data exchange standards. A testing infrastructure can support a broad spectrum of healthcare data exchange standards. It should consist of a set of reusable components that can be assembled to build specific test tools. Key functionality includes generation and validation of test objects, test agents, and communication infrastructure [8, 9]. A test harness can be employed to orchestrate the modules. Additional components to support test case development are also needed. The concepts presented in this chapter help drive and shape the testing infrastructure design discussion presented in Chap. 13.

Furthermore, this chapter focused on the distinct testing models and *what* could be tested in these models. Chapter 11 describes and expands on some of the topics introduced here. In particular, the test hierarchy organization is explained in-depth. Chapter 12 provides the underlying foundation for determining how requirements can be validated. Such assessments are built into the validation tools. In the testing architecture discussion (Chap. 13), a description of *how* test systems can be designed and built based on these models is given. Specific case studies describe existing testing frameworks that *implement* these design principles. Chapter 14 provides a sampling of conformance and interoperability test tools that are being used in practice. Chapter 15 describes how the tools are *used* for testing and certification.

References

1. ISO Reference - ISO/IEC 17000 Conformity assessment - Vocabulary and general principles, first edition 2004-11-02.
2. Glossary of Conformance Terminology, Interoperability and Conformance Technical Committee, OASIS. http://www.oasis-open.org/committees/ioc/glossary.htm
3. Institute of Electrical and Electronics Engineers. IEEE Standard Computer Dictionary: A Compilation of IEEE Standard Computer Glossaries. New York, NY: 1990.
4. Benson T. Principles of Health Interoperability HL7 and SNOMED. Health Informatics Series. Springer-Verlag London Limited 2010.
5. Woo J, Ivezic N, Cho H. Agile test framework for Business-to-Business Interoperability, Information Systems Frontiers, July 2012, Volume 14, Issue 3, pp 789-808.
6. HL7 EHR-S Functional Requirements: S&I Framework Laboratory Results Messages, Release 1, US Realm Draft Standard for Trial Use March 2016; http://hl7.org
7. Snelick R, Rontey P, Gebase L, Carnahan L. Towards Interoperable Healthcare Information Systems: The HL7 Conformance Profile Approach. Enterprise Interoperability II: New Challenges and Approaches. Springer-Verlag, *London Limited 2007 pp*. 659-670.
8. Gebase L, Snelick R, Skall M. Conformance Testing and Interoperability: A Case Study in Healthcare Data Exchange, 2008 Software Engineering Research and Practice (SERP08), WORLDCOMP'08 July 14-17, 2008, Las Vegas, NV.
9. Snelick R, Gebase L, O'Brien G. A Framework for testing Distributed Healthcare Applications. 2009 Software Engineering Research and Practice (SERP09), WORLDCOMP'09 July 13-16, 2009, Las Vegas, NV.

Chapter 11
Principles of Conformance Testing

11.1 Overview

This chapter focuses on the fundamental principles of conformance testing. Although the concepts of conformance testing are the key focal points addressed here, they can't be discussed in isolation; thus, we include related concepts when appropriate. A testing life cycle and process are presented along with their relationship to the standards development life cycle. An important principle in standards development is to integrate testing early in the process in order to obtain feedback for the authors of the standard. A testing methodology framework is introduced that provides a process for developing, organizing, and managing tests, as well as conducting testing and analyzing the results. A detailed description and example of a Test Plan is given. Since our focus is on communication between distributed applications, we discuss how sending and receiving applications can be tested, using a laboratory test results case study as the context. Next, we offer a set of basic principles for developing Test Plans and Test Cases. Finally, a comparison between capability testing and site-testing is presented. The conformance testing principles discussed in this chapter are applied in Chap. 13 and are examined in relation to test tool implementations in Chap. 14.

It is important to note that testing is not an exact science; a certain latitude is allowed in the strategy and approach, which are heavily influenced by what is being tested. The vast range of types of standards and conformance testing precludes having just one approach. This chapter describes methodologies that are based on the experiences of the authors (guided by common practice) and that have been proven to be valuable for testing distributed healthcare applications. Although we believe the concepts and the processes presented here are sound and effective, we do recognize there are viable alternative approaches. Often the test strategy needs to be adapted to the goal of the testing as well as what is being tested. In this sense, there is a touch of art intertwined with the science of the methodology. The Tester

F. Oemig and R. Snelick, *Healthcare Interoperability Standards Compliance Handbook*, DOI 10.1007/978-3-319-44839-8_11

uses what they consider to be the "best" and "most practical" approach to obtain the necessary evidence for their conformity assessment.

11.2 Conformance and Interoperability Testing

11.2.1 Conformance Testing

Conformance testing is a process that determines if an entity (message, document, application, system, etc.) adheres to the requirements stated in a specification. Since conformance testing is predicated on the specification, it is essential that the requirements are comprehensive and unambiguous. Conformance testing can only test to what is explicitly documented in a standard. Testing the full range of requirements is not always realistic, but the evaluation of specific requirements is feasible as well as useful. Practically speaking, conformance can't be proven. Only non-conformance can be determined, because the test space and the number of tests needed for testing conformance typically would have to be so large as to be unattainable, and proving that all of the needed tests have been included would be extremely difficult. In addition, there is no certainty that the included tests are correct. Therefore, conformance testing strives to establish a degree of confidence in the conformity of a given entity based on the quantity and the quality of the Tests performed (which, as stated, are directly dependent on the requirements).

Conformance testing is a multi-faceted operation that can range from a simple assessment of the validity of a message value to a nuanced determination of a system's reaction to a complex sequence of events. The ultimate goal of conformance testing is to enable interoperability among different system implementations. Conducting actual interoperability testing adds another dimension to the requirements for the testing environment, but conformance testing is seen as a means of increasing the likelihood that systems will be interoperable [1].

11.2.2 Interoperability Testing

Interoperability testing assesses whether applications (or software systems) can communicate with one another effectively and accurately, and whether they can provide the expected services in accordance with defined requirements. Such testing is critical, since many modern system architectures are designed as distributed systems and rely on seamless operation. The levels of interoperability testing include transport; syntax and data format compatibility; encoding mechanisms; and a common understanding and use of the data exchanged[1] (semantic).

[1]Both coded and un-coded.

Unlike conformance testing, which is performed in isolation,[2] interoperability testing is only meaningful in pairwise combinations of systems and is performed with multiple systems. For N interconnected systems, (N^2- N)/2 distinct system pair combinations *should be* tested. Therefore, for eight interconnected systems, 28 pair combinations are necessary to be tested.

An event such as the IHE Connect-a-thon [IHE-CONN] provides a venue for such interoperability testing for the set of IHE Integration Profile specifications. Because of limited time and resources, however, a system typically is tested with three to five systems at the IHE Connect-a-thon, with a minimum of three systems (per IHE policy) for each integration profile actor submitted by a vendor for testing.

11.2.3 Conformance and Interoperability Testing Relationship

Conformance and interoperability testing are related, and both are necessary to foster interoperability. The intent of conformance testing is to verify that a software system correctly implements to the established specifications of the standard. Interoperability testing is complementary and may be viewed as the next step in conformance testing, verifying that disparate software systems do indeed work together effectively to deliver expected functionality. During implementation, conformance to the standard is achieved first, and it should not be compromised during interoperability testing. Without conformance, two implementations can be made to interoperate while destroying interoperation with all other systems [2]; therefore, conformance testing should be performed simultaneously with interoperability testing if feasible. The Interoperability Test Bed (ITB) described in Chap. 13 embodies this principle. Events such as the IHE Connect-a-thon also should follow and enforce this policy. If vendors are making changes to their code to pass interoperability tests, the system has to be retested for conformance. This highlights why the tests should be conducted simultaneously.

A system under test that passes all conformance tests developed for a specification demonstrates that it is conformant to the requirements covered by those tests. The results of the tests do not prove that the system is conformant to the specification. The higher the quality and the greater the scope of the conformance tests, the more confidence the Tester can have in the system's degree of conformity. Therefore, the goal of the conformance tester is to provide a comprehensive (not necessarily or typically exhaustive) set of Test Cases, minimizing the number of Test Cases while maximizing the requirements tested.

[2]Meaning that there is only one system tested in isolation. Conformance testing may proceed multiple times until the system passes all Test Cases.

If system "A" passes all conformance tests for specification "X", and system "B" passes all conformance tests for specification "X", it ***does not*** necessarily follow that system "A" and system "B" are interoperable. Why not? It is a belief among some that if System "A" is conformant to specification "X" and system "B" is conformant to specification "X" then system "A" and system "B" are interoperable. It already has been established, however, that a specification is neither defined precisely to provide unambiguous requirements nor is it practical (nor possible) to develop an exhaustive set of conformance tests to prove that an entity is conformant given the unbounded test space[3]; therefore, interoperability testing is still necessary. Over time as systems are in production, problems will be identified and more tests will be added. This continuous process of refinement and testing puts the systems on the path toward working interoperability. The degree to which "out-of-the-box" interoperability can be achieved, however, is dependent on the industry's willingness to participate in the testing effort and to make improvements to the standards.

Systems may be "interoperable" or, perhaps more properly stated, may be able to exchange information in such a manner that their users' may conduct business as desired. Proving that two systems are actually interoperable, however, is not possible for the same reasons conformance can't be proven. The test space needed to conduct all such tests is too large, the tests are not guaranteed to be correct, and the finite set of tests that need to be performed can't be determined. Often, systems are referred to as being able to interoperate, but, again, only to a certain degree of confidence, and this confidence typically applies only to specific functioning capabilities. For most applications, this level of certainty is sufficient if the systems are able to conduct their business as desired and then issues are detected and resolved over time. In essence, the systems ultimately do achieve a state of *working* interoperability.

Systems can interoperate even though they have failed conformance testing, since failing conformance testing does not prevent systems from exchanging data. Two systems may not follow the conformance specification as given, but if the trading partners involved both agree upon how their systems will depart from the standard in order to suit their business needs, then the systems can still interoperate. By departing from such standards, however, these systems limit (or prevent) their capability of interoperating with other trading partners. Unfortunately, the decision to deviate from the standards might be caused not just by customer requests (business needs) but also by local regulations or the need to gain a perceived competitive advantage.[4]

Standards are developed to improve the feasibility of systems interoperating seamlessly without prior point-to-point agreements. The goal is for the industry to agree upon and implement standards, thus reducing the effort for interfacing. Often interface engines are employed to bridge different requirements (interface

[3]For all specifications except the most rudimentary; in the healthcare space most specifications are complex.

[4]If this is the case, interoperability initiatives may be impaired.

implementations) among systems. In theory, the need for interface engines could be eliminated[5] if a set of well-defined exchange standards are established and followed. Due to the enormous complexity and the diverse requirements in the healthcare domain, the industry is far from achieving this goal in practice—and it probably is unattainable; however, by following the standards development principles presented in earlier chapters, and by conducting conformance and interoperability testing along with certification, the industry can move closer to realizing this goal (in part by reducing the volume of translations needed). Progress in this direction will ultimately lead to increased efficiency, reduced errors, and lower costs of interface development.

11.2.4 Periodic Testing

In order to be effective, testing must be a periodic process; that is, testing is not a "one and done" proposition. Changes to the standard and the implementations make retesting necessary, including conformance testing and interoperability testing. When the standard is revised or errata are issued, implementations must be updated accordingly. The Test Suite must be revised as well, and conformance testing needs to be repeated. When implementations detect and fix errors or add new features, the specification should be updated and conformance needs to be retested. Whenever an implementation is modified and retested for conformance, interoperability retesting also must be performed. Trading partners have to ensure simultaneous updates, otherwise the interface is likely to be problematic (see Chap. 8). Having trading partners update their agreements, along with a plan for periodic testing and a testing platform to support it, significantly improves the chances of maintaining *working* interoperability.

11.2.5 Conformance Testing in Operational Environments

Conformance testing is not commonly thought of as an activity performed in operational (production) environments. Conformance testing usually occurs in the context of the assessment of a product (system) in an isolated, controlled setting (i.e., testing environment); however, systems developers or users may choose to incorporate conformance testing into an operational environment as a mechanism to verify data quality. Typically, though, data quality checks go beyond conformance testing. Based on the outcomes of data quality tests (and associated functional requirements), the system may decide not to process part or all of a message (or document).

[5]In the context of this discussion; interfaces engines serve other purposes as well.

Furthermore, operational systems conformance and data quality testing should be an on-going process used for monitoring an interface. Potentially, a trading partner could modify an existing interface, and monitoring could alert system administrators of resulting issues in data fidelity.

An important point to note is that conformance tests can be repurposed for an operational environment, but it does not necessary follow that failing conformance testing should prevent data exchange between systems. In instances where the data causing the failure are critical to processing the message or committing an entry to an electronic patient record, the non-conformance should prevent the data exchange. In other instances, where the data (in error) may be inconsequential to the application, non-conformance should not prohibit useful data exchange. Receivers will make the necessary determinations based on the requirements in their environments; however, they should be careful not to reject usable data and should work with the trading partner to resolve non-conformities. An example of this kind of situation would be the case of multiple-immunizations in which three out of four are conformant. The three valid immunization events should be processed, and an error should be returned for the invalid immunization in order to trigger a follow up action. Note, the invalid immunization event may or may not be processed depending on the severity of the error.

11.3 Standards Development Life-Cycle

Testing is an often overlooked aspect of the standards development life-cycle. Standards development can be thought of as a three-legged stool consisting of the standards development, implementation, and testing, in which all three legs are necessary for viability. Each aspect provides feedback to the others. When implementation and testing are initiated during the early stages of a stable standard, the quality of the standard is improved significantly, since ambiguities and issues are discovered early on in the process.

Figure 11.1 illustrates a high-level conceptualization of a typical information technology standards development life cycle [3]. Although the processes in the life cycle are successive, many of the processes can and should occur concurrently. During the first steps, a broad set of initial business requirements are obtained and a base standard is developed in accordance with those requirements. An example is the HL7 v2 base standard (e.g., HL7 v2.5.1), which is a framework standard covering many domains for healthcare data exchange. When more targeted requirements are obtained for a particular use case, specific profiles (refinements) are created. As discussed in Chap. 7, a profile hierarchy can be established to provide intermediary refinements until the level of a completely defined implementable profile is reached. An example of a profile is the laboratory results

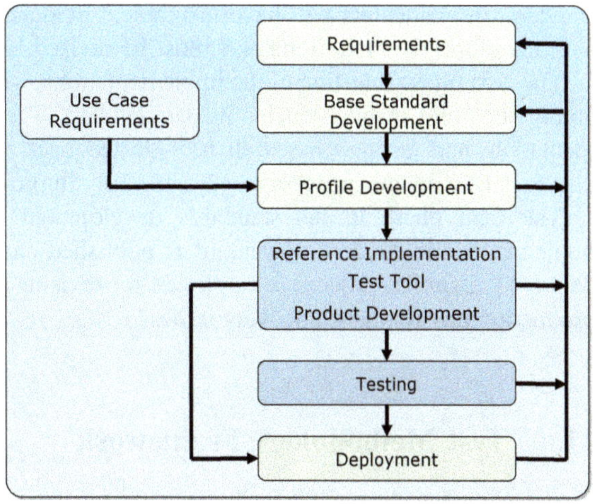

Fig. 11.1 Standards development life cycle [adapted, 3]

interface (LRI) profile [4]. This is a constrainable profile, i.e., not all requirements have been fully specified, and some optionality remains.

The next phase in the life cycle is implementation. This phase can include vendor implementations, reference implementations, and test tools. Pilots are implementations that are built early in the standards development life cycle to provide valuable feedback before the standard goes to final (normative) publication.

A reference implementation is a fully functional implementation[6] of a specification and assists in clarifying the requirements for that specification. The main purposes of a reference implementation are:

- to verify the specification is implementable
- to provide a definitive interpretation of the specification
- to uncover errors and ambiguities in the specification
- to help clarify the intent of the specification when the specification and conformance tests are not adequate for this purpose
- to aid in the validating a Test Suite
- to serve as a benchmark to which other implementations can be compared
- and to provide baseline source code that implementers can leverage

Reference implementations usually are developed by the extended SDO community and are likely to be in the public domain. Reference implementations should be developed along with the standard and the conformance Test Suites. Pilots can be vendor implementations or reference implementations.

The development of the test tools in conjunction with the standard also helps improve the standard, as specific test assertions are written based on the conformance requirements. If test assertions can't be derived from the requirements in the

[6]This is the goal; however, partial functionally is also desirable and useful.

standard, implementers will have insufficient guidance for correct implementation, and, therefore, the “requirements” must be revised.

The next phase is testing of the implementations, which often uncovers additional ambiguities and inconsistencies in the standard. The profile development, implementation, and testing phases all provide feedback to the standards development phase. Following this process can significantly improve the quality of the standard.

The final phase in the standards development life cycle is deployment of implementations. Once the standard is published and implementations have been deployed, a similar process is employed for revising the standard as its use in live production environment uncovers issues.

11.4 Test Methodology Framework

Chapter 10 gave a brief overview of the organization of a Test Suite and associated concepts and definitions. In this section we elaborate on those concepts and definitions and put them into context. Figure 11.2 illustrates a Test Methodology Framework that we will refer to during this discussion. This figure shows an example configuration but not necessarily the only possible approach. Other test methodology frameworks will include some or all of the components indicated, and the components may be organized differently depending on what is being tested. These differences are immaterial; the important aspects are that a process is established, and that this process is well defined and is used consistently throughout the entirety of the project where it is being applied. Definitions of Test Suites can be much more simplistic or elaborate than the example presented here; our goal is to highlight and describe the key features found in the real settings where such a framework is in use.

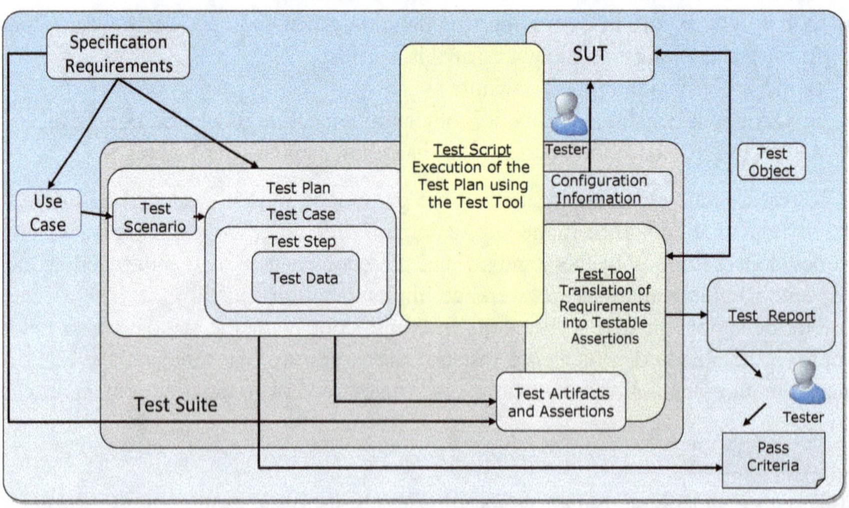

Fig. 11.2 Testing landscape

As described in Sect. 11.3, the process of developing standards, and utimately testing of the standards, follows a given life-cycle process. Aspects of this process are presented again here, but from a different perspective.

The planning of the Test Suite orginates from the requirements described in a specification. A Test Suite can contain a Test Plan, a Test Script, Configuration Requirements, and a Test Tool. The Test Plan is composed of one or more Test Cases. A Test Case is composed of one or more Test Steps and each Test Step can have associated Test Data. A Test Case is a specific instance of a Test Scenario and a Test Scenario is a specific path (instance) of a Use Case.

Figure 11.3 illustrates the relationship between a Use Case, a Test Scenario, and a Test Case along with examples for each. The broad Use Case may be creation of a lab result message based on an interoperability specification. A Test Scenario, or one possible path of that use case, might be creating a (valid) Lipid Panel lab result message. Another Test Scenario might be creating a rejected specimen lab result message. A specific instance of a Test Scenario is realized as a Test Case. One Test Case could provide Lipid Panel lab results for a specific patient, for example, for Donna Burden, along with associated data to be included in the message. Another Test Case for the Lipid Panel scenario might be for patient Connor Austin and could provide data to be included in the message associated with his lab results. In the latter instance, the lab result could include abnormal values, whereas in the former instance the lab result could include only normal values. Sometimes the line between what constitutes a different Test Scenario as opposed to a different Test Case related to a Test Scenario can become blurred. Determining what is to be a Scenario versus a Test Case often is a judgement call that depends on how the test developer wishes to organize the Test Plan.

The Test Script describes the steps necessary to carry-out (execute) the tests on the system-under-test (SUT) given the specific Test Plan, configuration requirements, and Test Tool. Testing Artifacts that contain the Assertions are derived from the Specification and Test Cases. The Test Tool produces Test Reports for each Test Case executed. A Test Case also can contain additional testable criteria not addressed by the Test Tool. The Test Plan provides the instructions on how to evaluate each criterion that is carried out by the Test Script. The results of such tests also are provided to the Tester for assessing conformance to the stated requirements.

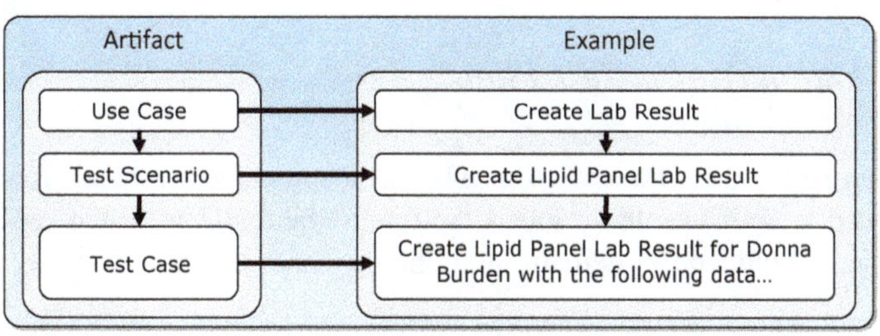

Fig. 11.3 Relationship between a Use Case, Test Scenario, and Test Case

A similar test methodology framework was established by NIST for the ONC[7] Health IT Certification Program for the HL7 v2 related certification criteria, and a Test Procedure document is provided for each criterion in addition to the HL7 v2 specification named in the criterion. Each Test Procedure document includes additional information from the ONC Final Rule about the HL7 v2-related certification criterion and provides a high-level script of the testing process and associated requirements. Inclusion of this document is a valid variation on the test methodology framework illustrated in Fig. 11.2.

Using tools to build use cases, capturing and profiling requirements, building Test Plans, and automating validation can facilitate the standard development and testing process while providing consistency and accuracy when moving from one phase to the next. The objective of such tools is to create models of data, so, when these data are changed in one phase specified in the standards document, those changes are either reflected automatically (if applicable) in other phases specified in the document, or the tool alerts the authors to the inconsistencies. Much work is still needed in this area, but significant progress has been made.

11.4.1 System-Under-Test (SUT)

The system-under-test (SUT) is the software system that is being tested. The Tester relies on existing capabilities of the SUT production (or candidate for production) version in order to examine its functionality. The Tester can't require or expect the product to be modified solely to support testing activities.

11.4.2 Anatomy of a Test Suite

A Test Suite can contain a Test Plan, a Test Script, Configuration Requirements (e.g., to connect to the test tool and SUT), and a Test Tool. Depending on what is being tested, some or all of these components may be included in the Test Suite. Typically, all Test Suites need to include, at minimum, a Test Plan and a Test Script.

11.4.3 Anatomy of a Test Plan

The objective of a Test Plan is to provide a documented approach for testing a system in order to ensure that it meets the requirements given in the specification. The approach should be systematic and should contain a test coverage analysis.

[7]Office of the National Coordinator.

A test coverage analysis gives a mapping of the Test Cases and requirements, indicating to the user the aspects that are to be tested and how to test them. It also provides a high-level explanation about the focus of a Test Case.

A Test Plan usually is organized as a set of Test Scenarios and Test Cases. A Test Scenario is a term usually reserved for a sequence of events that mimic real world workflow; that is, it is a use case instance, it represents a specific path through the use case, and it may involve testing of different but related standards. A Test Case is created to describe the specifics of how the Test Scenario is tested. More than one Test Case can be employed to test a Test Scenario.

11.4.4 Anatomy of a Test Case

A Test Case is created to target the specific requirements to be tested. These requirements can be high-level, such as use case instances, or low level, such as messaging requirements. A Test Case typically includes the following components:

- Test Story—Purpose and Description
- Pre-Condition
- Test Steps
- Test Data
- Post-Condition
- Test Objectives
- Evaluation Criteria
- Notes to the Test Administrators
- General Comments

It is advantageous to combine high-level and low-level requirements into single Test Cases. Section 11.7 discusses best practices for effective Test Case construction.

The Test Case must provide all information necessary to define, execute, and assess the outcome of a test. The evaluation criteria are critical components of the Test Case, since they indicate what constitutes success or failure and are the basis for determining the "verdict" of the test.

A Test Scenario is a higher-level notion that can be thought of as a way of grouping test cases and/or combining test cases into extended workflow testing.

11.4.5 Anatomy of a Test Step

Test Cases contain one or more Test Steps. A Test Step provides instructions or operations to be performed by the SUT, Test Tool, or test administrator. The test steps are created for a number of purposes, for example, for test set up or for SUT assessment. Test steps can be manual or automated. The granularity of a test step is subjective and is determined by the test case designer. Generally, a good dividing point is at a distinct actionable operational event; but exactly what "actionable operation event" means is debatable. Often this decision is influenced by what is being examined, and then *natural* partitioning points generally become apparent.

When testing messaging systems (the automated) test steps are typically associated with a single exchange (interaction). As described previously, an interaction is a single atomic exchange between two actors. An example of an interaction is Actor "A" sending a message to Actor "B". A transaction is a round trip exchange between two actors to enact a specific purpose. An example of a transaction is Actor "A" sending a message to Actor "B", followed by Actor "B" sending an acknowledgement message to Actor "A".

In the round-trip exchange, if the SUT is Actor "A", which is an EHR-S, a possible transaction would be for Actor "A" (EHR-S) to send a message containing immunization information to a registry (i.e., the Test Tool). The registry (Actor "B") is expected to send back an acknowledgement message to Actor "A", and this receiver is expected to *handle* it, which completes the transaction. A Test Case could be developed in which the first Test Step would test the immunization message instance. Test Step two would test the import of the acknowledgement message (which is likely a minimum test in this case). This level of granularity is a design choice, however, following the recommendation above, each interaction would be a Test Step.

11.4.6 Test Data

Data that are associated with the Test Case are designed to produce certain stimuli or responses from the SUT. The test data may be categorized to indicate the source and the expectations for their use within the testing process. For example, some data may be categorized as *system generated* where the expectation is that the system creates these data as a by-product of routine system operations. Generating the current time of day is one such case. Other data might be categorized as *test case fixed* data. Here, the Test Case is explicitly requiring exact data to be used in order to support the assessment. Other categories can exist at the discretion of the test developer. This topic is further expanded upon later in this chapter.

11.4.7 Test Script

The Test Script provides the glue that connects the Test Plan, Test Tool, and SUT for executing the tests. The test results provide the evidence such that an assessment can be performed. The Test Script indicates how the test materials provided in the

Test Plan and Test Tool are applied to test the SUT; and this script also describes the steps involved for the setup and execution of the tests, including the configuration of the SUT. Typically, configuration consists of networking and addressing configuration and the preloading of data. For example, to prepare for messaging, the Test Tool and the SUT will coordinate Internet Protocol (IP) addresses and port numbers. They also may have to coordinate application names. Data may have to be pre-loaded in the application database; for example, a patient record may be created so the SUT can consume an incoming message and associate the received data with an existing patient record. In certain circumstances large quantities of data must be preloaded. For example, a server that is to respond to queries must be *primed* before execution of tests. Testing of the IHE Patient Demographics Query (PDQ) server is an example of a testing situation that requires this priming. For this conformance testing, the SUT (PDQ Supplier) is pre-loaded with a set of demographics data. The Test Tool (acting as PDQ Consumer) is used to query the PDQ Supplier. The Test Tool, upon receiving the responses from the SUT, performs an analysis on the responses based on the query and the data that were loaded into the SUT. The details of such testing can be found in Chap. 13.

11.4.8 Inspection Documents

Many requirements can be tested via the automation provided by the test tool; but in some cases it is not feasible to automate testing, or it is not practical to do so because of the cost. Though it is always preferable to conduct automated testing, under certain circumstances the use of inspection is necessary or more appropriate. Inspection testing involves a human proctor using a check list of criteria to examine the results of the testing. The check list of criteria is referred to as an Inspection Document or a Juror Document. A Juror Document often is employed when testing a receiving system for incorporation of data. The criteria listed on the Juror Document are directly related to the stimulus provided to the SUT as part of the Test Case, e.g., a message that is sent to an electronic health record (EHR-S) system.

11.4.9 Test Artifact

A Test Artifact consists of materials used to evaluate a Test Object (e.g., a message or EHR-S display). Test Artifacts are derived from requirements stated in specifications such as implementation guides, conformance profiles, templates, or regulations. Test Artifacts contain the Test Assertions. The Test Artifacts typically are integrated with the Test Tool when such a tool exists.

11.4.10 Test Assertion

Test Assertions may be machine processable instructions or a check list in the form of a Juror Document. A Test Assertion is the question that is asked in order to confirm or refute a claim or an instantiation of a requirement. As an example, the requirement might be "MSH-9.2 (Event Type) SHALL be valued with the constant 'R01'", and the assertion for this requirement could be "Is the message element MSH-9.2 (Event Type) equal to 'R01'". A programmer may instantiate the assertion as:

assert(profile.messageElement(MSH-9.2) == 'R01');

The above statement makes an assertion about the requirement. This assertion is wrapped in a decision construct such as an ***if*** statement. If true, the claim is substantiated, and a passed indication is issued to the reporting mechanism. If false, the claim is refuted, and a failed indication is issued to the reporting mechanism. How the notice of the refutation is rendered to the end user may vary depending on the severity of the fault. For example, an assertion that is flagged as failed during testing could be considered an error, a warning, an alert, or some other level of severity depending on the specification. Leading practice dictates that assertions are atomic to enable managing assertion reporting in this manner, offering the end user the needed flexibility in reporting.

11.4.11 Test Tool

A Test Tool is an application (or utility or service) that can be used for conducting conformance or interoperability testing. A Test Tool can interact with users, the SUT, or other Test Tools (e.g., Test Agents). The Test Tool enables execution of the Test Cases and can be referenced by a Test Script.

11.4.12 Configuration Information

Configuration information is necessary for executing the Test Cases defined in the Test Plan. Configuration is necessary at two levels: the tool level and the Test Case level. At the tool level, connection information is necessary in order for the tool to communicate with the SUT. Test Case level configuration consists of a variety of actions, including loading the system with data, setting the system to a particular state, and loading and associating the appropriate test material needed by the Test Tool.

11.4.13 Test Report

A Test Report lists what was tested and the results of the test. It is used by the test assessor to make a judgment regarding the SUT with respect to the expected results and pass/fail criteria, or it is used by an implementer to correct issues.

11.5 Testing in Practice

Chapter 2 describes in detail the system architectures and exchange mechanisms for distributed applications. Distributed applications communication is enabled by interfaces. This architecture influences how the systems are tested. The testing can be separated into three categories; testing the sender interface, the receiver interface, and the functional requirements of the applications. These forms of testing often naturally go hand-in-hand. In what follows, some perspectives are given on testing the sending and receiving applications combined with functional requirements testing. Broadly speaking, testing the sender entails determining whether the application can construct an object (e.g., message) in accordance with the specification requirement based on a stimulus, which may or may not include specific test data. Testing the receiver focuses more on the extraction of content from the object (e.g., message) and incorporation of it into the business operation of the receiver to enact certain functionality. Such functional requirements are described in interoperability (messaging) specifications or application functional requirement specifications.[8]

11.5.1 Testing Sending Applications

When testing the ability of the SUT to create messages,[9] the focus of the conformance testing strictly centers on validating the message produced by the sending system (e.g., an EHR-S). When functioning as the *sender*, the SUT is treated as a "black box"—how the requirements are realized is not of interest; the content of the message is. To elaborate on this point, the technical aspect, i.e., what an implementer has done to achieve this functionality, does not matter; however, it does matter that the implementation functions correctly.

[8]Some messaging implementation guides include functional requirements; IHE integration profiles combine interoperability and functional requirements. In some cases, however, an interoperability specification is devoid of functional requirements; they are determined by the implementer's business operations.

[9]We explain concepts in this section in the context of HL7 v2 messages; however, the concepts apply equally to documents and other message protocols.

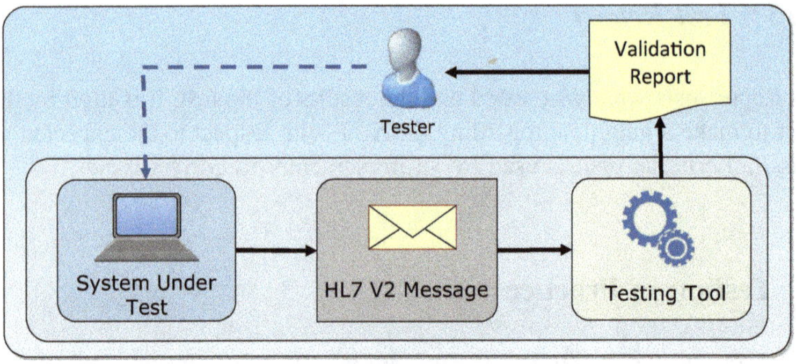

Fig. 11.4 Context-free validation test flow

Conformance test tools for validating sending systems can have two operational modes:

- Context-free
- Context-based

The context-free mode validates any message created by the SUT. It is not dependent on a specific use case instance, Test Case, or specific test data content. Figure 11.4 illustrates the context-free test flow.

The context-based (or context-sensitive) mode validates messages that are associated with a given use case instance and a Test Case that includes specific test data that are to be entered into the SUT. The SUT creates a message that corresponds to the test data provided in the Test Case. Testing assesses both the technical requirements and content-specific requirements specified in the Test Case. Context-based validation expands the test space, enabling more comprehensive testing (e.g., testing of conformance usage constructs such as "conditional" and "required, but may be empty"). Figure 11.5 shows the context-based test flow.

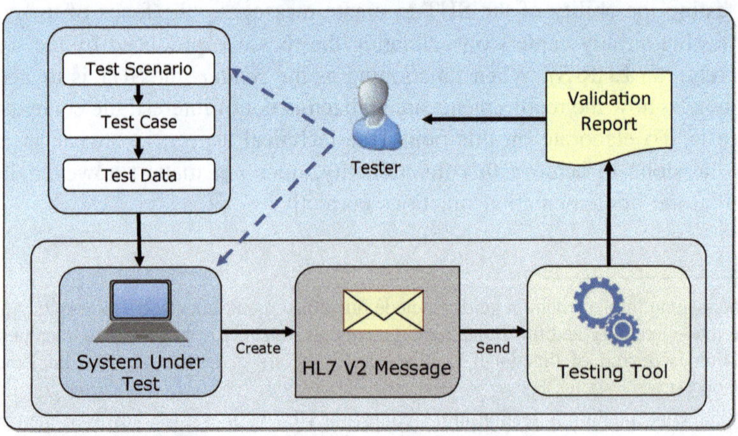

Fig. 11.5 Context-based validation test flow

Both context-free and context-based modes are useful for conducting message validation. Since context-free testing is not tied directly to test case data, any message instance can be validated. This suits site implementations well, enabling in-house testing to be performed on production messages (real-time or not) if desired. Context-based testing is driven by directed Test Cases. This targets specific Test Scenarios and allows for more precise testing. Context-based testing is the preferred method for the ONC Health IT Certification Program testing. The NIST HL7 v2 conformance test tools [5, 6, 7, 8, 9] support both modes of validation, although the ONC HIT certification testing is context-based. The context-free validation functionality provided in the Test Tool can be used to assist certification testing in certain circumstances, however, and has proven to be a useful tool for local installation testing. For example, many states require that physician practices and hospitals verify the ability of their HIT technology to produce conformant messages using the NIST validation tools before on-boarding with public health registries [10].

The development and use of context-based tests provides an added benefit in the interpretation and understanding of requirements. The Test Case Descriptions and associated test data provide a bridge between the concepts in the specification and real world application.

11.5.1.1 Context-Free Testing Versus Context-Based Testing

Context-free testing and context-based testing offer the Tester complementary instruments for conducting validation. The context-free validation utility of the test tool provides validation unrelated to any specific content; thus, providing a simple and cost effective method to conduct testing. Context-based validation provides a richer test space to evaluate. This is especially important for testing:

(1) The capabilities of a system and
(2) The appropriate use of such systems in accordance with requirements given in the specification (implementation guide) and local requirements.

For item (1) above, some of the conformance constructs can't be adequately assessed using the context-free methodology alone. Such constructs include certain usage requirements (e.g., RE, C), length, and cardinality. Consider the "RE" (Required, but may be empty) construct. From an implementation perspective, "RE" elements are required to be implemented. From an operational perspective the element may or may not be valued in the message depending on relevance or data availability.

When testing "RE" elements in a context-based environment, the validation is performed using the additional information provided by the Test Case. The test cases are designed with data provided for the "RE" elements. When data are available for "RE" elements, the validation testing effectively makes the "RE" element an "R" (Required) element for conformity assessment. See the section Test

Data Categories in this chapter for a classification of the type of content testing that can be assessed. See Chap. 12 for details on the test truth tables for the suite of conformance constructs.

Another method for assessing support for "RE" elements can be in the context-free validation mode when considering a set of messages (e.g., 1000) from the SUT. A collective analysis of the messages can be assessed, and if at least one message in that set contains data for the "RE" element analyzed then it can be surmised that the element is supported. If no messages exist with data for that element, it is likely that it is not supported, but this can't be determined definitely. Such testing is neither as directed nor precise. Additionally, obtaining a large enough set of messages might be challenging, since they are likely to be operational messages from which protected health information would need to be scrubbed. This situation is more likely used for in-house testing rather than for certification testing.

Requesting one or a few maximally populated messages is another approach that can be used in the context-free mode. When time and resources are limited this tactic can be an effective mechanism for a rudimentary assessment; however, a maximally populated message is unobtainable when the presence of some elements are mutually exclusive.

C (Conditional) elements can be tested in a similar fashion. In the context-based mode, targeted Test Cases are developed. Take for example the relationship between the Completion Status (RXA-20) element and the Substance/Treatment Refusal Reason (RXA-18) element in the Immunization Implementation Guide [11]. The RXA-18 element has a usage of C(R/X)[10] with the following condition predicate:

> *If RXA-20 (Completion Status) is valued "RE"*[11] *(Refused)*

This statement translates into:

> *If RXA-20 (Completion Status) is valued with the literal "RE" (indicating the Completion Status was Refused), then the RXA-18 (Substance/Treatment Refusal Reason) element SHALL be valued, otherwise the RXA-18 (Substance/Treatment Refusal Reason) element SHALL NOT be valued.*

With regard to context-based testing, a Test Case is developed where the patient refuses the vaccine, thus providing the context to test the RXA-18 (Substance/Treatment Refusal Reason) element. Another Test Case is needed to test the false predicate outcome (i.e., it was not refused).

Other conformance constructs, such as Cardinality, Length, Encoding, Vocabulary, and so on, can be tested in a similar manner. For example, if the cardinality constraint for an element is [1…3], a Test Case can be constructed in which three instances of test data are provided for that element.

---

[10]Usage is R-Required when the condition predicate is true and the usage is X-Not Supported when the condition is false.

[11]Not be confused with the "RE" usage construct.

Content testing is also supported in context-based testing. This capability allows the tester to test for specific content, which can be used to test a variety of requirements such as specific vocabulary content and functional requirements. As should be evident, context-based testing is necessary to test the full range of capabilities required in specifications.

Context-free testing provides a simple and cost effective method to conduct testing since targeted Test Cases are not created. A capabilities assessment can be obtained, fueled by a set of messages or by maximally populated messages. Conversely, context-based testing, although more costly, is the more revealing testing mode.

11.5.2 Case Study: Laboratory Results

In this section a case study for creating a laboratory results message is explored in order to explain the principles of context-based testing for a sending application. This case study addresses the ONC 2014 Edition certification criterion for the transmission of laboratory results. The criterion references the HL7 v2.5.1 Laboratory Results Interface (LRI) Release 1 Implementation Guide [4]. An example Test Case taken from the NIST Test Procedure is presented and the test process is explained.

For testing a sending system, the focus of the conformance testing strictly centers on validating the message. The SUT is treated as a "black box"—how the message is created or transformed is not in scope. If we consider a Laboratory Information System (LIS) or a Laboratory module that is integrated with an EHR-S (hereafter "lab component"), testing is not concerned with the detailed architecture of the lab component, but rather with what it produces (a message) based on a given set of inputs (i.e., the Test Case). The "black box" can be a self-contained lab component (upper half of diagram, Fig. 11.6) or be composed of multiple modules with a data flow between them, for example, a lab component and an integration engine; however, the "black box" must contain a lab component, and test case data must be entered into and originate from the lab component (see Fig. 11.6—lower half). In the diagram, an interface engine is used to transform the message created by the lab component.

The Test Cases listed in the certification Test Procedure documents [12], and described in detail in the downloadable PDF packages provided in the NIST conformance test tools, can be selected and used for automatic validation of messages in the Test Tools. For context-based testing, each Test Case describes the set of events that provide the context for the testing.

The Use Case for the transmission of lab results could consist of the following steps:

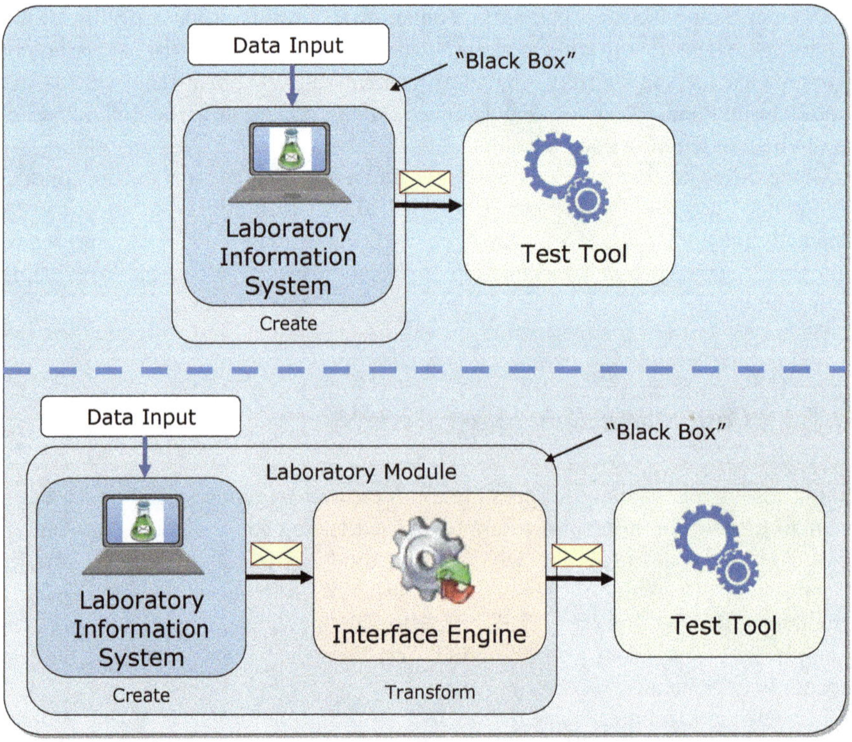

Fig. 11.6 Possible system architectures and black box testing

1. A lab test is ordered for a patient
2. The specimen is collected (if applicable), and is received and processed by the lab
3. The lab result is produced and entered into the LIS
4. **The lab result message is created**
5. The lab result is transmitted to an ambulatory electronic health record (EHR) system
6. The lab result is incorporated into the ambulatory EHR system

The scope covered by the transmission of the lab results criterion is step 4 above—the lab result message is created. Step 6—the lab result is incorporated into the ambulatory EHR—is covered by the incorporate lab results Test Procedure, which will be discussed later in a separate case study for testing receiving systems.

The Test Cases provide specific laboratory tests (test scenario) for which a lab result(s) message will be imported into the conformance test tool. For example, Test Case "LRI_1.0-GU_Final" uses "Erythrocyte Sedimentation Rate" as the lab test.

A Test Case consists primarily of a narrative Test Story (one possible path described by the Use Case) and a Test Data Specification. The Test Story gives a real

"Mr. William A. Jones is a 51 year old white male who presented with pain, swelling, and redness in several joints including his elbows, wrists, knees, and hips on March 31, 2011 at 2:05 PM PST. In order to rule out rheumatoid arthritis, Dr. Nicholas Radon ordered an erythrocyte sedimentation rate (ESR or Sed Rate) blood test to be performed, specifying that the laboratory was to draw the blood specimen from the patient. The final result of this test was 10 mm/hr, a normal value with the normal reference range being 0-17 mm/hr. The final result report for this lab test was generated by the LIS and transmitted to the patient's record in the ambulatory EHR used in Dr. Radon's office practice on March 31, 2011 at 4:28 PM PST."

Fig. 11.7 Erythrocyte sedimentation rate test story example

world situation that provides the context for the Test Case. Figure 11.7 shows an example Test Story for the creation of an Erythrocyte Sedimentation Rate lab result.

The Test Story also provides details associated with the Test Case, such as comments, pre-conditions, post-conditions, test objectives, and notes to testers. The Test Data Specification provides the data associated with the Test Story and consists of information that is typically available in the clinical setting. Figure 11.8 shows excerpts from the Erythrocyte Sedimentation Rate Test Data Specification related to the specimen information and the results of the lab test (for the complete Test Data Specification see [5]). Together the Test Story and the Test Data Specification provide sufficient information to be entered into the EHR-S (LIS Module)[12] for a particular Test Case such that a lab results message can be created.

Another artifact called the Message Content Data Sheet is provided to show a conformant message instance for the Test Case. The message content is organized in a table format that provides the HL7 v2 message elements and the data associated with the message elements for a given Test Case. Figure 11.9 shows an excerpt from the Erythrocyte Sedimentation Rate message content for the OBX segment. If necessary, the Message Content Data Sheet can be used to assist the Tester in loading the SUT with the Test Case specific data. It may also be used to provide assistance to the Tester and vendor to resolve issues discovered in conformance testing. In short, the Message Content Data Sheet can be thought of as the "answer" to the Test Case "question" articulated by the Test Story and the Test Data Specification. The testing program will determine whether the message content is revealed to the vendor of the SUT prior to the start of a testing session. The ONC Health IT Certification Program, in a concerted effort to be transparent, does reveal the expected message content to the vendors whose HIT is being tested.

For certified EHR technology (CEHRT), ONC policy is to make the testing transparent, because the focus is to assess the capabilities of a product. Site testing may be required by the end-user to assess correct usage of the installed product. This

[12]The case study is for ONC 2014 Edition Certification in which EHRs are being certified. The case study is showing an EHR-S with an LIS module. The testing can equally apply to independent LISs.

Specimen Information

Element Name	Data
Specimen Type	BLD
Alt Specimen Type	Blood
Specimen Original Text	Blood Specimen
Start date/time	Thu Mar 31 14:05:51 GMT-08:00 2011
Specimen Reject Reason	
Alt Specimen Reject Reason	
Reject Reason Original Text	
Specimen Condition	Cool
Alt Specimen Condition	Cool
Condition Original Text	Cool

Lab Results

Observation	Result	UOM	Range	Abnormal Flag	Status	Date/Time of Observation	Notes
Erythrocyte sedimentation rate	10	mm/h	0 to 17	N	F	Thu Mar 31 15:05:51 GMT-08:00 2011	

Fig. 11.8 Erythrocyte sedimentation rate test data specification example

OBX : Observation Results Segment

Location	Data Element	Data	Categorization
OBX.1	Set ID - OBX	1	IG Fixed Data
OBX.2	Value Type	NM	Test Case Fixed Data
OBX.3	Observation Identifier		
OBX.3.1	Identifier	30341-2	Test Case Fixed Data
OBX.3.2	Text	Erythrocyte sedimentation rate	Test Case Fixed Data
OBX.3.3	Name of the Coding System	LN	Test Case Fixed Data
OBX.3.4	Alternate Identifier	815117	Changeable Data
OBX.3.5	Alternate Text	ESR	Changeable Data
OBX.3.6	Name of Alternate Coding System	99USI	Changeable Data
OBX.3.9	Original Text	Erythrocyte sedimentation rate	Changeable Data
OBX.4	Observation Sub-ID		
OBX.5	Observation Value	10	Test Case Fixed Data
OBX.6	Units		
OBX.6.1	Identifier	mm/h	Changeable Data
OBX.6.2	Text	millimeter per hour	Changeable Data
OBX.6.3	Name of the Coding System	UCUM	Changeable Data
OBX.6.4	Alternate Identifier		
OBX.6.5	Alternate Text		
OBX.6.6	Name of Alternate Coding System		
OBX.6.9	Original Text		
OBX.7	Reference Range	0 to 17	Changeable Data
OBX.8	Abnormal Flags	N	Test Case Fixed Data
OBX.11	Observation Result Status	F	Test Case Fixed Data

Fig. 11.9 Erythrocyte sedimentation rate test message content example

type of testing likely would not be transparent, since the focus would be to ascertain whether users are able to make the product perform as required based on the provided use case. End-user education about the difference between certification testing and site testing is an important part of the testing process and should not be overlooked.

The information in the ***Location*** column in Fig. 11.9 indicates the canonical element location in the HL7 v2 message. For example, OBX-3.1 represents the 1st component in the 3rd field of the OBX segment. The ***Data Element*** column indicates the name of the data element as specified by the referenced standard. The ***Data*** column provides the expected data (if applicable) for that message element. The ***Categorization*** column indicates the classification of the data for validation. How the data are classified is directly related to how the message content is validated. In some cases, the validator tool is examining a message element for the presence or absence of data, whereas in other cases it is examining the message element for both the presence of data and exact content. See Table. 11.1 for a description of the data categorization and how each data class is being validated.

Figure 11.10 summarizes the test flow process for the Erythrocyte Sedimentation Rate Test Case and provides a specific example of the Context-based Validation Test Flow. The use case describes the general laboratory results workflow. The Test Scenario expresses a specific path related to that use case. The Test Case (consisting of, among other items, the Test Story and the Test Data Specification) provides the details of the Test Scenario. The Test Data Specification supplies the data necessary for input and represents what is typically available in a clinical setting for the given Test Story. For example, these data would include the name of the laboratory test being performed, but not the code (e.g., LOINC) that would be sent in the message (see Fig. 11.8).

Table 11.1 Description of data categorization and validation

Data Categorization	Description	Validation
Configurable	Data that are typically configured by the system (customer-definable). Example data is provided	Validate for the presence of data
System generated	Data typically generated automatically by the system, e.g., time of message. Example data are provided	Validate for the presence of data
Implementation guide (IG) fixed	Data that are fixed by the implementation guide; data can't be changed. Specific data are provided	Validate for the presence of data and data content
Test case fixed	Data that are specific and fixed by the test case; data can't be changed and are selectively[a] validated Specific data are provided	Validate for the presence of data and may validate data content
Changeable	Data where the specific content is not relevant for the Test Case; data can be changed. Example data are provided	Validate for the presence of data

[a]Such data should always be tested for specific content for this category. Insufficient granularity in the test data categories and tooling precipitated this compromise. Such deficiencies have since been addressed and used in NIST ONC 2015 Edition Health IT Certification testing. See the Sect. 11.6 in this chapter for an in-depth discussion

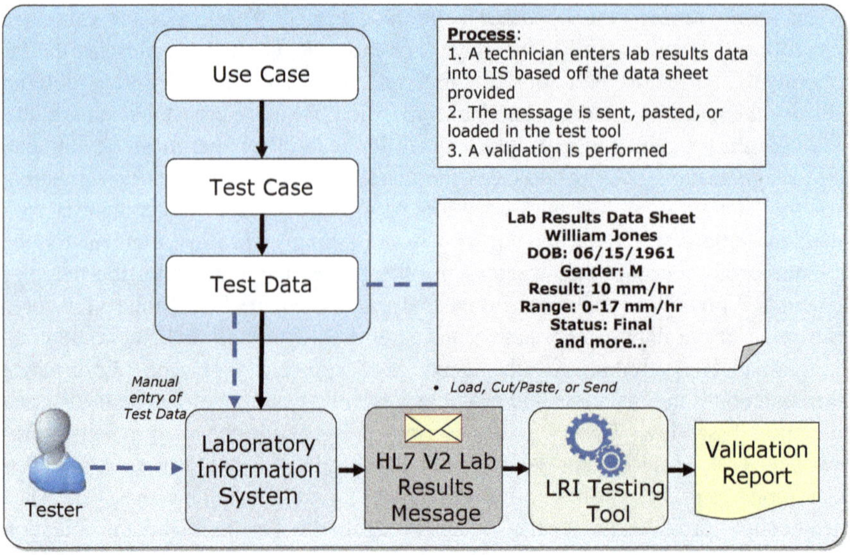

Fig. 11.10 Context-based validation test flow lab case study

The next step in the process is loading of the data into the LIS—for testing, this may be a manual process using the user interface (UI) capabilities of the LIS or may be accomplished via an EHR-LIS interface using the user interface capabilities of the EHR (i.e., the EHR-S has an LIS component). In the case of the name of the laboratory test, the system could provide a menu from which the user could select. Other elements of the message may be populated using free-text fields. Once all relevant test data are loaded into the LIS, a message is generated. The message is validated by selecting the corresponding Test Case in the Test Tool and then importing the generated message. The Test Tool provides a graphical user interface in which the validation results can be browsed and explored; reports also can be produced for archiving. See Chap. 14 for details about the operation of the Test Tool.

In addition to validating the technical requirements specified in the implementation guide, the Test Tool performs selective content validation based on the Test Story and Test Data Specification (and associated data categorization) provided. Deviation from the test data may cause the Test Tool to issue Errors. For this reason, the Tester should use the test data as specified.[13]

[13]In some cases, it may be necessary for the test tool to allow for variances, e.g., LOINC equivalencies. These exceptions are decided by the test administrator.

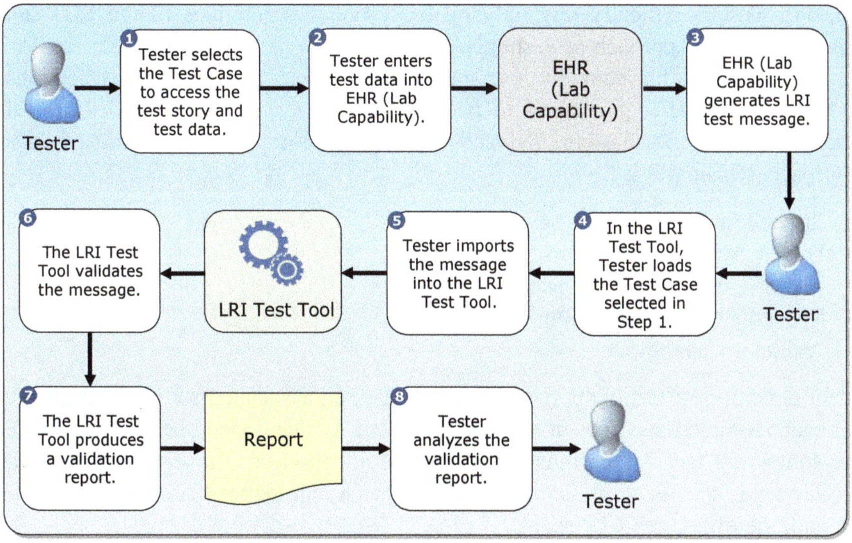

Fig. 11.11 LRI sending testing workflow

11.5.2.1 Test Procedure Workflow

The NIST MU 2014 Edition certification test tool is used in conjunction with the ONC Test Procedure document [12]. The test procedure workflow illustrated in Fig. 11.11 combines the steps in the test procedure with the expected method the Tester will use to verify the SUT's capabilities for meeting the ONC certification criterion. The testing process is composed of a series of steps that must be followed to ensure complete and accurate evaluation of the SUT. The diagram indicates the steps taken by the testing laboratories when certifying the EHR system (in this case the LIS is part of the EHR-S).

11.5.3 Testing Receiving Applications

Testing of receiving systems presents a set of challenges, because, typically, no artifact is produced for the Tester to assess directly. This situation is in contrast to testing of a sending system, in which an artifact (e.g., a message) is produced that can be assessed directly.

A key principle for Testers is to test a system as it currently exists (i.e., as released as a product—Testers shouldn't request for functionality to facilitate testing). Additional interfaces and functions specifically designed to facilitate testing are luxuries that usually aren't available. Even if they are available, such utilities would have to be verified by the Tester as functioning correctly. For these reasons, Testers typically rely only on the product capabilities of the SUT and design a testing approach accordingly.

The following list contains five approaches for testing receiving applications. Depending on the requirements to be tested and the system capabilities, not all approaches may be feasible. Typically, a combination of two or more of these approaches is employed.

- Inspection Testing
- Use of Acknowledgements
- Use of Query and Response Interfaces
- Related extended workflow requirements
- Artificial Capabilities

In order to test receiving systems adequately, an associated set of requirements for each required data element must be specified. As mentioned, these requirements are sometimes listed in an interoperability specification or in a separate functional requirements specification. In other instances, such requirements are not specified at all and, therefore, can't be tested.

11.5.3.1 Inspection Testing Approach

Inspection Testing relies on human investigation (a visual inspection) of the SUT in order to collect evidence for conducting a conformity assessment. Usually, the inspection testing process involves priming or knowing the state of the system; providing a known and documented stimulus to the receiving system; and evaluating the system's response to the stimulus against expected results based on the input and requirements. The inspection test approach, as shown in Fig. 11.12, is composed of a test tool and a human inspector.

The test tool contains the Test Case and associated test material such as the test message and Juror Document. The Juror Document is used to inspect the receiving

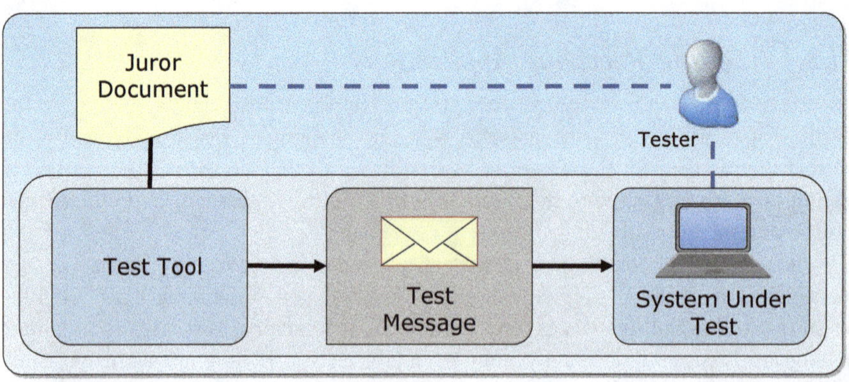

Fig. 11.12 Simple architecture for testing a receiver system

SUT. The information contained in the Juror Document is based on the data provided in the test message and the known state of the system. Details of the Juror Document and the level at which the information is inspected for incorporation of the message into the receiving system are discussed later.

During the inspection process, evidence of conformance can be obtained through a variety of methods, including viewing the system display, browsing the system data base, viewing the configuration files, or other mechanisms supported by the SUT.

11.5.3.2 Use of Acknowledgements Approach

The use of application level acknowledgements is a technique that can be employed to assess the system's capabilities with regard to content requirements. The Test Plan can include Test Cases designed with the intent to trigger content error responses (i.e., acknowledgement messages) from the receiving system. The triggers may include required elements that are missing from the message or an element that contains data the receiver can't process completely. Specific requirements must be provided in the specification to use this testing approach appropriately; when these requirements are missing, implementers just apply their own business rules however they see fit.

11.5.3.3 Query and Response Approach

The third of the five approaches listed above relies on the receiving system having the ability to support a standardized or non-standardized[14] query and response interface. A standardized interface is preferred since the Test Tool would need to support only one interface. In some cases, the requirement for the incorporation of data is accompanied by a broader set of requirements (i.e., a workflow) that includes query and response capabilities. Under these circumstances, the Tester can take advantage of these system capabilities and utilize them during testing to gain efficiency. This approach is employed in the IHE PIX/PDQ test cases, testing architecture, and the tool presented in Chaps. 13 and 14.

The query/response approach is used to assess the SUT's ability to incorporate data based on a given input. The system may or may not be primed with a known state before a stimulus is provided (e.g., a message or a set of messages are sent). After the stimulus is generated, a query of the SUT is performed, requesting the data provided in the stimulus for comparison to the expected results. At this point it must be assumed that the query/response mechanism in the receiving system is

[14]This is not desirable, but it may be useful if a vendor already supports a proprietary interface and not a standard interface.

operating correctly.[15] If a standardized interface is in place, it may be tested first (i.e., as part of the Test Plan, since it is a requirement of the specification). Data are extracted from the response message and compared to the expected results either via an automated (machine) process, a visual inspection, or a combination of both.

One example of an instance when this approach would be applicable is during testing of a patient registration system. In this case, the Tester starts with a *clean* system to be tested in which no patients exist in the data base. The Test Tool sends patient registration messages to the SUT, and then a query is performed to verify that the patient information was captured satisfactorily and stored by the system. The Tester determines if the SUT is functioning "satisfactorily" based on a set of requirements. The process of establishing such requirements and developing adequate Test Cases to examine the requirements can be a challenging undertaking. A further test may involve updating patient information that already is stored in the database of the SUT; then a subsequent query can be performed to verify that the update occurred in accordance with the requirements.

A second example of an applicable instance for this approach is recording of immunization information. Several vaccine administration occurrences for one patient can be sent as separate messages to an immunization information system (IIS). A query for the complete immunization history of the patient can be requested and the query results can be compared to the expected results. For testing the query/response interface of the IIS, preloading of the patient's immunization history into the system may be required.

11.5.3.4 Extended Workflow Approach

The fourth approach to assessing a receiving system is to leverage extended workflow requirements. These requirements may or may not be available, and, even when they are available, a Tester cannot rely on these requirements being correct. Cross-checking using the inspection test approach, however, can alleviate or mitigate concerns about their accuracy. The extended workflow approach by its very nature supports the notion of (extended) scenario testing, which, in itself, is often an end goal for testing.

In the extended workflow approach, a stimulus is provided to the receiving SUT, which has known state. Based on the stimulus and known state, the receiver is required (based on another related requirement) to produce an artifact. In cases where not all of the information is provided by the stimulus, additional information is entered into the receiving system, which can be achieved in the priming step. The output artifact is examined by the Tester using the methods described for testing sending applications. Specific content can be examined by the test system by correlating the input provided in the input artifact to the output artifact. This method

[15]Even without this assumption, the response only will deliver the correct responses if this interface is functioning correctly.

can be automated. For example, a lab results message for a whole blood lead test with an observation of 24 ug/dL is sent to an EHR-S and is to be incorporated per a requirement. The Test Case[16] instructs the EHR-S to create a lab result message based on the incorporation of the whole blood lead test that adheres to the standard for public health lab reporting. The test system examines the content in the message created by the EHR-S for public health lab reporting and compares it to the content sent to the EHR-S. This testing approach would work well for two separate EHR certification criteria that are included in the ONC Health IT Certification Program 2014 Edition. The two criteria are related in that one criterion addresses receiving a lab results message and incorporating the information, and the other criterion addresses generating a lab results message for public health (ELR).

Figure 11.13 illustrates the workflow and testing process for the example extended workflow approach described above using the incorporation of laboratory results test scenario. In this particular example, some of the information needed for the public health ELR message may not be available in the original stimulus; however, the Test Case could provide the additional information necessary (e.g., in a Test Data Specification for testing sending applications). The ELR message, generated from the incorporated lab results data plus any additional information provided via the Test Case, can be examined for specific content. This content is very important (as will be discussed further in the detailed lab result case study that addresses how the lab result is incorporated and managed in the receiving system). For example, if the date of birth (DOB) in the lab result message is different from the DOB in the receiving system's data base, what is the *appropriate* DOB value to

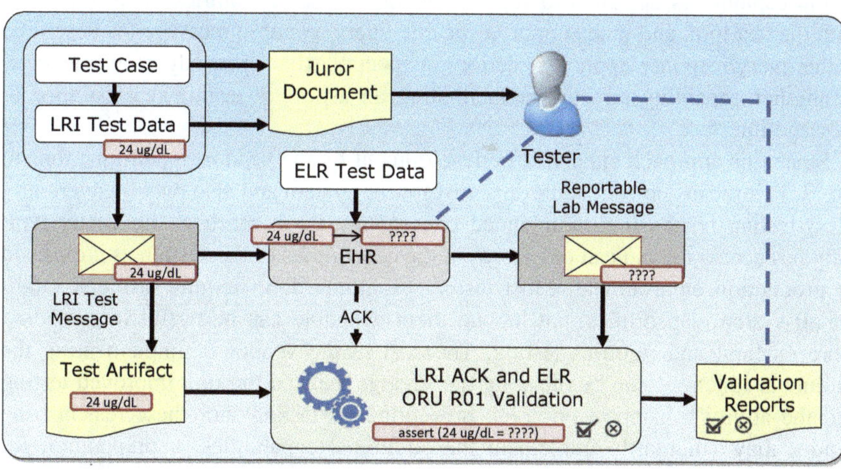

Fig. 11.13 Example of extended workflow testing

[16]Although this scenario is not typical it is valid. In most cases the EHR-S lab module would directly create the ELR message.

be sent to the public health agency? A functional requirement must specify this. If the receiving system incorrectly incorporated or used the DOB data, this error can be detected by examining the message generated for the public health agency.

Note that the protocol used in the input doesn't need to match the one used for the output. For example, the input may be an HL7 v2 message while the output could be a CDA document. The assessment can be performed even if these protocols are different.

Linking together multiple requirements as an extended workflow provides a number of benefits and brings additional rigor to the testing process. First, it is often desirable to test such a workflow to confirm that multiple standards do in fact work together to perform a given clinical task. This approach also provides a good test of the SUT, whether it consists of an integrated product from a single vendor or multiple products from different vendors. Secondly, the results of one test can be leveraged to assist in another test. In this case, the content in the ELR message is used to aid in assessing the incorporation of the LRI message. This testing approach is predicated on the SUT supporting the linked standards. IHE uses a form of this method of testing at their connect-a-thons in perpetration of workflow demonstration at the HIMSS Interoperability Showcase. In this setting, multiple vendors participate in the workflow.

11.5.3.5 Artificial System Capability Approach

To facilitate automated and cost-effective testing, the SUT may develop or use plugin capabilities designed to support testing. These capabilities directly interact with the test tool, and may support a specific query response message (as described in the query/response approach section), a specialized acknowledgement message, or another capability targeted at facilitating an aspect of testing (e.g., a specific message interface).

Since this approach entails extra development by the vendor to add functions to the SUT, it means upfront additional cost for the system and also may inadvertently affect testing results (i.e., unintended consequences). In practice, the Tester typically has access to, and can only rely on, the capabilities of the system as it exists in its production environment. Most testing programs don't require artificial (additional) system capabilities, but having them available can be useful in providing more efficient and rigorous testing. The cost to the vendor of implementing the additional functions can be offset by the savings realized through improved testing and the ability to support on-going or continuous testing. For these reasons, the vendor may voluntarily implement the additional capabilities in preparation for testing.

11.5.3.6 Combining Approaches

A combination of the approaches for testing receiving systems can and should be used to garner a more complete assessment of the implementation. Each approach has strengths and weaknesses. The Tester has at their disposal a set of methods in their toolbox, and they will decide which approach or combination of approaches work best to assess the SUT in terms of both rigor and resource effectiveness. In certain cases, one approach can be used to verify the value of another approach. For example, the inspection testing approach can be used to verify that the automated query/response approach is operating correctly, allowing the Tester to feel confident that this automated approach can be used for the majority of the testing.

11.5.4 Case Study: Incorporation of Laboratory Results

This case study is taken from the ONC 2014 Edition Incorporation of Laboratory Results certification criterion [12, 5]. This criterion focuses on incorporation of laboratory results, and it references the LRI implementation guide and other standards. This case study uses the inspection testing approach.

Testing the incorporation of laboratory results presents a set of challenges, because no output artifact (e.g., a message) is produced that can be assessed directly during the test. For this criterion, the ambulatory EHR-S, as the receiving SUT, is examined for evidence of the *incorporation* of laboratory results information from the received message and also for the ability to display seven types of information that are part of a laboratory results report (per requirements adopted from CLIA, the Clinical Laboratory Improvement Amendments, which are regulatory standards for clinical laboratory operations in the US). The ONC criterion specifies the Laboratory Results Interface (LRI) Implementation Guide for generating the laboratory results message. Conformance testing involves a Juror Document (inspection check list) and a human inspector. The content of the Juror Document is derived from the Test Case and test message. Figure 11.14 illustrates the testing flow when using the NIST conformance test tool for the incorporation of laboratory results test procedure.

The Test Tool interacts with the EHR SUT, simulating the function of an LIS (or a laboratory module) that would create the LRI message. Test Cases are developed for the various use cases described in the LRI implementation guide, and test data are created for each Test Case. Based on the Test Case and test data, a test message and Juror Document are generated automatically by the test tool infrastructure. The ambulatory EHR-S is primed with data (i.e., patient demographic information and test order information) to enable incorporation of the data elements in the lab result message with a specific patient's record. The Test Tool and EHR-S are configured (e.g., IP address and port number) to enable communication between the systems. The message is also configured (e.g., application name and facility) to match that of the receiving system (i.e., the EHR-S). The lab result test message is sent to the

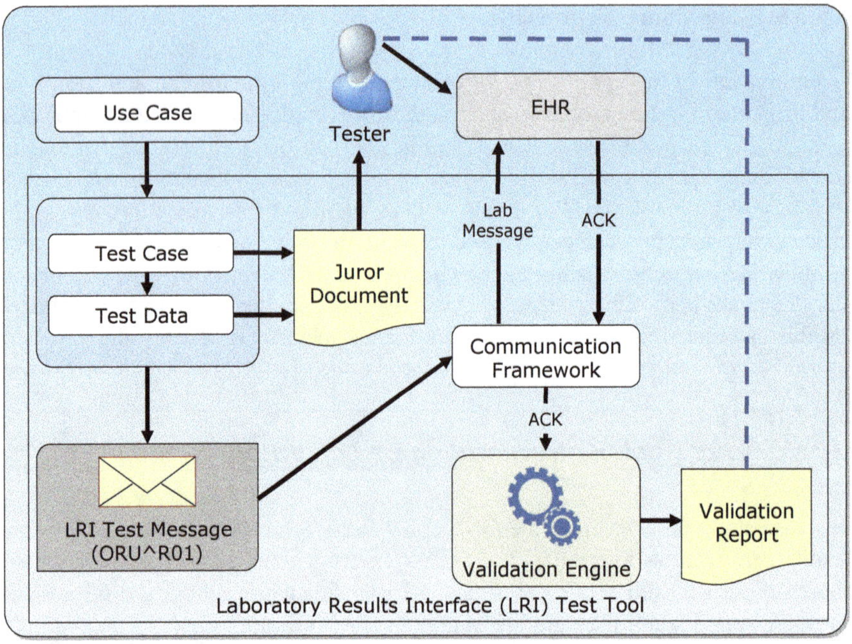

Fig. 11.14 Test flow for testing EHR-S receiving transmission of lab results

EHR-S, and the Tester uses the Juror Document to examine the EHR-S to verify incorporation of the data elements. The Juror Document is the test case-specific checklist the Tester uses to verify and document the presence or absence in the EHR-S of the data elements transmitted in the test message sent from the LRI Test Tool. The data elements are categorized in the Juror Document according to how they are to be verified. For example, some data elements are required to be displayed to the clinical user on the EHR-S screen as well as stored in the EHR-S, while other data elements are required to be stored or derivable only. Defining precisely the meaning of terms (e.g., display, store, and use) used for evaluation is essential. An effort in the ONC S&I Framework initiative is addressing this need through the development of the Laboratory Functional Requirements Specification [13]. Certain data elements sent in the test message need not be verified for incorporation, since they are not relevant to the incorporation of laboratory results (e.g., message processing elements).

The use case that describes testing of the creation of the lab results message is the same as the one used for testing of incorporation of lab results data. The testing in each instance focuses on a different aspect in the same use case. The description of the Test Case also is the same, except that the perspective of what is being tested is different. The use case is outlined in the following steps:

1. A lab test is ordered for a patient
2. The specimen is collected (if applicable), and is received and processed in the lab
3. The lab result is produced and stored in the LIS database
4. The lab result message is created
5. The lab result is transmitted to an ambulatory electronic health record (EHR)
6. **The lab result is incorporated into the ambulatory EHR (EHR-S Test Plan Scope)**

The ONC criterion that addresses transmission of electronic lab results is addressed in step 4 above—the lab result message is created. This step was discussed previously in this chapter. Step 6—the lab result is incorporated into the ambulatory EHR-S—is addressed in the incorporate lab results test procedure, which is the focus of this case study.

The testing process is composed of a series of steps that must be followed to ensure complete and accurate evaluation of the SUT. Figure 11.15 depicts the workflow for testing an EHR-S receiving transmission of laboratory results. As previously discussed, the Juror Document is the test case-specific checklist the Tester uses to assess and document the incorporation by the EHR of the data elements received in the message from the LIS Test Tool. The Tester will verify the presence or absence of the data elements in the EHR-S to determine if the incorporation meets the specified requirements. Table 11.2 shows an excerpt from a Juror Document used for assessing incorporation of lab results for ONC 2014 Edition certification testing. [5].

As illustrated in Fig. 11.14, validation for incorporation of lab results data elements has two components: (1) validation of the acknowledgement message,

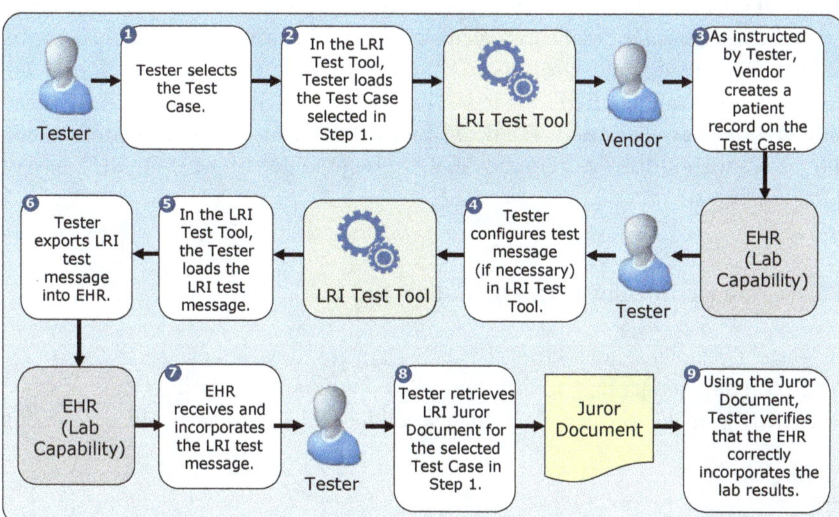

Fig. 11.15 LRI receiving testing workflow

Table 11.2 Data element incorporation categorization

Category	Description	Example
Display verification	Verify data are displayed on EHR user interface	Lab result (OBX-5)
Incorporate verification	Verify data are persisted in the EHR (e.g., inspection of the data base; however, a specific method for attestation is not prescribed); Note, display verification can be used for data classified as incorporate verification in the Juror Document	Unique patient identification (PID-3) including support for assigning authority (for the GU profile)
Implied verification	Verify the appropriate data associations and subsequent rendering if applicable	Linking of parent/child results (OBX-4—Sub ID)
No verification	Data verification not relevant	Processing of the message type (MSH-9)

which is an automated process in the test tool[17]; and (2) validation via inspection with the Juror Document as the assessment checklist.

For the first component, the lab result message is sent to the EHR-S from the Test Tool, and an acknowledgement (ACK) message is returned to the Test Tool. The acknowledgement is captured by the Test Tool and then forwarded to the validation engine where it is assessed. The assessment is based on the requirements specified in the LRI implementation guide for the ACK message. The Validation Report is the output of the validation engine. This report states whether the EHR-S has passed or failed this part of the test and identifies the points of failure.

The second, and more important, component of the validation is inspection testing. This process utilizes an inspector to ascertain if the lab result data elements sent in the test message are incorporated into the EHR system. As mentioned above, the Juror Document guides the inspector through the assessment process. Inspection may include viewing the EHR-S screens, browsing the EHR database, or examining configuration files. The results gathered by the inspector are used in combination with the Validation Report from the ACK message to determine if the SUT passed or failed the test.

11.5.4.1 Juror Document Interpretation and Use

The Juror Document categorizes the data elements received in the test message based on requirements that specify how incorporation of those data elements into the EHR-S is to be verified through inspection testing. A variety of verification

[17]Testing of the Acknowledgements is not part of ONC 2014 Edition certification testing; however, it is planned for future releases of the test tool (and should be included in testing).

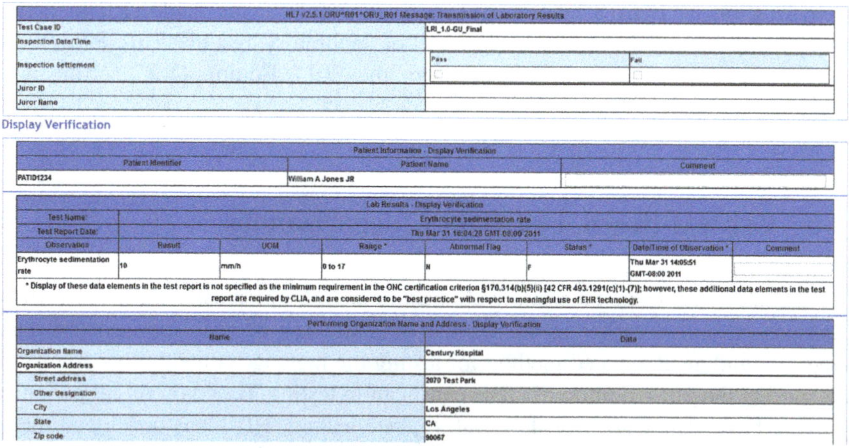

HL7 v2.5.1 ORU^R01^ORU_R01 Message: Transmission of Laboratory Results		
Test Case ID	LRI_1.0-GU_Final	
Inspection Date/Time		
Inspection Settlement	Pass	Fail
Juror ID		
Juror Name		

Display Verification

Patient Information - Display Verification		
Patient Identifier	Patient Name	Comment
PATID1234	William A Jones JR	

Lab Results - Display Verification							
Test Name:	Erythrocyte sedimentation rate						
Test Report Date:	Thu Mar 31 16:04:28 GMT-08:00 2011						
Observation	Result	UOM	Range *	Abnormal Flag	Status *	Date/Time of Observation *	Comment
Erythrocyte sedimentation rate	10	mm/h	0 to 17	N	F	Thu Mar 31 14:05:51 GMT-08:00 2011	

* Display of these data elements in the test report is not specified as the minimum requirement in the ONC certification criterion §170.314(b)(5)(ii) [42 CFR 493.1291(c)(1)-(7)]; however, these additional data elements in the test report are required by CLIA, and are considered to be "best practice" with respect to meaningful use of EHR technology.

Performing Organization Name and Address - Display Verification	
Name	Data
Organization Name	Century Hospital
Organization Address	
Street address	2070 Test Park
Other designation	
City	Los Angeles
State	CA
Zip code	90067

Fig. 11.16 Example excerpt of the lab results Juror Document

categories can be specified, each one defining a different threshold to be met by the SUT; and the rigor of testing can vary significantly based on the verification category assigned to each data element in the test message. The Juror Document used for ONC 2014 Edition certification testing provided a mid-level threshold the SUT had to meet for demonstrating incorporation of the lab results data elements. Table 11.2 describes the categorization used for 2014 Edition certification testing. Note that not all data elements sent in the test message require explicit verification; for this reason, data elements assigned to the "Implied Verification"[18] and "No Verification" categories do not appear in the current Juror Document.

The Juror Document is composed of two sets of tables listing the data elements that must be verified as incorporated for a given Test Case. The first set of tables (labeled "Display Verification" and shown in Fig. 11.16) contain the data elements that are verified by the Tester viewing the data elements displayed on a screen in the SUT as a clinician would view them. The second set of tables (labeled "Incorporate Verification" and not shown in Fig. 11.16) contain the data elements that must be verified by the Tester via inspection of the database, the tables, the configuration files, or other tools used by the SUT. Implied Verification is expressed (in some cases) by the structure of the Juror Document, for example, grouping of data. Not all data elements contained in the test message are subject to verification. These elements fall into the "No Verification" category and do not appear on the Juror Document.

Specificity of the requirements is essential for testing the incorporation of data, but, unfortunately, the requirements often are underspecified or do not exist at all. For future certification, the ONC Standards and Interoperability (S&I) Framework

[18]However, "Implied Verification" elements can have an impact on the juror document. For example, results related to parent-child linking have a certain organization that must be met.

is working on an EHR-S laboratory functional requirements guide [13] to better define the criterion for the incorporation of laboratory results. This effort is a positive outcome of lessons learned from the 2014 Edition ONC certification program.

11.6 Context-Based Test Data Categorizations

The case study for testing a sending application's ability to create laboratory results messages presented earlier in this chapter includes use of NIST-defined test data categories and an associated method for testing the message content. This approach was used in the 2014 Edition of ONC certification testing. Based on this experience applying basic data categories for conformance testing, NIST has developed more granular categories, which are used in the latest testing framework (including the 2015 Edition ONC certification test tools). Assigning test data and discrete assessment categories to elements provides a mechanism that enables expanded testing of a specification's messaging requirements and of the data element content as well. The data categories associated with the message elements are, in essence, an additional conformance assessment indicator that is focused on content.[19] Test case authors can use this method to create targeted test cases for probing a sending application's capabilities. The testing approach presented in this section pertains to the entity that created the object (e.g., a sending application that created a message). A similar set of test data categorizations and approaches can be applied for testing recipients. Additionally, the discussion and examples focus on positive test cases, and the approach applies equally to negative testing. Although the use of test data categorization presented here targets HL7 v2.x, the approach is applicable to other standards.

As explained earlier, a mechanism is needed to bind a specific test data category to test data and to show users which categories have been applied. In some cases, the test tool validator (based on the test data categorization) simply examines the message element for the presence of data, whereas in other cases the validator examines the message element for the presence of data and for exact content. For the HL7 v2.x conformance testing tools, a Message Content Data Sheet is used to show which categories are assigned to each data element. Figure 11.17 shows an example of the Message Content Data Sheet listing the location, data element, test data, and the associated test data categorization.

Table 11.3 shows descriptions of the test data categories (Indicators) and the testing implications associated with use of each category. The test data categories enable classification of the test data in order to extend and strengthen the rigor of

[19]Use of test data and the associated test data categories can be used to assess all of the requirements imposed by the various conformance constructs (including usage, cardinality, vocabulary, and length).

Location	Data Element	Data	Categorization
RXA-1	Give Sub-ID Counter	0	Value-Profile Fixed
RXA-2	Administration Sub-ID Counter	1	Value-Profile Fixed
RXA-3	Date/Time Start of Administration		
RXA-3.1	Time	20150624	Presence-Content Indifferent
RXA-5	Administered Code		
RXA-5.1	Identifier	49281-0560-05	Value-Test Case Fixed
RXA-5.2	Text	Pentacel	Presence-Test Case Proper
RXA-5.3	Name of Coding System	NDC	Value-Profile Fixed
RXA-6	Administered Amount	0.5	Presence-Test Case Proper
RXA-7	Administered Units		
RXA-7.1	Identifier	mL	Value-Test Case Fixed
RXA-7.2	Text	mL	Presence-Test Case Proper
RXA-7.3	Name of Coding System	UCUM	Value-Profile Fixed
RXA-9	Administration Notes		
RXA-9.1	Identifier	00	Value-Test Case Fixed
RXA-9.2	Text	New Record	Presence-Test Case Proper
RXA-9.3	Name of Coding System	NIP001	Value-Profile Fixed

Fig. 11.17 Example message content data sheet for RXA segment (immunization)

Table 11.3 Test data categorization: descriptions and testing implications

Indicator	Description	Testing implications	Comments
Indifferent	No test data are provided as part of the test case	No additional validation	The validation is indifferent to the presence of data or specific content in the message element **Meaning**: Value or don't value this data element
Presence	Test data are provided as part of the test case; content indifferent	Validated for the presence of data.	The specific content is not pertinent to the test cases for the purpose of testing. The test data can be modified **Meaning**: Value this data element
Presence-length	Test data are provided as part of the test case; minimum[a] length of the content is expected	Validated for the presence of data to a minimum length	The specific content is not pertinent to the test cases for the purpose of testing, but the length of the content is. The test data can be modified as long as the minimum length of the test data is maintained **Meaning**: Value this data element to a minimum length
Value	Test data are provided as part of the test case; specific content is provided and expected	Validated for the presence of data and for specific content.	The specific content (or choice of content) is provided and is expected to be present

(continued)

Table 11.3 (continued)

Indicator	Description	Testing implications	Comments
			in the message. The test data can only be modified with data in the allowable data set. In some cases, the set is a single constant **Meaning**: Value this data element with the test data options provided
Non-presence	No test data are provided as part of the test case and no content for this message element is expected	Validated for the non-presence of data	Content is not specified in the test case and is not expected to be present in the message **Meaning**: Don't value this data element

[a]Maximum length should also be addressed

the testing. For each category, the table lists the criteria that are used by the test tool to assess the test data that populate each element in a message. These criteria in turn tell the tester whether or not the test data in a specific element can be changed, the source of the test data, and to what level of precision the validation tool will assess the data. A common example for extending the testing capability involves message elements specified with a Usage of RE (Required, but maybe Empty). Context-based testing must be used when the tester wishes to assess the system's ability to support these elements, because without context (test data provided) an automated validation tool has "limited ways of knowing" whether the data needed for the RE data element are available for use in the message or not. Using a test case and associated categorized test data, the tester can inform the validation tool (and the user) of the conformance expectations for this message element. In the case of assessing an application's ability to support an element with RE usage, the category assigned would be "Presence", which notifies the tester and validation tool that data shall be present in the message for this element.

The test data categories provide a classification scheme for defining the impact that the test data given in a test case have on the validation of message instances. The use of test data expands the scope of message validation. For each test case, test data are given that coincide with the test story. The test case developer uses the test data categories as an aid to assess vendor product capabilities required by the implementation guide in the context-based testing operation mode (such requirements can't be tested easily in a context-free environment). The Qualifier (Table 11.4) provides a refinement of the test data category and provides additional information about the source of the data and expectations of the data element. The Qualifier does not have an impact on the validation of the data element.

Table 11.4 Test data categorization with qualifiers and more details

Indicator	Description	Qualifier	Description
Indifferent	No content is specified	*None*	None
Presence	Example content is specified	*Content indifferent*	Content is expected to be present in the message, but not a specific value
		Configuration	Content is expected to be present in the message, but not a specific value. The value is usually determined at installations
		System generated	Content is expected to be present in the message, but not a specific value. The value is system generated
		Test case proper	Content is expected to be present in the message, but not a specific value. However, content is expected to be consistent with the clinical test story
Presence-length	Example content is specified to a minimum length	*Same qualifiers as for presence*	Content of a minimum length is expected to be present in the message, but not a specific value
Value	Specific content is specified	*Profile fixed*	Content is defined as a constant in the conformance profile. The constant is specified in the test data
		Profile fixed-list	Content is defined as a set of allowable values in the conformance profile. One value from the allowable set is specified in the test data
		Test case fixed	Content that is defined as a constant in the test case
		Test case fixed-list	Content is defined as a set of allowable values in the test case. One value from the allowable set is specified in the test data
Non-presence	No content is explicitly specified	*None*	None

To keep this discussion brief, the test data categories presented here address only data elements with R (Required) and RE (Required, but may be Empty) usages. The method applies equally to other usage indicators, however, most context-based testing focuses on elements with R and RE usage. Elements with C (Conditional) usages resolve to either R, RE, O, or X usages based on the outcome of the condition predicate. The test case developer will provide (or not provide) data to trigger the various conditional outcomes, hence, data elements with C usage for a specific test case resolve to another usage and are handled as described above for that specific usage. The test case developer can use this mechanism to ensure that each conditional will be triggered.

Table 11.5 provides additional information about the testing implications the test data categorization has on the conformity assessment. The notion of "R → None" indicates that the usage for the element is "R-Required" and that the test data category assignment doesn't add any more constraints that don't already exist from the requirements documented in the profile; therefore, no additional assertions are needed. An example where a test data category assignment does generate an additional assertion is in the case of the Presence, "RE → Validates for the presence of data". The table also provides insight regarding when a particular category should be used.

Table 11.5 Test data categorization: testing implications and use

Test data categorization assessment indicators	
Indifferent	
Testing implications	None R → None RE → None
Use/examples	Data are not provided as part of the test case. No assessment of the data element is made beyond that specified in the standard. Usually applies to elements with RE usage in which valuing the element, or not, is not of interest for the test case
Presence	
Testing implications	1. The presence of content is being assessed by the validation tool 2. Specific content is not being assessed by the validation tool R → None RE → Validates for the presence of data
Use/examples	R: Indicates the characteristic of the test data given and expected in the message RE: Data are provided for use in the test case to test whether the SUT supports the element. Indicates the characteristic of the test data given and expected in the message The characteristic type of the data is further described by the qualifier
Presence-length	
Testing implications	1. The presence of content is being assessed by the validation tool 2. The length of the content is being assessed by the validation tool 3. Specific content is not being assessed by the validation tool R → Validates the length of the data for a minimum value RE → Validates for the presence of data and the length of the data for a minimum value
Use/examples	Example data are provided for the test case, specific content is not of interest, but the minimum length of the content is Example use: Tests that the SUT supports the PID-5.3 (Second and Further Given Names or Initials Thereof) element to a certain length to ensure that more than a middle initial is supported

(continued)

Table 11.5 (continued)

Test data categorization assessment indicators	
Value profile-fixed	
Testing implications	1. The presence of content is being assessed by the validation tool 2. Specific content is being assessed by the validation tool as specified in the conformance profile R → None RE → Validates for the presence of data
Use/examples	The value is defined as a constant in the conformance profile. That constant is provided in the test data. The validation of the content is accounted for in the profile constraints; no additional assertion is needed for Required elements. For RE elements, a presence check is required. A typical use is when the constant is required when an RE element is present
Value profile-fixed list	
Testing implications	1. The presence of content is being assessed by the validation tool 2. Specific content is being assessed by the validation tool as specified in the conformance profile R → None RE → Validates for the presence of data
Use/examples	The value is defined as a set of allowable values in the conformance profile. One value in this set is provided as the test data. The validation of the content is accounted for in the profile constraints; no additional assertion is needed for Required elements. For RE elements, a presence check is required. A typical use is when the constant is required when an RE element is present
Value test case fixed	
Testing implications	1. The presence of content is being assessed by the validation tool 2. Specific content is being assessed by the validation tool as specified in the test case R → Validates for specific content RE → Validates for the presence and data specific content
Use/examples	A specific value for this data element is specified in the test case and that specific value is expected in the message. The test case developer is requesting a specific value to assess support for a certain value that is in the scope of the defined requirements (e.g., a specific coded value); to trigger a certain workflow or function; or to enable subsequent test steps in a test case
Value test case fixed list	
Testing implications	1. The presence of content is being assessed by the validation tool 2. Specific content is being assessed by the validation tool as specified in the test case R → Validates for specific content RE → Validates for the presence and data specific content
Use/examples	A specific value from a set of values for this data element is specified in the test case and one of the values from that set is expected in the message (not necessarily the specific value given in the test data). The test case developer is requesting one value from a set of values to assess support for a certain set of values that is in the scope of the defined requirements (e.g., a coded value defining a concept); to trigger a certain workflow or function; or to enable subsequent test steps in a test case

(continued)

Table 11.5 (continued)

Test data categorization assessment indicators	
Non-presence	
Testing implications	1. The non-presence of content is being assessed by the validation tool R → None RE → Validates for the non-presence of data
Use/examples	Content is not specified in the test case and is not expected to be present in the message. Typically applies to data elements with RE usage for which the test case developer wishes to ensure that the implementation doesn't provide a default value in the message when no data is available

11.6.1 Data Content Conformity Assessment Examples

Table 11.6 shows how the test data categories can be applied in practice. For example, the first row indicates that the usage is "RE" and the test case provides "Donna" as the test data. Since the test category is "Presence Content-Indifferent" there is an expectation that the element be valued. If that element is not valued in the message, then the validation result is "Fail". The second row indicates that a value is present, therefore, the result of the validation is successful. To emphasize the point of Presence Content-Indifferent, the third row shows that the data in the message is "Sue", and the result of the validation is successful (because, the assessment indicator is looking for only presence, not exact content).

Table 11.6 Test data categorization: testing implications and examples of use

Element	Usage	Test data	Test data category	Conformity assessment	Data in message	Validation result
PID-5.3 (middle name)[a]	RE	Donna	Presence content-indifferent	Required	<Empty>	Fail
PID-5.3 (middle name)	RE	Donna	Presence content-indifferent	Required	Donna	Pass
PID-5.3 (middle name)	RE	Donna	Presence content-indifferent	Required	Sue	Pass
PID-5.3 (middle name)	RE	Donna	Presence-length content-indifferent	Required min length = 5	Victoria	Pass
PID-5.3 (middle name)	RE	Donna	Presence-length content-indifferent	Required min length = 5	Sue	Fail
PID-5.3 (middle name)	RE	Donna	Value-test case fixed	Required value = Donna	Donna	Pass

(continued)

Table 11.6 (continued)

Element	Usage	Test data	Test data category	Conformity assessment	Data in message	Validation result
PID-5.3 (middle name)	RE	Donna	Value-test case fixed	Required value = Donna	Sue	Fail
PID-5.3 (middle name)	RE	<Empty>	Indifferent	Indifferent	<Empty>	Pass
PID-5.3 (middle name)	RE	<Empty>	Indifferent	Indifferent	Donna	Pass
PID-5.3 (middle name)	RE	<Empty>	Non-presence	Forbidden	Donna	Fail
MSH-9.2 (trigger event)	R	V04	Value-profile fixed	Required value = V04	V04	Pass

[a]The example used is for HL7 v2.x. For brevity, "middle name" is used instead of the actual element name (second and further given names or initials thereof)

In contrast, when examining the sixth and seventh rows of the table, the assessment indicator is now set to Value-Test Case Fixed for the same usage/test data scenario. In the case where "Donna" is expected (seventh row), the message with content of "Sue" now fails. As shown in these examples, use of the test data categories and their associated assessment implications provides a systematized method for expanding testing capabilities, not only for the technical requirements but also for specific content. For an instantiation of this method and more examples see the NIST Immunization Conformance Testing Tool [7].

Table 11.7 presents an example of how a coded element can be tested using test data categories. Based on the test story, data for a newly administered immunization for Pentacel using the NDC code system (instead of CVX) are entered into the SUT. The Identifier "49281-0560-05" is expected to appear in the message exactly as given, the associated Text needs to be equivalent to the concept of "Pentacel", and the Coding System must be exactly "NDC".

Table 11.7 Use of test data categorization for coded elements

Element[a]	Test data	Test data category	Conformity assessment
RXA-5.1 (identifier)	49281-0560-05	Value-test case fixed	Content must be present and exactly "49281-0560-05"
RXA-5.2 (text)	Pentacel	Presence-test case proper	Content must be present and indicate a value equivalent to "Pentacel"
RXA-5.3 (coding system)	NDC	Value-profile fixed	Content must be present and exactly "NDC"

Element is RXA-5 (administered code—in this case an immunization)

11.6.2 Testing Cardinality and Other Conformance Constructs

As demonstrated, the test data category methodology addresses the conformance constructs of usage, length (minimum), and content[20] (specifically, vocabulary). Support of multiple occurrences is tested in a similar fashion using test data, and no additional special mechanism is necessary. If the cardinality of an element is, e.g., [0…3], test data can be provided for 0, 1, 2, or 3 occurrences. The test data and associated test data category assessment indicators provide sufficient information such that a validation can be performed. For example, if the specification indicates a cardinality of [0…3] for phone number, a test case could be created in which data for two phone numbers were given. Additionally, test data can be provided to violate the conformance boundaries (e.g., 4 instances in the prior example), such negative testing is equally as important positive testing.

11.7 Strategies and Best Practices for Test Case Development

The creation of the Test Plan (i.e., set of Test Cases) starts with an analysis of the test space. The test space may include many dimensions, such as use cases, negative testing, and data requirements. The dimensions are determined by the requirements in the specification.[21] Once the test dimensions are established, a Test Case matrix can be developed. One approach for developing this matrix is to list all of the requirements categorized by the test dimensions, which can become a set of rows in the matrix. This initial matrix can be initially populated with the extractable requirements derived from the specification. Test Cases can then begin to be developed to address each requirement. A given Test Case can and should address more than one requirement; in fact, for efficiency in terms of time and cost, a good Test Suite will contain a relatively small number of Test Cases for a given set of requirements. Another strategy involves leveraging an existing Test Case by making small changes to address a particular requirement or requirements. For example, in negative testing it may be desired to determine if a receiving system responds to certain errors sent in a message. A simple initial message with no errors can be created and used to test and confirm that the SUT can handle it correctly, which sets the baseline. This message can then be modified to introduce errors to

[20]Testing of content should also include the handling of encoding characters.

[21]It is important to note that the set of requirements are drawn from the specification and any specification it references or is derived from. For example, in HL7 v2 a conformance profile is defined that is based on the underlying HL7 v2 standard. Requirements from the base standard are brought forward and must be supported unless they are replaced (profiled) by the conformance profile definition.

target specific interests to test. It is important not to perform "equivalent" tests. In our message example, it is sufficient to determine if a receiving system correctly handles a missing required element (field) that is selected arbitrarily without examining all such elements. Of course, this testing approach does not prove that all such elements are correctly implemented; it is assumed that they are, based on testing the general mechanism. If there is reason to believe that a particular element is troublesome (or critical), then additional targeted probes may be included. It also may be appropriate to test a number of such dimensions over the test space to better ascertain the quality of the implementation. Again, this decision usually is left up to the Test Suite developer based on the time and resources available to test the system, the cost of additional testing, and the importance of the tests. The goal is to cover all requirements, but when resources are limited the strategies presented can optimize the test space covered. However, for certification testing an "*adequate*" amount of tests—including negative test cases—should be performed.

Another strategy is to develop a comprehensive set of Test Cases, depending on available resources; then the Tester can select a subset of the Test Cases for the actual testing. This is a viable strategy for certification testing, because the vendor needs to be prepared to pass all of the Test Cases, but during administration of testing, the Tester will select a subset at random. This tactic can dramatically reduce the number of tests that must be performed, which improves the efficiency and reduces the cost of the certification program. Implementers, however, should always be prepared to demonstrate the ability to pass all of the conformance tests.

When developing a set of Test Cases, it is important to start by addressing the breadth of Test Cases needed before concentrating on one specific area. Figure 11.18 represents a contrived test space for a given specification. The "dots" represents areas in the test space that have been targeted to be tested. Akin to

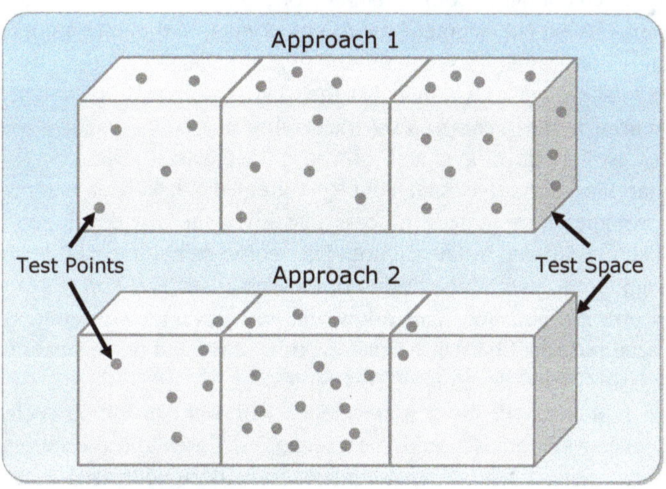

Fig. 11.18 Strategic sampling of the test space

Table 11.8 Mockup requirements traceability matrix

	Prem.	Final	Corrected	Amended	…	Req. N
Test Case 1	X	X				
Test Case 2		X	X			
Test Case 3		X	X			
Test Case 4	X	X		X		
…						
Test Case N	X	X	X	X		

statistical sampling, it is important to select strategic tests that have broad coverage. A Test Plan design, as shown in approach 1, is preferred over approach 2; however, knowledge of the specification may direct testing to a more concentrated area, if that area is known to be particularly complex or troublesome to implementers. Determining the best option often requires a judgment call be made based on the test case developer's experience and knowledge of the specification.

An essential tool that can help map the coverage space is a Test Case requirements traceability matrix. Table 11.8 provides a mockup of a simple Test Case traceability matrix in which requirements (normative statements) are on one axis and the list of Test Cases is on the other axis. Often multiple levels of matrixes must be created in a Test Plan to cover high-level and low-level requirements. If we revisit our laboratory results case study, we may want to create a traceability matrix for each lab result Scenario covered in the use case. The requirements axis might include entries such as single lab result with final result, single lab result with corrected result, a rejected specimen, a panel result, a reflex test, and a microbiology lab result with a parent-child relationship. This approach describes a traceability matrix at the *scenario level*. Another traceability matrix could be created at the message requirement level. For example, one axis would contain a list of all required elements (at the segment, field, component, and sub-component levels), the cardinality constraints for segments and fields, the length for primitive elements, and so forth. The other axis would list the Test Cases, some of which would be those referenced in the *scenario level* traceability matrix.

As Test Cases are developed and assertions are created, a check mark is used to indicate that the normative statement (requirement) has been addressed. This approach promotes a systematic process that gives the test developers a map of what has been tested and what has not. The requirements traceability matrix provides a visual tool to help in the design of the Test Plan. The Test Cases also could be given a priority indicator. This allows the test developers to address the most important requirements first. Unfortunately, time, cost, and resources often become restraining issues when developing Test Suites.

To be comprehensive, the test developer will want to create such matrixes, identify *all* such requirements, and then create Test Cases to test each requirement. Test Cases are created until *all* requirements have been addressed by at least one Test Case; however, usually it is not practical to list *all* possible requirements at a fine grained level, so it may be useful to create groupings of requirements and test a subset within those groupings. For example, a Value Set that contains 250 codes might be bound to a particular data element. It is not practical or especially useful (see earlier discussion on equivalent testing) to create 250 separate Test Cases to ensure that a system can handle all of these codes. Using an arbitrary subset of the 250 codes is more suitable for testing purposes; and if some codes are more prevalent in the real-world setting than others, then these codes definitely should be included. The subset selected for one Test Case can be used for different Test Cases that target other requirements. This tactic speaks to the concept of testing as many requirements as possible via a single Test Case as long as the test objectives still are met. In addition, to further increase testing efficiency, it is advantageous to target requirements in other dimensions concurrently in the Test Cases.

Below is a list that highlights some key points a test developer should consider during the development of a Test Plan.

1. Make a Test Case requirements traceability matrix or matrixes.
2. Attempt to produce the fewest number of Test Cases necessary to cover the core (or crucial) requirements in the test space.[22] However, do not overload a single test case such that it is not realistic or it is so complicated that it makes evaluation difficult.
3. Include a simple Test Case or a few simple Test Cases for participants to use when becoming accustomed to the mechanics of testing (a smoke test).
4. Reuse/leverage existing Testing Cases. Create simple tests that establish a base set in which modifications can be made to target specific requirements; then creation of entirely new Test Cases is kept to a minimum through just making the required delta in existing Test Cases.
5. Leverage sender and receiver Test Cases—i.e., use the same test data for testing the creation of the message and the incorporation of the message whenever possible.
6. Avoid duplicate (equivalent) Test Cases.
7. Make Test Cases real-world relevant whenever possible. Example test data/messages are useful for understanding requirements and have a much broader impact than just serving as a part of the Test Cases.
8. Prioritize Test Cases—reality dictates that the cost will prohibit/limit creation of needed Test Cases as well as what can be tested by implementers and testing bodies. Therefore, target high-impact issues and common mistakes first, if known.
9. Group Test Cases and provide levels.
10. When time and resources are limited always choose quality over quantity. Conformance tests must be correct and complete.

[22]The recommendation is not to determine core (or crucial) requirements arbitrarily, but to test a functionality without being completely exhaustive for every possible instance. A simple example is cardinality, for which it is sufficient to test to 10 instances of an element if the requirement is to support 10 instances. It is of little value to test that it can support exactly 8 instances or exactly 9 instances. (Please see boundary testing later in this chapter.)

11.8 Capability, Site, and Interoperability Testing

Chapter 7 introduced the concepts of profiling and the profile hierarchy. A relationship can be drawn between the profile level and the type of testing that can be performed, as illustrated in Fig. 11.19. The relationships shown are not the only relationships possible, but they are the typical ones. SDOs that create implementation guides often do so at the national (realm) level. These constrainable profiles defined within an implementation guide express a minimum core set of capabilities that each implementer must meet. Beyond this core functionality definition, flexibility still exists for data elements not fully qualified in the implementation guide, i.e., some optional elements remain.

The established *baseline* ensures a consensus level of functionality that satisfies the targeted use cases. Vendor and local implementations further constrain and define requirements that are compliant with the national level requirements. The methodology presented in Chap. 7 explains how an implementation profile is created. Local, that is site[23] specific, variations are denoted explicitly.

National certification programs (such as the ONC Health IT Certification Program in the US) develop and/or reference national level profiles for their certification criteria. The focus of certification testing is to assess whether the

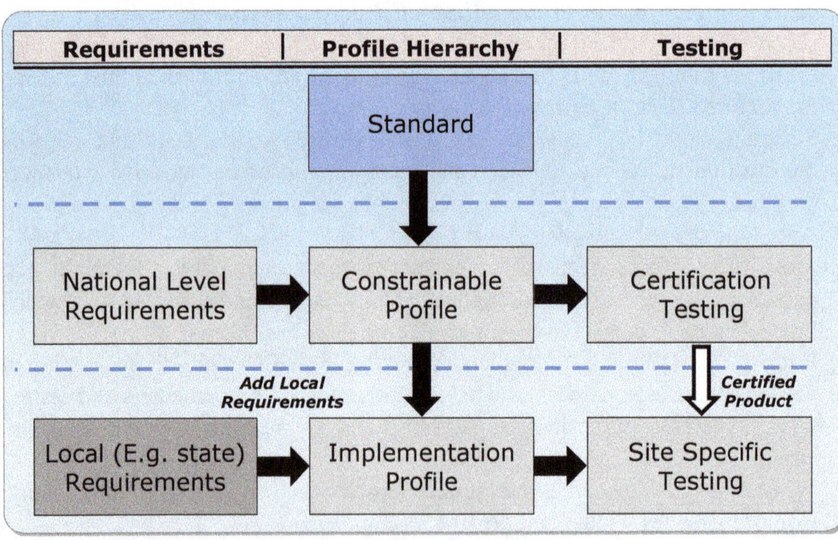

Fig. 11.19 Profile level and testing relationship

[23]The term "site" in this context can mean a single site, multiple sites, or a group of sites that define the same (implementation) profile requirements.

capabilities in each vendor's product meet the requirements defined by the specified profile. Capability Testing is the type of testing used for ONC certification and based on constrainable profiles as depicted in Fig. 11.20. A key point to bear in mind for Capability Testing is that the purpose of this type of testing is to verify that a product has the required capabilities, not to verify how the product might be used when installed in a production environment. Once additional local requirements (if any) are established and documented, site testing is performed using an implementation profile (i.e., a completely defined specification). Site specific testing targets the capability of a product for its intended use at an actual installation, which may be based on partner agreements.

Certification seeks to ensure that every product that is certified supports the capabilities defined by the national level standard. National level certification brings a set of stakeholders one step closer to achieving interoperability, but it is only the first step (see Fig. 11.20). It is incorrect to conclude that having certified products will lead to "*out of the box interoperability*" when interfacing two or more certified products. ONC certification scope is phase 1. After Capability Testing of vendor products in a test environment is performed, a second round of Capability Testing should follow that includes local requirements; we refer to this as Site Capability Testing (see Fig. 11.20).

At the national standard profile level, local requirements and variations have not been taken into account. Once local agreements are defined and the profiles documented, site specific testing can occur. The distinction between the different profiles and the associated levels of testing is important. Capability Testing occurs

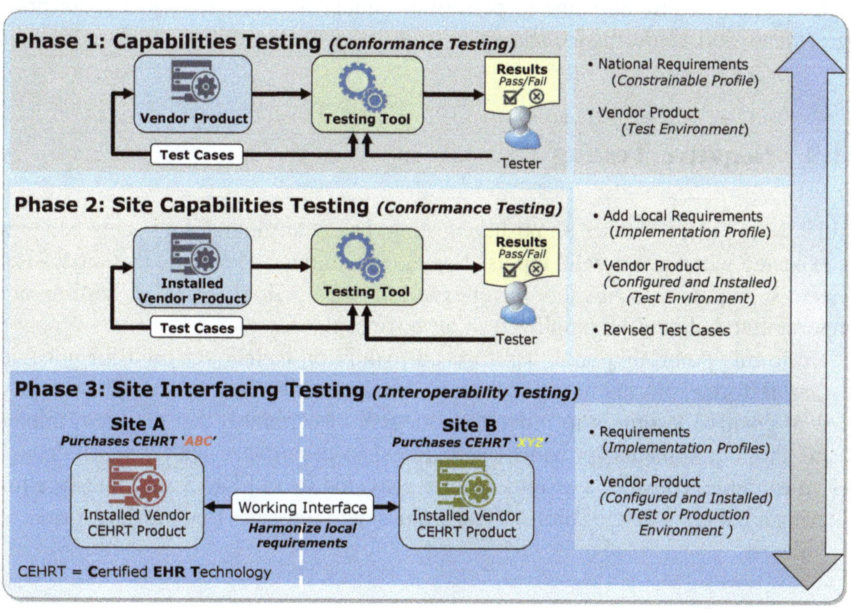

Fig. 11.20 Capability, site capability, and interoperability testing distinction

in phase 1 of the process and focuses on conformance testing. For site installations, the baseline requirements are customized to meet local requirements, and additional conformance testing needs to occur. Conformance testing is still required to ensure that the local requirements are implemented and that the national level requirements have not been compromised (think of this as a form of "regression" testing). Test cases developed in phase 1 can be leveraged and modified to meet the local variations. Once all parties participating in the site installation have completed this second round of conformance testing, then interoperability testing can proceed.

Phase 3 focuses on interoperability testing and ideally should incorporate conformance testing into the process. This is especially true if the implementations are being modified to achieve interoperability. It is important that conformance is not compromised to obtain interoperability. It is anticipated that the sites wishing to interoperate have purchased certified products that have been customized to meet site requirements and have tested those implementations accordingly. Site Interface Testing is applied to determine that data exchange and use meet business requirements. Such testing addresses the question: Does the interface work for the intended integration? Site Interface Testing can be performed in a test environment that mimics a production installation.

Although the testing steps are presented as a group, the concepts of conformance and interoperability testing are orthogonal. Conformance testing is performed on the various profile levels in the hierarchy. In this setting, the product is tested in isolation. Interoperability testing is performed among a set of products, be it in a test environment (such as the IHE Connect-a-thons) or at a production site. Although orthogonal in nature, the sequence in which testing should occur is logical. There is limited value in performing interoperability testing without prior agreements and conformance testing.

11.9 Negative Testing

Initial testing often focuses on positive testing, i.e., determining if a system behaves as expected when given valid inputs. Negative testing is a technique that analyzes a system's response to invalid or unexpected input. Both types of testing are important and should be employed in all testing plans.

Up to this point, this book has focused mainly on techniques used for positive testing. Before exploring negative testing, positive testing is reviewed. The primary goal of positive testing is to prove (to a degree of certainty) that a system implements the requirements (provides capabilities) in accordance with a specification. As an example, consider a textbox feature provided in an EHR-S user interface for entering a patient's date of birth.[24] The requirement indicates that the data format is as follows:

[24]For simplicity of the example, required precision for the date of birth is to the day.

MM/DD/YYYY

where:

MM	represents a two digit positive integer in the range of 01–12
DD	represents a two digit positive integer in the range of 01–31[25]
YYYY	represents a four digit positive integer expressing the year
/	represents a delimiter

This functionality could be implemented in a number of ways,[26] but for this example we assume it is a simple textbox. For a positive test, the tester would enter valid data into the textbox (e.g., 05/19/1994). Upon submission of this information, the system should validate the entry and process the data accordingly[27] (e.g., store it in the patient record for subsequent use). A test may assert that the system captured the data from the user interface, placed the data into the data base correctly, and that normal operation of the system continued.

A goal of negative testing is to expand the test coverage to determine how robustly the system handles an invalid stimulus. For a negative test, the tester would enter invalid data into the textbox (e.g., 05/**32**/1994). Upon submission of these data, the system should verify the entry and detect an error. A test may assert that the system detected an error, notified the user of the error, and did not accept the data into the patient's record. This example demonstrates the basic characteristics of negative testing.

Both positive and negative testing is necessary to adequately assess the system. Negative testing must not be omitted. A system must be able to account for errors and react appropriately. A common deficiency in standard specifications, however, is that the requirements are not provided or are not detailed enough to perform negative testing to a level/granularity that is necessary. In the case of date, it is obvious, but in other cases it is not obvious. Testers cannot conjecture, the requirements must be explicit.

11.9.1 Message and Document Incorporation

Maybe the most important use of negative testing is for assessing a system's response upon receipt of an invalid message or document. This kind of test is of significant importance when testing the binding of a system's data interface and the system's internal capabilities. In messaging testing, errors can be implanted into the messages to determine how a system reacts to the invalid stimulus. As previously discussed, to

[25]Additional requirements would also be specified to account for the number of days that can occur for a given month.

[26]For example, a calendar dialog could be used to select a date, or a series of drop down boxes that restrict the user's input to valid entries could be used.

[27]In conformance to another set or sets of requirements for handling and use of the date.

adequately test a system's response to invalid data, associated functional requirements must have been defined. For example, depending on the error, a system may be required to reject the message, or the system may be required to respond with an acknowledgment indicating that an error was detected while continuing to process the data. The severity of the error determines whether the receiving system rejects the message completely or processes the data after generating an error type of acknowledgement. In either case, specific conformance requirements related to the expected behavior must be available to the Tester, whether these requirements are the vendor's business rules or standardized requirements.

Another simple example of negative testing is creation of a message in which a required element that is critical for understanding the content of the message is missing. An example of this kind of element would be the abnormal flag or the reference range for a quantitative laboratory result. Since this information is critical in the interpretation of the results, the system must be able to detect the omission error and act accordingly. Depending on the requirements that have been specified, this error may be one that needs to be addressed at the interface (system) level or at the application level.

Workflow requirements may also be assessed through negative testing. One example might be where a Tester creates a sequence of messages containing changes in the status of a lab result; that is, the lab results status might be preliminary followed by a status of final (with the same order filler number identifying both instances of the test result as belonging to the same order). In a positive test, the Tester would create two lab result messages. The first message indicates a preliminary result and the second a final result (note that the Tester ensures that the preliminary result is received before the final result). In a negative test, the Tester would create two messages, the first of which indicates a final result and the second a preliminary result (note that the Tester ensures that the final result is received before the preliminary result). The functional requirement that serves as the basis for the test would reference a state diagram where a preliminary result can change to a final result, but a final result cannot change to a preliminary result (Note: a final result could change to a corrected result). Hypothetically, such an error could occur at the lab processing center.[28] In the negative test scenario, the Tester verifies that the system detected the error and issued an alert in some manner.

Opportunities abound for the Tester to create negative tests; in fact, so many opportunities exist that the tests likely won't be exhaustive. The invalid test space typically is larger than the valid test space; however, the Tester, through their real-world experience and their knowledge of the standard, can select scenarios that are more likely to reflect potential problems seen in the production setting or would

[28]A contrived example might be that the LIS was configured so the Preliminary result required verification by a pathologist before it could be released for transmission to the EHR-S, and the pathologist did not verify it, so it was not transmitted; then, the Final result was produced, the pathologist verified it, and this Final version of the result was transmitted to the EHR-S. The pathologist then realizes s/he hadn't verified the Preliminary version of the result, and now they verify it, and it is transmitted to the EHR-S AFTER the Final version of the result was transmitted.

incur patient safety issues. The mere fact that such test cases are made available to the implementers raises the awareness of potential errors and the consequences of those errors. The test cases' availability can aid implementers in their testing or confirm their existing testing.

11.9.2 Boundary Testing

Boundary testing means that the test probes the lower and upper limits of a requirement. One example of boundary testing would be validation of the length of a text string for a comment contained in an observation note (e.g., an NTE segment in HL7 v2). An implementation guide may state that a system must support (store and display) at least 10,000 characters.[29] A test can then be crafted to create a message with a 10,000-character string in the observation note. The Tester would verify that the receiving system stored the data and displayed the text string correctly (again, according to documented requirements).

Boundary testing is related to both positive testing and negative testing. For example, a particular standard may constrain the cardinality of a data element to "[2…6]", meaning that the system must be able to handle 2, 3, 4, 5 or 6 occurrences of the data element in a given message. Test cases can be developed to test for 1, 2, 6, and 7 instances of this data element in the message. The valid boundary of 2 and 6 instances are positive boundary tests and the invalid boundary of 1 and 7 are negative boundary tests. Both of these tests are equally important.

Typically, testing would not test every intermediate point in the range exhaustively (unless the system and test tool can completely automate the process and the in-scope range is not extraordinarily large, or a compelling reason existed to make it necessary). The endpoints would be tested, both in the positive and negative space. In addition, depending on the in-scope range, one or more intermediate points would be tested (e.g., 4 occurrences in the cardinality example might be tested in addition to 1, 2, 6, and 7). This strategy promotes efficiency in testing especially in large ranges.

11.9.3 False Positive and False Negative Test Results

False Positives and False Negatives can occur in testing. Figure 11.21 shows a truth table of possible outcomes of testing. A true positive refers to the case when the implementation is correct and the validation indicates that it (the entity that is being tested) is correct (by testing and in its reporting). A true negative occurs when the implementation is incorrect and the validation indicates that it is incorrect.

---

[29]In HL7 v2, this is expressed as the conformance length in a constrainable profile.

	Implementation is Correct	Implementation is Incorrect
No Failure Reported	True Positive	False Positive
Failure Reported	False Negative	True Negative

Fig. 11.21 Truth table of validation results (actual vs. reported) (the "true" and "false" indicators are given from the perspective of the validation tool)

A false negative occurs when the validation result indicates an error condition when no error exists (for the entity being tested). That is, the implementation (SUT) is correct, but the validation reports a failure. A problem exists in the testing process or the testing tool that produced the test report. This situation can happen because of a misinterpretation of a requirement or an incorrect implementation by the tool developer. Reported failures should be evaluated so false negatives are detected and eliminated.

A false positive test result occurs if the testing does not report a failure when an actual non-conformity has occurred. This situation can happen simply because a test has not been developed to include a particular requirement, and it quite often occurs in testing complex systems. False positives are more problematic, because they mislead implementers into thinking that their implementation is correct. As discussed previously, testing will not prove conformity—it simply tries to detect non-conformance.

False positives are harder to detect, because a Tester may have difficulty knowing what to look for. Complete and unambiguous requirements are essential to reduce false testing results. For example, in the case of negative testing related to date of birth, if no test was created to verify that a system could detect input and storage of an invalid date of birth, then the user may incorrectly assume that the system can handle invalid input for these data. In this circumstance, a false positive has occurred, which accentuates the importance of conducting negative testing and also highlights the need for comprehensive requirements and a test plan that provides broad coverage of those requirements. Employing a requirements traceability matrix as described earlier can aid in reducing false positives.

11.10 Other Types of Testing

Other types of testing and terms are often used when discussing conformance testing, interoperability testing, and testing in general. In this section, common test terms are provided for reference and for comparison to the concepts discussed in this chapter and throughout the book. This list is not exhaustive.

11.10.1 Smoke Testing

Smoke testing uses a series of preliminary Test Cases to conduct trial runs before the onset of more rigorous, formal testing. Smoke testing is used to ascertain if basic functions have been implemented correctly in a software product. Often, these initial tests are pre-requisites to completing other tests. A well designed Test Plan will indicate the sequence in which the tests should be run as well as the dependencies for running each test (i.e., no value can be obtained from running a certain test unless another test has been completed successfully first). The term "smoke testing" may have originated in the electronics industry where, if the equipment functioned properly without creating smoke, it passed the "smoke" test [14].

11.10.2 Communication Testing

In the tele-communication industry, a set of tests are used to identify the location of a problem. This approach is comparable to "smoke testing" mentioned before, but the focus is on the different levels of the communication stack.

When establishing communication between two trading partners, the entire stack must be tested. The lower layers (1–4) are usually available in computational environments, so the fact that we do have a communication stack is commonly overlooked. Sometimes, when network problems occur, "long-standing" tools such as *ping*, *ipconfig*, and communication sniffers are used to check that the communication is working, at least in principle, at the lower layers, which are represented by the red circles 1–4 in Fig. 11.22.

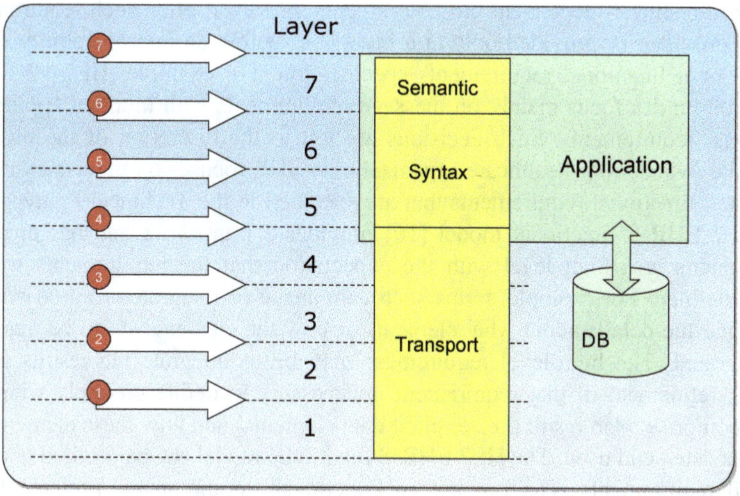

Fig. 11.22 Testing the communication stack (ISO/OSI Stack [15])

In order to test interoperability among applications, communication testing must be pursued on the higher levels as well. This notion is indicated by the red circles 5–7. In the context of this book, the establishment of fundamental communication and testing is expected and is worth mentioning. Beyond basic communication and communication testing are syntax and semantic testing of a specific application layer protocol (e.g., HL7 v2), which is the main focus of this book.

Inspection testing is conducted within the application, i.e., level 7, while message instances testing is performed at level 5 where the representation of the data is taken into account. Therefore, the way the data flows from the message instance into the application must be tracked.

As an example to consider is the use of character sets: if the application is utilizing the ASCII character set, but the message should use Unicode with a UTF-16 representation, some character codes must be changed and converted to a two byte representation. Hence, testing must be conducted to ensure that the represented characters are handled correctly during the encoding process and that a proper conversion occurs. This conversion should happen on level 6.

HL7 v2 is another very good example; it is specified on ISO level 7—hence, the name. It has two different representations: ER7 (i.e., "the pipe and hat" format) and XML. Different representational formats, for example, the two mentioned, require different tests for special characters like *ampersand* ("&") to verify that data are handled correctly. Section 5.9 in Chap. 5 provides background information.

11.10.3 Application Functional Testing

Application functional testing examines the system's ability to provide a capability (function) based on either a functional or business process requirement. Application functional testing is dependent on requirements; however, often such requirements are not provided or provided only at a high-level within an interoperability specification or a functional requirements specification. For example, HL7 v2 implementation guides focus mainly on message requirements with minimal application functional requirements. Such decisions are left to the discretion of the business entity (i.e., vendors or healthcare organizations). IHE focuses on the use cases and associated functional requirements that are specified in the Technical Frameworks. The HL7 EHR-S functional model [16] provides a framework and has provided requirements at a high level with the expectation that the requirements will be further defined. For example, terms such as manage or integrate are used without specifying the details about what elements or how the elements are to be managed or integrated. The high-level requirement may be to integrate lab results in the EHR-S; refinement of that requirement is necessary to define precisely what elements comprise a lab result (i.e., explicit data elements) and how these elements are to be persisted and used. The HL7 EHR-S functional model can be profiled to create detailed requirements. The Laboratory Functional Requirements implementation guide [13] is an example. This implementation guide initiative was prompted by the high-level ONC 2014 Edition certification criterion for incorporate laboratory results that provided little insight on what exactly constituted a laboratory result (which message elements) and what data had to be incorporated and displayed. NIST, working with subject matter experts, had to determine the requirements (which never should be the role of the test tool builders and Testers).

Interoperability specifications shouldn't be created in a vacuum; however, these specifications often are created in this manner. A best practice is to obtain the business requirements that drive the application functional requirements. Interoperability specifications can be developed then. The associated functional requirements are necessary to link the data being communicated with their intended business use. It is preferable to separate interface and functional requirements, because either can exist independently. For example, for a given functional requirements specification, two or more protocols may be applicable (e.g., HL7 v2 and NCPDP SCRIPT for prescriptions). Unfortunately, many interoperable specifications are created without functional requirement standards (or even guidelines).

Functional testing typically involves the use of scenarios to help determine whether the system can perform the function as intended. Various workflows can be developed from the bottom up to create elaborate end-to-end business processes. The methods described in this chapter for testing sending and receiving applications can be employed.

11.10.4 Data Quality Testing

Data exchange standards enable exchange of data in a structured way and provide limited assurance of correct content for use in real world settings. Conformance testing is bound by the requirements stipulated in a specification. Data quality analysis reaches beyond the requirements typically found in data exchange standards and bleeds into the functional requirements of the application.[30] Data quality checks that result in error may trigger application level error acknowledgements in messaging environment (because a business rule was violated). In other environments, other error notifications may be reported.

There are data dependencies that typically are not described in the data exchange specification but are relevant in the clinical setting. For example, data elements A, B, and C may all be required and the interoperability specification may prescribe certain constraints on the data; however, these requirements generally focus on the structure, usage, content, and so on, while the content of A, B, and C as a group may be very important for a given use. Such data dependency requirements are

[30]This is a grey area, and it is not always clear where the delineation should occur. Often such requirements do belong not in the interoperability specification but in functional requirement guides or defined as business rules. Where such requirements are defined is not of concern; that such requirements are specified and tested is important.

likely outside the scope of the interoperability specification, but they are important from the application perspective. This case is one type of a data quality issue.

An example of this issue in the immunization domain is when an immunization history is reported, and the vaccine administration date is prior to the date that vaccine was made available. A similar vaccine may have been the actual vaccine administered, but the system is not able to transmit a message containing an inactive (historical) vaccine. Another example is the pairing of the vaccine manufacturer and a specific vaccine lot number. These instances illustrate typical data quality issues related to immunization messaging implementations. Data quality testing focuses on this type of content testing that extends the requirements typically found in the interoperability specifications. The interoperability specification only cares that a valid vaccine code and a valid date are messaged for these elements. Data quality checks verify that the related content pairs are valid. Interoperability specifications have data element dependency requirements, but these specifications typically are focused on data consistency. For example, if an observation is of type Numeric, then the associated Unit of Measure is required. If the observation is of type String, then the Unit of Measure is not required. Data quality testing is generally more applicable for site installation testing of production systems.

An example of a data quality tool is the Immunization Data Quality Assurance (DQA) Tool [17]. This tool has been used to assess data transmitted to immunization registries. Providers and registries can retrieve and view summaries on a number of data quality issues, including support for immunization core elements. The results generated by the tool can be used by registries to alert providers about data quality issues.

11.10.5 Usability Testing

Usability testing is performed to evaluate an application from the human factor perspective. Metrics include how easy the software is to use in terms of navigation, layout, and speed. Other factors include how intuitive the software is and how closely the application relates to the workflow it is intended to support. Usability testing should help determine if the software supports the workflow or changes the workflow. Key components of usability testing (as described by [18]) include the following:

1. **Learnability:** How easy is it for users to accomplish basic tasks the first time they encounter the design?
2. **Efficiency:** How fast can experienced users accomplish tasks?
3. **Memorability:** When users return to the design after a period of not using it, does the user remember enough to use it effectively the next time, or does the user have to start over again learning everything?

4. **Errors:** How many errors do users make, how severe are these errors and how easily can they recover from the errors?
5. **Satisfaction:** How much does the user like using the system?

The end goal of usability testing is to ensure that the software provides the intended services in an easy to use and intuitive manner. Even if all of the requirements are met from a functional perspective, users must be able to access and apply the services in a way that best accomplishes the business objectives of the workflow.

The National Institute of Standards and Technology (NIST) Information Access Division has developed an EHR Usability Protocol (EUP) that establishes procedures for evaluating an EHR user interface from clinical and human factor's best practices perspectives. The validation focuses on studies of user interfaces with representative user groups performing realistic tasks. This work is documented in the publication "*Technical Evaluation, Testing and Validation of the Usability of Electronic Health Records*" [19]. This study provides an overview of usability testing and the EUP, and includes check lists for conducting usability tests of EHR user interfaces.

11.10.6 Load Testing

In the context of distributed applications communicating via interfaces, load testing is performed to determine if an interface (application) can process a large quantity of messages in a given timeframe. The process subjects the interface to a large volume of messaging traffic to establish the limits at which the system performance is significantly degraded or fails. The Tester seeks to simulate, typically in controlled lab conditions, real-world loads for a targeted application. Load testing can reveal the system's operating capability bandwidth and uncover bottlenecks.

11.11 Summary

The focus of this chapter is to provide an overview of the basic principles of conformance testing and related topics, such as interoperability testing. Conformance testing is an essential action for the successful interoperation of distributed systems. It is important that conformance testing is an explicit part of the standards development life cycle. Many benefits are garnered by including conformance testing in this activity, and clarification of the requirements specification is at the top of the list. The most effective conformance testing is conducted using a well-designed and organized process. We have presented one such approach.

Conformance testing is not an overly challenging technical discipline; however, it is an activity that must be performed with a great deal of diligence, discipline, precision, and completeness. Unfortunately, conformance testing is often overlooked, and the importance of it is not always recognized. We hope our readers will internalize the concept that conformance testing is crucial to the success of system interoperability.

The impact of conformance testing is contingent on the quality of the specification, that is, how well the requirements are written. Requirements are the key; they must be clear and unambiguous, not only for the benefit of conformance testing but also for implementers. The goal is to reduce the number of ways implementers can interpret a requirement. To improve requirement specifications, conformance constructs must be used and conformance testing needs to be built into the process of standards development. Ideally, conformance tests and test artifacts are developed as the standard is being developed. This process forces an interpretation of the requirement in a concrete manner. If a test can be written to support the requirement, then it is safe to say that the requirement is clear and unambiguous. Unfortunately, conformance testing often is not part of the standards development process, even though standards that are developed in association with conformance testing or pilot tests are much more likely to achieve greater success than standards that are not.

Conformance testing is aided by a well-designed and organized Test Plan. The Test Plan is composed of many parts, each of which describes in detail how to specify, manage, and organize the approach for testing a system. A Test Plan is part of the Test Suite that provides all of the necessary components and instructions to the Tester to carry out the testing.

When testing distributed applications, two perspectives need to be considered: testing the sending application and testing the receiving application. Each aspect has approaches that promote effective testing. There are two modes for testing the sending application: context-free and context-based. Context-free testing validates any message created by the SUT and is not dependent on any use case instance, Test Case, or specific test data content. The context-based mode validates messages that are associated with a given use case instance and a Test Case that includes specific test data. Context-based validation expands the test space, enabling more comprehensive testing. Testing of the receiving applications may be accomplished via a number of testing approaches, and using a combination of two or more of the approaches is most effective. In all cases, use of inspection testing is a key step in evaluating a receiving application.

Conformance testing can be conducted at many levels. It is important to have a strategy when developing the tests in order for as many requirements to be tested as possible using the minimum number of tests. Often, the quantity of testing is subject to time and resources, so testing must be performed efficiently. The tools presented in this chapter, such as traceability matrixes and strategies for creating effective test cases, help in this endeavor. Keep in mind that conformance can't be proven; only non-conformance can be detected. Conformance testing provides just a degree of certainty, and this level of certainty is based on the quality and quantity of the tests performed. Careful consideration is imperative, therefore, when planning and developing the test strategy and plan.

References

1. Gebase L, Snelick R. Testing Environments for Assessing Conformance and Interoperability. 2010 Software Engineering Research and Practice (SERP10), WORLDCOMP'10 July 12-15, 2010, Las Vegas, NV.
2. Monkewich O: Tutorial on Conformance and Interoperability Testing. International Telecommunication Union (ITU), December 8th, 2006.
3. Hogan MD, Fang Liu, Sokol AW, Tong Jin. NIST-SP 500-291, NIST Cloud Computing Standards Roadmap. August 10, 2011; http://www.nist.gov/manuscript-publication-search.cfm?pub_id=909024
4. HL7 Version 2.5.1 Implementation Guide: S&I Framework Lab Results Interface interoperability standards (DSTU), July 2012; http://www.hl7.org
5. National Institute of Standards and Technology (NIST): Lab Results Interface (LRI) DSTU Release 1 HL7 v2 Conformance Test Tool. http://hl7v2-lab-testing.nist.gov
6. National Institute of Standards and Technology (NIST): Immunization *Messaging*, Release 1.4 HL7 v2 Conformance Test Tool ONC 2014 Edition Certification Testing. http://hl7v2-iz-testing.nist.gov
7. National Institute of Standards and Technology (NIST): Immunization *Messaging*, Release 1.5 HL7 v2 Conformance Test Tool. ONC 2015 Edition Certification Testing http://hl7v2-iz-r1.5-testing.nist.gov
8. National Institute of Standards and Technology (NIST): PHIN Messaging Guide For Syndromic Surveillance: Emergency Department and urgent Care Data HL7 v2 Conformance Test Tool. Contact: rsnelick@nist.gov; http://hl7v2-ss-testing.nist.gov
9. National Institute of Standards and Technology (NIST): *Electronic Lab Reporting* (ELR), Release 1 HL7 v2 Conformance Test Tool. http://hl7v2-elr-testing.nist.gov
10. Meaningful Use Immunization On-Boarding Instructions; State of Arkansas. http://www.healthy.arkansas.gov/programsServices/MeaningfulUse/Documents/ImmunizationOn-BoardingInstructions.pdf
11. HL7 Version 2.5.1. Implementation Guide for Immunization Messaging. March 2014. http://www.cdc.gov/vaccines/programs/iis/technical-guidance/downloads/hl7guide-1-5-Mar2014.pdf
12. National Institute of Standards and Technology (NIST): Meaningful Use Stage 2, 2014 Edition, Approved Test Procedures http://healthcare.nist.gov/
13. HL7 EHR-S Functional Requirements: S&I Framework Laboratory Results Messages, Release 1, US Realm Draft Standard for Trial Use March 2016; http://hl7.org
14. Smoke Testing (Software) https://en.wikipedia.org/wiki/Smoke_testing_(software)
15. DIN ISO 7498. Informationsverarbeitung Kommunikation Offener Systeme, Basis-Referenzmodell. DIN EN ISO 7498-1 ISO/OSI-Modell, Beuth Verlag, 1982
16. HL7 EHR-S Functional Model Specification. http://www.hl7.org
17. Bunker N. Data Quality Assurance (DQA) Test tool for Immunization. https://openimmunizationsoftware.net/dataQuality/dataQuality.html
18. ISTQB Exam Certification. http://istqbexamcertification.com/what-is-usability-testing-in-software-and-its-benifits-to-end-user/
19. Lowry SZ, Quinn MT, Mala Ramaiah, et al. Technical Evaluation, Testing and Validation of the Usability of Electronic Health Records. February 12th, 2012. NIST Interagency/Internal Report (NISTIR) – 7804
20. HL7 Version 2.5.1 Implementation Guide: Electronic Laboratory Reporting to Public Health, Release 1 (US Realm); February 2010. http://www.hl7.org

21. Test Procedure for §170.314(b)(5)(A) Incorporate laboratory tests and values/results. http://www.healthit.gov/sites/default/files/170.314b5aincorporatelabtests_2014_tp_approved_v1.4_onc.pdf
22. Test Procedure for §170.314(f)(4) Inpatient setting only – transmission of reportable laboratory tests and values/results. http://www.healthit.gov/sites/default/files/170.314f4transmissionreportablelabs_tp_2014_approved_v1.3.pdf

Chapter 12
Conformity Assessment

12.1 Overview

The preceding chapters, especially Chap. 5, describe conformance constructs used in message profiles or document types. Chapter 7 describes in detail the different relationship among profiles. This chapter seeks to clarify the use of the conformance constructs by providing a context in which the requirements can be assessed. An example conformity assessment is presented for the usage, cardinality, and vocabulary conformance constructs. The example takes into consideration both the possible states of data-presence with regard to the specific attribute each conformance construct addresses as well as the conditional outcomes (if applicable). The result is a set of truth tables that will aid readers in interpreting the meaning of the conformance constructs. Similar assessments can be performed for the other constructs. The information provided in this chapter can serve as a guide when conducting conformance testing.

The conformance constructs are evaluated with regard to their roles in a sending or receiving application as they would appear in a referenced constrainable profile, which is illustrated in Fig. 12.1 (marked by the red arrows).

The conformity assessment tables in this chapter include a representative set of conformance constructs taken from the HL7 v2.7.1 [1] conformance model. As mentioned previously, although the various standards represent and define conformance constructs differently, the underlying concepts are the same; therefore, the analysis presented in this chapter is applicable to other standards as long as the appropriate translation of the concepts as defined in the standard of interest is used. Additionally, this chapter focuses on message processing, but the assessment tables apply equally as well to documents.

The conformity assessment tables presented in this chapter can be used as the logic behind implementation of conformance testing tools. As described in Chap. 11, the NIST HL7 v2.x test tools developed for the ONC Health IT

F. Oemig and R. Snelick, *Healthcare Interoperability Standards Compliance Handbook*, DOI 10.1007/978-3-319-44839-8_12

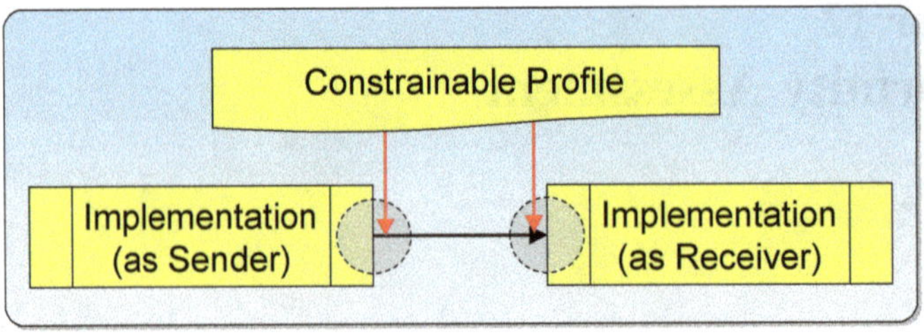

Fig. 12.1 Assessment for sender/receiver applications

Certification Program employed context-free and context-based testing for assessing sender implementations. These tools implement the logic given here.

In many cases, determining if the observed outcome or behavior of a system is "conformant" or "non-conformant" is a straight-forward process. In other words, the observed result is deterministic. A good example of a deterministic result is the presence of a given element for a sending application. If this element SHALL be present according to the referenced profile, and if this element IS present in the created instance, then the element is deemed "conformant". If the element is absent, then the element is deemed "non-conformant". This determination is easy to make for a sending application, because the expectation is that the provided data is sent according to the requirement of the conformance construct, as is described in the tables to follow.

On the receiving side, this determination is much harder to make and is not always clear. The requirements for the consumption of the data from an instance are not always specified or specific. Some conformance constructs are easy to interpret and realize, such as the use (processing) of a required element. If an application must (SHALL) process an element, some evidence of whether this capability is supported or not will be observable in this application.[1] In many situations, the data for this element will be displayed in some way to the user; but other mechanisms also can be used to find evidence that the application has executed the required operation for this element, e.g., storing it in a record, exporting it to another system, or some other observable processing.

Other conformance constructs are intentionally defined using a range, e.g., cardinality. This range is interpreted as a specific capability that is expected of an application. Consider the cardinality example of "0..n" which represents a requirement to receive and process up to "n" elements, but it does not imply that the application WILL always receive and process "n" elements (because "n" elements may not be sent). In most cases, the user has an expectation of what the system should—and most probably will—do with the data it receives. For example, if the receiver is sent "n" or fewer instances, the expectation is that these instances will be

[1]At least for consequential data elements.

"processed"; however, this "processing" expectation typically is neither documented nor manifested precisely in a specification. In other words, the particular specification may not formulate the expected behavior precisely enough in the form of requirements. For most assessments, clear guidance regarding "conformance" versus "non-conformance" can be found, but, in the absent of specific requirements, some cases will produce, and must be declared as having, "Non-deterministic" results. One such case arises when ">n" instances is sent; without a clear indication of specific requirements, what behavior must the receiver demonstrate in order to be considered conformant? For example, should the receiving system stop processing after "n" elements or process every element in order to select the most *suitable* "n" elements.

An important point to note in the assessment tables that follow is that a determination of conformance and non-conformance is being made for observations created under controlled circumstances and based on the requirements of the conformance constructs. The controlled elements are the availability of the indicated data, the requirements for the conformance constructs, the expected outcomes, and the presumed observable outcomes. In the case of a non-conformity, no guidance is provided as to what the remedy or remediation should be, because this action is determined by the application and is dependent on the severity of the non-conformity issue as it applies to the use case.

Additionally, the analysis provided in the assessment tables is predicated on the conformance requirements as defined in HL7 v2.7.1 Chap. 2B (Conformance) [1]. This version contains the latest definitions. One exception is that of the vocabulary; this analysis follows the generalized vocabulary definitions and requirements expressed in Chaps. 5 and 7. This chapter provides one set of assessment tables for the Usage, Cardinality, and Vocabulary conformance constructs. The other constructs have been omitted. Additionally, only one view (mostly following HL7 v2) is given. This assessment is representative only, and it does not follow that the conformance constructs in other standards are the same as those shown in the examples, although, in many instances they are the same. The purpose here is to provide an approach for conducting an assessment and to give a perspective on the meaning and impact the conformance constructs have on implementations (and how they may be tested). These assessment tables are necessary to create meaningful conformance validation tools.

This assessment is also predicated on the condition that the implementer has made a claim of conformance to a specification. Additionally, the claim must be assessed from a purely unbiased basis, that is, does the implementation meet the stated requirement? It does not matter how significant or insignificant a requirement is thought to be.

12.2 Processing Aspects (for Receiving Applications)

This chapter provides assessments for the different conformance constructs with regard to conformant behavior for processing (or not) of such an element. As mentioned earlier, in some cases the observed behavior does not match the expectations. This chapter does not prescribe how a system should behave in cases where a violation is detected. In some cases, it is absolutely necessary for an exception to be generated, which may be true for a missing required element if the value of this element is a precondition for proceeding to process the data. In other cases, simple warnings could be helpful to identify possible problems, or the system may behave agnostically to the absence an element. For example, how is a forbidden element handled when it is present? If this element conveys sensitive data, then an error may be indicated. In other cases, the sender may transmit more data than are needed to a set of different receivers to cover a set of different use cases while a specific receiver is not yet capable of managing every element. The demographic data broadcasting in HL7 v2 ADT messaging is one example of this approach (see Chap. 7). In this case, no error or warning should be raised; but, again, this behavior is tied to the actions a receiver might take in reaction to a non-conformity, and it does not change the fact that a non-conformity exists. A receiver application needs to recognize that non-conformity and react appropriately based on its functional requirements, whether the reaction is agreed upon with the sending application or independently established.

The remainder of this chapter does not address the appropriate reaction of an application to non-conformities; it concentrates only on whether the observed processing, when compared to the expected behavior, can be deemed "conformant" or not.

12.3 Usage/Optionality

The first set of assessments examine the usage/optionality declarations for "R-Required", "RE-Required but may be Empty", and "X-Forbidden" as taken from HL7 v2.x product family (specifically the definitions in HL7 v2.7.1). "Optional" is not considered, because, as mentioned in the previous chapters, this declaration is a placeholder that is to be replaced ultimately with an R, RE, or X usage. Without such a declaration, the "Optional" usage indicator is not testable directly. It is often the case, however, that test tools will test implementations (where optional usage does not exist) with requirements obtained from a constrainable (e.g., National Level) profile. In such cases, the assessment is non-deterministic at a discrete level. How conditional usage is handled is addressed later.

12.3.1 Sender Usage Conformity Assessments

The following tables present the truth tables that provide the expectation of sending applications for implementation of the usage conformance construct. The following information provides an explanation of the heading columns.

Usage indicator: Usage that is declared in the conformance profile for the element.

Test data provided: Indicates whether or not data were provided for this element in the test data set.

Conformity assessment indicator: Indicates the valid (expected) result the sender should provide when populating the message element.

Actual data sent: Indicates the possible (real) result, i.e., whether or not the sender populated the element with a value.

Conformity assessment: Indicates the result of the conformity assessment.

Comments: Provides additional insight about the assessment.

As an example, the first entry in Table 12.1 can be interpreted as: The sender profile specified the element usage as required (R). Data are available to the sender; therefore, the requirement for the sender is to populate the element (i.e., the element shall be present in the message). If the data are present for the element, then the application is conformant with respect to the element usage. If the data are not-present for the element, then the application is not conformant with respect to usage of the element.

A similar analysis applies to the required, but may be empty (RE) usage (Table 12.2). A source of much confusion for participants in the ONC Health IT Certification Program was the validation of elements with RE usage. A surprisingly large number of implementers and users interpreted this construct to mean optional. The context-based testing approach specifically addressed testing of elements with RE usage. Test cases were developed that provided data for these elements, meaning that, in terms of the conformity assessment, they are equivalent to that of required elements. The truth tables presented here demonstrate this analysis.

The "No message part sent" could result in the entire message not being sent. The message part is referring to a coherent group of data, for example, a message containing three sets of laboratory results in the form of three segment groups. If one of the required elements in one of the segment groups is unable to be satisfied, then the remaining message part should be sent and be considered conformant. If there is only one segment group, however, and data are missing, that makes the group, and therefore the message, nonsensical, then the entire message should not be sent in order to be considered conformant.

Conformance assessment for elements with conditional usage (i.e., C(a/b) is dependent on the result of the condition predicate). For example, if conditional usage for an element is specified as C(R/X) and the result of the condition

Table 12.1 Conformity assessment of the required usage code for sending applications

Usage indicator	Test data provided	Conformity assessment indicator	Actual data sent	Conformity assessment	Comments
R	Valued	Present	Present	Conformant	Affirmative
			Not-present	Non-conformant	Application does not send the required element when a value is provided
R	Not-valued	None—expected behavior is that no message part is sent	Present	Non-conformant	Application sends a value even though it does not have a valid value to send[a]
			Not-present	Non-conformant	Application sends a message with a required element not populated.
			No message part sent	Conformant	Application correctly detects that it does not have data for a required value and doesn't send the message part. See note below table.

[a]Such "negative" testing is necessary. For example, an application may incorrectly populate an element with a default value

evaluation is true, then the usage for the element is R and the conformity assessment table for R-required applies (Table 12.1). Likewise, when the result of the condition evaluation is false, then the usage for the element is X and the conformity assessment table for X-not supported applies (Table 12.3).

When testing elements with conditional usage, both the true and false scenarios need to be examined. The conformity assessment table below (Table 12.4) shows an example for the case C(R/X) for a sending application. Note that when the condition evaluates to true, the assessment is the same as the R-required assessment table (Table 12.1); and when the condition evaluates to false, the assessment is the same as the X-not supported (Table 12.3). Similar tables can be built for all other combinations, such as C(R/RE) and C(RE/X).

Some standards (e.g., HL7 v2.5) define conditional usage indicators explicitly and have pre-defined true and false outcomes, e.g., C and CE. These indicators resolve to C(R/X) and C(RE/X). More recent versions of HL7 v2.x (2.7.1 and later) replaced[2] the explicit conditional usage indicators with a generic construct C(a/b) where a and b can be a non-conditional (i.e., R, RE, O, or X) usage indicator [1 Chap. 2B]. Regardless of the conformance construct defined by the conditional usage indicator, the conformity assessment is based on the usage indicator to which

[2]In the constraint model defined in the conformance chapter (i.e., not the base standard).

Table 12.2 Conformity assessment of the required but may be empty usage code for sending applications[a]

Usage indicator	Test data provided	Conformity assessment indicator	Actual data sent	Conformity assessment	Comments
RE	Valued	Present	Present	Conformant	
			Not-present	Non-conformant	Application does not send the required element when a value is provided
RE	Not-valued	Not-present	Present	Non-conformant	Application sends a value even though it does not have a valid value to send[b]
			Not-present	Conformant	Application sends a message without the element populated

[a]There are multiple interpretations of "RE" when a value is known. One is "the capability must always be supported and a value is sent if known", the other is "the capability must always be supported and a value may or may not be sent even when known based on a condition external to the profile specification. The condition may be noted in the profile but cannot be processed automatically". This is what can be interpreted from the "relevant" part of the definition. Regardless of the interpretation, for the permutations presented here, external conditions that may affect a value being sent or not are eliminated from consideration. Test cases can be developed such that these situations won't exist. For example, a common example of when an element may not be sent is when a patient doesn't authorize it to be sent; in this scenario, the patient having authorized consent is a pre-condition in the test case (Another—and preferred—option is to define separate profiles for the different contents.). Regardless of the interpretation the "RE" usage code, a set of test circumstances can be developed to sufficiently test the "RE" element. That is, the external condition can't always prevent an element from being sent, otherwise it is not a condition. Hence, "RE" elements can in fact be fully tested in the manner described.

[b]Such "negative" testing is necessary. For example, an application may incorrectly populate an element with a default value.

the predicate resolves. This key point is depicted in the example in Table 12.4. Since all such conditional usage analysis tables can be derived, no further assessment tables are provided.

12.3.2 Receiver Usage Conformity Assessment

The following tables present the truth tables that provide the expectation of receiving applications for implementation of the usage conformance construct. Below are explanations of the heading columns.

Usage Indicator: Usage declared in the conformance profile for the element.

Test Data Sent: Indicates whether or not the element was populated in the test message.

Table 12.3 Conformity assessment of not-supported usage code for sending applications

Usage indicator	Test data provided	Conformity assessment indicator	Actual data sent	Conformity assessment	Comments
X	Valued	Not-present	Present	Non-conformant	Non-conformant because value was sent for a not-supported or forbidden element
			Not-present	Conformant	Test case results confirm correct usage of X element by providing data and the application did not send value
X	Not-valued	Not-present	Present	Non-conformant	Non-conformant because value was sent for a not-supported element
			Not-present	Conformant	Confirms expected behavior

Conformity Assessment Indicator: Indicates how the receiver should respond to the test message with regard to an element.

Receiver Action: Indicates what action the receiver took in response to the test message.

Conformity Assessment: Indicates the result of the conformity assessment.

Comments: Provides additional insight about the assessment.

As an example, the first row in Table 12.5 can be interpreted as: The receiver profile has specified an element usage as required (R). A test message is created in which the element is populated with a value. The requirement for the receiver is to process the element. If the receiver processed the element, then the application is conformant with respect to the element usage. If the application did not process the element, then the application is not conformant with respect to the element usage. Tables 12.5 (R), 12.6 (RE), and 12.7 (X) provide the conformity assessment tables for usage for receiving applications.

It is a common belief among implementers and users of data exchange standards that required elements can be ignored at the discretion of the receiver.[3] In terms of conformance, this behavior is not correct. The authors hope that, throughout this book, sufficient mechanisms have been provided—specifically, the profiling

[3]A required data element is defined as required because of its importance for a specific use case. Otherwise it would be sufficient to mark such an element as "required but may be empty". Therefore, if such an element is missing it should always lead to an appropriate exception.

Table 12.4 Example conformity assessment of conditional usage code C(R/X) for sending applications

Usage indicator	Test data provided	Condition predicate result	Conformity assessment indicator	Actual data sent	Conformity assessment	Comments
C(R/X)	Valued	True (R)[a]	Present	Present	Conformant	
				Not-present	Non-conformant	Application does not send the required element when a value is provided
C(R/X)	Not-valued	True (R)	None—expected behavior is that no message is sent	Present	Non-conformant	Application sends a value even though it does not have a valid value to send[b]
				Not-present	Non-conformant	Application sends a message with a required element not populated
				No message sent	Conformant	Application correctly detects that it doesn't have data for a required value and doesn't send the message
C(R/X)	Valued	False (X)	Not-present	Present	Non-conformant	Non-conformant because value was sent for a not-supported element
				Not-present	Conformant	Test case results confirm correct usage of X element by providing data and the application did not send value
C(R/X)	Not-valued	False (X)	Not-present	Present	Non-conformant	Non-conformant because value was sent for a not-supported element. Value sent when condition is false and no value provided
				Not-present	Conformant	Confirms expected behavior

[a]The notation of (R) and (X) as indicated here represents the equivalent presence indicator as the result of the condition predicate. For example, if the condition predicate is true, then the same analysis as a "Required" element is given
[b]Such "negative" testing is necessary. For example, an application may incorrectly populate an element with a default value

Table 12.5 Conformity assessment of the required usage code for receiving applications

<table>
<tr><th>Usage indicator</th><th>Test data sent</th><th>Conformity assessment indicator</th><th>Receiver action</th><th>Conformity assessment</th><th>Comments</th></tr>
<tr><td rowspan="2">R</td><td rowspan="2">Valued</td><td rowspan="2">Process element</td><td>Processed</td><td>Conformant</td><td></td></tr>
<tr><td>Not-processed</td><td>Non-conformant</td><td>Application does not process the required element received</td></tr>
<tr><td rowspan="2">R</td><td rowspan="2">Not-valued</td><td rowspan="2">Raise exception</td><td>Processed or not-processed; application raises an exception</td><td>Conformant</td><td rowspan="2">The application shall raise an exception when a required element is not sent. The application makes a determination of what parts of the message, if any, are processed (see the text below this table for elaboration on this analysis) In all cases the application should acknowledge the non-conformity</td></tr>
<tr><td>Processed or not processed; no exception raised</td><td>Non-conformant</td></tr>
</table>

Table 12.6 Conformity assessment of the required but may be empty usage code for receiving applications

<table>
<tr><th>Usage indicator</th><th>Test data sent</th><th>Conformity assessment indicator</th><th>Receiver action</th><th>Conformity assessment</th><th>Comments</th></tr>
<tr><td rowspan="2">RE</td><td rowspan="2">Valued</td><td rowspan="2">Process element</td><td>Processed</td><td>Conformant</td><td>Affirmative test result</td></tr>
<tr><td>Not-processed</td><td>Non-conformant</td><td>Application does not process the required element received</td></tr>
<tr><td rowspan="2">RE</td><td rowspan="2">Not-valued</td><td rowspan="2">Process message</td><td>Not-processed and/or the application raises an exception</td><td>Non-conformant</td><td>Application should process the message when this element is omitted. In this case the application did not process the message and/or raised an exception</td></tr>
<tr><td>Processed; application does not raise an exception</td><td>Conformant</td><td>Application processes the message</td></tr>
</table>

concepts—to enable interfaces to be defined precisely such that the requirements and responsibilities are clearly specified, and, perhaps, to be defined for senders and receivers separately. If such requirements are not part of a use case, then they should not be included in the form of required elements.

Table 12.7 Conformity assessment of not-supported usage code for receiving applications

Usage indicator	Test data sent	Conformity assessment indicator	Receiver action	Conformity assessment	Comments
X	Valued	Don't process the element[a]; raise exception	Element processed	Non-conformant	Non-conformant because data were processed for a not-supported element; correct behavior is to not process the element[b]
			Element not-processed	Conformant	Application did not process not-supported element
X	Not-valued	Process message	Application raises an error	Non-conformant	Application should process the message without raising an exception
			Processed	Conformant	Confirms expected behavior

[a]*Note* stricter conformance may apply based on business rules associated with the element. For example, the trading partner's conformance agreement may have included a privacy requirement that forbids sending the patient name for this application. The sender sent the patient name in error. If it is strictly prohibited in this agreement to send the patient name, the receiver should reject the message, and then raise an exception to notify the sender of the error and that the message was not processed. In circumstances where business rules are indifferent for this element, the receiver can choose to ignore the data with or without raising an exception. In either case, the receiver shall not process the information. It is important to recognize that, for a receiver not-supported element, there is no way to distinguish between a strict "shall not receive" and "indifference" within the framework of the message profile. Documented business rules are necessary, and lack of them prevents straight forward analysis and processing

[b]It is often the case in practice that when this situation occurs it turns out to be an error in the interface documentation. This assessment is based on what is documented

That being said, a determination of when a receiver should out-right reject, partially process, or completely process a message should be defined in a separate functional requirements document (or local business rules if non-existent).

An important point here is that non-conformance should not necessarily prevent data-exchange of usable data. Although an in-bound message may be missing required data according to the specification, the decision to process the message or partially process the message must be determined by local business rules or functional requirements.

A number of factors come into play for making this determination. The importance of a missing element and relevance with respect to the entire message content are two significant considerations. In the immunizations domain, for example, more than one immunization record can be sent in the same message. A particular immunization record may be missing the vaccine code, which is an essential element for identifying the vaccine administered, however, other immunization records in the message are complete. An appropriate behavior might be to record the valid records and return an acknowledgement with an error for the record with the missing vaccine code. Using this approach, even though the message is non-conformant, useful information is communicated. Conformance is not necessarily the strict determinant of data exchange. In fact, a large percentage of working interfaces are likely non-conformant. This fact, however, in no way means that non-conformant interfaces are considered (purposely) acceptable practice, and one goal of this book is to reduce the incidence of such interfaces. Knowledge of non-conformities in a message is valuable information that can be acted on. The goal of conformance testing is to detect such faulty implementations, and applications should be prevented from creating a message in which this essential information is missing (e.g., regarding a missing vaccine code, the application could be designed to require the selection of a vaccine at the user interface level to support the process of documenting immunization administration).

As another example, a number of immunization records can be sent in a message in which the patient name is missing. Under this circumstance, the appropriate behavior of an Immunization Information System can be to reject the entire message, since this information is essential for processing and linking the patient records. Such requirements may be described by local business rules or realm-specific functional requirements. This situation describes one where non-conformance is fatal to the transaction.

On the other end of the spectrum is the case where a completely inconsequential element is omitted (e.g., in HL7 v2.x Set ID for the PID segment in which the PID segment is required and constrained to one in an implementation guide). In this case, the appropriate behavior is to process the entire message and possibly respond with a warning that alerts the sender of the non-conformity. Even though the message is technically non-conformant (and a conformance test will issue an error), it should not prevent the exchange of useful information.

Having said all this, the overall obligation is to ensure that an element that is marked as required in the referenced (constrainable) profile is present in a message and that it is processed by the receiver. Whether this element is *correctly* marked as required is out of scope for this discussion, and whether an element must be required for the sender AND receiver is debatable as well; but if an element is designated as required, this requirement has an impact on the receiving application.

A reasonable distinction also must be made between a (implementable) profile that documents an interface for a receiving application and a profile defined at the constrainable (e.g., national level), as is shown in Fig. 12.2. If the interface for the receiving application is not conformant against an implementer's own local (implementable) profile, then an update to either the implementation or documentation is necessary because one or the other (or both) is incorrect. Most likely the

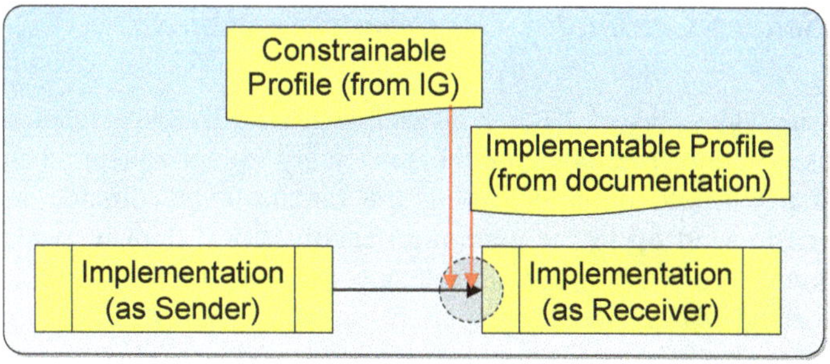

Fig. 12.2 Assessment for receiver applications on required elements

implementation, i.e., the interface, operates as intended but the documentation is outdated and does not correctly reflect the interface behavior. In this case, the documentation itself is wrong and is of limited use for evaluating the interface behavior against the higher (national) level requirements (using the interface itself is more appropriate). But if the conformance violation is against the profile on the national level, and, given that the national level profile only declares elements as required if they are absolutely necessary to fulfill the underlying use case, then the interface for the implementation in question is deemed non-conformant to the constrainable profile and is not suitable to fulfill this intended use case.

A discussion that is analogous to raising an exception for a missing required element is a discussion about the presence of a non-supported element. From a conformance perspective, the element shall not be present in the message, and the receiver is obligated to inform the sender ("the contract has been broken"). The severity can range from inconsequential to requiring rejection of the message. An example in which rejection of the message would be appropriate is when patient identification information is sent to a public health agency along with an HIV laboratory result.

Careful consideration should be given regarding prohibiting elements in national level specifications in view of the impact on conformance.

12.4 Cardinality

Cardinality defines the minimum and maximum number of occurrences that must be supported for an element and, therefore, identifies the allowable range for an element to occur in a message instance. Conformity assessment is determined by creating the possible combinations of cardinality specification, and then exercising each combination with various test data realizations. This analysis is provided for both sending and receiving applications.

12.4.1 Sender Cardinality Conformity Assessment

The following tables present the truth tables that provide the expectation of sending applications for implementation of the cardinality conformance construct. **The analysis is predicated on interpreting the maximum cardinality as a strict requirement to send up to the maximum cardinality if data is available.** This interpretation is a common and reasonable one, but it is not always explicitly stated as such in standards (and is not explicitly stated in HL7 v2.x, on which these assessments are based).

The following information provides an explanation of the heading columns.

Card.: Cardinality declared in the conformance profile for the element. Also, the usage associated with the cardinality is indicated (e.g., (X)).

Test data provided: Indicates the number of instances provided for this element (or in general whether the element is valued or not) in the test data set.

Conformity assessment indicator: Indicates the valid action the sender should take when populating the message element.

Actual data sent: Indicates the possible behavior, i.e., whether or not the sender populated the element with a value (or values).

Conformity assessment: Indicates the result of the conformity assessment.

Comments: Provides additional insight of the assessment.

As an example, the first entry in Table 12.8 can be interpreted as: The sender profile specified the minimal and maximal cardinality as zero (0). Data are available to the sender for this element; however, the requirement for the sender is to not

Table 12.8 Conformity assessment of cardinality [0..0] for sending applications

Card.	Test data provided	Conformity assessment indicator	Actual data sent	Conformity assessment	Comments
0..0 (X)	Valued	Not present	Present	Non-conformant	Application sends the message with the value(s)
			Not-present	Conformant	Application sends a message without the element populated
0..0 (X)	Not-valued	Not present	Present	Non-conformant	Application sends a value when it is required to be empty. It may be the case where the application incorrectly applies a default value for this element
			Not-present	Conformant	

populate the element (i.e., the element shall be empty in the message). Hence, if the data are present in the message for the element then the application is non-conformant with respect to the element's cardinality. If the data are not-present for the element, then the application is conformant.

The cardinality conformity assessment in Table 12.9 applies to elements with "RE" usage; O-Optional usage elements are not included in the analysis. In all implementations, optional elements are "profiled" to a definitive usage, so for any real implementation such analysis is not applicable. It is often the case, however, that conformance test tools will test to a constrainable (e.g., national level) profile, because this profile is the only one available. Such assessment outcomes for discrete elements are non-deterministic, because the actual requirement is not known at the time of the evaluation, and, therefore, conformance can neither be confirmed or refuted.

Table 12.9 Conformity assessment of cardinality [0..1] for sending applications

Card.	Test data provided	Conformity assessment indicator	Actual data sent	Conformity assessment	Comments
0..1 (RE)	Single value	Single value	Single value present	Conformant	Application sends the message with a value
			Not-present	Non-conformant	Application sends a message without the element populated although it is requested to send it
0..1 (RE)	Multiple values	Single value	One value present	Conformant	Application sends the message with a value. Any value out of this set is fine if there is no additional guidance
			Multiple value present	Non-conformant	Application sends more than one value whereas maximum cardinality is 1
			Not-present	Non-conformant	Application sends a message without the element populated although it is requested to send it
0..1 (RE)	Not-valued	Not present	Present	Non-conformant	Application sends a value when it is required to be empty. It may be the case where the application incorrectly applies a default value for this element
			Not-present	Conformant	

Table 12.10 provides the cardinality conformity assessment when the range is zero to many. For analysis purposes, "n" is considered to be greater than 1. Tables 12.11, 12.12, 12.13, and 12.14 complete the conformity assessment tables for cardinality for sending applications.

Table 12.10 Conformity assessment of cardinality [0..n] for n > 1 for sending applications

Card.	Test data provided	Conformity assessment indicator	Actual data sent	Conformity assessment	Comments
0..n (RE)	Single value	Single value	Single value present	Conformant	Application sends the message with a single value to match data provided
			Not-present	Non-conformant	Application sends a message without the element populated although it is requested to send it
0..n (RE)	Multiple values, but less than or equal to n	Multiple values	One value present	Non-conformant	Application sends the message with a single value populated for this element although it is requested to send all values provided
			Some[a] values present	Non-conformant	Application sends more than one value but not all of the values provided
			All values present	Conformant	
			Not-present	Non-conformant	Application sends a message without the element although all values should be sent
0..n (RE)	Multiple values, but more than n	n values[b]	Single value present	Non-conformant	Application sends the message with a single value although "n" values should be sent
			Some values present	Non-conformant	Application sends the message with more than one value although "n" values should be sent
			n values present	Conformant	The application has selected n values out of the given set
			All values present	Non-conformant	The application sends more than n values whereas maximum cardinality is n
			Not-present	Non-conformant	Application sends a message without the element populated although it is requested to send "n" values
0..n (RE)	Not-valued	Not present	Present	Non-conformant	Application sends a value although the element should stay empty
			Not-present	Conformant	

[a]"Some" in this context means that multiple instances provided (available) are sent, but not all are sent (as indicated by the test data provided)

[b]Guidance as to which subset the sender selects should be provided

Table 12.11 Conformity assessment of cardinality [1..1] for sending applications

Card.	Test data provided	Conformity assessment indicator	Actual data sent	Conformity assessment	Comments
1..1 (R)	Valued	Present	Present	Conformant	
			Not-present	Non-conformant	Application does not send the required element when a value is provided
1..1 (R)	Not-valued	None—expected behavior is that no message part is sent.	Present	Non-conformant	Application sends a value although no value is available to send
			Not present	Non-conformant	
			No message part sent	Conformant	

Table 12.12 Conformity assessment of cardinality one to many for sending applications

Card.	Test data provided	Conformity assessment indicator	Actual data sent	Conformity assessment	Comments
1..n (R)	Single value	Single value	Single value present	Conformant	Application sends the message with a value
			Not-present	Non-conformant	Application sends a message without the element populated although it is requested to send the value
1..n (R)	Multiple values, but less than or equal to n	Multiple values	Single value present	Non-conformant	Application sends the message with a single value although all values provided should be sent
			Some values present	Non-conformant	Application sends more than one value but not all of the values provided
			All values present	Conformant	
			Not-present	Non-conformant	Application sends a message without the element although all values should be sent

(continued)

Table 12.12 (continued)

Card.	Test data provided	Conformity assessment indicator	Actual data sent	Conformity assessment	Comments
1..n (R)	Multiple values, but more than n	n values[a]	One value present	Non-Conformant	Application sends the message with one value although "n" values should be sent
			Some values present	Non-conformant	Application sends the message with more than one value although "n" values should be sent
			n values present	Conformant	The application has selected n values out of the given set
			All values present	Non-conformant	The application sends more than n values whereas maximum cardinality is n
			Not-present	Non-conformant	Application sends a message without the element populated although it is requested to send "n" values
1..n (R)	Not-valued	None—expected behavior is that no message part is sent	Present	Non-conformant	Application sends a value although there is no value to send
			No message part sent	Conformant	

[a]Guidance as to which subset the sender selects should be provided

Table 12.13 Conformity assessment of cardinality many to many (1 < m <= n) for sending applications

Card.	Test data provided	Conformity assessment indicator	Actual data sent	Conformity assessment	Comments
m..n (R)	Single value	None—expected behavior is that no message part is sent	Present	Non-conformant	Application should not send the message because less than "m" values are available to send
			Not-present	Non-conformant	Application should not send the message because less than "m" values are available to send
			No message part sent	Conformant	

(continued)

Table 12.13 (continued)

Card.	Test data provided	Conformity assessment indicator	Actual data sent	Conformity assessment	Comments
m..n (R)	Multiple values, but more than or equal to m and less than or equal to n Call it x where m <=x <=n	Multiple values, x	Single value Present	Non-conformant	Application sends the message with a single value although "x" values should be sent
			Less than m values present	Non-conformant	Application sends less than "m" values although "x" values should be sent
			More than m but not x	Non-conformant	Application sends more than "m" values, but not "x" values ("x" values should be sent)
			x values present	Conformant	
			Not-present	Non-conformant	Application sends a message without the element populated although it is requested to send "x" values
m..n (R)	Multiple values, but more than n	Multiple values, n	One value present	Non-conformant	Application sends the message with a value although n values shall be sent
			m values present	Non-conformant	Application should send n values
			More than m, but less than n values present	Non-conformant	Application should send n values
			n values present[a]	Conformant	The application has selected n values out of the set that is greater than n
			All values present	Non-conformant	The application sends more instances than the number that is allowed to be sent
			Not-present	Non-conformant	Application sends a message without the element populated although it is requested to send the values

(continued)

Table 12.13 (continued)

Card.	Test data provided	Conformity assessment indicator	Actual data sent	Conformity assessment	Comments
m..n (R)	Not-valued	None—expected behavior is that no message part is sent	One or more values present	Non-conformant	Application sends a value when it is required to be empty. It may be the case where the application incorrectly applies a default value for this element
			Element not valued but message part sent	Non-conformant	
			No message part sent	Conformant	Application should not send the message part because not enough values are available to send

[a]Guidance as to which subset the sender selects should be provided

12.4.2 Receiver Cardinality Conformance Assessment

Tables 12.15, 12.16, 12.17, 12.18, 12.19, 12.20, 12.21, and 12.22 present truth tables for assessing cardinality for receiving applications. **The analysis is predicated on interpreting the maximum cardinality as a strict requirement to receive and process up to the maximum cardinality if data is available.** This interpretation is a common and reasonable one, but it is not always explicitly stated as such in standards (and is not explicitly stated in HL7 v2.x in which these assessments are based on).

In the case of cardinality "0..1", the receiver is always responsible for processing this element. At minimum, this responsibility includes scanning the element, evaluating it, and making a decision about what to do with the data. It may happen that, after evaluation, the receiver determines the data are not needed, e.g., the receiver already has the information or cannot use it for some reason (the outcome of this evaluation is out-of-scope for the conformity assessment). The receiver cannot simply ignore the data and be considered conformant.

Another option to consider is for the receiver to announce in some manner the number of elements they can process if the information is taken. In the case of cardinality "0..1", the receiver may only take a single element. At this point no statement is made, whether any single element is checked and processed or whether the first element is taken. It may be that the receiver scans all occurrences and decides to take the 3rd element out of a set of 5. This action may occur if, for example, the receiver is searching for a mobile phone number in the set of contact

Table 12.14 Conformity assessment of cardinality one to unlimited for sending applications

Card.	Test data provided	Conformity assessment indicator	Actual data sent	Conformity assessment	Comments
1..* (R)	Single value	Single value	Present	Conformant	
			Not-present	Non-conformant	Application sends a message without the element populated although it is requested to send the value
1..* (R)	Multiple values	Multiple values	One value present	Non-conformant	Application sends the message with a single value although all values should be sent
			Some values present	Non-conformant	Application sends more than one value, but not all
			All values present	Conformant	
			More than the number of values given	Non-conformant	The application sends more instances than were provided
			Not-present	Non-conformant	Application sends a message without the element populated although it is requested to send the values
1..* (R)	Not-valued	None—expected behavior is that no message part is sent	Present	Non-conformant	Application sends a value when it is required to be empty. It may be the case where the application

(continued)

Table 12.14 (continued)

Card.	Test data provided	Conformity assessment indicator	Actual data sent	Conformity assessment	Comments
					incorrectly applies a default value for this element
			No message part sent	Conformant	Application should not send the message part because not enough values are available to send

data, with the goal of storing the first one that is detected in case a mobile phone number is sent. Vice versa, a cardinality of “0..n” can be interpreted to mean that the receiver will scan multiple occurrences of the data without raising an error.

If there is no guidance for cardinality 0..1 for a given element, then this element shall be processed. From a logical point of view both reactions are acceptable. Taking into account the expectation that data exchange occurs in order to gather new information, one would assume that the processing of this element is the preferred, i.e., desired behavior. This phenomenon is designated as “**non-deterministic**”, because, in principle, the element is allowed to be either processed or not processed.

In the optimal situation, a use case analysis and specific requirements can (and should) be created to indicate the expected behavior. Once this information is known, a deterministic conformity assessment can be performed.

Below are explanations of the heading columns.

Card.: Cardinality declared in the conformance profile for the element.

Test data sent: Indicates whether (how many) or not the element was populated in the test message.

Conformity assessment indicator: Indicates how the receiver should respond to the test message with regards to an element.

Receiver action: Indicates what action the receiver took in response to the test message.

Conformity assessment: Indicates the result of the conformity assessment.

Comments: Provides additional insight into the evaluation scenario.

As an example, the first row in Table 12.15 can be interpreted as: The receiver profile has specified that an element is not-supported (0..0). A test message is

Table 12.15 Conformity assessment of cardinality [0..0] for receiving applications

Card.	Test data sent	Conformity assessment indicator	Receiver action	Conformity assessment	Comments
0..0	Not valued	Process message	Not-processed	Non-conformant	Application should process the message when this element is omitted. In this case the application did not process the message and/or raised an exception
			Processed	Conformant	Application processes the message
0..0	Valued	Don't process the element	Element processed	Non-conformant	Non-conformant because data were processed for a not-supported element; correct behavior is to not process the element
			Not-processed	Conformant	Application does not process the provided element

created with no data for this element. The requirement for the receiver is to process the message (with respect to this element[4]). If the receiver does not process the message, then the receiver is non-conformant. If the receiver processed the message, then the receiver is conformant.

The cardinality of "0..1" does not clearly indicate that a receiver is or is not capable of checking for multiple occurrences (repetitions) of this element in an instance, although this cardinality does indicate the receiver must be capable of storing a single value. Some vendors interpret a cardinality of "0..1" as "no occurrences allowed"; therefore, they do not scan for repetitions (i.e., anything instance beyond the first), and, thus, do not check whether a more "appropriate" element may occur in subsequent repetitions. In other cases, multiple occurrences of an element are interpreted as an error and indicated as such (Table 12.16).

Instances of an element's presence in a message exceeding the specified upper cardinality limit is a conformance violation; however, this violation does not necessarily mean that the data are not to be processed. The receiving system should indicate an exception of some degree based on published functional requirements or local business rules.

[4]The assessment is based on the action of the receiver for the element in the analysis. There may be other reasons why the message is not processed (i.e., non-conformity of other elements).

Table 12.16 Conformity assessment of cardinality [0..1] for receiving applications

Card.	Test data sent	Conformity assessment indicator	Receiver action	Conformity assessment	Comments
0..1	Not valued	Process message	Message processed	Conformant	
			Message not processed	Non-conformant	
0..1	Single value	Process the element	Element processed	Conformant	
			Not-processed	Non-conformant	
0..1	More than 1 value	Process an element	First element processed	Conformant	Without specific requirements, this situation is non-deterministic. The assessment made here is based on common expectation. However, explicit requirements should be documented based on the particular use case analysis
			One element processed, but not the first one	Conformant	
			More than one element processed	Non-conformant	
			Not-processed	Non-conformant	Without specific requirements, this situation is non-deterministic. It is conceivable that a specification could request such processing and therefore this could be conformant

An upper limit for the cardinality normally indicates that the receiving application can only handle a specific number of elements, which raises the question as to how the receiver should handle a message in which more elements than are permitted by the upper limit of the cardinality are sent (Table 12.17). Without having further requirements, which is often the case, the conformity assessment for this circumstance is non-deterministic. What might be a common expectation? One expectation is that the application will handle the first “n” elements while the rest are ignored. Another expectation is that the receiver inspects all instances and makes a determination as to which instances are best to process. A specification should, however, explicitly state what the receiver must do.

Table 12.17 Conformity assessment of cardinality [0..n] for receiving applications

Card.	Test data sent	Conformity assessment indicator	Receiver action	Conformity assessment	Comments
0..n	Not valued	Process message	Message processed	Conformant	
			Message not processed	Non-conformant	
0..n	Single value	Process the element	Element processed	Conformant	
			Element not-processed	Non-conformant	
0..n	Multiple values, but less than or equal to n	Process all elements	One element processed	Non-conformant	
			Some elements processed	Non-conformant	The common expectation is that all of the elements are processed
			All elements processed	Conformant	
			Not-processed	Non-conformant	
0..n	Multiple values, but more than n	Process n elements	First n elements processed	Conformant	The common expectation is that the application processes the first n elements if more than n elements are present. However, other rules may determine which elements are selected
			Any n elements processed	Conformant	
			More than n elements processed	Non-conformant	
			Less than n elements processed	Non-conformant	
			Not-processed	Non-conformant	

Table 12.18 Conformity assessment of cardinality [0..*] for receiving applications

Card.	Test data sent	Conformity assessment indicator	Receiver action	Conformity assessment	Comments
0..*	Not valued	Process message	Message processed	Non-conformant	
			Not processed	Conformant	
0..*	Single value	Process the element	Processed	Conformant	
			Not-processed	Non-conformant	
0..*	Multiple values, with a "high value"	Process all elements	Some elements processed	Non-conformant	
			All elements processed	Conformant	
			Not-processed	Non-conformant	

The unlimited (upper) cardinality means that all occurrences for a data element are to be processed; however, in reality, testing is impossible without limitations, as is creating test messages with endless data (Table 12.18). To overcome these challenges, tests have to be conducted using messages with a very high number of elements. The number of elements should be in the hundreds or thousands, at least, not just a few dozen in order to have a meaningful test of this construct. The decision as to how many elements are needed for a test may differ for various elements. Based on a use case analysis, specifications can create testing limit guidelines for each element with unlimited cardinality (e.g., see [2]).

Note for Table 12.19: Most (if not all) base standards are silent on the expectations under these circumstances (described for the case of "Multiple Values" in Table 12.19). The expectation might be to process the first element, any element, or perhaps no elements. This situation is technically non-deterministic without having further requirements in a derived specification. For the purpose of this analysis, processing the first or any element is considered conformant; however, without specific requirements, a receiver that does not process any element and issues an exception could argue (or claim) to be conformant as well.

Note for Table 12.20: Most (if not all) base standards are silent on the expectations under these circumstances (described for the case of "Multiple values, but more than n" in Table 12.20). The expectation might be to process the first "n" elements, any "n" elements, or perhaps no elements. This situation is technically non-deterministic without having further requirements in a derived specification. For the purpose of this analysis, processing the first "n" elements or any "n" elements is considered conformant; however, without specific requirements a

Table 12.19 Conformity assessment of cardinality [1..1] for receiving applications

Card.	Test data sent	Conformity assessment indicator	Receiver action	Conformity assessment	Comments
1..1	Not valued	Raise exception	Exception raised	Conformant	
			Exception not raised	Non-conformant	The receiver should indicate in some fashion the non-conformity, however, the indication may be informational, a warning, an error, or result in a rejection of the message entirely
1..1	Single value	Process the element	Processed	Conformant	
			Not-processed	Non-conformant	
1..1	Multiple values	Process the first element (**See note for this table**)	First element Processed	Conformant	Technically non-deterministic
			One element processed, but not the first one	Conformant	Technically non-deterministic. The selection of this element may be controlled by business requirements so that this behavior is conformant
			More than one element processed	Non-conformant	
			Not-processed; exception raised	Non-conformant	Technically non-deterministic

receiver that does not process any element and issues an exception could argue (or claim) to be conformant as well.

Note for Table 12.22: Most (if not all) base standards are silent on the expectations under these circumstances (described for the case of "Multiple values, but more than n" in Table 12.22). The expectation might be to process the first "n" elements, any "n" elements, or perhaps no elements. This situation is technically non-deterministic without having further requirements in a derived specification. For the purpose of this analysis, processing the first "n" elements or any "n" elements is considered conformant; however, without specific requirements, a receiver that does not process any element and issues an exception could argue (or claim) to be conformant as well.

Table 12.20 Conformity assessment of cardinality [1..n] for receiving applications

Card.	Test data sent	Conformity assessment indicator	Receiver action	Conformity assessment	Comments
1..n	Not valued	Raise exception	Exception raised	Conformant	
			Exception not raised	Non-conformant	The receiver should indicate in some fashion the non-conformity, however, the indication may be informational, a warning, an error, or result in a rejection of the message entirely
1..n	Single value	Process the element	Processed	Conformant	
			Not-processed	Non-conformant	
1..n	Multiple values (x), but less than or equal to n	Process x elements	First element processed	Non-conformant	
			Some (<x) elements processed	Non-conformant	
			Multiple elements (x) processed	Conformant	
			Not-processed	Non-conformant	
1..n	Multiple values, but more than n	Process n elements (**See note for this table**)	First n elements processed	Conformant	Technically non-deterministic.
			Any n elements processed	Conformant	Technically non-deterministic.
			More than n elements processed	Non-conformant	
			Less than n elements processed	Non-conformant	
			Not-processed	Non-conformant	Technically non-deterministic.

Table 12.21 Conformity assessment of cardinality [1..*] for receiving applications

Card.	Test data sent	Conformity assessment indicator	Receiver action	Conformity assessment	Comments
1..*	Not valued	Raise exception	Exception raised	Conformant	
			Exception not raised	Non-conformant	The receiver should indicate in some fashion the non-conformity, however, the indication may be informational, a warning, an error, or result in a rejection of the message entirely
1..*	Single value	Process the element	Processed	Conformant	
			Not-processed	Non-conformant	
1..*	Multiple values, with a high value (x)	Process (x) elements	One element processed	Non-conformant	
			Some (< x) elements processed	Non-conformant	
			All (x) elements processed	Conformant	
			Not-processed	Non-conformant	

Table 12.22 Conformity assessment of cardinality [m..n] for receiving applications, with m greater than one

Card.	Test data sent	Conformity assessment indicator	Receiver action	Conformity assessment	Comments
m..n	Not valued	Raise exception	Exception raised	Conformant	
			Exception not raised	Non-conformant	The receiver should indicate in some fashion the non-conformity, however, the indication may be informational, a warning, an error, or result in a rejection of the message entirely

(continued)

Table 12.22 (continued)

Card.	Test data sent	Conformity assessment indicator	Receiver action	Conformity assessment	Comments
m..n	Single value	Raise exception	Exception raised	Conformant	
			Exception not raised	Non-conformant	The receiver should indicate in some fashion the non-conformity, however, the indication may be informational, a warning, an error, or result in a rejection of the message entirely
m..n	Multiple values (x), but less than or equal to m	Raise exception	Exception raised	Conformant	
			Some (<x) elements processed and/or Exception Not Raised	Non-conformant	
m..n	Multiple values (x), but more than or equal to m and less than or equal to n	Process (x) elements	(x) elements Processed	Conformant	
			The number of elements processed is other than (x)	Non-conformant	
m..n	Multiple values, but more than n	Process n elements (**See note for this table**)	First n elements processed	Conformant	Technically non-deterministic
			Any n elements processed	Conformant	Technically non-deterministic
			More than n elements processed	Non-conformant	
			Less than n elements processed	Non-conformant	
			Not-processed	Non-conformant	Technically non-deterministic

12.5 Vocabulary Conformance and Assessment

Chapter 5 described how to specify vocabulary, and Chap. 7 described how to constrain vocabulary in subsequent specifications. The discussion of vocabulary continues here with an overview of vocabulary conformance and vocabulary assessment. Please refer to Chaps. 5 and 7 for background information on the example value sets used in this section.

12.5.1 Vocabulary Conformance

The conformance and compliance for vocabulary usage indicators were discussed in Chap. 7. The following three figures present specific examples of vocabulary specifications and the associated conformance, compliance, and testing implications. The conformance and testing implications are only meaningful for bindings with a strength of "Required" (however, validation tools could issue warnings or alerts when binding strength is "Suggested"). The analysis in this section applies to both sender and receiver.

Figure 12.3 indicates for conformance that "F" and "M" must be supported and "A", "N", and "O" must not be supported. "U" and other codes may or may not be supported depending on their specification in a derived profile. These options are given in the compliance row. The Testing row presents observations about what can be tested based on the requirements that are known at the time of testing. In this case, all that is known is a constrainable profile, which is not the full set of requirements for an implementation. Therefore, the evaluation for some codes is non-deterministic (this is the case for "U"—the requirement for this code is not known, so no direct test is meaningful). To elaborate, if the code "U" or "X" is present in a message, no determination can be made with regard to its validity. It is unknown whether "U" was constrained to "R" or "E" and it is unknown if a new

Constrainable	
Value	Usage
A	**E**
F	**R**
M	**R**
N	**E**
O	**E**
U	**P**
E = Open	
S = Static	

Conformance Requirements	❖ **The implementation SHALL support the codes F and M.** ❖ **The implementation SHALL NOT support codes A, N, and O**
Compliance: Specification Options for a Derived Profile	❖ **In a Constrainable Profile the usage for code U MAY BE further specified as R or E, or remain P** ❖ **In an Implementation Profile the usage for code U SHALL BE further specified as R or E** ❖ **Additional codes are allowed to be added to the value set**
Testing	❖ **Support for codes F and M can be tested** ❖ **Non-support for code A, N, and O can be tested** ❖ **U cannot be tested because the usage requirement is unknown** ❖ **Additional codes cannot be tested because the usage requirement is unknown**

Fig. 12.3 Vocabulary specification implications—Example 1

code of "X" was added to the value set (and if so, with what usage) in the derived profile that was implemented. It is important to note here that the validation is being performed based on a constrainable profile but the message that is being validated was created for an implementation (using an implementation profile that may or may not have been documented and is likely to differ from the constrainable profile).

Figure 12.4 shows a derivation of the previous example. In this case, the Extensibility changed from "open" to "closed", resulting in a derived specification for which no additional codes can be specified. Any additional code found during testing of an instance would be deemed a non-conformity.

Figure 12.5 shows a derivation of the previous example. In this case, the profile is documented as implementable and the code "U" has been profiled to "R". Now, a definitive statement can be made with regard to conformance and testing outcomes. A similar analysis can be determined if "U" had been profiled to "E".

The impact of the stability being "dynamic" is discussed in the Vocabulary Conformity Assessment section that follows.

Constrainable	
Value	Usage
A	**E**
F	**R**
M	**R**
N	**E**
O	**E**
U	**P**
E = Closed	
S = Static	

Conformance Requirements	❖ **The implementation SHALL support the codes F and M.** ❖ **The implementation SHALL NOT support codes A, N, and O**
Compliance: Specification Options for a Derived Profile	❖ **In a Constrainable Profile the usage for code U MAY BE further specified as R or E, or remain P** ❖ **In an Implementation Profile the usage for code U SHALL BE further specified as R or E** ❖ **Additional codes are NOT allowed to be added to the value set in any derived profile**
Testing	❖ **Support for codes F and M can be tested** ❖ **Non-support for code A, N, and O can be tested** ❖ **U cannot be tested because the usage requirement is unknown** ❖ **Additional codes CAN be tested because the usage of all other codes is E**

Fig. 12.4 Vocabulary specification implications—Example 2

Implementable	
Value	Usage
A	**E**
F	**R**
M	**R**
N	**E**
O	**E**
U	**R**
E = Closed	
S = Static	

Conformance Requirements	❖ **The implementation SHALL support the codes F, M, and U.** ❖ **The implementation SHALL NOT support codes A, N, and O**
Compliance: Specification Options for a Derived Profile	❖ **No additional specification is possible** ❖ **The usage for code U is specified as R**
Testing	❖ **Support for codes F, M, and U can be tested** ❖ **Non-support for code A, N, and O can be tested** ❖ **Additional codes CAN be tested because the usage of all other codes is E**

Fig. 12.5 Vocabulary specification implications—Example 3

12.5.2 Vocabulary Conformity Assessment

Vocabulary conformity assessment is dependent on a number of factors, including the type of the profile, the binding, binding strength, extensibility, and stability. In general, a simple determination is made as to whether the code that is present in the message or document is part of the valid codes allowed as defined by the vocabulary binding. For the discussion that follows, the binding strength is Required. There is no enforceable requirement for a binding strength of Suggested, because a derived profile must specify definitive requirements. For constrainable profiles where the binding strength of Suggested is possible, however, a validation tool may report violations in the form of an informational alert or warning.

12.5.2.1 Conformity Assessment for Senders

When testing vocabulary in the data instance testing model, an assessment is rendered simply by comparing the element content in the object (e.g., a message) against the vocabulary specification requirements. The assessment is made on an object created by an implementation; however, the assessment may be based on requirements documented in a constrainable or implementation profile. In essence, the artifact created by the implementation is for an implementation profile, whether it is documented or not. This is often the case in certification testing, since the specifications are usually constrainable profiles (e.g., the specifications named in the ONC Health IT Certification rule are national level implementation guides that contain constrainable profiles). These conformance test tools are built to test against constrainable profiles, but are used for testing implementations. If implementation profiles are provided, then testing against the implementation profile can be performed, and a deterministic assessment can be made.

Table 12.23 shows the assessment for the various vocabulary specification combinations shown in Fig. 12.3 (i.e., for various settings of Extensibility for different profile types). If "F" or "M" is found in the instance, then the implementation is conformant. On the other hand, if "A", "N" or "O" is found, then the implementation is non-conformant, because those values are excluded. The

Table 12.23 Vocabulary conformity assessment–sender

Usage indicator	Data in message	Constrainable open	Constrainable closed	Implementation closed
R	F, M	Conformant	Conformant	Conformant
E	A, N, O	Non-conformant	Non-conformant	Non-conformant
P	U	Non-deterministic	Non-deterministic	Not-possible
?[a]	Any other code	Non-deterministic	Non-conformant	Non-conformant

[a]"?" indicates that the usage indicator is unknown for any other code in the case of "open" extensibility

assessment for constrainable profiles can't be determined for "U", since the requirement is not known. Having "P" usage for code "U" in an implementation profile is not possible and would be a specification error. The code "U" in an implementation would have to have been profiled to usage "R" or "E". If the implementation profile is available to the assessment and "U" has been profiled to "R" or "E", a definitive assessment can be made. The last row presents the situation in which a code that is not in the value set is found in the message. For open extensibility, all other codes are considered permitted, therefore, the same analysis for the code "U" would apply. On the other hand, for closed extensibility, the conformity assessment for codes not in the value set is non-conformant.

The assessment in Table 12.23 holds true regardless of the Stability setting. For dynamic, the assessment is made on the version of the value set in use, and therefore the assessment is made against a specific version. This version has to be communicated in some manner, either to the test tool or in the object being tested, otherwise false outcomes are possible. To reiterate, meaningful assessments can only be performed according to a known set of requirements.

In controlled testing environments such as ONC Health IT Certification, the approach and implications differ. The ONC rule specifies a "minimum" version of a code system, but "newer" versions can be supported. During testing, the version of the code system must be indicated in order for a completely meaningful[5] assessment to be conducted. In essence, the assessment for a value set with stability of dynamic-documented is the same as for static stability—it is a "snapshot" in time.

As an edge case, specifications may allow for unexpected codes at runtime (although, as indicated previously, no current standard provides sufficient mechanisms to disambiguate the specification of allowing unexpected codes from the existing mechanisms). If a specification was defined that allowed for unexpected codes, then testing in operational systems would have to allow for it. In controlled testing environments, only an assessment of what is known can be performed; however, the tester can determine whether the implementation supports the capability to include a code that is not in the defined value set by asking the implementer to create a message with an unspecified code.

In the assessment indicated in Table 12.23, the content of the object (e.g., a message) is evaluated without context. A different method of assessment is available in a controlled testing environment. The tester can have direct inquires to assess support of the vocabulary specification. For example, a test case could indicate the expectation of the concept defined by code "M". The tester could request that the SUT enact this condition (for example, via a dropdown list in a GUI), and create an object. This object can then be assessed for the specific code. Likewise, for an excluded element, the tester could investigate to see if an excluded code is available in a dropdown list. If it is selectable, then the tester would require that an object be generated. If the message is generated with the code, then the implementation is non-conformant. If the application utility (e.g., GUI) does not

[5]Only codes in the delta are problematic (which may or may not be addressed in the test set).

include the code for selection, or indicates an exception when a message is attempted to be generated, then it can be surmised that the application is conformant. The mechanism used to ensure nonsupport of codes is not important; however, the fact that the application doesn't support the use of the code for the specified profile is important. In the absence of an implementable profile, no determination can be made for permitted codes.

12.5.2.2 Conformity Assessment for Receivers

Conformity assessment for a receiver evaluates whether the implementation supports required codes and does not support excluded codes. Table 12.24 focuses on constrainable profiles with Extensibility of "open". The assessment for an implementation profile is the same as a constrainable profile, except that the assessment of permitted usage is not applicable.

Exactly what action should be taken by a receiver when they receive an excluded or an unexpected code? Specific requirements should be defined in a specification based on the use case analysis. The actions that could be taken range from no action to rejection of the message.

Table 12.24 Vocabulary conformity assessment–receiver–open extensibility

Usage indicator	Test data sent	Conformity assessment indicator	Receiver action	Conformity assessment	Comments
R	F, M	Process	Processed	Conformant	
			Not-processed	Non-conformant	Should raise an exception
E	A, N, O	Don't process	Processed	Non-conformant	Processed or no exception raised
			Not-processed	Conformant	Should raise an exception
P	U				Not meaningful to test
? Static	Any other code	Don't process	Processed	Non-conformant	Processed or no exception raised
			Not-processed	Conformant	Should raise an exception
? Dynamic	Any other code	Don't process	Processed	Non-conformant	
			Not-processed	Conformant	Should raise an exception
Unexpected code (documented)	Any other code	Process	Processed	Conformant	
			Not-processed	Non-conformant	

A few observations need to be shared here about performing a conformity assessment when an unknown code is received and the specification indicates a dynamic value set. Strictly speaking, this circumstance is no different from receiving an unknown code when the value set is static. Dynamic indicates that the implementations need to communicate with trading partners on the version of the value set that is being used. In this context, there is no difference from when the value set is static; it is a "snapshot" in time. An analogy would be the task of evaluating a software package for trading stocks online; the requested test was to be performed on the current release (version 5.3) of the software package, however, the tester was given access only to an old release (version 4.1). How much useful information can be derived, and how much confidence can the requester have in the result of the assessment?

If the specification allows for unexpected codes (and states that unexpected codes are allowed at runtime) for a particular coded data element, then the implementation must be prepared to accept unexpected codes (and be tested for it).

12.6 Summary

This chapter presents a set of assessment tables to illustrate conformant and non-conformant states of an implementation based on systematic test situations for the usage, cardinality, and vocabulary conformance constructs. The conformity assessment tables provide a basis for evaluating implementations. They also provide a definitive statement on the interpretation of the conformance constructs. It is important to note that this assessment is focused on determining conformity based on stated requirements and is not a prescription for real-world applications. As stated before, strict conformance is not a pre-requisite for useful data exchange. The views in the truth tables are literal interpretations, which they must be. These tables are necessary for determining the outcomes of validations used in conformance testing tools.

References

1. Health Level 7 (HL7) Standard Version 2.7.1, ANSI/HL7, July, 2012, Chapter 2B – Conformance http://www.hl7.org.
2. HL7 Version 2.5.1 Implementation Guide. S&I Framework Lab Results Interface interoperability standards (DSTU), Release 2, September 2015; http://www.hl7.org
3. Snelick R. HL7 v2 Value Set Specification Proposal. Profiling Vocabulary in HL7 v2 Implementation Guides. Original September 2013; last update June 2015. http://hl7v2tools.nist.gov (Publications/Presentations and Technical Documents).

Chapter 13
Testing Architectures

13.1 Introduction

Chapter 10 described the various testing models from a conceptual perspective as well as the types of testing that could be performed in each model. Chapter 11 presented principles of conformance testing that explained the testing life cycle, test plan, and a methodology for testing both sending and receiving applications. In this chapter, the realization of the concepts and methodologies is presented as testing architectures, including descriptions of a testing infrastructure, testing frameworks, and test instantiations (one of which is an interoperability test bed). Case studies are provided to emphasize the utility of the modular approach. Chapter 14 builds upon this theme by providing a sampling of test tools created using the approaches explained in this chapter. Finally, Chap. 15 describes how the tools are used in testing and certification programs, such as the IHE connect-a-thon [1] and the ONC Health IT Certification Program [2].

Figure 13.1 depicts the foundation for the discussions in this Chap. 14. One approach to building a test system is, first, to develop a testing infrastructure that provides components that perform a specific focused task, such as validation. The components can be delivered as a service or library. The important aspects for the components are that they are independent and able to perform a certain function that allows for their reuse. The components of the testing infrastructure can then be used to build a domain-specific testing framework, and the framework can support one or more testing models (as described in Chap. 10). Typically, the framework will support data instance testing first, and then isolated system testing, and finally peer-to-peer testing. This progression is natural, and each layer provides foundational components upon which additional testing capabilities can be built. Once a testing framework is established, specific testing tools are developed that leverage the framework's components. The concept of reusability allows for rapid development of test tools.

F. Oemig and R. Snelick, *Healthcare Interoperability Standards Compliance Handbook*, DOI 10.1007/978-3-319-44839-8_13

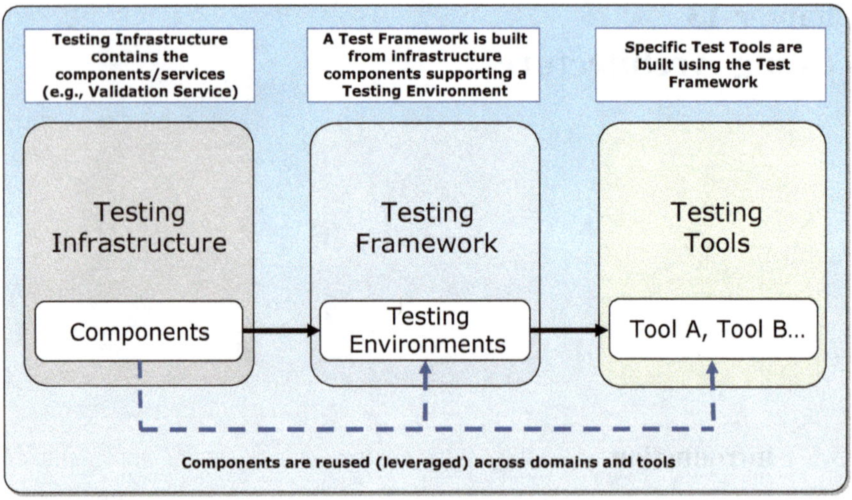

Fig. 13.1 Tool development process

The concepts in this chapter are presented using an instantiation of an HL7 v2.x testing infrastructure and testing framework. The HL7 v2.x-centric implementation provides concrete examples to explain the key ideas; however, the general principles apply broadly to data exchange standards. In fact, many components of the testing framework (for HL7 v2.x) described in this chapter were leveraged to develop ONC 2014 Edition and 2015 Edition certification test tools for ePrescribing (NCPDP SCRIPT) [3].[1] Additionally, many of the concepts also apply to document-based standards such as CDA. This chapter, however, does not seek to cover the other possible test architectures and approaches, nor does it claim that a component-based testing infrastructure is the best approach. Rather, the intent is to give the reader a flavor of the various core components needed for testing and one approach for the organization and use of those components.

13.2 Testing Infrastructure

The central design principle behind the construction of a test system is a modular and flexible approach afforded by a testing infrastructure. This testing infrastructure provides reusable components with well-defined interfaces that can be utilized in a test system as needed. The obvious advantage of this approach is that the user can combine

[1]The architecture described here was developed by the National Institute of Standards and Technology (NIST) and used to create the HL7 v2.x and ePrescribing ONC EHR Certification Test Tools.

the components of the test system into whatever configuration is most suitable for solving the problem at hand. In addition to being flexible, such a system is easily extensible. Since each test system component runs independently, adding new services to the test system can be accomplished readily. The architecture of a testing infrastructure can be contained in a single system or can be distributed across multiple discrete systems. The testing infrastructure is also scalable, since the components are independent and can be distributed. The test systems described and referenced in this work, including the Interoperability Test Bed (ITB), use this approach.

The testing infrastructure is composed of three types of high-level components: the services (including network functions), the test harness (services composition), and resource repository. Additionally, a test management system may be employed, but it is not central to the test infrastructure—it is likely a separate system. Services provide the testing features and functions. For this model to be used effectively in conducting testing, the interactions that occur between the user and the supported testing services must be facilitated using several mechanisms. A test harness is necessary to orchestrate the services for conducting a test; a resource repository is used to manage the needed test artifacts; and a network function, which may include logging and proxy capabilities, is deployed to route messages.

A test management system (e.g., IHE Gazelle [22]) can be used to assign, manage, and track each set of tests. A certification testing lab may utilize such a system in their process, however, it is considered a peripheral component of the testing infrastructure.

Services provide a portfolio of testing-related capabilities that are designed to perform unique functions within the testing infrastructure. Each service has well-defined responsibilities and authorities, and they work together in collaboration with other services to support the execution of test cases. The service portfolio will support functions such as the validation of testing objects, logging of procedure steps and test results, deployment of test agents, and generation of test reports. To keep the discussion brief, only a few pivotal services pertinent to the case study to follow are presented here.

A testing infrastructure is simply a collection of related components, each of which provides a function, and which, when combined, perform a specific testing task. Figure 13.2 illustrates the concept of a testing infrastructure based on services. One essential idea behind a Service Oriented Architecture (SOA) is that functionality is aggregated into groups for the purpose of providing a collection of well-defined services. These services are made available to users locally or over a network, allowing the services to be combined in ways that best suit the user's development requirements. The model provides an architecture for development that scales well and is both modular and flexible. The services can be loosely or tightly integrated with testing tools and can have various access interfaces.

The testing infrastructure is composed of three parts: the resource repository, the test harness, and the services. The resource repository contains the artifacts necessary for conducting tests and facilitating test execution processing. A test harness is necessary for orchestrating the services to conduct a test and to analyze the collective test results. Many test orchestration (engine) instantiation choices are

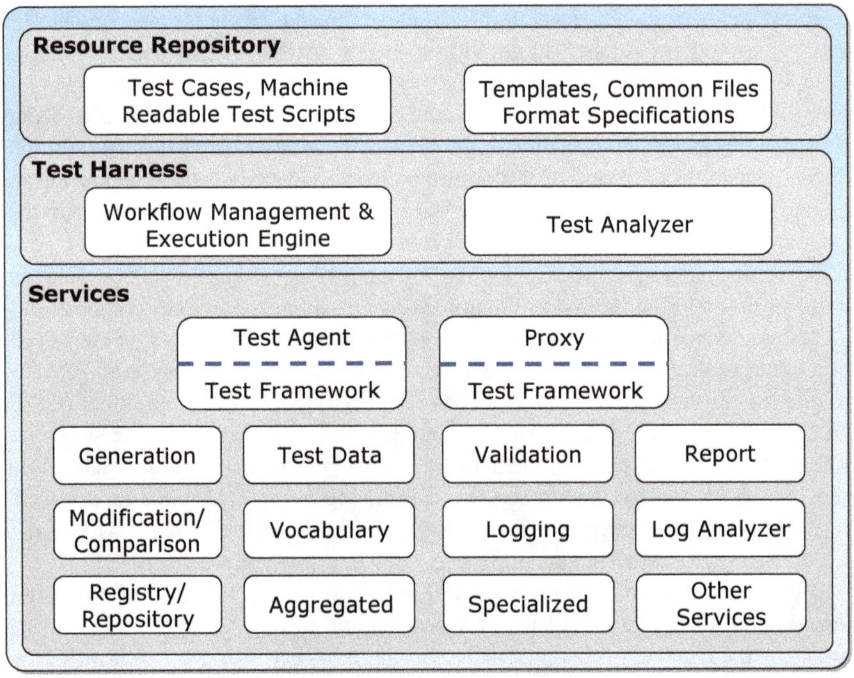

Fig. 13.2 Testing infrastructure services

available—ranging from an ad hoc test driver to powerful process execution languages. In some cases, it may be appropriate for a testing infrastructure to support multiple test engines that are tailored to the particular domain it is servicing. Services provide the testing and testing-related functionality. In an SOA design, services are autonomous, and they hide implementation details. For this model to be used effectively in conducting testing, the interactions between the user and the supported testing services must be facilitated.

Another important aspect of the overall design of the testing infrastructure is the development of interfaces that connect the components—an Enterprise Service Bus (ESB). For example, a common interface between the services composition component and the test agents is essential. This design supports additional test agents seamlessly through the common interface.

In line with the philosophy of SOA, the testing infrastructure is not meant to be a single purpose system, but to provide components that can be reused and/or repurposed in a testing framework or test tools. For example, a generic HL7 v2 Validation Service can be provided and can be used in many contexts. The input to the validation service (in the form of profiles) provides the details of the context. For example, for a specific ONC HIT Certification immunization messaging test case, the conformance message profile, value set requirements, and test case-specific validation requirements are provided along with the message to be tested. The context could easily have been a lab result message just by changing the input profiles. The goal is to allow the service to be easily incorporated into various test systems. The service can be used for data instance testing, isolated system testing, and peer-to-peer testing. Examples of test tools for each testing model are provided in the next chapter. Data instance testing can be a web-based application where the user selects the conformance message profile and uploads the message. For isolated system testing, the validation service handles multiple message types and is integrated into the test framework. Input is directed by the test cases. The validation service could also be incorporated in an interoperability test bed controlled by a test case management system such as IHE Gazelle [22]. These examples demonstrate how the testing infrastructure can be used. In the sections that follow, a detailed explanation of each test framework is given.

13.2.1 Key Objectives of a Testing Infrastructure

The key objectives for developing a testing infrastructure include the following:

- Provide a variety of testing services to health information technology stakeholders
- Support conformance and interoperability testing for numerous healthcare messaging and document data exchange standards
- Provide a set of reusable components and services
- Support different delivery mechanisms including application programming interfaces (API), desktop applications, web applications, and web services
- Integrate with existing testing frameworks and tools
- Provide a platform to support collaboration and harmonization with other tooling efforts
- Roll out tools and resources incrementally
- Provide consistency in testing

In the following sections we elaborate on each of the testing infrastructure components. The components given provide a sampling of what may constitute a testing infrastructure. A given testing infrastructure may be constructed with whatever components are necessary to support the testing activities desired. Additionally, the description provided for each of the components is not rigid, merely emblematic.

13.2.2 Resource Repository

The *resource repository* contains the artifacts necessary for conducting tests and facilitating test execution processing. Artifacts that support test case execution typically include the test execution script, test case descriptions, test data specifications, test data, and test specifications. Certain test specifications, such as those used for content testing, usually will reside in the testing infrastructure resource repository, because it is specific to the test case. Test specifications for a particular standard (e.g., an XML conformance message profile for the HL7 v2.5.1 ORU R01 message type) could be associated with the v2 validation service or in the resource repository. Additional artifacts may also be contained in the resource repository to facilitate the test execution process. These artifacts include templates with common file formats. Such templates can be used to dynamically construct test specifications.

The purpose of the resource repository is to enable users (ranging from domain experts to testing organizations) to access and post materials, such as use cases, test cases, and machine-readable test scripts, for use within the testing infrastructure; and to access specifications to develop materials for use within the testing infrastructure, such as artifact templates and common file formats. This component may be accessed directly by end-users or utilized by the infrastructure while establishing a test case.

13.2.3 Test Harness

The test harness is composed of a test engine and a test analyzer. The test engine is a workflow management tool used to direct the execution of defined test cases through the orchestration of testing services. A test analyzer is also integrated into this component to compile and analyze the results of test object validations throughout the lifecycle of a test case.

An important aspect of the SOA is the composition of the services into an executable process. Services are assembled in a particular order and follow a set of rules to carry-out a business process—a test scenario, for example. Arbitrary composition of services supports a broad range of test requirements in a straightforward and flexible manner. Additionally, the complexity of the services composition is at the discretion of the user of the services. Modifications to test execution are handled easily in this model—allowing for quick adaptation to changing requirements in test scenarios.

The *test engine* orchestrates services to produce an executable implementation of the testing workflow. A test management control system may provide input (test execution scripts—residing in the resource repository) that directs the actions of the test engine. The test engine carries out the instructions by employing the services.

There are many choices available for implementing the test engine. These options include powerful process execution languages such as BPEL (Business Process Execution Language) [4], a web browser client with scripting language support, or a high-level programming language such as Java. The testing infrastructure may contain any number of test engine implementations. Multiple test engines within a testing infrastructure might be appropriate to support the various types of testing required. Experience has shown that attempting to build a universal (general) test engine is complex.

The test case will typically consist of numerous steps, possibly for multiple applications under test. This creates many individual validation reports. A *test analyzer* is necessary at this level to make a collective determination of the test results. The test analyzer can use the test script for navigating, linking, and analyzing the array of validation reports.

13.2.4 Services

Services provide a portfolio of testing-related capabilities that are specified to perform unique functions within the testing infrastructure. Each service has well-defined responsibilities and authority, and they work together in collaboration to support the execution of test cases. The service portfolio will support functions such as the validation of test objects, logging of test results, instantiation of test agents, and generation of test reports.

In the sections that follow, we present a set of typical service categories. This list is not exhaustive and not all services need to be included in a testing infrastructure. The testing requirements determine the need for a service. Also, a testing infrastructure may contain multiple instances of a service category. For example, a testing infrastructure could contain validation services for HL7 v2, HL7 CDA, and NCPDP SCRIPT. In addition, it may contain multiple validation services for the same protocol, i.e., multiple HL7 v2 validation services. There are no limitations on the set of services included in a testing infrastructure.

13.2.4.1 Generation Services

Generation services support the creation of test objects such as messages and documents, for example, HL7 message instances [5]. Figure 13.3 illustrates a typical work flow for accessing and integrating a generation.

In the case of HL7 v2, the generation service can build a message using the XML conformance message profile as the message template. The test data retrieved from the Test Data service can be overlaid onto the message template to create a message instance. Various settings to the Test Data and Validation services are provided for tailoring the message to accommodate the requirements in the test case. Such a service can be used to support dynamic creation of test messages that can be used in a variety of settings (Table 13.1).

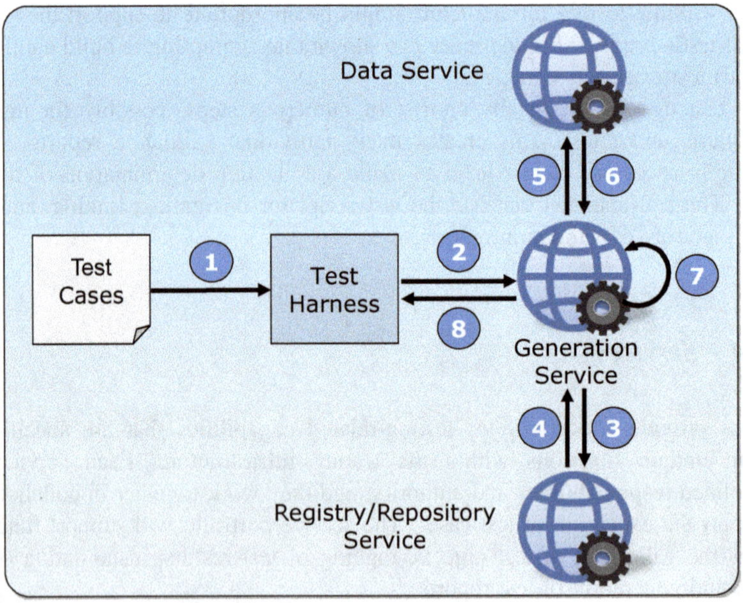

Fig. 13.3 Generation service

Table 13.1 Steps for using a generation service

Step	Description
1	Information about the test case, including configuration information and possibly references to test artifacts are passed to the test harness for execution
2	The Test harness orchestrates testing activity based on the selected test case. Information is sent to the generation service to generate a test object (e.g., a message)
3	The generation service requests referenced test artifacts from the registry/repository service—such as generation context files[a]
4	The registry/repository service sends requested test artifacts to the generation service for test object generation—such as generation context files
5	The generation service requests the test data sets required for test object generation. The data service itself may have accessed a value set service to retrieve and/or verify coded data
6	The data service returns requested test data sets for the generation of a test object
7	The generation service conducts internal processing to generate a test object (based on information from the test harness, registry/repository service, and data service)
8	The generation service sends the test object back to the test harness to initiate the testing sequence The generation service may also be accessed via test agents or other software

[a]Generation context file refers to an artifact (e.g., an XML file) that contains instructions and data that, when combined with a profile, can be used to create a message instance

13.2.4.2 Validation Services

A validation service provides an evaluation function for a given protocol, for example, validation of an HL7 v2 message instance against an HL7 v2 conformance profile [6, 7]. Figure 13.4 illustrates a typical work flow for accessing and integrating a validation service. Table 13.2 provides a description for each step.

In the case of HL7 v2, the validation service can validate a message using an XML conformance message profile. The message profile contains the requirements, such as the message structure, usage, cardinality, and so on. Additional requirements may be captured in other testing artifacts that go beyond what can be validated in a conformance message profile. For example, specific data content is typically examined in test cases in order to determine if there is support for certain message elements (e.g., those specified with RE usage) and functional capabilities.

The validation service can also access other validation services, such as a Value Set Validation service (not shown). In instances where a specification requires the support of a large value set, it may be more appropriate to create a specific validation service for this purpose. In addition, the specific value set validation service could be used to support multiple protocols, such as CDA and HL7 v2, since this service is an independent function. Additionally, such a service is best provided by the maintainers of the vocabulary. This example demonstrates the utility and importance of partitioning services at a granular level to support broad reuse.

13.2.4.3 Test Agents

Test agents (also referred to as simulators) are implementations of actors (or applications) that support the functionality of the underlying specification of the actor. The test agent does not have to be a complete reference implementation; it

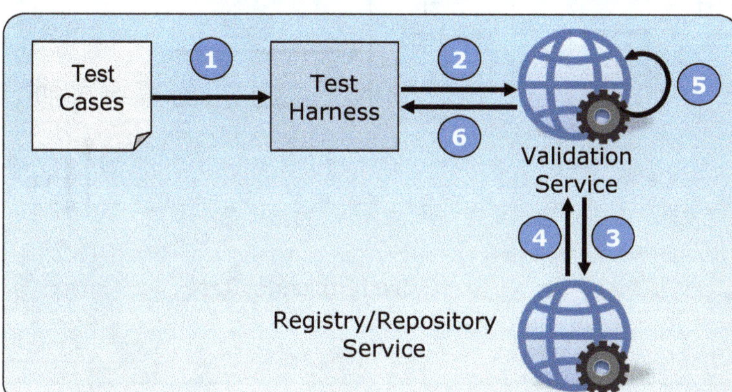

Fig. 13.4 Validation service

Table 13.2 Steps for using a validation service

Step	Description
1	Information about the test case, including the test object, configuration information, and possibly references to test artifacts, is passed to the test harness for execution
2	The test object and test artifacts (or references) are sent to the validation service
3	The validation service requests test artifacts from the registry/repository service—such as validation context files
4	The registry/repository service sends requested test artifacts to the validation service for processing—such as validation context files
5	The validation service executes its internal validation processes with information from the test harness and registry/repository service
6	The validation service returns the test object validation results to the test harness The validation service may also be accessed via test agents or other software. (i.e., this example shows one access point)

only needs to support the functionality of the actor to support testing of applications. Test agents are stand-in *applications* with which the SUT would normally interact; however, over time a test agent may become a reference implementation. Potentially, many actors will exist in a testing infrastructure—although for any given test, typically three or fewer will be incorporated. The distributed nature of the SOA allows for test agents to be built independently and maintained at different locations. Figure 13.5 shows how a test agent interacts with the test harness and SUT. Table 13.3 provides a description for each step.

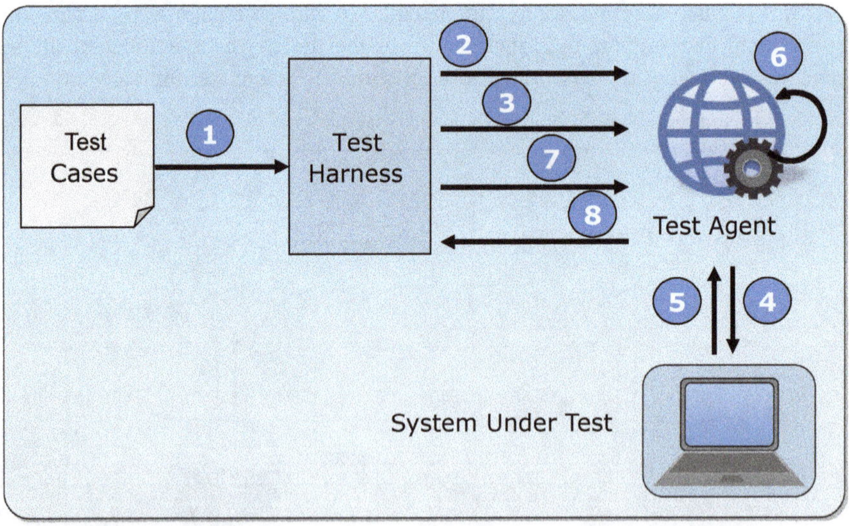

Fig. 13.5 Test agent service

As mentioned previously, the complexity of a test agent can vary significantly. On one end of the spectrum, the test agent can have predetermined responses (*canned*) to an interaction or request. This approach is perfectly valid, since the goal of the test agent is to take the place of the system that the SUT would normally interact with for the given transaction and to respond accordingly. It does not matter to the testing system or the SUT whether the response is *canned* or created dynamically; however, predetermined responses have limited utility and flexibility since they are tied to specific test cases and test data. The more actor functionality a test agent can provide, the more useful it is for support of testing. At the other end of the spectrum is a reference implementation, which is a complete implementation of the actor. Typically, each test agent occupies a position between the two endpoints that is most effective in terms of utility and cost, depending on factors such as the sophistication of the type of testing being performed and the resources needed to develop additional functionality.

Note that this case is one possible use and work flow of a Test Agent—many more uses and workflows are possible. For example, in a peer-to-peer test model there may not be any interaction between the test engine and the test agent. The test agent can be a reference implementation and be deployed to interact with one or more SUTs or other test agents. Here, a centralized proxy may intercept, capture, and forward message exchanges. The test harness (test engine and test analyzer) can assimilate the test objects (e.g., messages) to construct the results of the test.

Table 13.3 Steps for using a test agent service

Step	Description
1	Information about the test case is communicated to the test harness
2	The test harness initiates the first test step by instantiating and configuring a test agent (as specified by the test case)
3	The test harness then sends test case instructions and associated test artifact references to the test agent
4	The test agent processes instructions from the test harness and its internal application functionality and interacts with the system under test (SUT)
5	The system under test (SUT) responds back to the test agent
6	The test agent processes the response(s) according to its internal application functionality
7	The test harness requests the test agent's processing information (e.g., a message received by the test agent from the SUT)
8	The test agent responds to the test harness

13.2.4.4 Registry/Repository Services

A repository contains testing artifacts needed in testing. The registry provides mechanisms to index, organize, and retrieve the artifacts. The registry may first be used to locate a particular artifact that is later accessed in the Repository. The Registry/Repository service may be a combined service or separate services. The Registry/Repository can potentially maintain the specifications, schematron rules, conformance profiles, test messages, value sets, etc., to support testing. The generation and validation workflows shown in Figs. 13.3 and 13.4 illustrate a typical use and incorporation of the Registry/Repository service in a service composition.

13.2.4.5 Test Data Services

The Test Data Service provides test data that have broad applicability in testing. The test data can be standard-agnostic or structured (customized) to a specific standard. For example, a test data service could provide patient demographic data that includes patient name, address, and contact information. The service could return a general XML format (or other representations) that can be adapted to the standard of interest. Alternatively, the test data service can be specific to a particular standard, for example, the superset of patient demographic data for HL7 v2 with mappings to the appropriate data elements. One implementation of this service could be to return complete PID segments in which the data is interrelated (i.e., sensible).[2] The end user of the service can filter the data as appropriate to meet the specific testing need. The test data service can be used by related services, for instance, a generation service to create test objects such as HL7 v2 messages or CDA documents. The use of templates (e.g., a conformance message profile) is essential for binding data to a structure object. The test data service itself can use other services, such as the value set service. Here, data for coded elements can be obtained and verified prior to inclusion into a data set.

A test data service can support testing tools in various ways. It can provide structured data sets that have been verified for common concepts or data groupings (such as patient demographics). This convenience allows test developers to create test case-specific data sets quickly. The service can also be used to support dynamic data. For example, a test case may have a fixed data set and, just prior to execution of a test case, the patient demographics can be substituted. In addition, the service could provide data randomization features that help in data creation.

[2]However, the preferred approach is to create the data sets as standard agnostic and then map to standard specific structures.

13.2.4.6 Report Services

The Report Service enables the generation and formatting of assorted reports. This service can provide the ability to produce low-level domain-specific validation reports (e.g., an HL7 v2 Validation Report) as well as high-level reports that summarize the results of an executed test case.

13.2.4.7 Consistent Time Service

Ensuring that the system time is aligned is important in the execution of certain tests. A consistent time service provides the current time of day using a reference time service, such as that provided by NIST [8]. The service guarantees that SUT(s) and the test system's time are synchronized and provides an authoritative reference time for all functions within the test system.

13.2.4.8 Proxy Service

A Proxy Service captures all related information to support viewing, debugging, and analyzing messages within the test system where it is deployed. The primary functions of a proxy are to capture, store, and forward messages. Stored messages are associated and analyzed by the test system. The need for proxies primarily exists in the peer-to-peer testing model since communication is between multiple SUTs. A test system may deploy a centralized proxy, in which all messages pass through, or distributed proxies bound to each SUT. A Proxy Service may support multiple protocols, for instance, HL7 v2, HL7 V3, NCPDP, and DICOM [9], communication protocols (See the next section), and a viewer module to preview messages. The viewing capabilities could support parsing and searching capabilities. An example of how a proxy is deployed and used is described in the interoperability test bed discussion. Among its other capabilities, Mirth [10] is a well-known software product that provides proxy capabilities.

13.2.4.9 Communication Infrastructure

A test system instantiation will need to support an array of communication protocols (MLLP, SOAP, etc.) to aid message exchange with test agents, proxies, and the systems-under-test. The communication infrastructure module provides such capabilities; Mirth [10] is one example. Figure 13.6 illustrates a design of a communication infrastructure that provides support for an assortment of transport protocols as well as an interface that allows the test agents and proxies to interpret the payload.

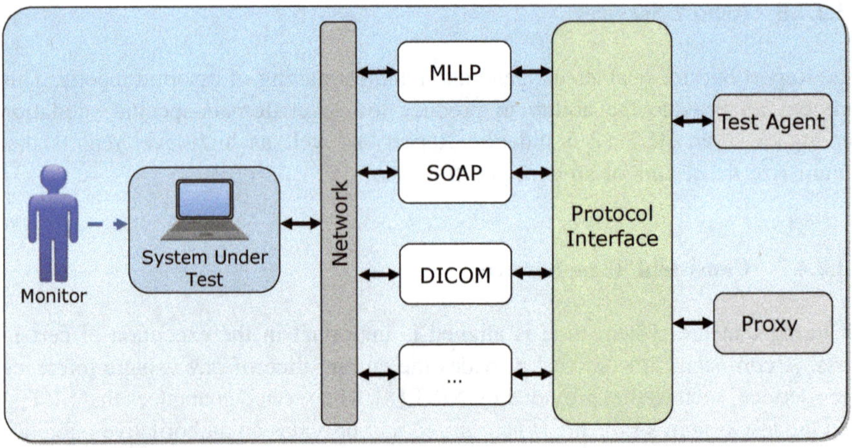

Fig. 13.6 Communication infrastructure

13.2.4.10 Terminology Service

A Terminology Service provides access to vocabulary or terminology in the form of code systems or value sets. The service may support multiple models for accessing the terminology and may be locally (tightly-integrated) or remotely connected to the testing infrastructure or test system. The service may have a standardized interface such as CTS2—Common Terminology Services [11] as offered by OMG as WSDL and WADL files for the CTS2 functional model.

One use of a Terminology Service is in conjunction with a Validation Service. The Validation Service uses the value set retrieved from the Terminology Service. For example, in the IHE Patient Care Device (PCD) domain, test cases require validation against the Rosetta nomenclature[3] (value set). A Terminology Service includes a mechanism to access value sets needed for the execution of Test Cases in various domains. The Validation Service may be pre-populated with value sets or may check the Terminology Service periodically to update the Validation Service for dynamic value sets. The way in which the service is composed and used will depend on the testing needs of the user.

Alternatively, rather than having a validation service access and incorporate value sets, the terminology service can have a validation component. A test client can provide a code and a value set, and the terminology service would return whether or not the code is a member of the value set. The client determines the

[3]IHE-PCD has developed an infrastructural profile known as 'Rosetta Terminology Mapping' (RTM) that harmonizes standard nomenclature as defined in the ISO/IEEE 11073-10101 Medical Device Communication standard. Such information is carried as content, providing semantic value, within the defined HL7 message.

value set by inspecting the binding of the value set to the data element in the specification.

A validation service may perform additional checks beyond simple membership. For example, in IHE-PCD with Rosetta Terminology Mapping (RTM) not only is validation accomplished per the defined value set, but additional testable assertions can be executed based on co-constraints (e.g., where a particular term has associated units of measurement, body sites, and enumerations).

One important aspect with regard to testing is the manner in which the value sets are bound to the requirements in the specification. The caller of the service needs this information to uniquely identify the appropriate value set. It is important that authors of specifications narrow the scope of the value set for the element (for a specific use) to which it is bound. That is, there is limited value to binding an element to a large value set (or an entire code system) in which only a few of the codes in the value set are applicable to the element to which it is bound. Chapters 5 and 7 address this issue.

13.2.4.11 Aggregated Services

Services may be aggregated. For example, an implementation of a workflow may become a service itself. Services may use other services—test agents may choose to invoke a validation service directly. Other utilities for the support of test harness instances include templates—for example, a web browser client. This approach will allow for uniform creation of web sites for a particular set of tests, for example, IHE pre-connect-a-thon tests. This method could be applied at the organization level or at a testing event level.

Aggregated Services are the integration of existing infrastructure services to improve system efficiency, performance, or usability. For example, in some circumstances system performance may be improved by combining the Generation Service, Test Agent Service, and Validation Service. An aggregated service does not replace independent services, rather it provides a convenient bundling of services.

13.2.4.12 Other Services

As previously mentioned, only a sampling of potential services that a testing infrastructure might include is being presented, along with insight into the makeup of each service. The testing infrastructure is not bound to a defined set of services; the set is determined by the objectives of the testing goals and system. Additional services, such as ones that support security and logging, may be suitable to incorporate in a testing infrastructure.

13.2.5 Infrastructure Components

Tangential to the core components, are infrastructural components that aid in specification of artifacts and the operational aspects of the testing infrastructure. These include well-defined component interface definitions that enable usability and provide a flexible design for third-party users. A common and effective method for achieving this goal is the use of the Enterprise Service Bus (ESB) architecture paradigm. Examples of the interface definitions include the application programming interface (API) to the validation service and the web service definition to the external validation service.[4]

Another important aspect is the definition of common file formats or templates. In some cases, these formats are defined elsewhere, such as in the standard. One example is the schema for the HL7 v2 conformance message profile. It provides a standard way to define the requirements in the conformance profile. For artifacts that are not standardized, the Testing Infrastructure should define them, and, if appropriate, promote them to the SDO as a standardized format. Such adoption will encourage the creation and use of tools for development of the artifacts and subsequent reuse of the artifacts. Common file formats enable interoperability among the testing infrastructure functional components. Typical artifacts that can use common file formats include (demographic or clinical) test data, results reports (at various levels), generation context files, validation context files, and configuration files.

13.2.6 Testing Infrastructure—A Broader Context

Figure 13.7 illustrates how the core components (from Fig. 13.2) of a testing infrastructure can be applied in a broader context to support a testing platform. This broader context includes support for, and integration with, stakeholders, a test management system, tool access and delivery, development components, and external tools and services.

13.2.6.1 Test Management Systems

As mentioned previously, the test management system is not necessarily part of the testing architecture, but it is an important ancillary system. The management system is responsible for setting up test cases, and reporting and maintaining results. Auditing services can also be included. Testing entities, such as the ONC Accredited Testing Laboratories (ATLs) and IHE, will likely employ a test

[4]The NIST HL7 v2.x message validation web service provides an example [7].

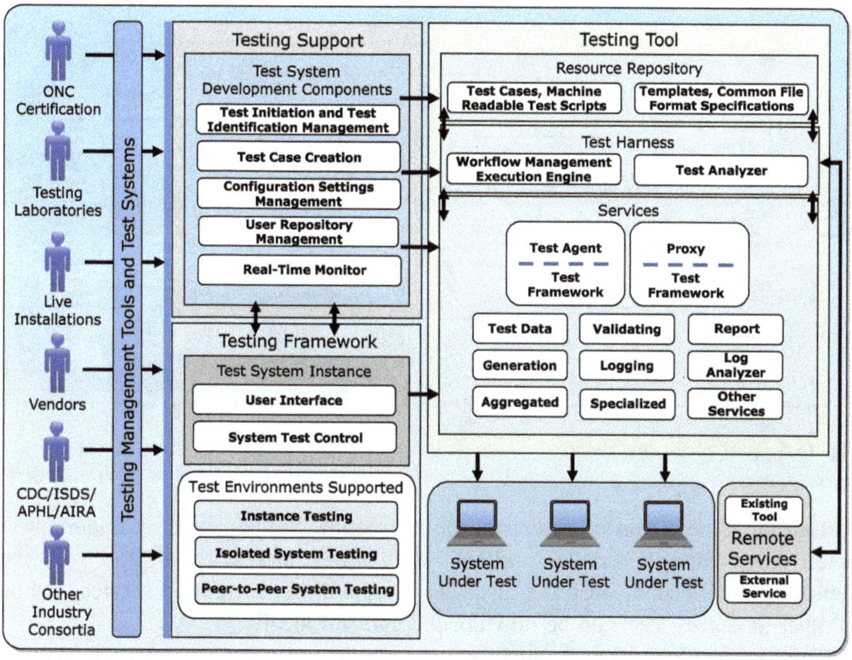

Fig. 13.7 Testing infrastructure—a broader context

management system. For example, at IHE Connect-a-thons, the Gazelle [22] test management system is used to set up and organize all tests.

13.2.6.2 Tool Access and Delivery

A testing infrastructure should accommodate multiple access points. Figure 13.8 illustrates several possibilities. End-users (e.g. vendors, implementers) may access the (1) Test System (Tool) User Interface directly to configure, execute, and monitor test cases. Configuration information entered into the Test System User Interface will inform the Test Harness to orchestrate services from the Service Portfolio (via the Web Services Interface or Java APIs) to support the execution of test cases.

End-user organizations (e.g., Accredited Testing Laboratories—ATLs—and industry consortia) may develop and utilize (2) third-party software to access or integrate various components of the testing infrastructure to meet their individual testing needs. Third-party software may be a web-based client or desktop application that utilizes one or more of the infrastructure components, or it may be a

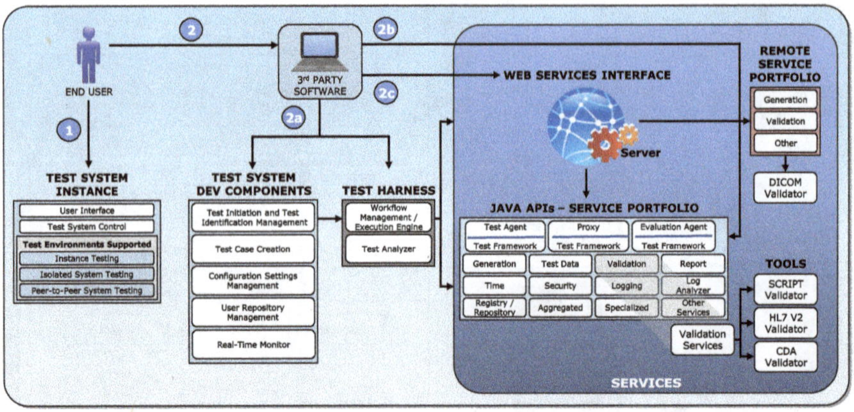

Fig. 13.8 Tool access and delivery

custom implementation of an existing infrastructure component. It is important to note that testing services within the infrastructure portfolio will be deployment-dependent; in some instances, they will be active web services, while in other instances they can be downloaded and run locally.

Third-party (2a) software, such as the Gazelle test management tool, may be customized to access the Test System Development Components or Test Harness directly. The Test Harness will then orchestrate services from the Service Portfolio (via the Web Services Interface or Java APIs) to support the execution of test cases.

Implementers may download the Java APIs for integration (2b) into a custom application in order to utilize the various service-based testing functionality.

Third-party software, such as a vendor's web-based client (2c), may be customized to access the Web Services Interface directly. The Web Services Interface then utilizes the Java APIs to call various service-based testing functionality.

13.2.6.3 External Tools and Services

A test infrastructure will often need to incorporate external tools or services, for example, to gain access to a large vocabulary. A standardized interface[5] may be available or a customized interface may be used to accommodate the external service, and transformation of the results to the format needed by the testing infrastructure may be necessary. A testing infrastructure should accommodate the incorporation of external resources to leverage existing functionality.

[5]For example, the Object Management Group (OMG) provides the official Common Terminology Services 2 (CTS2) WSDL specification for the abstract HL7 CTS2 specification.

13.2.6.4 Development Components

Auxiliary tools and utilities live outside the boundaries of the testing infrastructure. These *development* components facilitate use of the testing infrastructure and provide testing artifacts for the testing infrastructure. An example is test case authoring tools. The resultant artifacts, i.e., test cases, are used by the testing infrastructure.

13.2.7 Testing Infrastructure Observations

A testing infrastructure will generally be composed of the three parts presented. However, the make-up of each part can differ significantly depending on the targeted need of the testing infrastructure. For example, perhaps services listed in the testing infrastructure example presented are not necessary, while other services that are not listed are necessary. Likewise, there may not be a need for a test analyzer. The testing infrastructure is a conceptual notion that will be realized depending on the testing needs.

The services in a testing infrastructure can be loosely-coupled (distributed) via web services. Various organizations may have specialty services that they expose in a pool of resources. Common services include validation which may include message, document, and value set validation services. For example, in certain circumstances, it may be more manageable and efficient for a conformance test tool to validate coded content via an external value set validation service. The value set may be extremely large and dynamic. Incorporating such capabilities into a testing tool is costly (because of unnecessary duplication) and error prone (due to synchronizing with a source value set).

13.3 A Test Scenario

In this section, we describe an example case study and associated workflow that demonstrate typical transactions among disparate healthcare information technology systems. This test scenario is intended to serve as a case study to assist in describing the testing architectures to follow. Aspects of the test scenario are utilized for explaining relevant points of the testing architecture under consideration. First, an overview of the applications, including the functional role played by the application, is presented. An application is generally made up of a single actor, but it may include multiple actors. The Integrating the Healthcare Enterprise (IHE) organization defines an actor based on the functional components supported by the actor. IHE publishes integration profiles that describe many healthcare workflows [12]. In our use case example, an actor can be equated with a healthcare application, such as the patient identifier cross-referencing manager (PIX Manager).

Note that a PIX Manager actor may exist within a hospital's healthcare information technology (HIT) system or other HIT systems, such as an Immunization Information System (IIS). We describe a typical workflow of cooperating patient identifier and document management systems. The scenario is supported by the IHE Information Technology Infrastructure Integration Profile [13]. The data exchange standard used in this case study is HL7 v2 (but could be others such as HL7 V3). For the purposes of demonstrating the test execution of the testing architectures, the scenario focuses on the HL7 v2 messaging PIX aspects.

It is important to note that a simple and succinct patient management scenario is given for explanatory purposes. The example is valid, however, it does not convey the entire complexity possible nor the optimal solution for patient management implementations. For further explanation and a better solution, see [14]. What is important, though, is that the same testing approach can be applied to test a simple use case or complex.

Healthcare systems can be divided into various administrative domains, each responsible for managing a set of patient information. Patients may require services provided in different healthcare settings. When this situation occurs, different electronic health records for the same patient may exist in more than one setting. It is clearly desirable to be able to recognize when multiple records exist belonging to the same patient. IHE has addressed this problem by delegating the responsibility for determining when two patient identifiers belong to the same patient, and, hence, there are two records belonging to the same patient to the PIX Manager actor. Our example examines a healthcare system made up of a Patient Identifier Cross-referencing (PIX) Domain and a Cross-Enterprise Document Sharing (XDS) system. We examine a typical PIX domain made up of three disparate actors: a PIX Source, a PIX Manager, and a PIX Consumer. A PIX Source is used for adding and modifying patient demographic data; a PIX Manager is used for managing and cross referencing patient identifiers from different domains; and a PIX Consumer is used for querying a PIX Manager for patient identifiers. All communications among the actors are accomplished through the exchange of HL7 v2 messages. An XDS system supports registering and retrieving documents across enterprises within an administrative domain.

Our case study examines some of the data points the PIX Manager must consider; for example, when it is determined that two patients are actually the same patient, how will the information be propagated across the healthcare organizations The resolution is important, since a single patient identifier is typically used to retrieve documents about a patient from a repository.

The workflow in Fig. 13.9 illustrates the integration not only among applications within a system, but also between systems. This example assumes that an appropriate information sharing policy agreement exists, and that appropriate security and privacy protocols are used.

The scenario is predicated on a family physician at Practice Y seeking pertinent medical documents for patient Donna Bee. Practice Y relies on Hospital X's patient management and document repository systems. However, before the physician can retrieve the documents from the repository, he must obtain the patient identifier for

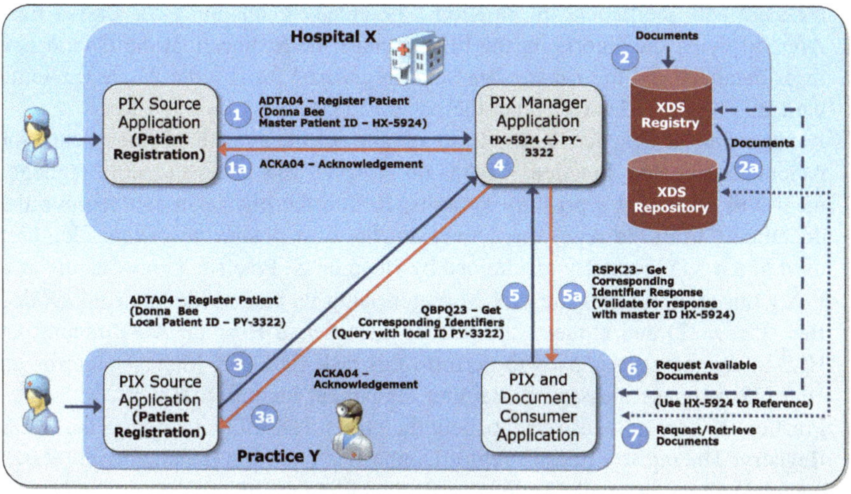

Fig. 13.9 Patient identification cross-referencing workflow

the corresponding setting used by Hospital X's document repository (which could be an implementation of the IHE XDS Registry and Repository). Practice Y acting as a PIX Consumer queries the PIX Manager using its patient identifier for Donna Bee (PY-3322) and requests the patient identifier in Hospital X's domain. An HL7 query message is used to perform this task. The PIX Manager returns an HL7 response message containing the patient identifier (HX-5924). Once the patient identifier is acquired, it can be used to query for available documents in the registry and retrieve these documents from the repository.

1. Hospital X has a patient administration system (ADT) that includes a PIX Source actor. When a new patient, Donna Bee, is registered through the system, the PIX Source generates a patient identifier (HX-5924). Using the identifier and demographic data, an HL7 message (Patient Identity Feed—PIF) is constructed and sent to the PIX Manager that is part of Hospital X's health information technology system.
2. Documents pertaining to patient Donna Bee are registered and uploaded into a repository (XDS) from various document sources (internally, at Hospital X, or externally). This repository maintains a master patient identifier for accessing the documents. For the purposes of this example, this identifier is HX-5924 established in the previous step.
3. Donna Bee now visits Practice Y for a medical procedure. Practice Y has a patient registration system (ADT) that includes a PIX Source actor, and a PIF message is sent to the PIX Manager. Donna Bee's patient identifier at Practice Y is PY-3322.
4. The PIX Manager, upon receiving the message from Practice Y for Donna Bee, applies its cross referencing algorithm to compare the demographics data in this

message with the patient information it is already maintaining for Donna Bee. After applying the algorithm, the PIX Manager determines that the *Donna Bee* in its database and the *Donna Bee* being registered for Practice Y are the same patient. The PIX Manager links the patient identifiers for Donna Bee.
5. A physician at Practice Y wants to obtain pertinent medical documents for patient Donna Bee. Practice Y relies on Hospital X's patient identity management and document repository systems. Before the physician can retrieve the documents from the repository, however, he must obtain the patient identifier used in the XDS Registry maintained by Hospital X. Practice Y, now acting as a PIX Consumer, queries the PIX Manager using its patient identifier for Donna Bee (PY-3322) and requests the patient identifier in Hospital X's domain. An HL7 query message is used to perform this task. The PIX Manager returns an HL7 V2 response message containing the patient identifier (HX-5924).
6. Practice Y can now use the patient identifier HX-5924 to query the XDS Registry. The registry doesn't return Donna Bee's clinical documents; it returns metadata about the available documents, including the identifiers and location to retrieve them. Note that the registry manages documents created in Hospital X and other document sources (potentially other hospitals, clinics, etc.).
7. The physician at Practice Y reviews the information and can use the references to retrieve the desired documents from the Document Repository.

Successful completion of the above case study requires that each application involved in the process correctly performs certain tasks that can be measured based on the application's externally observable behavior. The requirements on the application's external behavior can be formulated as a set of conformance and interoperability testing requirements. Among others, they include message validation and functional behavior validation. Each system involved in a message exchange must send messages that adhere to the message construction requirements defined by the associated standard. Additionally, HL7 messages are further constrained based on the use case, and must also validate against the corresponding message conformance message profile [6, 15]. Assessing functional requirements necessitates evaluation of message content. Although no explicit interoperability requirements have been defined, successful completion of all of the steps in the workflow provides a prima facie demonstration of interoperability among the systems.

In the following example, specific test steps for a test case are derived from the above scenario. Although the test case is simple, it provides a representative set of applications and steps that have to be accounted for in testing and supported by a test system. One patient (Donna Bee) is registered in different domains. The registration messages are sent to a Cross Reference Manager. A PIX Query is sent to resolve a reference to patient Donna Bee in a specific domain. Patient Donna Bee is expected to be found.

Step 1: Hospital X PIX Source sends a registration message (ADT^A04) to register patient Donna Bee in domain HOSP-X. Patient ID is HX-5924.

The PIX Manager shall register the patient and send an Acknowledgement (ACK) message back the PIX Source.

Step 2: Practice Y PIX Source sends a registration message (ADT^A04) to register patient Donna Bee in domain PRAC-Y. Patient ID is PY-3322. The PIX Manager shall register the patient and send an ACK message back to the PIX Source.

Step 3: Practice Y PIX Consumer sends a query message (QBP^Q23) to ask for Donna Bee's ID in domain HOSP-X using their ID PY-3322 in domain PRAC-Y. The PIX Manager is expected to respond to the query with Donna Bee's ID HX-5924 in domain HOSP-X.

13.4 Testing Frameworks

In a previous section, we discussed the concept of the testing infrastructure that provided an unfastened collection of components that can be used to support testing. The infrastructure provides the foundation for building testing frameworks and, ultimately, specific test tools. Testing frameworks can be realized for each of the testing models described in Chap. 10. The sections that follow present the test frameworks that support the data instance, isolated system testing, and peer-to-peer test models.

13.4.1 Data Instance Test Framework

Data instance testing has a specific focus: validating a test object (e.g., message) with respect to a specification (e.g., an HL7 V2.5.1 ORU R01 conformance profile). Figure 13.10 presents a representative model of a testing framework design to support the *data instance* testing model. This is one realization of the data instance testing model; other testing frameworks can be built to support the model.

The test framework utilizes a test execution engine and various services. Figure 13.4 (in the Sect. 13.2.4.2) shows the sequence of events for conducting the validation. The framework is designed to handle any version of the standard, message type, and constraint variations (conformance profiles). For instance, a test framework for supporting validation of HL7 v2.x messages can be built using this model. The repository contains the set of XML HL7 v2.x conformance message profiles of interest. When a new profile is to be tested, it is added to the repository. The framework could handle all versions of the standard, all message types, and all levels of conformance profiles for each message type. Similarily, the framework can support validation of CDA documents or NCPDP SCRIPT (ePrescribing) messages. The test framework provides a modular and flexible architecture that can be adapted to suit the testing need.

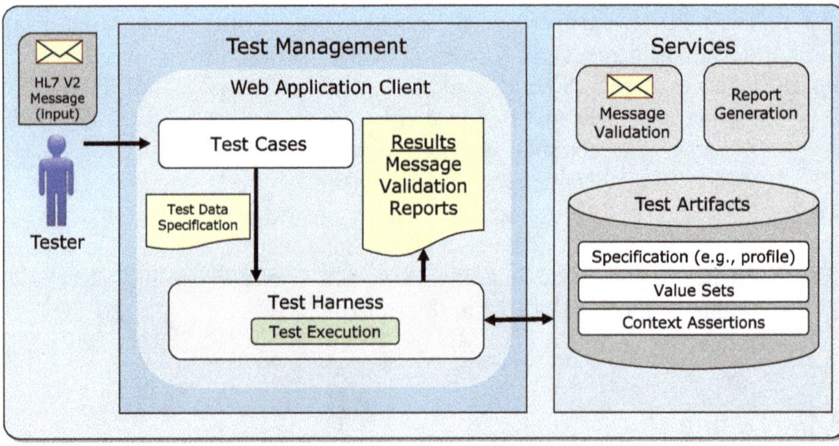

Fig. 13.10 Data instance test framework

A distinction between context-free and context-based testing can be made in this testing model. In context-free testing, the specification requirements are all that is needed. In context-based testing, an additional validation specification (context assertions) is needed for testing the content associated with a test scenario (e.g., the registration message in Step 1 for the test scenario given in Sect. 13.3).

In the context of our test scenario, a message produced by a system can be tested. This is usually the first step in the assessment of the system, but does it meet the requirements specified in the standard for a message? For example, for PIX Source, does it create a conformant registration message (ADT A04) in accordance to the IHE PIX Integration Profile specification? As described in Chap. 11 for context-free testing, not all requirements can be tested, for example, the RE-required but maybe empty usage construct. In order to extend the testing coverage, context-based testing is employed. Here a test data specification is given, which is used as input for creating a message in the system and to codify the additional requirements. This becomes supplementary input to the validation engine. In terms of the test scenario, support for RE and Conditional (C) data elements can now be assessed. For example, Patient Address is RE,[6] and, thus, to test for support of this element, data are provided as part of the test case.

A number of NIST 2014 and 2015 Edition ONC Certification test tools (see Chap. 14 for more details) are a realization of the data instance test framework. The test framework is used to instantiate the laboratory results interface, reportable laboratory results, immunization, syndromic surveillance, and ePrescribing test tools. For each domain, an implementation guide describes the requirements. These

[6]Actually IHE defines this concept as R2.

requirements are codified in an XML conformance message profile (see Chaps. 7 and 8). The validation engine processes and interprets the specific requirements and performs an assessment based on the rules established in the underlying standard. The conformity assessment tables provided in Chap. 12 express in detail the outcome of the analysis. An obvious advantage of this approach is that requirements are captured in a standardized, codified format that can be interpreted uniformly in a machine-processable manner. The validation engine is based on a rule interpreter that can process the standardized machine-processable format. Separation of the requirements (rules) specification and requirements (rules) interpretation provides a powerful and flexible approach for accomplishing validation.

13.4.2 Isolated System Test Framework

As described in Chap. 10, in the isolated system testing model a test is conducted with the SUT and a test tool. Conformance testing, including data exchange and functional testing, is the main objective in using this model. Functional testing is achieved with a test scenario in which a sequence of orchestrated transactions is created to probe certain requirements. The test framework simulates (or includes) functionality of an application (i.e., test agent) that an SUT would typically interact with in an operational environment. Once a system has successfully undergone conformance testing, interoperability testing usually proceeds more easily.

An example testing framework to support isolated system testing is illustrated in Fig. 13.11. The test framework utilizes additional components to accommodate interaction with the SUT—in particular, a proxy, communication capabilities, and test agent functionality. The test framework as shown incorporates a user interface depicted in the form of a web application. This example test framework model can be used to build test systems.

The test framework employs a number of services provided by a testing infrastructure, including message generation and validation, a data source, test agents, report generation, communication (transport) support, and a repository to maintain artifacts needed for testing. A Proxy is employed to intercept, persist, and forward message exchanges. The test manager is a web application that provides the functionality to present and manage test cases and results. Additionally, a test execution component is employed to control the operation of the test execution. The test management module provides a template for the user interface aspects of the test framework. The communication module is used to support message exchange among the test agents and the SUT. The SUT provides its own communication infrastructure. The framework can be developed to support multiple communication protocols (e.g., SOAP and MLLP). Messages and documents are routed through the Proxy and are stored such that validation can be performed at the direction of test harness.

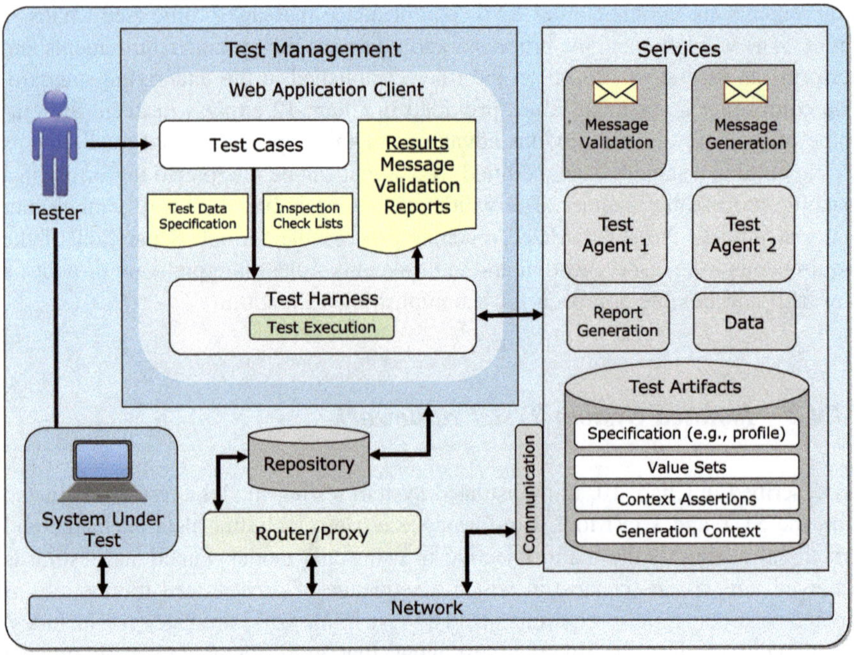

Fig. 13.11 Isolated system testing framework model

The foremost design principle for developing a test framework is the use of modular components that allow for reuse and flexibility for building specific test tools. The test framework provides a core set of capabilities that can be leveraged. The communication infrastructure is used to support transport for a number of protocols. The test agent design provides an API and utilities, enabling specific test agents to be built. For instance, an HL7 v2.x generic test agent is built that provides an API to access functions, parse messages, map data to a common internal object representation, and provide control. For a specific test agent, the actor (application) functionality still needs to be provided; however, the import, export, and transformation to an information model is provided by the testing framework. This approach expedites the creation of a test agent for developers.

13.4.3 Peer-to-Peer Testing Framework

Peer-to-peer system testing is designed to test interoperability among one or more systems. The peer-to-peer system testing model poses different and significant challenges in testing from that of isolated system testing. In this environment, data exchange occurs among a group of systems, and the testing tool no longer has direct interaction with the systems under test. Here, an intermediary or a proxy can be employed to intercept, log, and route messages to their intended destination. Peer-to-peer system testing may include some or all of the conformance testing described for isolated system testing. When conformance testing is conducted in advance, peer-to-peer testing specifically targets both syntactic interoperability testing and semantic interoperability testing. The conformance test cases that were developed for isolated system testing can be leveraged in peer-to-peer testing. The abstract test cases could be identical; however, execution of the test steps, configuration requirements, and assertion assessment will differ. By ascertaining that the conformance requirements are now met in an environment where the SUTs are interacting, we can make a declaration of the interoperability capabilities of the systems.

As with the Isolated System Testing, frameworks to support peer-to-peer testing can be built by leveraging the components of a testing infrastructure. The IHE Gazelle toolkit is an example for such testing framework [22]. Figure 13.12 illustrates an example model for a peer-to-peer testing framework. In many aspects it is similar to the Isolated System Testing framework. Section 13.5.3 demonstrates an instantiation of the Peer-to-Peer Testing Framework in the form of an Interoperability Test Bed (ITB).

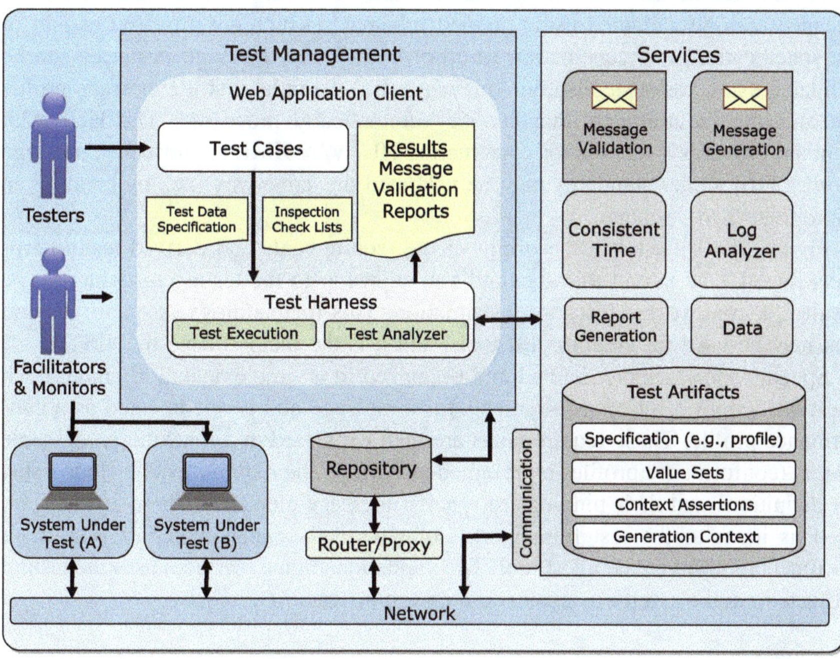

Fig. 13.12 Peer-to-peer testing framework model

13.5 Instantiation of Test Tools

Section 13.1 presented an approach for designing and organizing test system architectures. Various testing frameworks that support the testing models described in Chap. 10 can be built from the testing infrastructure. This section describes the final step of the approach, which leads to specific test tool creation. The goal of presenting the possible conformance and interoperability testing architectures in this manner is to show typical constituent parts, organization, and design. This approach for designing and building test architectures is not the only suitable approach. Chapter 14 shows examples of test tool instantiations.

13.5.1 Data Instance Testing Test Tool

Once the framework is established, specific tools can be built. A key step in this process is the creation of the test artifacts. For simple context-free data instance testing, this step involves capturing the requirements and expressing them in a machine-processable format. As previously discussed, this format can be XML files that codify the requirements such that assertions can be made during testing. Examples include CDA (XML documents) and HL7 v2.x message profiles. CDA instances can be validated using defined schemas[7] (which are provided as part of the specification) and schematron assertions. HL7 v2.x message instances can be validated using various constraint languages. It is essential that the message profile contains the requirements that can be automatically processed. The HL7 v2.x standard provides a schema for constructing HL7 v2.x XML conformance message profiles [16]. Other standards may be validated the same way, i.e., by creating an appropriate XML schema.

Figure 13.13 illustrates the origin of the requirements and derived testing artifacts for HL7 v2.x, and this standard's relationship to the testing machinery. The result is a context-free test tool instantiation. This methodology is one of several that may be used for creating test tools, and it is the method used by NIST.

Specific use cases are defined and organized in an implementation guide. Each use case defines a set of requirements for a message and is documented as a conformance profile. These requirements are then expressed in a machine-processable format (conformance profiles represented as XML). The requirements include value set definitions and their bindings to specific message elements. These artifacts are used as input to the test framework along with associated materials (e.g., user documentation) to create a test tool. The validation engine (service) uses the testing artifacts to make assertions against a message instance.

[7] The XML schemas provided are considered informative, because, although they are created according to the specification, they may contain errors. Therefore, the published standard is normative, while XML schemas are for convenience.

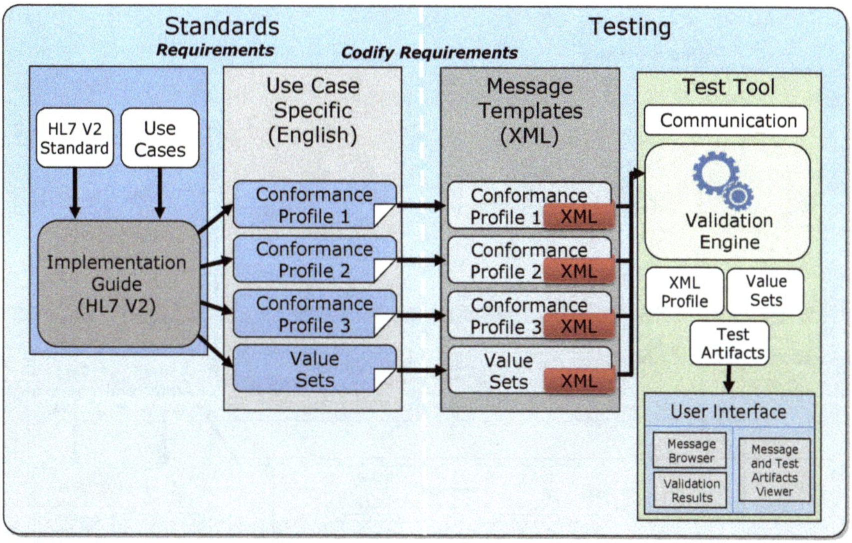

Fig. 13.13 Generic context-free HL7 v2 test tool instantiation

A second instantiation of the data instance testing model is that of context-based testing (Fig. 13.14). To support context-based testing, specific test cases and test data are needed. Various use cases defined in an implementation guide are identified, and selected scenarios are determined. For each scenario one or more test cases can be developed along with the associated test data. Depending on what the Tester wishes to test, additional assertions are created and communicated to the validation service. As indicated previously, providing test data allows Testers to expand the scope of testing, for example, verifying that the SUT supports a specific coded value or conditional elements. The testing process and system described for context-based testing support assessment of both sender and receiver (by creating inspection documents) applications. See Chap. 11.

The design goal of the testing infrastructure and test framework is to build specific test tool instances for a targeted implementation guide. Chapter 14 presents examples of test tools that follow this approach.

13.5.2 Isolated System Testing Test Tool

From the information provided above, it follows that the Isolated System Test Framework can be leveraged to construct domain-specific conformance testing tools for this testing model. A central design principle of the testing framework is

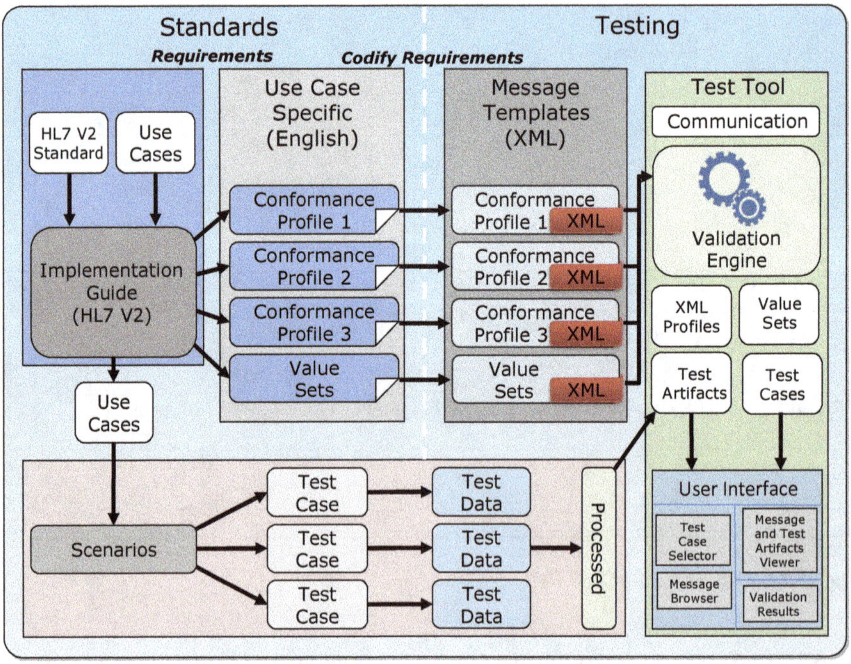

Fig. 13.14 Generic context-based HL7 v2.x test tool instantiation

that it leverages components from the testing infrastructure, and, once built, the testing framework can be leveraged to build specific test tool instances. For example, the testing framework described (in Sect. 13.4.2) is used to build the NIST PIX/PDQ and PCD (Patient Care Devices) IHE pre-connect-a-thon test tools [17, 18]. Figure 13.15 shows a test tool instantiation, focusing on the components for testing the IHE PIX integration profiles for both HL7 v2 and V3. The process of creating the test artifacts that was described for data instance testing is equally applicable in this case, and it is indicated in the figure as the "Test Artifacts" component.

Many of the core components in the test framework are reusable. For example, the same test agents are used for PIX v2 and V3, since the functional requirements are the same, although a different protocol is used to exchange messages. The HL7 v2 message generation and message validation services are again key components in this tool. Additionally, since this test tool supports the IHE HL7 V3 PIX/PDQ integration profiles, the test tool accesses the HL7 V3 message generation and message validation services. Associated test artifacts specific to the PIX/PDQ domain are created for both the HL7 v2 and V3 environments (e.g., an XML representation of the HL7 v2 ADT_A04 registration message conformance profile specific for PIX). The framework allows tool builders to concentrate on the domain-specific aspects, such as development of the test cases and providing the functionality of the test agents.

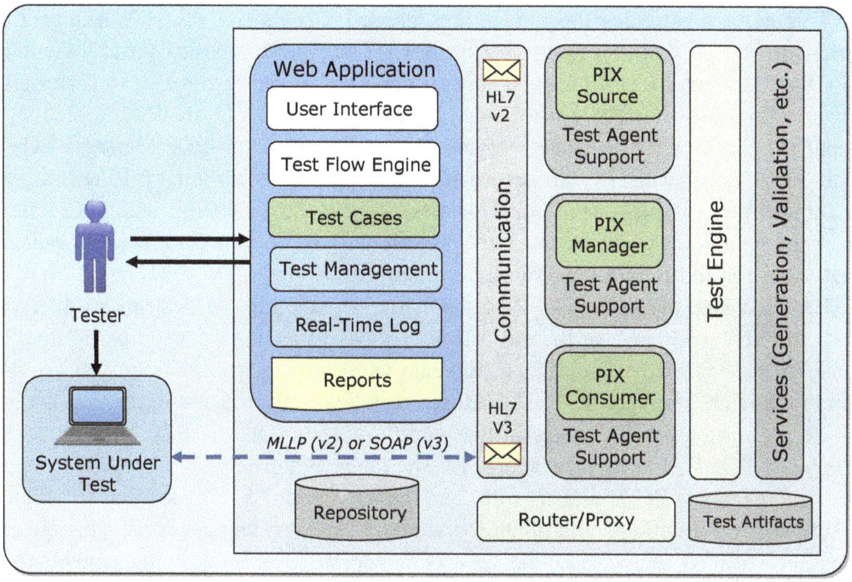

Fig. 13.15 PIX/PDQ pre-connect-a-thon testing tool

Figure 13.16 depicts an abridged test system and its interaction with a PIX Manager application (the SUT) for the transactions described in the test scenario given in Sect. 13.3. Note that steps (2), (4), (6) and (7) are not included in this illustration because these steps involve an internal PIX Manager operation or XDS transactions (i.e., are not HL7 v2 transactions, which are the focus of PIX/PDQ test tool).

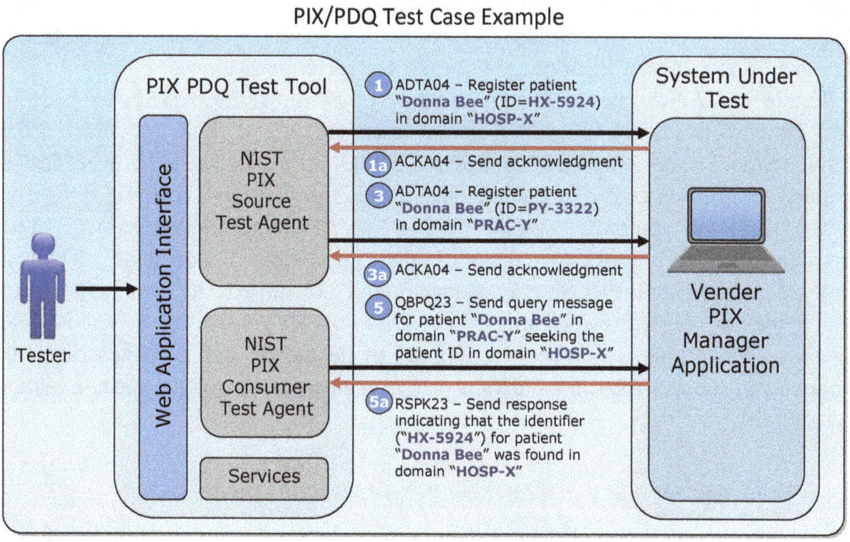

Fig. 13.16 PIX test case workflow

This system provides the capabilities needed to evaluate the PIX Manager's behavior. The PIX Source and PIX Consumer Test Agents are deployed by the test tool for this scenario. Once the test agent is deployed, it can be directed to perform a given action. For example, for the first step in our use case (1), the PIX Source test agent can be directed to send a registration message to the PIX Manager SUT. The PIX Manager SUT, in accordance with its specification, will return an acknowledgement message (1a). The message can be evaluated using the HL7 message validation web service. The response will depend on the message content that was sent and is indicated by the test script.

For each step along the way, the test harness directs the test agents to interact with the SUT and can use the validation services to evaluate responses. Message generation services can be utilized to create valid messages, which the test agents send to the PIX Manager SUT. The test script indicates the content of the data given to the generation service. Later in the workflow, testing of the PIX Manager will employ a PIX Consumer test agent. As shown in Fig. 13.16, the PIX Consumer queries (5) the PIX Manager with one patient identifier, requesting a patient identifier for the same patient in another domain. The test harness creates the query message with assistance from the generation service. The harness then directs the PIX Consumer test agent to send the query message to the PIX Manager. The PIX Manager is expected to send a response message (5a) back to the PIX Consumer. The test harness now can request the message from the PIX Consumer so the message can be evaluated (this method uses the Test Agent for proxy services, alternatively a central proxy can be used to capture all messages). The test harness knows the context of the use case, which aids in evaluation of assertions (i.e., it will know exactly the patient identifier that should be returned). The results of the evaluations can be displayed to the user via the browser interface. Seeing the method used for evaluating the PIX Manager SUT, it follows that the approach can be used to evaluate the other actors described in the workflow. It should be noted that use of the web browser client and test harness model for controlling the test is just one option chosen from many possible service compositions.

Figure 13.17 illustrates an excerpt of the test flow of the Isolated System Testing Test Framework for the PIX test scenario described in Sect. 13.3, specifically, the derived Step 3 (Query the PIX Manager) in the test scenario. Table 13.4 provides a detailed description of the individual steps needed to execute a test step.

By using the approach presented above for providing testing services, it is possible to test each application (actor) in the test scenario independently. The test tool supports testing a PIX Source, Manager, and Consumer. The perspective from which the test steps are interpreted is based on which application is the SUT. Likewise, the test agents evoked are imposed by the SUT. Chapter 14 describes the front-end of the test tool and shows how a user interacts with it to execute tests.

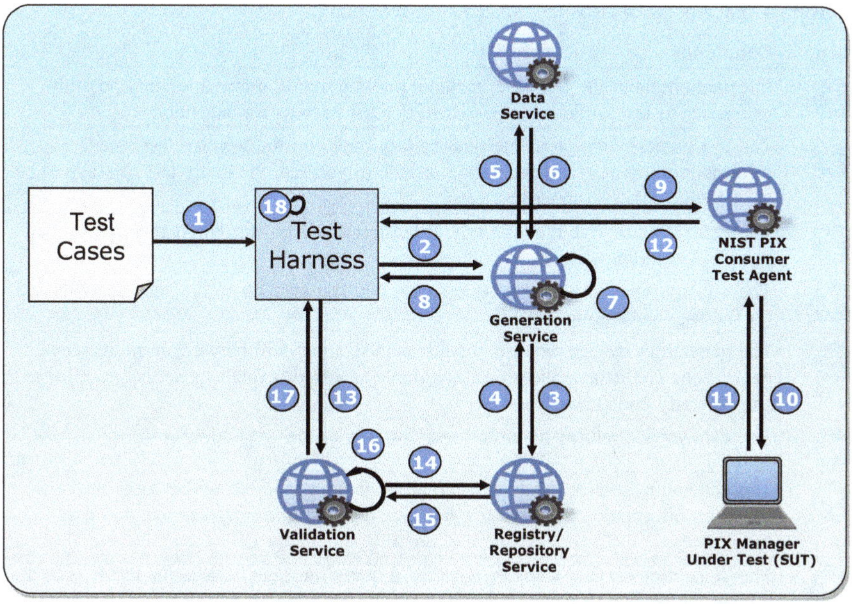

Fig. 13.17 Isolated system testing—test flow excerpt

13.5.3 Interoperability Test Bed

The next step in the evolution of the testing system is the interoperability test bed, as described in [19]. The interoperability test bed supports the peer-to-peer testing model that accommodates multiple systems under test. Most of the components of the testing framework that support isolated system testing can be leveraged. Key technical challenges that arise in peer-to-peer testing are coordinating the actions of the multiple systems being tested, intercepting interactions for evaluation, and assessing how systems incorporated and use the data. The testing framework functionality is expanded to address these challenges.

Figure 13.18 depicts a scaled-down design of the architecture that employs a set of fundamental components and operating procedures necessary to conduct testing. A description of each component and its capability is provided followed by an abbreviated step-by-step test flow.

13.5.3.1 Operational Functions

The interoperability test bed has a number of logical operational divisions including scheduling, configuration, test setup, test execution, results reporting, and analysis. A summary of these functions are given below.

Table 13.4 Excerpt set of steps for isolated system testing

Step	Description
1	Information about the test case, including configuration information and possibly references to test artifacts are passed to the test harness for execution
2	The test harness orchestrates testing activity based on the selected test case. Information is sent to the generation service to generate the query test message to be used by the PIX consumer test agent
3	The generation service requests referenced test artifacts from the registry/repository service—including generation context files
4	The registry/repository service sends requested test artifacts to the generation service for message generation
5	The generation service requests the test data sets that will be used in the message generation. The data service itself may have accessed a value set service to retrieve and/or verify coded data
6	The data service returns requested test data sets to the generation service
7	The generation service conducts internal processing to generate the query message based on information from the test harness, registry/repository service, and data service
8	The generation service sends the generated query message back to the test harness to initiate the testing sequence Alternatively (not shown), the generation service may also be accessed via test agents or other software
9	The test harness sends the query message generated previously to the PIX consumer test agent
10	The PIX consumer test agent sends the query message to the PIX manager SUT
11	The PIX manager SUT processes the query message according to its internal logic and sends a response message to the PIX consumer test agent
12	Upon receipt, the PIX consumer test agent sends the response message created by the PIX Manager SUT to the test harness
13	The test harness sends the response message along with references to testing artifacts to the validation service
14	The validation service requests referenced testing artifacts from the registry/repository service
15	The registry/repository service sends the requested testing artifacts to the validation service
16	Using the response message and the testing artifacts, the validation service validates the message
17	The validation service returns the results of the validation to the test harness
18	The test harness will communicate results to the calling application and continue with the next test step if applicable

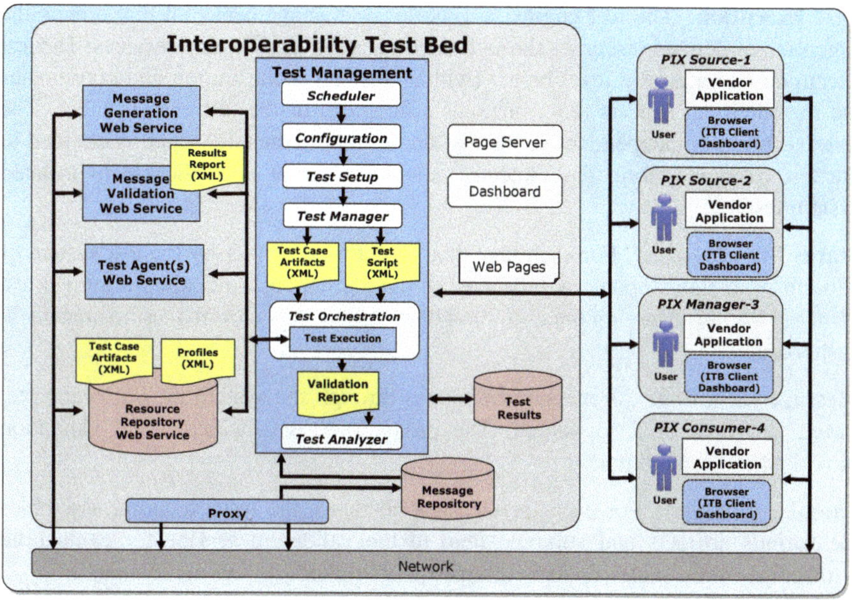

Fig. 13.18 Interoperability test bed architecture

Scheduling: A scheduling system is required to coordinate the vendors that participate in the testing. The system matches up testing partners based on their test selection, actors, and time availability. Vendors input their testing interests, product capabilities, and times they're available, and the scheduler pairs-up aligned requests and notifies the participants.

Configuration: The configuration utility records the connection and addressing information required for communicating with each participant's product. This information is necessary for the ITB to prime the proxy to handle intercepting and forwarding of messages.

Test Setup: Test setup includes informing each of the participants of the test instructions associated with the test case, which includes their roles, actions required, data requirements, and system configuration (e.g., loading test data in the data base).

Test Management: The test manager controls the overall operation of the ITB. These activities include managing simultaneous test executions and initiating test case instance executions.

Test Orchestration: The test management system relies on a test orchestration component to organize and coordinate the collective activities of the vendors and the test system. Information (e.g., instructions and status) is disseminated through a common shared user interface and a participant-perspective user interface. A test script encapsulates the choreographed steps and participant actions.

Test Execution: The test engine is a workflow management tool that directs the execution of defined test cases through the orchestration of testing services. The test execution operates at a level below (within) the test orchestration and coordinates the measurement aspects (e.g., message validation) of the test case instance. The test execution is independent of the test orchestration since its scope is coupled to the test case; therefore, the same test execution script is applicable to isolated system testing.

Status Broadcasting: For each task that is performed either by the test system or participant, a status update is broadcast to the participants, including a human test manager who is observing the execution of the test instance from a test management dashboard.

Message Handling: As messages progress through the system they are captured, stored, analyzed, and forwarded. The proxy, message database, and validation provide these capabilities.

Singular Analysis: For each interaction (message), the test execution assembles the various artifacts and submits them to the validation service for evaluation. A machine-processable report is returned and rendered to the participants.

Collective Analysis: A test case instance consists of numerous steps for the applications being tested, and it creates many individual validation reports. A *test analyzer* is necessary to make a collective determination of the test results. The test analyzer can use the test script for navigating, linking, and analyzing the array of validation reports.

Storing Test Results: Upon completion of the test instance execution, the test results are stored for analysis and auditing purposes.

13.5.3.1.1 Simulating a Vendor System

The ITB includes the capability to supply a simulated vendor system(s) as a testing partner when the participating systems needed for testing are not available or are not available at the desired time. This feature of the system provided by the ITB includes message generation and test agent services. Having one SUT and all test agents is essentially equivalent to isolated system testing provided by the pre-connectathon testing tools. The ITB encapsulates this model.

13.5.3.2 Test Flow

The test flow describes each of the actions required by the ITB and the participants to perform the test case instance. The test case calls for four applications (as indicated in the example test scenario) or application modules. There are two PIX sources (PS-1 and PS-2), a PIX Manager (PM-3), and a PIX Consumer (PC-4). The

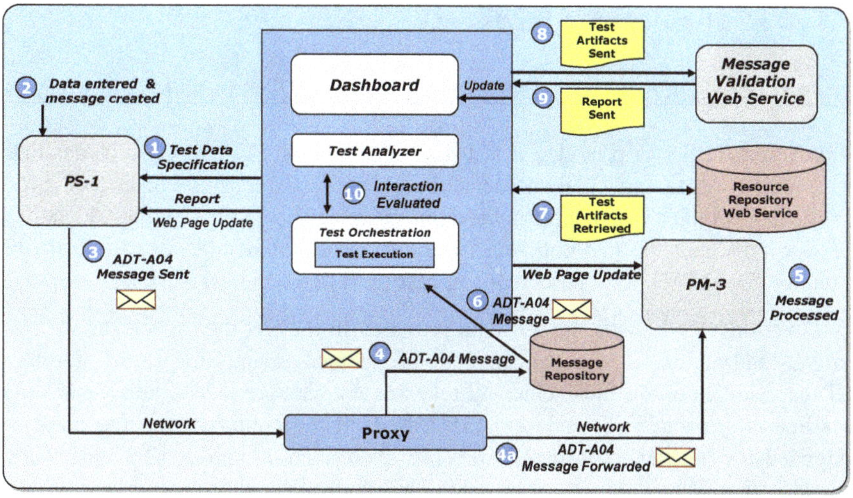

Fig. 13.19 Test flow for transaction 1, interaction 1

sections that follow focus on the operational aspects of the test instance. Figure 13.19 illustrates the events as they progress through the ITB for the Transaction 1 and Interaction 1 described below. The example test case presented is a "happy path" scenario; test cases for "exception paths" equally apply and can be demonstrated.

13.5.3.2.1 Scheduling and Configuration

The Scheduler is an independent operational component of the ITB and is part of the test management. For the purpose of discussion here, it is assumed that the scheduling, configuration, participant assignment, and test selection have been completed.

13.5.3.2.2 Test Execution Status Evaluation and Progress Display

A common shared display is a key feature of the ITB, and it is used to inform the participants in a timely manner of an action that is required by them and to provide visual progress of the test case instance execution. As each event occurs, the display updates, and test execution analysis is performed. A fine level of granularity is needed (e.g., interaction level) to track progression of the test execution or provide notification of failure.

13.5.3.2.3 Orchestration of Events

Transaction 1, Interaction 1—PIX Source 1 sends ADT message to PIX Manager

ITB Action: PS-1 is provided a test data specification (1),[8] which includes data (e.g., patient name and DOB) associated with the test story and consists of information that is typically available in the administrative and clinical settings. Together, the test story and the test data specification provide sufficient information to be entered into the SUT for a particular test case such that a message can be generated.

PS-1 Action: PS-1 loads the test data provided in the test data specification; typically, loading is a manual process performed using the user interface (UI) capabilities of the SUT. Once all relevant test data are loaded into the PS-1, a message is generated (2) and sent (3). Based on the configuration, the message (intended for the PM-3) is sent to the ITB proxy. PS-1, via the ITB dashboard, indicates that it has sent the message. This controlled execution eases the test instance navigation for the test execution engine.

ITB Action: The ITB proxy captures and stores the message in the message repository (4) along with pertinent message meta-data (some of which is provided by the test execution based on context) that provide sufficient information to map the message to the interaction (i.e., associate the PS-1, the test case instance, and the message).

ITB Action: The ITB test execution polls (or alternatively, the test execution subscribes to the message repository for events, and the message repository pushes events accordingly) the message repository for the interaction of interest. The ITB test engine retrieves the message from the message repository (6) and the conformance validation artifacts from the resource repository (7) and invokes the validation service to validate the message (8).

ITB Action: The ITB test analyzer evaluates the interaction along with validation results to determine if any detected errors would prevent the test from continuing (10). Note, inconsequential conformance issues are not pertinent at this point; the focus is on the delivery of the message and key data elements that might prevent other participants from completing their tasks. If a severe fault is detected, the test orchestration notifies all participants accordingly via the common shared display capability and then ends the test instance.

ITB Action: The ITB proxy forwards the message to the PM-3 (4a). Note that there are two design choices for handling this operation, each with pros and cons. The proxy could automatically forward messages upon receipt or wait for instructions from the test execution. We'll choose the former option for discussion purposes here.

[8] Represents the point in the Test Flow for Transaction 1, Interaction 1 diagram.

Post Interaction 1—Instructions and Status

ITB Action: The test orchestration reports that Interaction 1 is completed, and the common user interface display is updated accordingly. The validation report for the interaction is made available to the participants (9). The ITB now instructs PS-2 to begin Interaction 2. Note that the ITB also updates the status at intermediate events, for example, when the message is received by the proxy or forwarded.

Transaction 1, Interaction 2—PIX Manager processes ADT message

PM-3 Action: PM-3 receives, parses, and evaluates the message for acceptance (5). Based on its internal system evaluation, it creates and sends an appropriate acknowledgement message.

ITB Action: The ITB proxy captures and stores the message in the message repository. The ITB retrieves the message and validates it as described previously.

ITB Action: The ITB analyzer evaluates the interaction along with validation results to determine if any detected errors would prevent the test from continuing. In this instance, an obvious error that would halt the process would be the PM-3 rejecting the message.

PM-3 Action: Upon determining that the message is able to be processed, the PM-3 extracts the relevant data elements and assimilates the data into their system. The PM-3 enacts its patient matching algorithm to determine if this patient already exists in its database, and, if so, PM-3 links the patient. Since the test setup did not include this patient, no match is found.

ITB Action: The acknowledgement message is forwarded to PS-1.

PS-1 Action: PS-1 receives, parses, and processes the acknowledgement message. If there is an indication that the message was processed by PM-3, the transaction is completed.

Post Transaction 1—Instructions and Status

ITB Action: The test orchestration reports that Transaction 1 is completed and the common user interface display is updated accordingly. The validation reports for the transaction are made available to the participants. The ITB now instructs PS-2 to begin Transaction 2.

Transaction 2—PIX Source 2 sends ADT message to PIX Manager

Transaction 2 transpires much like Transaction 1. One significant difference is that PM-3 should be able to link the patient Donna Bee based on the information it received from PS-1 and PS-2; however, this capability is a functional aspect that is internal to PM-3. From the test case processing point of view, Transaction 1 and Transaction 2 are the same; therefore, we will not explicitly explain this transaction.

Post Transaction 2—Instructions and Status

ITB Action: The test orchestration reports that Transaction 2 is completed and the common display is updated accordingly. The ITB now instructs PC-4 to begin Transaction 3.

Transaction 3, Interaction 1—PIX Consumer queries the PIX Manager

ITB Action: PC-4 is provided a test data specification that includes relevant data elements to construct the query request in accordance with the test case data.

PC-4 Action: PC-4 loads the test data provided in the test data specification. Once all relevant test data are loaded by the PC-4, a message is generated and sent. Based on the configuration, the message is sent to the ITB proxy (intended for the PM-3). PC-4, via the ITB dashboard, indicates that it has sent the message; this controlled execution eases the test instance navigation for the test execution engine.

ITB Action: The ITB proxy captures and stores the message in the message repository. The ITB retrieves the message and validates as described previously.

ITB Action: The ITB test analyzer evaluates the interaction along with the validation results to determine if any detected errors would prevent the test from continuing.

ITB Action: The ITB proxy forwards the query message to the PM-3.

Post Transaction 3, Interaction 1—Instructions and Status

ITB Action: The test orchestration reports that Transaction 3 and Interaction 1 are completed, and the common user interface display is updated accordingly. The validation report for the interaction is made available to the participants.

Transaction 3, Interaction 2—PIX Manager processes query message

PM-3 Action: PM-3 receives, parses, and evaluates the query message for acceptance. Upon determining that the message is able to be processed, the PM-3 extracts the relevant data elements to find out if a master patient identifier exists based on the request. Given the test setup, the PM-3 should find the master patient identifier. The PM-3 constructs and sends a response message to the proxy (intended for PC-4).

ITB Action: The ITB proxy captures and stores the response message in the message repository. The ITB retrieves the message and validates as described previously. An important aspect in the validation not mentioned before is the evaluation of specific data content. In this particular operation, the validation checks for a specific patient identifier based on the test case data specification, and, therefore, the PM-3 functional behavior is assessed.

ITB Action: The ITB analyzer evaluates the interaction along with validation results to determine if any detected errors would prevent the test from continuing. In this instance, an obvious error that would halt the process would the PM-3 rejecting the message.

ITB Action: The response message is forwarded to PC-4.

PC-4 Action: PC-4 receives, parses, and processes the response message. At this point PC-4 can use the master patient identifier for the purposes of retrieving documents or other actions (out of scope for this example).

ITB Action: At this stage, Transaction 3 and the test case instance are complete; and the status is updated accordingly.

13.5.3.2.4 Analysis and Results Reporting

Upon completion of the test case instance, the test analyzer evaluates the collective results and determines the outcome of the test instance. This information, along with the individual interaction validation reports, is provided to the participants. The vendors can use these test results, as well as logging information and the observed behavior of their system, to further assess the performance of their product. A test manager can review the reports to assess the test instance. If desired, all related test instance data are stored in the test management system for auditing purposes.

13.5.3.2.5 Discussion

Although we have presented here a simplified portrayal of the architecture and case study, it still should be evident that the ITB provides the capabilities to conduct conformance and interoperability testing in support of distributed healthcare applications for a broad assortment of test cases essential for comprehensive testing. For example, an interoperability test may stipulate incorporation and display of laboratory results into an EHR. In this case, completely automated black box testing is unattainable; however, an inspection document based on the test data would be created dynamically and provided for this test step. Screen shots of the vendor's display and/or data base can be captured and submitted to the test system for visual evaluation by a monitor. A monitor will use the inspection document to verify expected behavior.

Also, different variations to the normal ("happy path") test scenario should be tested to ascertain how implementations perform under error conditions. Examples include missing required elements, incorrect coded information, or differences in syntactical representations that are allowed by the underlying standard.

13.5.3.3 Need for the ITB

IHE testing employs a number of incremental testing methods. First, vendors conduct conformance testing of their products. This task involves testing in isolation to determine if the system implements the requirements specified in the standard. These tests are labelled pre-connect-a-thon tests and correspond to the isolated system test model. Interoperability testing (peer-to-peer testing) is conducted at an event called a connect-a-thon in which scores of vendors bring their products to a central site, and live-monitored tests are performed over a period of a week [1]. Such concentrated events are useful, as a vendor can interact with many other vendors in a short period of time; however, connect-a-thons occur infrequently (once a year in the United States, Europe and Asia-Oceania) and are costly. One objective of the Interoperability Test Bed (ITB) is to provide an intermediate format in the form of an on-line virtual connect-a-thon in which interoperability testing is always available at any time.

In the connect-a-thon environment, participants indicate what they want to test and publish their availability. Once testing partners reach agreement, their systems are configured in the test bed and they can proceed with testing. The ITB leverages the testing infrastructure and implements the peer-to-peer testing model.

The NIST IHE Patient Identification Cross-referencing (PIX)/Patient Demographics Query (PDQ) [17] and Patient Care Devices (PCD) [18] pre-connect-a-thon test tools are examples of production implementations of the isolated system test model. The ITB is intended to extend this class of tools to a virtual connect-a-thon environment relying on the testing infrastructure as the anchor.

The ITB isn't fundamentally that different from the test system for the pre-connect-a-thon isolated test model. The main divergent point is testing multiple real systems instead of one, i.e., replacing some or all of the test agents in the isolated system environment with vendor products. This difference does, however, present noteworthy technical challenges including the scheduling of participants, sequencing of events and notification to the participants, and capturing/forwarding messages and then mapping the messages to the corresponding test case interaction.

13.5.3.4 Multiple Domain Test Scenarios and Testing

The test systems presented demonstrate how testing can be performed for a scenario that involves one data exchange protocol (HL7 v2 in the examples presented); often, however, broader scenarios need to be tested, such as those expressed in some of the IHE integration profiles. These scenarios include workflows that link HL7 v2 and XDS (the scenario presented), HL7 v2 and CDA, HL7 v2 and DICOM, etc.); and Test systems need to accommodate such test scenarios. The strategic design of the testing infrastructure and subsequent testing framework can support these requirements.

13.6 Summary

In practice, there are a variety of testing architecture approaches, but, in many respects, they have a common set of capabilities. The key capabilities were presented here. Many organizations and individuals have built tools to support testing a specific standard or a domain-constrained use of that standard. Although much fragmentation exists among the tool builders, each tool realization boils down to certain required functionality and, therefore, core components (e.g., message and document validation). This chapter attempts to add structure to those core components and defines an approach to the systematic development of tools. The approach is applicable to an array of healthcare data exchange standards including HL7 v2.x, HL7 V3, NCPDP SCRIPT, HL7 CDA, and others. The testing architectures presented focused on HL7 v2.x for a detailed test scenario.

The core of the approach is the testing infrastructure that is based on the SOA model, which allows the stakeholders to employ and combine testing services in arbitrary ways. The central design principle leverages components from the testing infrastructure and, once built, the testing framework can be leveraged to build specific test tool instances. This approach gives the stakeholders the capability to formulate solutions to problems based on the most effective use of the available services. The approach described herein is extensible and flexible, providing a framework that can support an expansive set of testing requirements. The stakeholder is afforded the flexibility to select the interface and environment in which they want to conduct testing. It is extensible, since services can be added and the composition of services can be built independently. Additionally, the framework scales well, since the set of services are independent, and services composition and test execution can occur spatially.

The test framework approach supports rapid test suite development, which can be accomplished independently and simultaneously. Stakeholders, such as certification testing laboratories or vendors testing in-house, can build the testing system that meets their requirements. Such an approach has been developed and adopted by NIST in the creation of HL7 v2.x tools used for ONC Health IT certification [3].

References

1. IHE Connect-a-thon, http://www.ihe.net/Connectathon/
2. ONC Certification Programs to Help Providers Choose EHR Technology; http://www.healthit.gov/providers-professionals
3. NIST Resources and Tools in Support of Health IT Standards and the ONC Meaningful Use certification program. http://healthcare.nist.gov/
4. Business Process Execution Language (BPEL), http://docs.oasis-open.org/wsbpel/2.0/wsbpel-v2.0.html
5. Snelick R, Gebase L, Henrard S. Dynamically Generating Conformance Tests for Messaging Systems. 2006 Software Engineering Research and Practice (SERP06), WORLDCOMP'06 June 26–29, 2006, Las Vegas, NV.

6. Snelick R, Rontey P, Gebase L, Carnahan L. Towards Interoperable Healthcare Information Systems: The HL7 Conformance Profile Approach. Enterprise Interoperability II: New Challenges and Approaches. Springer-Verlag, London Limited 2007 pp. 659–670.
7. NIST HL7 v2.x Validation Web Service. http://hl7v2.ws.nist.gov/hl7v2ws
8. NIST Special Publication 250-59. NIST Computer Time Services: Internet Time Service (ITS), Automated Computer Time Service (ACTS), and time.gov Web Sites http://www.nist.gov/calibrations/upload/sp250-59.pdf.
9. Digital Imaging and Communication in Medicine (DICOM), http://medical.nema.org.
10. MIRTH Connect; https://www.mirth.com/
11. Common Terminology Services 2 (CTS2), http://www.omg.org/spec/CTS2/1.0/
12. Integrating the Healthcare Enterprises (IHE). Technical Frameworks. http://www.ihe.net/Technical_Frameworks/
13. IHE IT Infrastructure (ITI) Technical Framework Integration Profile. http://www.ihe.net/Technical_Frameworks/#IT
14. Oemig F, Bender T. Was ist eine Domäne? und wie spielen sie zusammen? (What is a domain, and how do they interact?). In: eHealth 2015 - Informationstechnologien und Telematik im Gesundheitswesen, Eds: Prof. Dr. Frank Duesberg. medical future verlag. http://www.e-health-2015.de
15. Snelick R, Gebase L, O'Brien G. A Framework for testing Distributed Healthcare Applications. 2009 Software Engineering Research and Practice (SERP09), WORLDCOMP'09 July 13–16, 2009, Las Vegas, NV.
16. Health Level 7 (HL7) Standard Version 2.7. ANSI/HL7, January, 2011. http://www.hl7.org. Chapter 2B – Conformance.
17. NIST PIX/PDQ Pre-connect-a-thon Conformance Testing Tool. http://pixpdqtests.nist.gov:8080/
18. NIST IHE Patient Care Devices Pre-connect-a-thon Conformance Test Tool. http://ihe-pcd-precon.nist.gov/PCD-HL7WebPreCon/
19. Snelick R: An Interoperable Test Bed for Distributed Healthcare Applications. Enterprise Interoperability VI: Interoperability for Agility, Resilience and Plasticity of Collaborations. Springer International Publishing Switzerland 2014 pp. 489–499.
20. Gebase L, Snelick R, Skall M. Conformance Testing and Interoperability: A Case *Study in Healthcare Data Exchange*. 2008 Software Engineering Research and Practice (SERP08), WORLDCOMP'08 July 14–17, 2008, Las Vegas, NV.
21. Gebase L, Snelick R. Testing Environments for Assessing Conformance and Interoperability. 2010 Software Engineering Research and Practice (SERP10), WORLDCOMP'10 July 12–15, 2010, Las Vegas, NV.
22. Gazelle eHealth Test Framework for Interoperability. http://gazelle.ihe.net/

Chapter 14
Testing Tools

14.1 Introduction

The previous chapters described various approaches for models, frameworks, and architectures to support conformance and interoperability testing. This chapter provides an overview of tool instantiations. Many tools exist in the industry that provide testing capabilities related to the healthcare data exchange standards discussed in this book. A representative set of these tools is provided here. The tools in some fashion employ the concepts presented previously. When applicable, a link between the methodology used and the tool is given. Some of the production tools presented are used as part of testing and certification programs. In some cases tools are presented in detail, while in others a brief overview is given. The intent is not to provide an exhaustive catalogue and explanation of the tools, rather it is to provide a survey of the tooling landscape. The conformance testing concepts that were discussed in previous chapters are in many cases embodied in these tools.

The tools described include:

- NIST HL7 v2.x Test Tools
- Messaging Workbench (MWB) HL7 v2.x Message Validation
- CDC Messaging Quality Framework
- Australian Healthcare Messaging Laboratory (AHML)
- CDA Test Tools
- IHE Gazelle Testing Suite
- NIST e-Prescribing
- DVTk—DICOM Validation Toolkit

The National Institute of Standards and Technology (NIST) provides a suite of tools to support HL7 v2.x conformance testing. The tools are widely used and are integral to ONC Health IT Certification, the IHE Pre-connect-a-thon and Connect-a-thon test program, the CDC testing program, public health on-boarding, and public health registry testing. The MWB has a feature that performs HL7 v2.x

F. Oemig and R. Snelick, *Healthcare Interoperability Standards Compliance Handbook*, DOI 10.1007/978-3-319-44839-8_14

message instance testing based on the conformance profiles developed in the tool. The CDC provides message instance testing for public health use. The Australian Healthcare Messaging Laboratory (AHML) provides a context-free HL7 v2.x conformance testing service for a variety of profiles used in Australia. Testing tools for CDA are provided by five organizations including ART-DECOR, Lantana's Trifolia, MDHT, NIST, and eHealth Suisse. IHE provides an assortment of testing tools that include solely IHE-developed tools but can also leverage external tools by accessing them with their test management tool called Gazelle. NIST provides a test tool for the SCRIPT (e-Prescribing) standard that is used for ONC Health IT Certification and supports both EDI and XML message validation. The DICOM Validation Toolkit (DVTk) supports analyzing and testing against the DICOM Standard and IHE integration profiles.

Many other tools exist, publically available or privately developed for internal use, and they are at various maturity levels. The above list provides a sampling of mature tools in wide use and is not intended to be comprehensive. For newer standards, most notably HL7 FHIR, test tools are just emerging and do not warrant a discussion at this time, as any information provided would become dated quickly. The last section in this chapter provides links to the organizational sites that maintain the tools.

14.2 NIST HL7 v2.x Test Tools

NIST provides a portfolio of testing tools to conduct conformance and interoperability testing of HL7 v2.x messages. The tools are based on many of the concepts and testing infrastructures discussed in previous chapters of this book. The NIST HL7 v2.x test tools are used to support a number of certification and testing programs including the ONC Health IT certification in support of CMS Meaningful Use, IHE Pre-connect-a-thon and Connect-a-thon testing events, and various public health testing activities. NIST, as an agency of the US Government, provides the tools and source code as public domain resources. A summary of the NIST HL7 v2.x test tools is provided below:

- Immunization (2014 and 2015 Edition ONC Health IT Certification)
- Syndromic Surveillance (2014 and 2015 Edition ONC Health IT Certification)
- Reportable Labs—ELR (2014 and 2015 Edition ONC Health IT Certification)
- Reportable Labs Release 2—ELR R2
- Lab Results Interface—LRI (2014 ONC Health IT Certification)
- Lab Results Interface Release 2—LRI R2
- Lab Orders Interface—LOI
- Lab Compendium—eDOS
- Vital Records Death Reporting
- Height and Weight
- Patient Identification Management—PIX (IHE Technical Framework)

- Patient Demographics—PDQ (IHE Technical Framework)
- Patient Care Devices—PCD (IHE Technical Framework)
- Generic HL7 v2.x Message Validation
- Web Service Validation (EVS—External Validation Service)
- Support for testing of local implementation guides

NIST has developed a testing framework that supports testing of messaging data exchange standards in general. The framework has been applied to HL7 v2.x and NCPDP SCRIPT (e-Prescribing) standards. Chapter 13 described many aspects of this framework. A detailed explanation of the most recent NIST Immunization Suite (released in 2016) is provided in this section. This test tool is explained in detail to describe the features of the NIST test tools in general. The other NIST test tools have comparable capabilities, therefore these tools are not presented here. See [1] for a complete list of the NIST HL7 v2.x test tools, the targeted standards, use in testing programs, and access points.

14.2.1 NIST Immunization Test Suite

In collaboration with the CDC and AIRA, NIST developed a testing suite to support end-to-end testing of immunization systems. The test suite was built using the NIST healthcare data exchange testing infrastructure and framework. The test suite supports testing of transport standards, HL7 v2.x messaging, and testing of EHR-S and IIS functional requirements associated with immunization messaging. An overview of testing the HL7 v2.x messaging aspects and functional requirements is presented. The transport testing feature is not included since it is not within the scope of this book. The tool tests both sending and receiving applications used for immunization messaging and follows the principles described in Chap. 11.

14.2.1.1 General Tool Capabilities

The main features of the NIST tools include the validation capabilities and the rendering of the requirements that are in the specification. As described in previous chapters, HL7 v2.x specifications are organized as implementation guides containing use cases that can have multiple transactions. Transactions are made up of interactions. Interactions equate to an HL7 v2.x (conformance) message profile. The test tool validates to the requirements in the message profile. Validation includes context-free and context-based (i.e., associated with test data) operational modes. The requirements for each profile, along with the associated vocabularies, are displayed as separate utilities. Below is a summary list of the key capabilities in the NIST HL7 v2.x message validation tools:

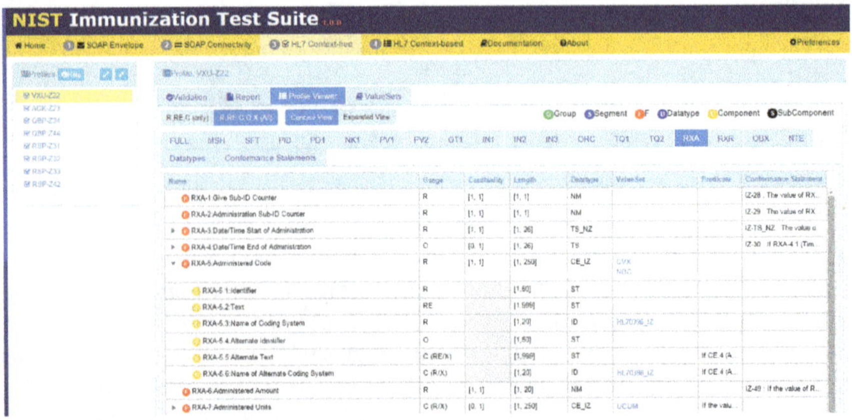

Fig. 14.1 Profile viewer

- Context-free Validation
- Context-based Validation (with associated test plans)
- Profile Viewer
- Value Set Viewer
- Communication Framework to Support Transport

Figure 14.1 shows a screen shot of the Context-free validation version of the Profile Viewer that provides the user with a browse-able version of the requirements specified in the implementation guide. Each of the segments is listed with their constituent fields and associated requirements for usage, cardinality, etc. Each element can be delved into further to examine requirements for child elements. On the left-hand side of the Profile Viewer is a navigation window in which each of the message profiles in the implementation guide is listed. On the right-hand side are tabs that equate to structures in the profile. For example, FULL represents the message structure and RXA represents the RXA segment (which is the active tab shown in the screenshot).

Each column indicates the requirement type as defined by the conformance constructs used in HL7 v2.x. See Chaps. 5 and 7 for the meaning of the construct and methods for applying constraints. As can be seen, the Profile Viewer provides a convenient mechanism for the user to browse requirements on-line and to troubleshoot issues when errors are reported by the validation.

One of the requirement types is Value Set, which indicates the coded options allowed for an element and the value set to which it is bound. The test tool provides a listing of each value set (see Fig. 14.2) for the selected profile.

Shown below is the value set collection, by sub-categories, for the VXU-Z22 profile (the CDC-IZ sub-category tab is selected in the screenshot). When a specific value set is selected, the details of that value set are displayed on the right-hand side of the Value Set window. The screenshot shows the details for the CVX value set.

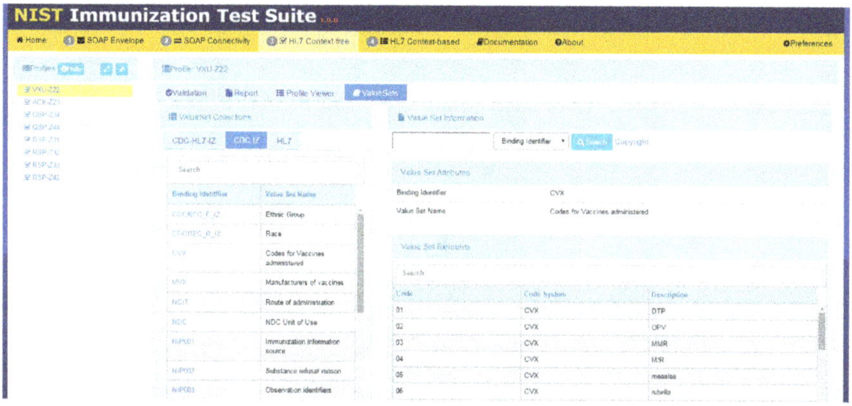

Fig. 14.2 Value set viewer

14.2.1.2 Testing Sending Applications in the Tool

When testing the ability of the System Under Test (SUT) to create messages, the focus of the conformance testing is on validating the message produced by the sending system (e.g., an EHR sending an immunization event message). As described in Chap. 11, there are two operational modes for validating sending systems: (1) Context-free and (2) Context-based. Validation is performed at the message profile (interaction) level. The Context-free mode validates any HL7 v2-based message created by the SUT for the given subject (e.g., immunization messaging, lab result messaging). It is not dependent on a specific use case instance (i.e., Test Case), or specific test data content. The Context-based mode validates messages created by the SUT that are associated with a given use case instance and a Test Case that includes specific test data, which are entered into the SUT. This validation assesses the technical requirements and content-specific requirements specified in the Test Case. Context-based validation expands the test space, enabling more comprehensive testing (e.g., testing of conformance usage constructs such as "conditional" and "required, but may be empty").

The NIST test tools support both validation operational modes. Figure 14.3 depicts a screenshot of the Context-free validation panel in the test tool.

Use of the tool in the context-free mode is straight-forward. The user selects the Context-free tab and then the desired message profile and imports the message into the test tool. The message can be uploaded using one of three mechanisms, including copy/paste into the message editor window, file upload, or directly via a communication portal. Once the message is imported, the message validation is performed automatically. The left-hand panel gives the user a tree structure view of the message where individual data-content can be examined. The upper-right panel is the message content window. The user can edit the message directly in this window to experiment with the data-content and observe the consequences such

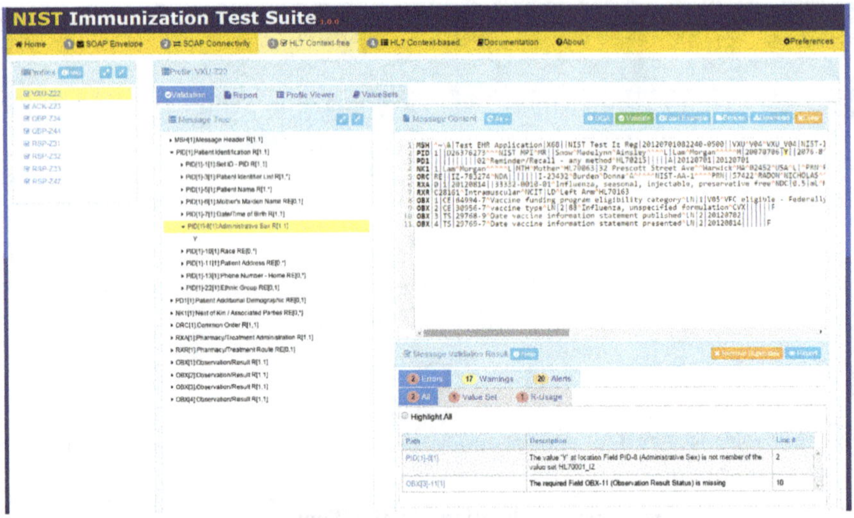

Fig. 14.3 Context-free validation

modifications have on the validation results. The validation results are displayed in the lower-right panel of the Validation window and include a description of the error and the location. Selection of the location indicator navigates the user to the place in the message where the error is located. Various detection categories are given, such as Errors or Warnings. Additionally, sub-categories are provided to further catalog the information; for example, Errors can be filtered by type such as R-Usage, Value Set, and Format. A validation report can be viewed and saved in a variety of formats.

The Context-based mode of the test tool uses the same validation panel as the one illustrated for Context-free testing. Figure 14.4 depicts a screenshot of the Context-based test selection panel for displaying the test plan and test cases.

On the left-hand side is a representation of the Test Plan that contains a number of Test Case Groups, Test Cases, and Test Steps. The user selects a Test Step to set the context of the validation. The validation is based on the profile associated with the Test Step and the data requirements specified in the test data specification. The tool provides all of the information necessary to carry out the test. Additionally, an example message is provided in both the ER7 encoding and a *pretty print* format (Message Content tab). In the Message Content sheet is an indication of how certain message elements are being validated.

Test Cases are provided for the specific domain targeted by the test tool—in this case immunization. A Test Case consists primarily of a narrative Test Story (one possible path described by the Use Case) and a Test Data Specification. The Test Story describes a real-world situation and provides the context for the Test Case. The Test Story also provides details associated with the Test Case such as pre-conditions, post-conditions, test objectives, and notes to testers. The Test Data

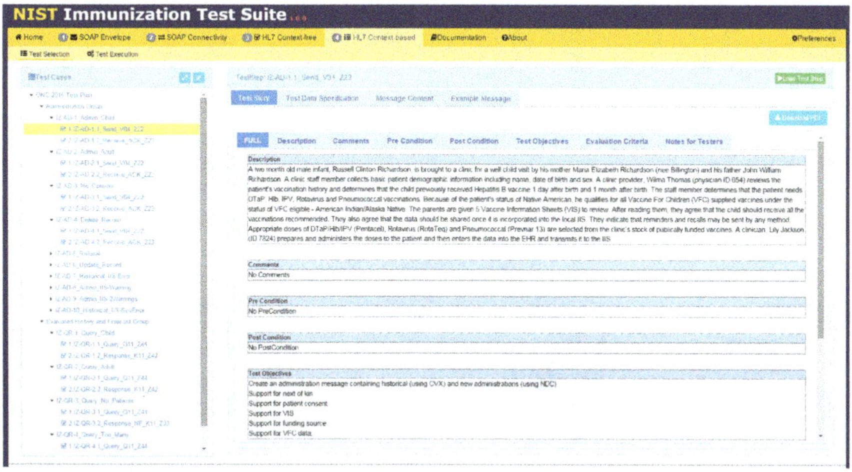

Fig. 14.4 Context-based validation test selection panel

Specification provides the data associated with the Test Story and consists of typically available information in the clinical setting. Together the Test Story and the Test Data Specification provide sufficient information to be entered into the SUT for a particular Test Case, e.g., sending a newly administered immunization. A Message Content Data Sheet is provided to show a conformant message instance for the Test Case. It also lists a testing category for each message element that indicates the kind of data and the expected source, which are based on the test case and test case objectives. How the data are categorized is directly related to how the message content is validated by the Test Tool. In some cases the validator is examining a message element for the presence or absence of data, and in other cases it is examining the message element for both the presence of data and exact content. The Message Content Data Sheet provides the evaluation criteria (expectations) and can be thought of as the "answer" to the "question" given in the Test Story and the Test Data Specification. This mechanism allows for the creation of test plans that can target a wide range of not only messaging requirements but also functional requirements. For a complete description of the makeup of a Test Case see Chap. 11 . The NIST tools implement the approach described in that chapter. An example message in ER7 encoding is also provided (Fig. 14.5).

To validate a message instance bound to the particular test step, the user selects the "Load Test Step" button. The tool then displays the validation panel as explained before in the Context-free Validation description. A key difference for Context-based is that the validation requirements are expanded according to the specifics in the test case definition. That is, the test coverage is broader and can include testing of specific content and support for "RE" usage elements.

Figure 14.6 shows a screenshot of validation results in which specific content assertions are listed based on the test case. The "Content" prefix shown with the Description indicates the detection type. For element PID-11.5 (Zip or Postal Code)

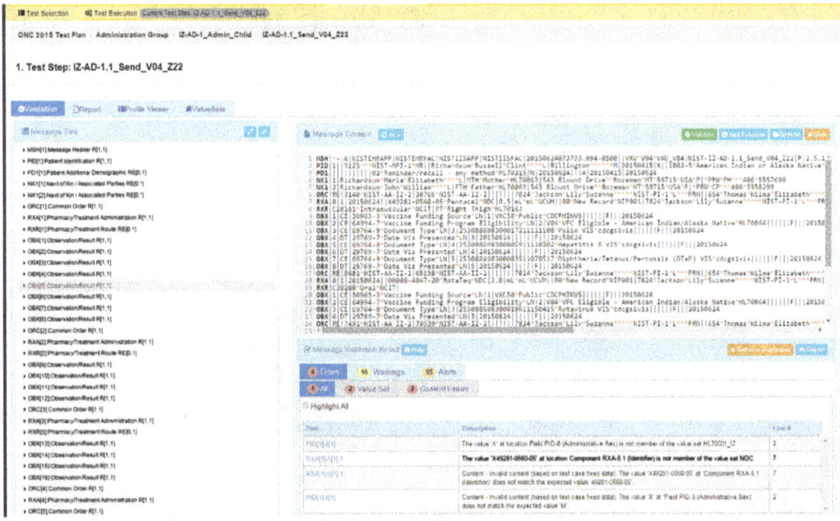

Fig. 14.5 Context-based validation panel

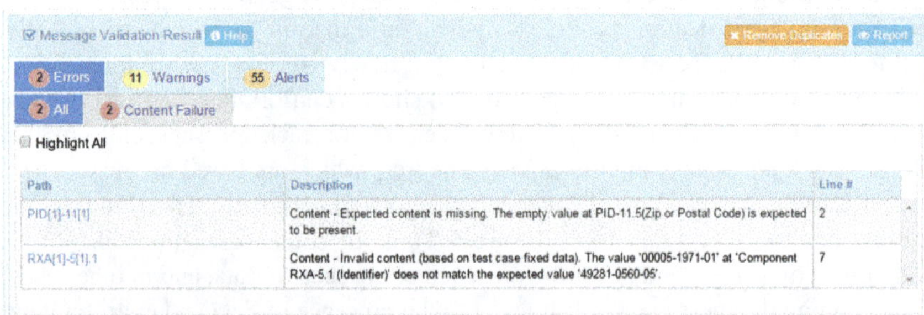

Fig. 14.6 Validation results with content violations

the element's usage is "RE". Test data are provided, therefore, the element is expected to be populated. This method can be used to test for the SUT's support of the element. For RXA-5.1, a specific NDC code is expected based on test data that indicates a particular vaccine. The NDC code provided is valid in general, but it is not valid based on the test story. This example illustrates the difference between how Context-free testing and Context-based testing are handled in the tool.

14.2.1.3 Testing Receiving Applications in the Tool

Testing a receiving system that is consuming the message is a challenge, because the SUT does not produce a tangible object (e.g., a message) for the Tester to assess

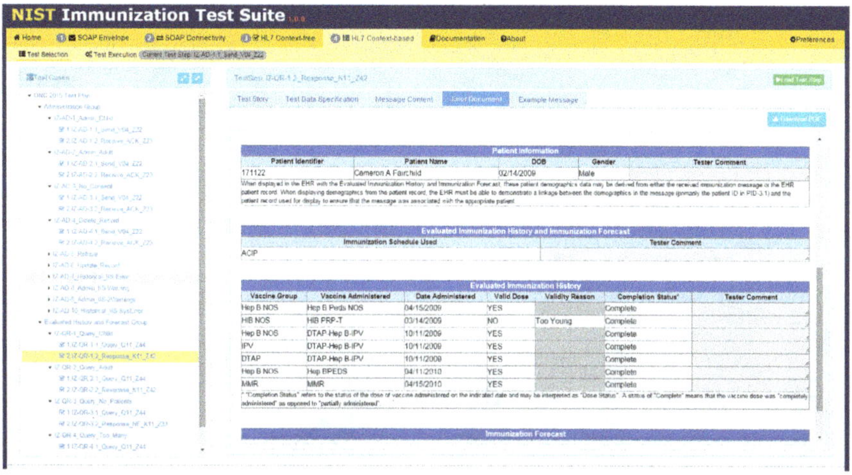

Fig. 14.7 Juror document (inspection check list)

directly. From the available testing approaches used for testing receiving systems, one approach is Inspection Testing, which has been proven suitable for various testing purposes. If the receiver is a server, automated testing can be employed. This approach is described in the next section on testing functional requirements.

Inspection Testing relies on human validation (a visual inspection) of the SUT in order to collect evidence for the conformity assessment. Usually, the Inspection Testing process involves priming or knowing the state of the receiving system; providing a known and documented stimulus to the system; and evaluating the system's response to the stimulus against expected results based on the input and requirements. The NIST test tools support this approach to testing by creating the stimulus and a corresponding inspection check list called a Juror Document.

Inspection testing uses the components described in the Context-based validation framework. Figure 14.7 shows that a response-oriented test step has been selected. In this use, the tool is a "test harness" that provides the Test Case and associated test material, such as the test message and a Juror Document (shown in Fig. 14.7). The Juror Document (a test case-specific inspection check list) is used by the Tester to inspect the receiving SUT for conformance to a set of requirements. The information contained in the Juror Document is based on the data provided in the test message, the known state of the system, and requirements listed in the given test criterion. During the inspection process, evidence of the SUT's conformance can be obtained through a variety of methods, including viewing the system's display screens, browsing the system's data base, viewing the configuration files, or other mechanisms supported by the SUT.

Figure 14.8 illustrates how the test tool can be used to test a query and response test case. In this case, the EHR is the SUT and the NIST test tool is simulating the Immunization Information System (IIS). The Test Case is designed to test the query

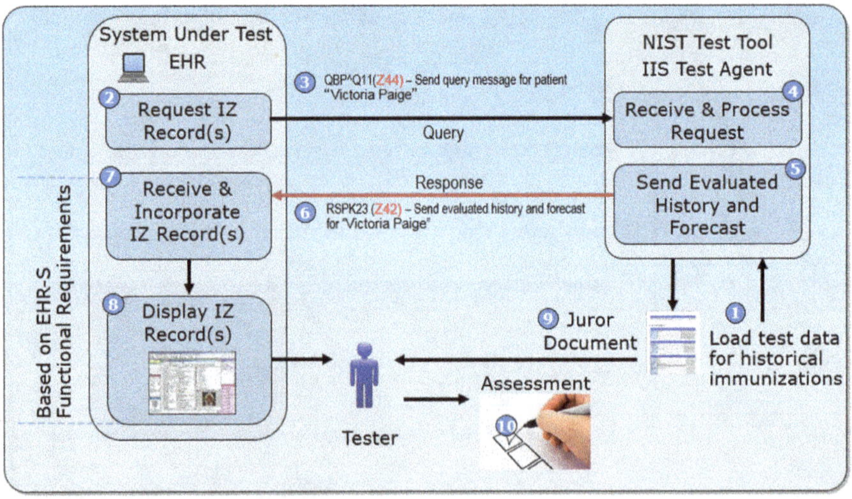

Fig. 14.8 Inspection testing using the tool

message created by the EHR (using the Context-based testing capability) as well as the EHR's ability to receive and display relevant content returned in the response message (as indicated by the Juror Document). The test tool provides the response message. In the example shown in Fig. 14.7, the requirement is to receive a response message from the IIS (simulated by the tool) and to display an evaluated history and forecast based on the content of the response message.

14.2.2 Testing Functional Requirements with the Tool

Functional testing examines the SUT's ability to provide a capability (function) based on either a functional or business process requirement. The test tool framework is capable of testing functional requirements in scenario-based test cases. The Context-based feature of the tool supports this capability through the Test Plan definition. Test cases are developed to enact a sequence of transactions that assess functional capabilities (when the SUT is a server). Figure 14.9 provides a scenario to test an IIS's capability of processing, linking, and subsequently returning an amalgamated patient's immunization evaluated history and forecast.

The first three interactions are used to *set the stage* of the test. The first is to send the immunization history of the patient as known by the EHR. For this test case, the IIS has no previous records of the patient. The NIST test tool is used to send a valid message to the IIS. The IIS is expected to return an acknowledgement to the test tool. Upon receipt, the acknowledgment message is validated. The second transaction sends a new immunization for the patient. The IIS is expected to link this

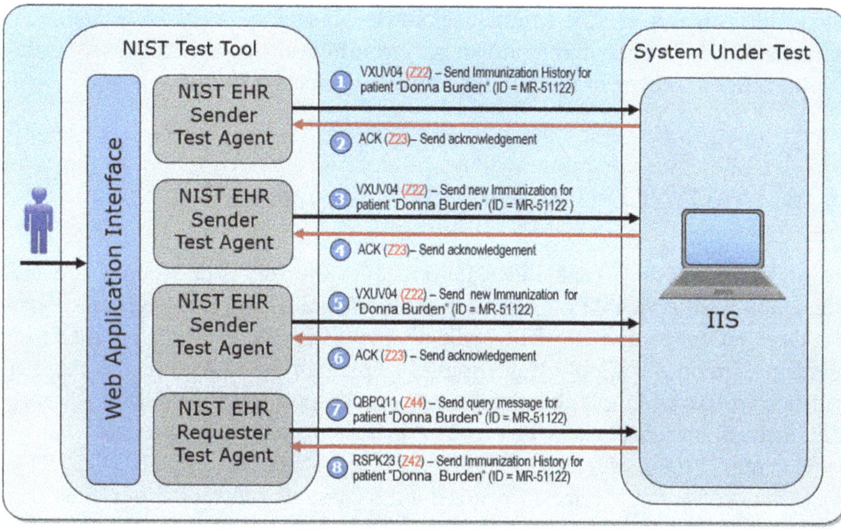

Fig. 14.9 Scenario to test functional requirements

new immunization event to the existing history. A third transaction updates the IIS record containing the immunization sent in the previous step. At this point, the IIS has an expected state based on the known stimuli. A number of functional requirements can be examined, for example, the IIS's ability to consume an immunization history of a patient, to associate and link new immunization events to an existing patient record, to update an existing record, to create an evaluated history and forecast, and to message that evaluated history and forecast according to the interoperability specification.

The test tool can be used to query for the patient's information in the IIS. Upon receipt, the test tool will first validate the message for conformance against the interoperability specification. Additionally, the test case definition includes assertions to assess the functional requirements, for example, the number and type of immunizations in the history for the patient. The expectation is for the IIS to include all of the events in the initial history load plus the new vaccine administration. Another function that can be tested is the ability to update a patient record. All such inquiries are made in the test case via the test data assertions as specified by the test data categories. See Chap. 11 for a description of the test data categories and how they are used for testing content, and, indirectly, functional requirements.

It is important to note that the same framework is used to conduct all of the testing within the test tool. What changes are the specifics of the test plan and the test case definitions, enabling any sort of scenario to be created, including test cases that assess the SUT's behavior in response to invalid input. For example, NIST has created a test plan that assesses the IISs ability to respond to immunization messages that are incorrect, not only from a conformance perspective, but also from a data quality perspective. The returned acknowledgement messages are examined to see what the IIS detected and reported. A screenshot for the scenario-based testing with transport is shown in the NIST e-Prescribing section in this chapter.

14.2.3 NIST HL7 v2.x Testing Web Services API

The underlying testing capabilities described in the previous sections are also offered as a web service API to enable users to integrate conformance testing easily into their processes locally. The validation WSDL (Web Service Description Language) provides a simple validation API in which the caller supplies the conformance profile, or simply the identifier (if pre-loaded), and the message instance. Additional parameters can also be provided to set the vocabulary or to test against a specific context (i.e., test case). The web service has been used by IHE Gazelle as an external validation service in connect-a-thon testing and by various sites with HL7 v2.x interfaces installed (including many in the public health arena). In addition to the web service, the NIST validation backend can be accessed directly via REST calls in the web-application tools that use the newer framework.

14.3 Message Workbench (MWB)

As explained in Chap. 9, the Messaging Workbench (MWB) is a tool for specifying and maintaining conformance profiles. The MWB also provides additional functionality including validating message instances. The validation capability is built directly into the profiling tool.

14.3.1 Message Instance Validation

Figure 14.10 shows the MWB context-free message instance validation utility. The user loads a profile (which may have been previously created by the MWB) and a message instance (see Message Capture tab). The user then selects Parse Message, which parses the message and provides a tree view of its content. Once parsed, the message can be validated. The popup dialog shows the results of the message validation. Various options allow the user to view the message results in different ways.

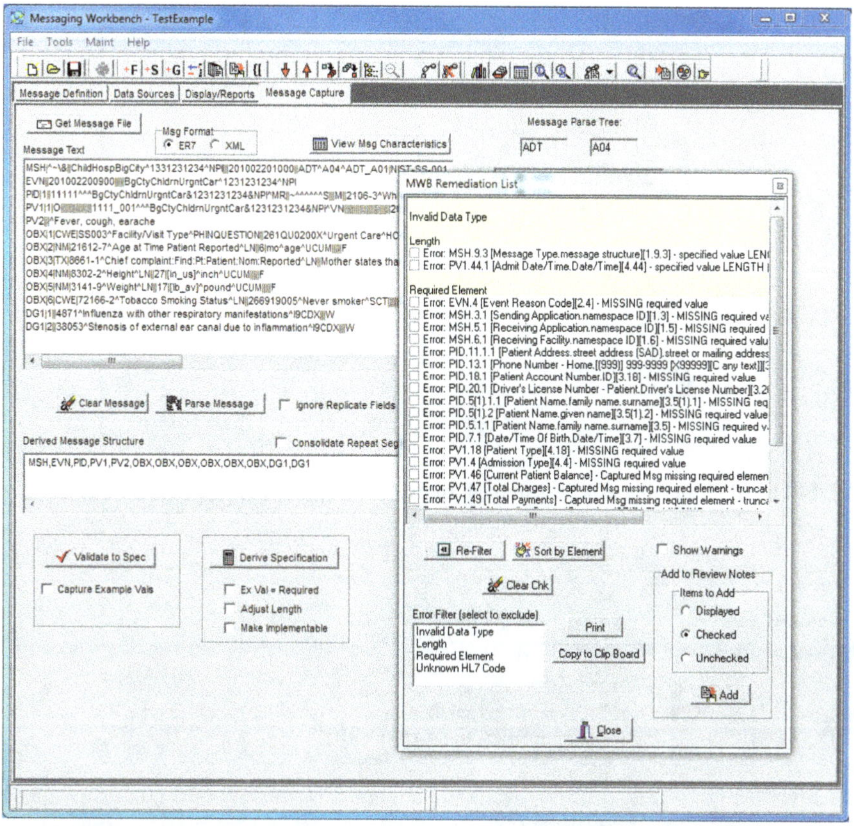

Fig. 14.10 MWB message validation

14.3.2 Message Validation via a Proxy-Server

Figure 14.11 demonstrates the MWB running as a Pass-Through Server. In this mode, the MWB routes the messages to another server without any modifications or adjustments to the messages; however, the MWB scans the messages, determines the correct profile (depending on the information found in the message header), and validates the message instance against the profile. The results are saved allowing for subsequent viewing of validation assessment.

14.3.3 MWB Validation Server

Another option is to run the MWB as a validation server using MLLP for transporting the messages (Fig. 14.12). This option allows MWB to be used remotely by

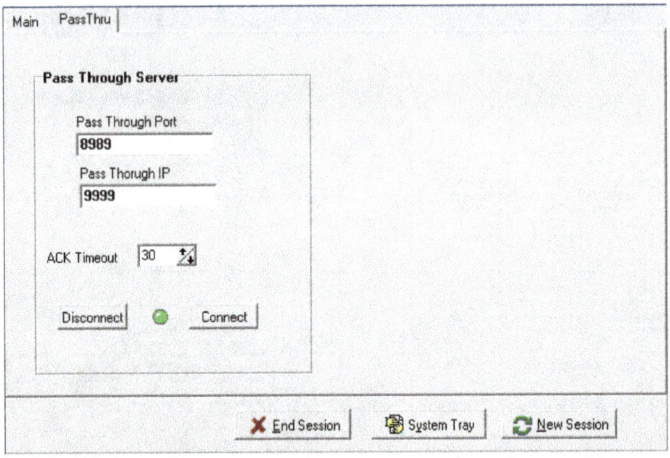

Fig. 14.11 MWB running as a pass-through (proxy) server

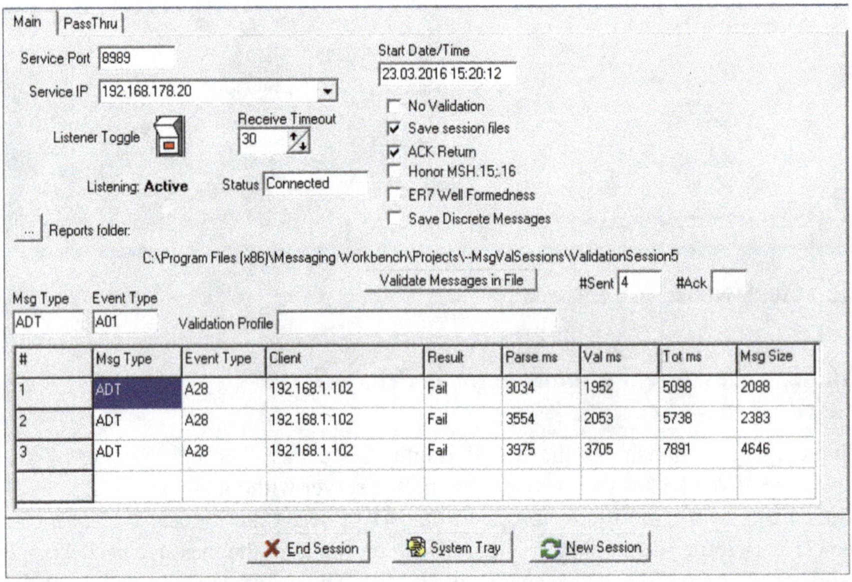

Fig. 14.12 MWB running as a validation server

other systems as a testing service. In this mode, the MWB listens on a specific port for incoming messages and responds with appropriate acknowledgements. The MWB performs validation checks against the currently loaded profile, or loads the corresponding profile according to the message profile identification sent in the message header. It also can furnish the reply message with the result (including errors) of the validated message.

14.4 CDC Message Quality Framework

The Centers for Disease Control and Prevention (CDC) provides the Message Quality Framework (MQF), which is an HL7 v2.x validation tool that supports testing of various conformance profiles for public health [CDC-MQF]. The public health profiles include case reporting, immunization, reportable labs, syndromic surveillance, and influenza. The test model of MQF is context-free data instance testing and is similar to the NIST context-free testing tools. The tool is a web-based application and provides a simple and easy-to-use interface. The user simply selects a conformance profile to validate against, uploads the message, submits it for validation, and, finally, views the validation report. The validation tool provides structural and vocabulary testing.

Figure 14.13 illustrates the user interface for requesting a validation, and Fig. 14.14 depicts an MQF validation report.

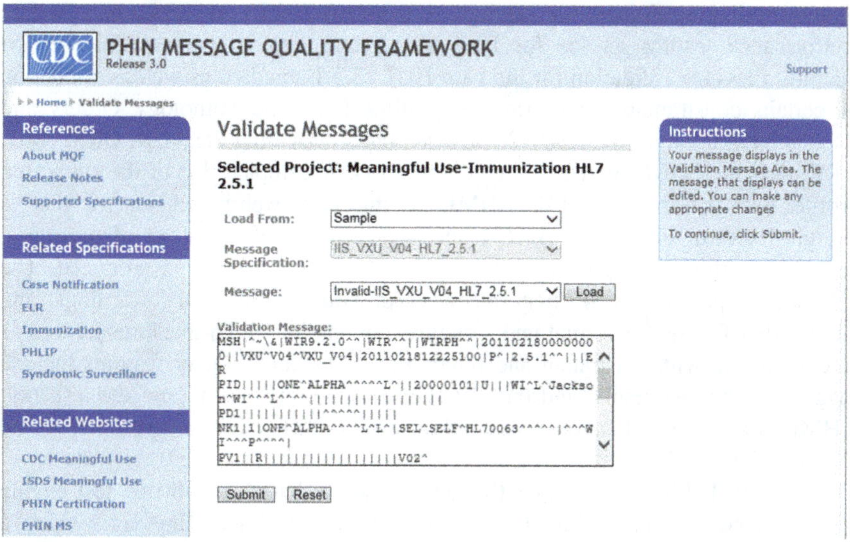

Fig. 14.13 CDC MQF validation HL7 v2.x tool [2]

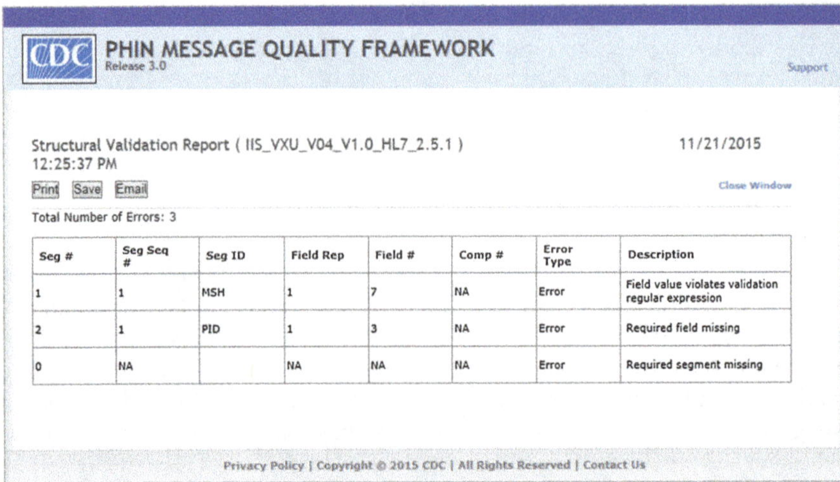

Fig. 14.14 Sample CDC MQF validation report HL7 v2.x tool [MQF]

14.5 AHML-Australian Healthcare Messaging Laboratory

The Australian Healthcare Messaging Laboratory (AHML) provides a context-free conformance testing service for HL7 v2.3.1 and v2.4 messages. This service includes message validation for the base HL7 v2.3.1 standard as well as validation of certain constrainable conformance profiles (e.g., the Pathology Orders and Results integration profile HL7 v2.3.1, AS4700.2—covering the ACK, ORM_O01, ORR_O02, and ORU_R01 message definitions). A complete list of the supported profiles can be found at [3]. AHML testing is a web-based service that is straight-forward to use (Fig. 14.15); the user simply uploads a set of messages, selects a conformance profile to validate against, and a report is produced. The validation report provides three categories of notification: errors, warnings, and alerts. AHML tests for format and structure, content, and high-level business rules in compliance with Australian and International standards. Other features include logging of the test results and the capability for a user to configure the test tool. AHML is also a certification organization; more information on this topic can be found in Chap. 15.

The AHML Message Testing Engine is a server-based, automated test engine that can receive many different types of electronic healthcare messages using a variety of transmission protocols [3]. The on-line web-based design allows users to access the service continuously. In addition to the web-based user interface, users can submit messages using HTTP (Hypertext Transfer Protocol). This capability supports the validation of a large quantity ("bulk") of messages. The users have an account and can log into browse and analyze the test results.

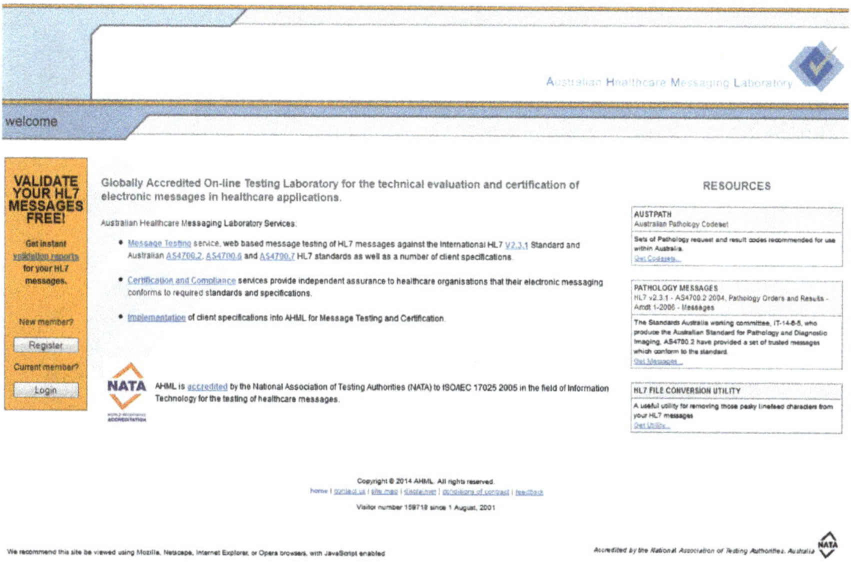

Fig. 14.15 AHML homepage [3]

14.5.1 Message Testing Process

The testing service supports three levels of testing:

- Format and Structure
- Content
- Functional Requirements (Business Rules)

Format and structure testing determines if the message adheres to the construction rules established by the conformance profiles. These rules include correct sequencing of segments, use of data types, message element Usage, and so forth. Limited content testing is also provided via lookup tables or specific databases. The testing service can support validation of specific business rules; here, the user provides the specific requirements, and the rules are imported into the testing engine. Figure 14.16 [3] illustrates the methodology for providing greater specificity of requirements and, thus, of the testing capabilities. In essence, AHML employs the profiling concepts discussed in Chap. 7. AHML depicts their approach to testing in a chart that shows the relationship of the profiling levels (requirements specification) to the types of testing, as illustrated in Fig. 14.16 (adapted from [3]).

The profiling levels indicate the degree of specificity required for a particular circumstance. The foundational level is the base standard, in this case HL7 v2.x. Beyond that, additional constraints, variations, or extensions can be indicated. These requirement specifications can be for structural, content, and functional (business rules) types of testing. Various requirement specifications—as well as

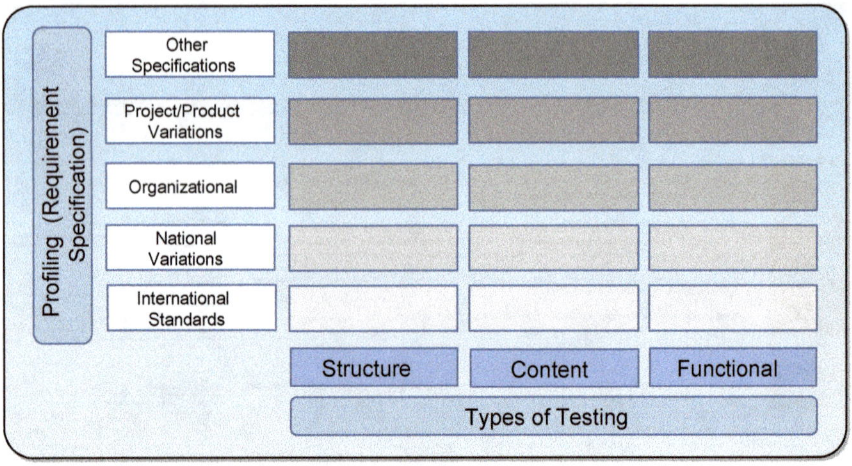

Fig. 14.16 AHML testing against profiling levels [3]

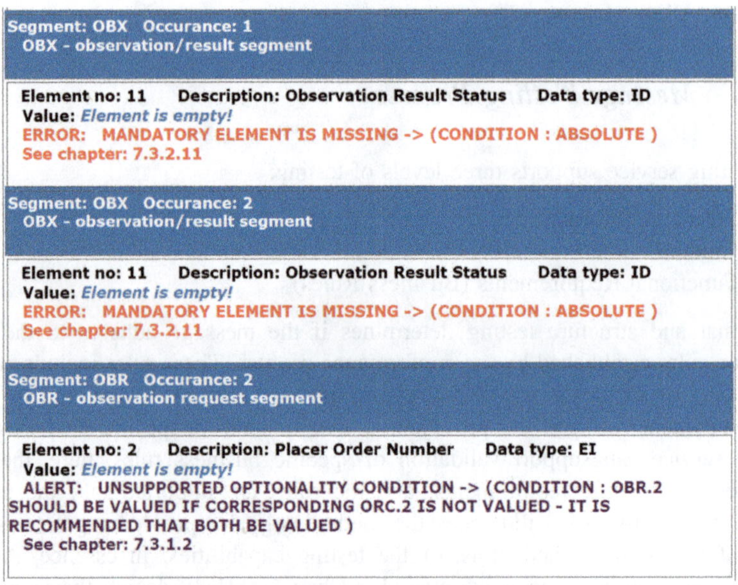

Fig. 14.17 AHML summary message validation report [3]

rules related to structure, content, and functions—can be imported into the service, thus providing a range of testing capabilities (Fig. 14.17).

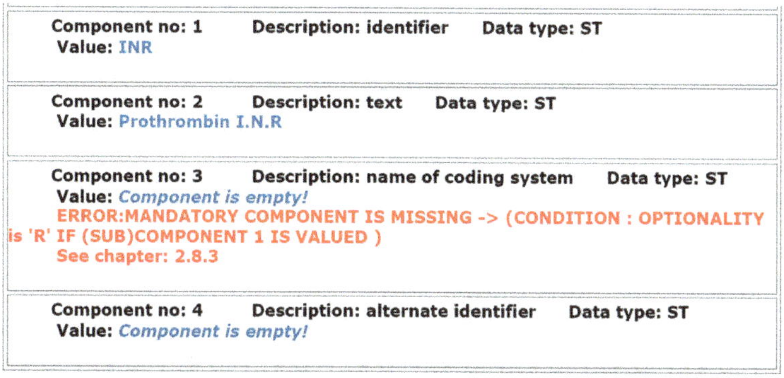

Fig. 14.18 AHML detail message validation report [3]

14.5.2 Reporting

AHML provides various levels of test reports, including summary, details, and historical. All tests and results are stored, so users can perform additional analysis such as comparison, aggregate result analysis, or general diagnosing of problems. Figure 14.18 shows a summary report that indicates just notifications (i.e., errors, warnings, and alerts). A detail report indicates the findings for all message elements; thus, in addition to failures, it reports affirmatives both when data are present and not present (see Fig. 14.18).

14.6 CDA Test Tools

This section summarizes the most prominent tools that provide testing functionalities for CDA-based documents. CDA validation includes checks for XML well-formedness, structure, and semantic content. CDA schema validation allows implementers to ensure generated templates are valid based on the underlying information model (CDA R-MIM for CDA templates).

14.6.1 ART-DECOR

The testing process with ART-DECOR works in a way that is different from "normal" tools because the testing itself is not accomplished within the tool. ART-DECOR creates a set of Schematron files based on the template definitions that are maintained. The process starts with downloading a compiled version of a project. A specific XML translation (XSLT) provided with DECOR2schematron. xsl converts the project definition into a set of rules that can be processed with any

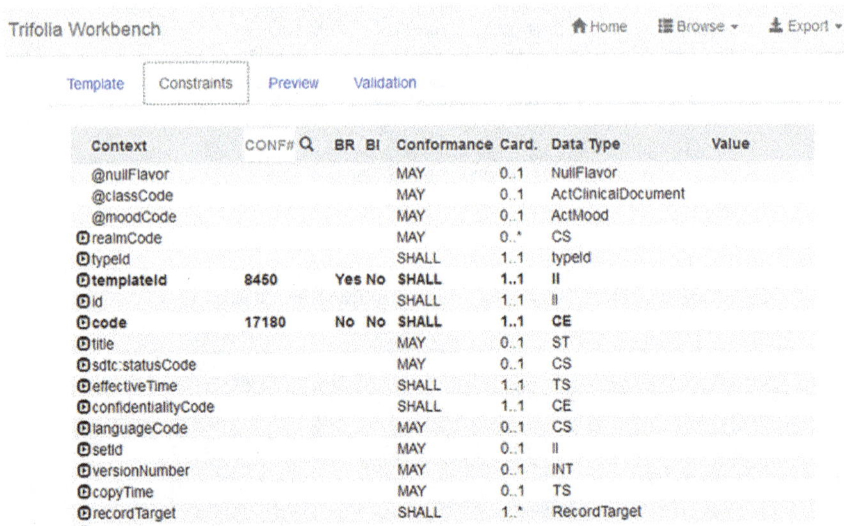

Fig. 14.19 Trifolia template editor—constraints

Schematron[1] engine that comes with most professional XML tools. Therefore, the validation part is separated from the toolkit and can be used at installed sites.

14.6.2 Lantana Trifolia

The Lantana's Workbench Trifolia for creating CDA implementation guides also provides testing capabilities. Trifolia is a schema-based tool and, therefore, facilitates the generation of templates that conform to the CDA XML schema by:

- Prohibiting the selection of invalid data types on elements
- Automatically generating the correct wording for constraints (see Fig. 14.19)
- Generating links to value sets and code systems when binding to value sets or code systems
- Versioning templates and Implementation Guides
- Automatic generation of XML fragments to represent a template and its constraints

Trifolia helps by exporting the Schematron and the XML vocabulary file for the relevant Implementation Guide into the same directory as the example CDA instance.

Within the IG development process, implementers can generate Schematron validation rules once a template is created within Trifolia. The generated Schematron files help to identify errors in the IG and related example CDA instance files.

[1]Schematron is a schema language that allows implementers to express rules and check an XML document against those rules.

"Schematron Quality Assurance" refers to the process of using Schematron-compiled rules to perform quality checks on an IG and its associated templates and sample file.

Schematron validation steps that Trifolia supports are:

1. Create good test sample files
   - These files test whether the template is created correctly and that sample files contain all of the expected values. If the constraints are modified, the Schematron will reflect those changes when regenerated.
2. Create bad test sample files
   - These files test the SHALL and SHOULD conformance statements, hard-coded values and STATIC bindings when bad data are purposely entered into the sample file.
3. Validate sample files against the Schematron to ensure Schematron is generating the correct errors and warnings
4. Fix all Schematron issues

The Lantana CDA Validator is a free-to-use online application that allows implementers to validate various flavors of CDA documents against a collection of different IGs as shown in Fig. 14.20. During the IG development cycle, implementers can use the CDA Validator to identify and debug inaccuracies within common types of CDA documents.

14.6.3 NIST CDA Testing

NIST has independently and in collaboration with IHE, Alschuler Associates, LLC (now Lantana), and CCHIT (now disbanded) created a tool that validates CDA/CCD-based specifications. The tool supports testing of the HITSP and IHE specifications and the ONC Health IT Certification Program.[2] The tool provides a web-application and a web-service interface. The underlying methodology of the validation is the development of Schematron rules (assertions) for CDA implementation guides. That is, individual XPath expressions are written and used to assert that the implementation conforms to a rule in a given context.

Figure 14.21 depicts the NIST CDA validation selection panel for Healthcare Surveys that is used for ONC 2015 Edition certification testing. The user simply uploads the document and validates. Figure 14.22 illustrates the validation results panel. An overview and details of the errors are given.

The NIST CDA validation tool supports in excess of 75 document types.

[2]Note: some of the CDA-based specification validation for ONC are supported by non-NIST tooling.

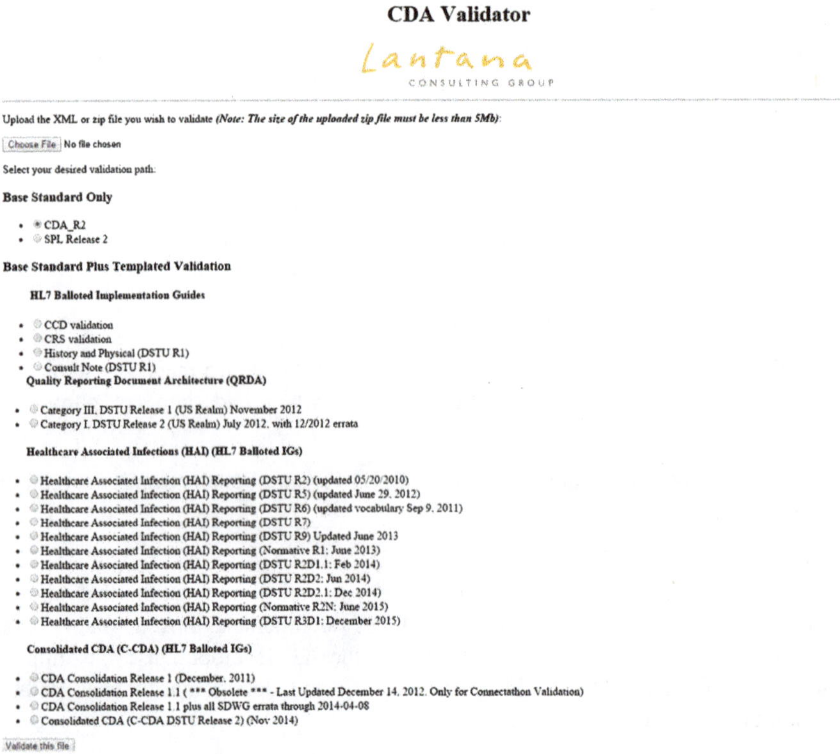

Fig. 14.20 Trifolia CDA validator

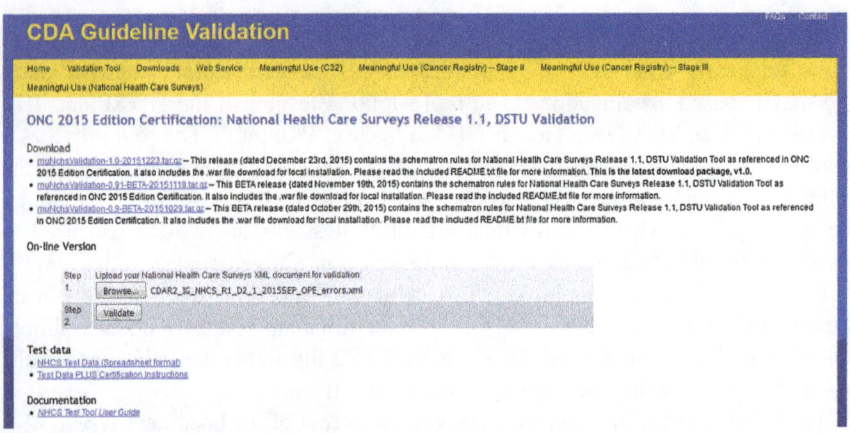

Fig. 14.21 NIST CDA validation selection panel example

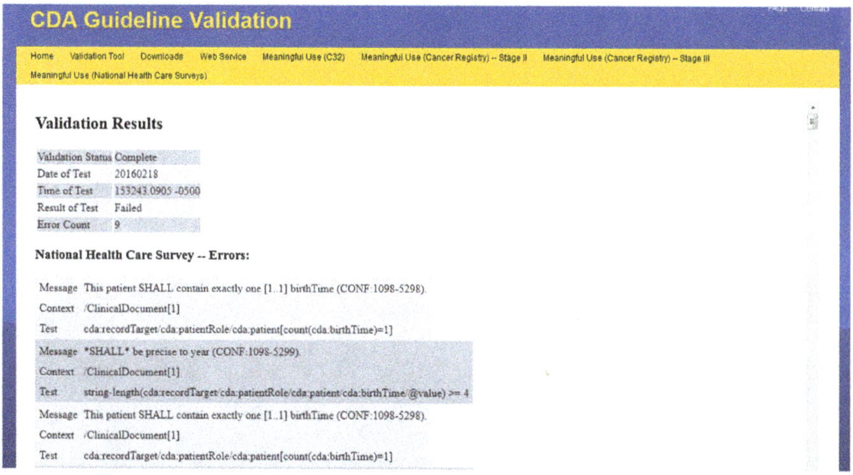

Fig. 14.22 NIST CDA validation results panel example

14.6.4 eHealth Suisse

eHealth Suisse provides a CDA validator for use in Switzerland. The primary objective is to validate CDA instances according to the Swiss implementation guides (Fig. 14.23).

At the time of this writing, eHealth Suisse provides testing capabilities against the following detailed specifications:

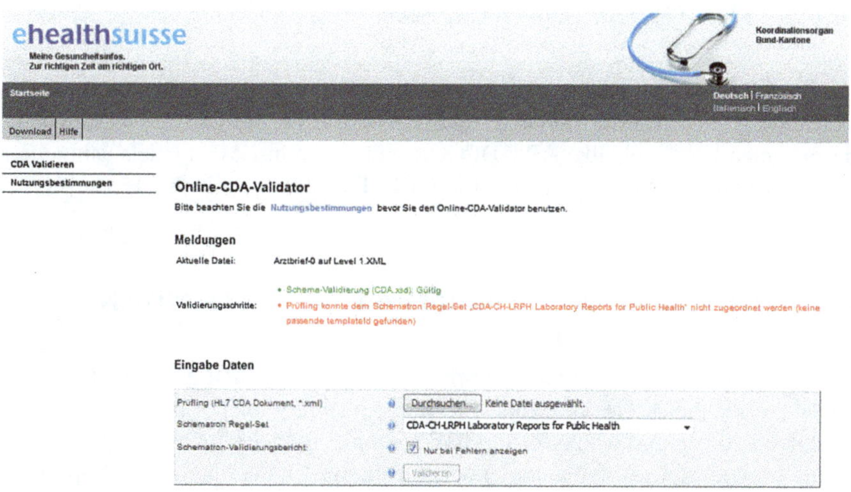

Fig. 14.23 eHealthSuisse CDA validation

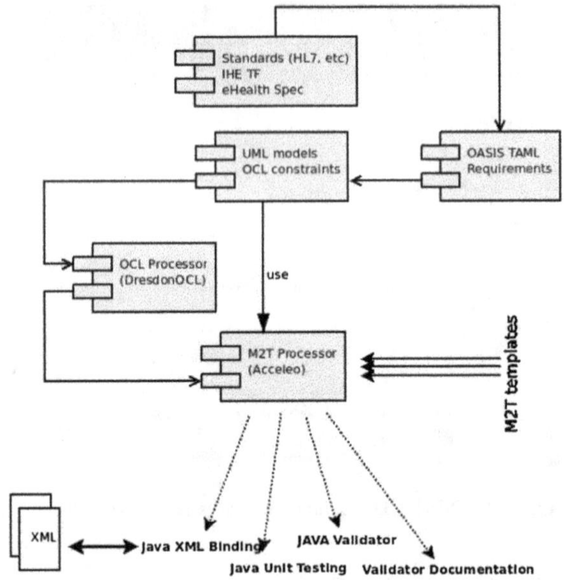

Fig. 14.24 Gazelle object checker methodology

- CDA-CH-LRPH Laboratory Reports for Public Health
- CDA-CH-LRTP Laboratory Reports in the Transplantation Process
- CDA-CH-VACD eVACDOC

HL7 Switzerland is currently working on extending the set of IGs and the associated testing.

14.6.5 IHE Gazelle Object Checker

The Gazelle Object Checker aids in testing CDA instances against CDA implementation guides. The methodology is illustrated in Fig. 14.24. The requirements are extracted from tools like ART-DECOR and stored in UML models using class hierarchies and constraints expressed in OCL. For more details please see [4].

14.7 IHE Conformance and Interoperability Test Tools

IHE has developed a number of conformance and interoperability test tools in their Gazelle eHealth Test Framework for Interoperability platform [5]. The main objective is to support testing of the IHE technical frameworks as part of the IHE testing programs. As is explained in detail in Chap. 15, Gazelle is a multi-purpose test bed that combines test management with a suite of conformance and interoperability testing capabilities. Gazelle has its own testing capabilities, but IHE also designed it to leverage tools created by other organizations via its external validation service interface. Gazelle is used to conduct and manage IHE testing events such as the Pre-connect-a-thon and Connect-a-thon. More information on this testing program and Gazelle's test management capabilities can be found in Chap. 15. The focus of this section is on the Gazelle conformance and interoperability test tools.

During testing, a vendor's system will create certain artifacts, such as HL7 v2 messages or CDA documents. These artifacts can be linked to a test case, and a validation report can be generated. Some of these capabilities are automated and some are manual (i.e., an artifact is copied from Gazelle and pasted into another tool). Automated capabilities include capturing and validating message instances during a Connect-a-thon and linking the tester to a specific test case. For HL7 v2.x message validation, the Gazelle validation engine can be used or an external validation services (EVS), such as the NIST validation web service, can be called via Gazelle. As Gazelle continues to evolve, more validation processes will be automated.

Gazelle also provides test agents (called simulators in Gazelle) that substitute for a given IHE actor (application). The PAM (Patient Administration Management) Simulator [6] mimics the actor's handling of patient demographics and visits. The PAM simulator can act as a test partner for a host of actors (e.g., Patient Demographic Supplier). Other tools provided by Gazelle are the data generation tools, for example, a service that randomly retrieves a person's demographics. This type of service facilitates testing when used in conjunction with test tools.

Gazelle also provides an interface to perform data instance testing for a particular test object (e.g., message or document) related to an integration profile. The tooling supports a number of standards including HL7 v2.x, HL7 V3, HL7 CDA, and DICOM. Figure 14.25 shows the External Validation Service (EVS) Front-end, which lists the services supported and provides a drop-down menu from which the HL7 v2.x validation is selected.

Upon selection of the HL7 v2.x validation, the user is presented with a text-box to enter or upload a message instance and a list of available conformance profiles to validate against that correspond to a given interaction (e.g., ITI-8) for a given actor (e.g., Patient Identity Source) in an integration profile. The user simply uploads the message and selects the conformance profile they wish to validate against. Figure 14.26 shows the validation panel for v2.x where the validation results are given as well as detailed errors and warnings (not shown in the figure). A similar interface and process is provided for other test objects, such as DICOM messages and CDA documents.

Gazelle has a vast collection of validation tools and support utilities available to aid users in testing. A small sampling has been provided here; the reader should explore Gazelle to gain an understanding of the full set of capabilities offered.

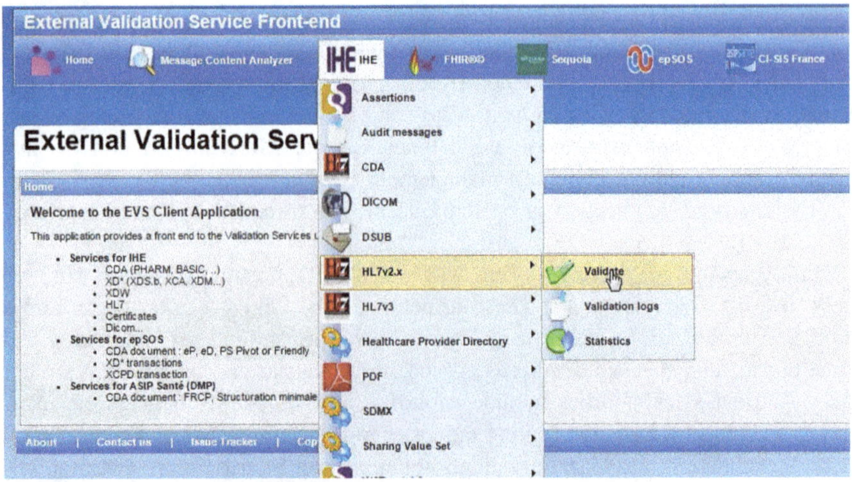

Fig. 14.25 Gazelle external validation service (EVS) front-end

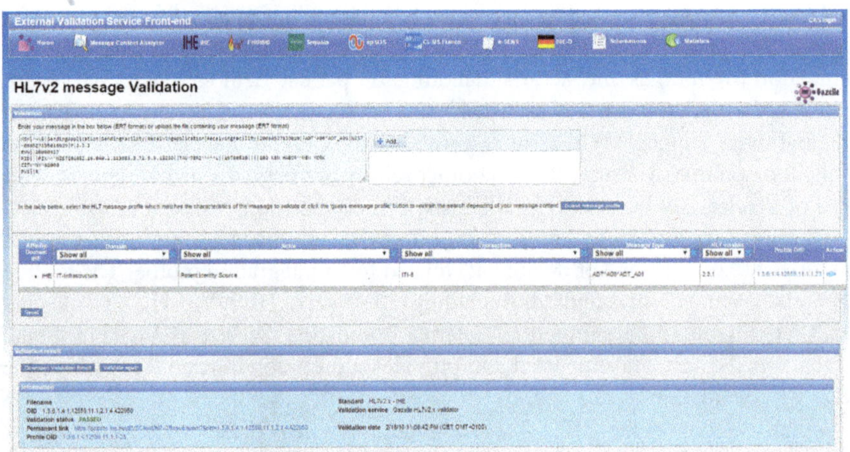

Fig. 14.26 Gazelle HL7 v2.x validation results panel

14.8 e-Prescribing (e-Rx) Tools

The two prominent conformance testing tools for e-Prescribing in the US are from Surescripts and NIST. Public information about the Surescripts test tools is not available. See Chap. 15 for an overview of the Surescripts certification. This section describes the NIST e-Prescribing conformance test tool. As of this writing, NIST and Surescripts are deliberating about transferring the NIST test tool technology to Surescripts.

14.8.1 NIST e-Prescribing Test Tool

The NIST conformance test tool for e-Prescribing is modelled after the NIST HL7 v2.x test tools. Both sets of tools use the same underlying testing framework. The NIST e-Prescribing tool validates against the NCPDP SCRIPT standard version 10.6 and supports validation of both EDI and XML encodings. There are two instances of the tool, and both support ONC Health IT Certification (2014 Edition and 2015 Edition).

Use of the test tool is the same as that described for the NIST Immunization test suite. Context-free and Context-based validation are provided along with Profile and Value Set viewers. The test plans in Context-based testing for e-Prescribing are elongated scenarios, and the tool is setup to communicate directly with the SUT via SOAP. The four general test scenario categories include Change, Cancel, Refill, and Medication History. The New Prescription message is part of the Change, Cancel, and Refill scenarios.

Figure 14.27 shows a screenshot of a test case for e-Prescribing using the multi-message (step) mode in which the EHR-S is tested for creating a new prescription, approving a change request, and receiving a fill status message from the pharmacy. The EHR-S under test communicates directly with the NIST test harness. In this case, the tool is simulating the pharmacy system. The upper part of the screenshot provides a table that lists the test steps and, during test execution, progress and validation result indicators. To the right of that table is a log of the communication exchange. For each step, the message instance being validated is displayed in the validation panel (shown at the bottom). Upon completion of the test case, a summary of the test is given. The user can navigate to any test step to view

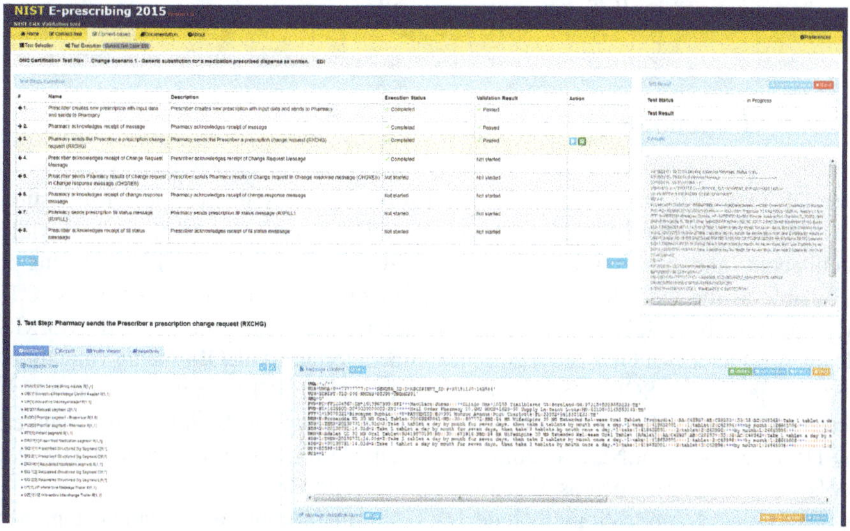

Fig. 14.27 e-Prescribing scenario base testing screenshot

results of the step for post analysis. As with the NIST immunization test tool, the e-Prescribing testing can be executed in a scenario-based fashion with automated transport, or as individual "unit" tests via cut/paste or file upload.

14.9 DVTk—DICOM Validation Toolkit

14.9.1 History

The history of DVTk goes back to 1997. The first version of the Validation Test Suite (VTS) was developed within the *Architecture Re-use and Communications* (ARC) group of Philips [7]. This application was a DICOM Validation tool with a command line interface. The subsequent Agfa DICOM Validation Tool (ADVT) was created based on this version and was the first tool with a Graphical User Interface (GUI), which made DICOM validation more user-friendly.

Philips and Agfa wanted to join forces, and their collaboration became a reality in 2001. The first version of DVT (v1.2) was born in 2002. After major redesign and improvements, DVT v2.1 was released in a vendor-neutral form in June of 2005. This version was the transition of the application from the Philips-AGFA cooperation project to the Open Source community. In 2006, *ICT Automatisering* [8] joined the DVTk Open Source project as the third participating company beside Philips and Agfa. Other parties, such as Medical Communications (UK) and NIST (US), have contributed TCP/IP capture-to-file and HL7 v2 validation capabilities. In 2007, DVTk began participating in the IHE Gazelle project by supplying an External Validation Service (DICOM Validation Web Service). In 2008, Services for the DVTk Open Source project was introduced. [9] Today, this toolkit is primarily maintained by ICT Automatisering, NL.

14.9.2 Functionality

The DICOM Validation Tool (DVT) is a software utility that can assist in testing conformance to the DICOM standard. The DVT test framework is a flexible architecture and uses service–object pair (SOP) class definition files, making it adaptable as the DICOM standard evolves in supporting a set of modalities (CT, MR, X-Ray, NM, RT, US, etc.), workstations, archives, printers, and HIS/RIS devices. It includes a GUI and a command line interface, DICOM media validation, service class user (SCU) and service class provider (SCP) emulators, and a rich scripting language. For more advanced testing, VBScript or JScript can be executed by DVT, and a set of.NET assemblies is available for developing stand-alone test tools with languages such as Visual Basic.NET and C# [10].

DVTk-based applications include DVT, the main application, which, together with the core, forms what is now referred to as the DICOM Validation Framework

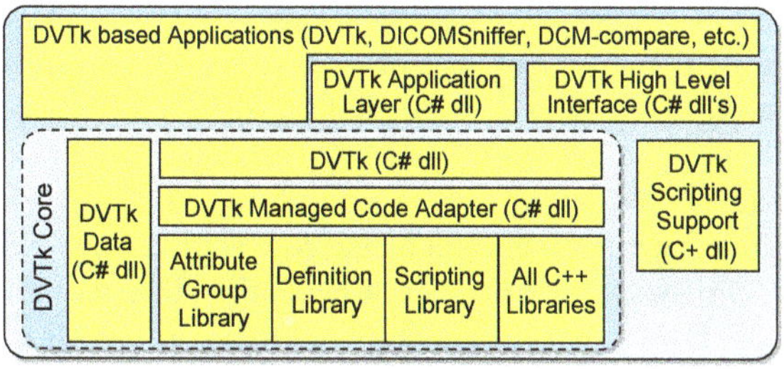

Fig. 14.28 DVTk validation framework [10]

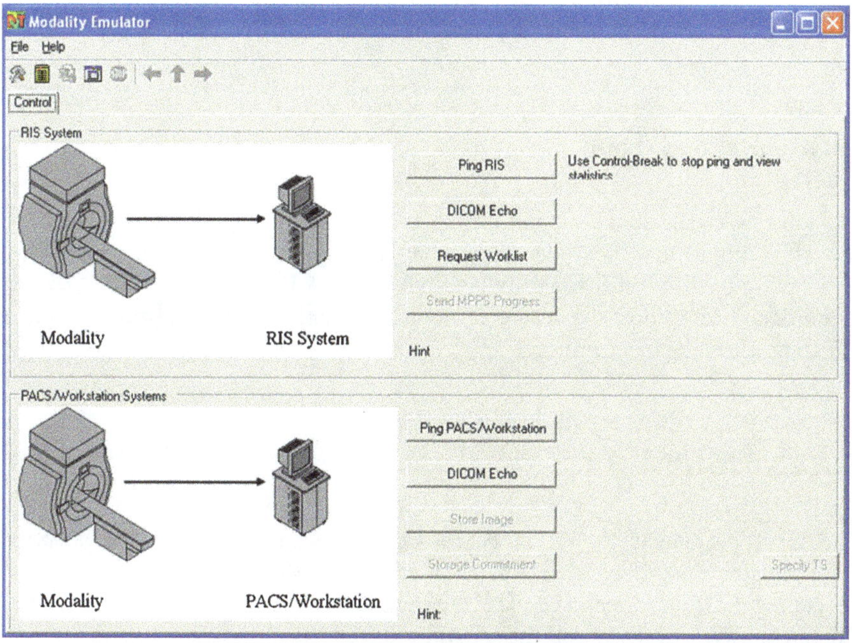

Fig. 14.29 DVTk modality emulator [11]

(Fig. 14.28). The core includes a DICOM testing data model and object-oriented class structure. The DVTk and DVTkData libraries provide access to this data model and class structure via the managed code adapter. The core includes the DICOMScript language that is supported by DVT. This language can be separated into basic programming, which includes the SEND and RECEIVE commands for simulating DICOM SCPs and SCUs (shown in Fig. 14.29), and advanced programming. The advanced programming language includes commands such as SYSTEM, for executing operating system native applications, and a number of commands for working with the Data Warehouse feature [10].

A DVT project is a container for one or more test sessions. A session is a container for the configuration of one or more tests to be performed against a system under test (SUT). [10]DVT is designed to work on a single project at a time, although multiple views of the project may be opened from which multiple tests may be simultaneously executed.

Other DVTk-based applications built on the core and currently available on dvtk. org include: DICOM Network Analyzer, a network sniffer and DICOM protocol analyzer; DICOM Editor, for displaying and editing DICOM files; DICOM Compare Tool, for comparing the attributes and values of two DICOM files; DICOM Attribute Validator, for validating DICOM files, including Structured Report objects, against definition files; DICOM File Stripper, for removing all but mandatory attributes from a DICOM file; and DICOM File Anonymizer, for removing patient and physician information from a DICOM file [10].

14.10 Related Tools

The tools described above support testing of interfaces and applications; other tools provide utilities that help developers in creating and maintaining interfaces. A sampling of these other tools are presented here. A high-level overview is given to introduce each tool; the reader is invited to explore each one further before initiating a development project.

14.10.1 HAPI

The most prominent toolkit is HAPI—an abbreviation for *HL7 Application Programming Interface*. It is a Java-based toolkit that allows for parsing and generating HL7 v2.x messages [12]. Originally, HAPI was built from the HL7 Comprehensive Database [13] that provides the entire v2.x standard in a relational database. The HAPI generator converted the HL7 v2.x data from the database into Java classes. Subsequent versions of HAPI provided a GUI to help with manually modifying the underlying structures in order for a user to influence and control the Java class generation more easily (Fig. 14.30).

Another HAPI feature works with XML-based conformance profiles as specified by the HL7 v2 standard. The test panel allows validation of HL7 v2 message instances against the underlying profiles. HAPI also has features that aid in maintaining tables and their values. The test panel provides an edit function to define and populate tables with values.

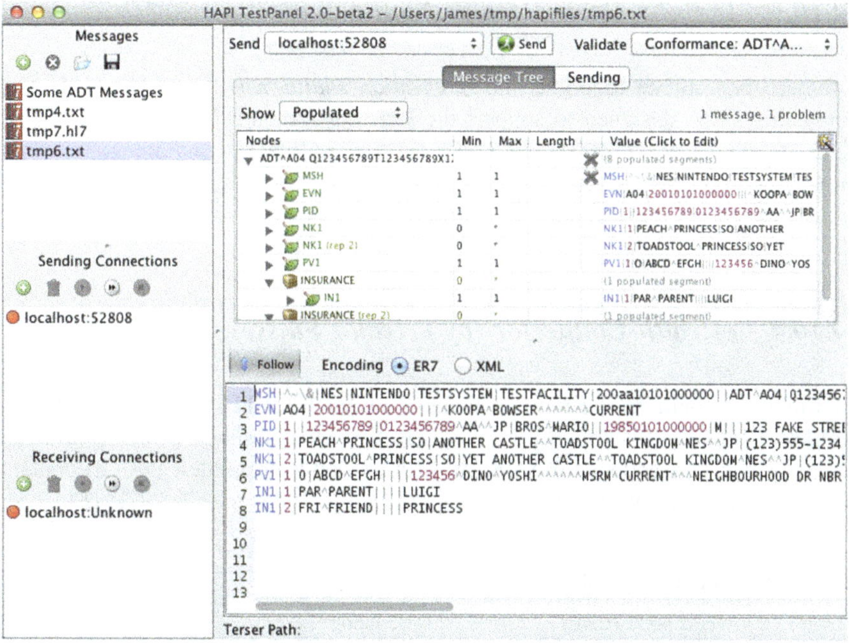

Fig. 14.30 HAPI test panel [12]

14.10.2 MDHT

The Model Driven Health Tools (MDHT) is an initiative hosted inside the Eclipse Modeling Project. Authors of healthcare interoperability standards, validators, and software developers are supported by the following MDHT capabilities:

- Definition of UML profiles
- Publishing tools to generate documentation. e.g., in DITA
- Model transformation, facilitating Eclipse Modeling Framework (EMF) and Object Constraint Language (OCL)
- Editing and Maintaining Clinical Terminology
- Editing and Maintaining Clinical Information Models
- Generation of Java classes for Templates, Profiles, and Archetypes

The primary asset of MDHT is probably a Java library that helps in creating valid CDA instances. The Java library is based upon UML models generated from the HL7 Version 3 Model Interchange Format (MIF) files providing the HL7 Version Reference Information Model (RIM) and Vocabulary.

14.10.3 IPF (by Open eHealth Foundation)

Another open source toolkit is the *Integration Platform* (IPF) of Open eHealth Foundation. It is designed to support the IHE integration profiles like PIX/PDQ, XDS, XCA and a few others. Its OSGi foundation enables easy integration into Java-based applications. As such, it facilitates use of HAPI and MDHT, and it aids in providing a scripting engine to simplify CDA instance generation.

14.10.4 eHealth Connector (by eHealth Suisse)

This toolkit is built on the runtime libraries of MDHT HITSP and the OHT IHE profiles. It supports developers by providing an API that abstracts from the complex details of IHE transactions for XDS and MPI as well as from the CDA-CH content profiles as specified in the national implementation guides for CDA-CH [14] [15].

Table 14.1 List of testing tools and access points

Tool(s)	Access point (URL)	Description
NIST	http://healthcare.nist.gov/NIST-TOOLS/	Tool Portal for all of the NIST related Healthcare conformance and interoperability test tools. Tools for HL7 v2.x, HL7 V3, CDA, e-Prescribing, and transport
MWB	http://www.hl7.org/ (download)	Messaging Workbench (MWB); general tool to support HL7 v2.x profiling and conformance testing
AHML	http://www.ahml.com.au	Australian Healthcare Messaging Laboratory tools for HL7 v2.x message validation
CDC MQF	https://phinmqf.cdc.gov/	The Centers for Disease Control and Prevention (CDC) Message Quality Framework (MQF); HL7 v2.x message validation for public health
Art decor	http://art-decor.org	Main project website
Trifolia	https://trifolia.lantanagroup.com/	Lantana's web-based workbench to create Implementation Guides for CDA
MDHT	https://projects.eclipse.org/proposals/model-driven-health-tools	Plug-ins for Eclipse using UML, EMF and OCL as foundation
eHealth Suisse	http://www.e-health-cda-validator.ch/validation.xhtml	A webpage provided by eHealth Suisse to validate uploaded CDA documents against the basic CDA XML schema and specific Schematron rules
IHE gazelle	http://gazelle.ihe.net/	A test management and conformance tool from IHE to support testing of the IHE technical frameworks
DVTk	http://www.dvtk.org/	A tool suite to support DICOM data exchange testing

14.11 Table of Tools and Access Points

Table 14.1 provides a sample of conformance and interoperability test tools, the URL for accessing the tool or suite of tools, and a brief description of what the tool or tool set is used for.

14.12 Summary

As mentioned many times throughout this book, testing is a vital aspect for assessing implementations and also for improving the quality of standards. Previous chapters discussed principles and architectures for conformance testing. This chapter presented a sample of tools that have instantiated many of these techniques. Test tools are essential instruments in certification processes; therefore, it is critical that test tools are comprehensive in order to provide broad coverage of the requirements being tested. Tools that support context-based testing are best for certification. Context-free testing is valuable for site installations. Chapter 15 focuses on testing and certification programs and provides details about the role test tools play in the certification process.

References

1. NIST Tool Portal of HL7 v2.x Conformance and Interoperability Test Tools: http://healthcare.nist.gov/NIST-TOOLS
2. Center for Disease Control (CDC) Message Quality Framework (MQF). https://phinmqf.cdc.gov
3. Australian Healthcare Messaging Laboratory. http://www.ahml.com.au/
4. Gazelle Object Checker. http://gazelle.ihe.net/content/gazelle-objectschecker
5. Gazelle eHealth Test Framework for Interoperability. http://gazelle.ihe.net/
6. Patient Administration Management Simulator: http://gazelle.ihe.net/content/patientmanager
7. Philips ARC group (Architecture Re-use and Communications). http://www.medical.philips.com/main/
8. ICT Automatisering, http://www.ict.nl/en/healthcare, last accessed January 2016.
9. DVTk, http://en.wikipedia.org/wiki/DVTk
10. Potter G, Busbridge R, Toland M, Nagy P. Mastering DICOM with DVTk. In: Journal of Digital Imaging, Vol.20, Suppl.1, 2007, pp. 47–62.
11. DVTk Eye2Eye Meeting. Oxford, Feb. 8th, 2008.
12. HL7 API. http://hl7api.sourceforge.net/, last accessed February 28th, 2016.
13. Oemig F: The Comprehensive HL7 Database, www.oemig.de/hl7/, last accessed February 28th, 2016.
14. HL7 Switzerland. CDA-CH. http://www.hl7.ch/publikationen0.html
15. eHealth Suisse. eHealth Connector. https://sourceforge.net/p/ehealthconnector/wiki/Home/
16. http://www.healthcare.philips.com/main/about/connectivity/dicom_validation_tool.wpd
17. DICOM Validation Toolkit. www.dvtk.org

18. eHealth Suisse. CDA Validator. http://www.e-health-cda-validator.ch/validation.xhtml
19. HL7 Version 2: XML Encoding Syntax, Release 1. ANSI/HL7 V2 XML-2003; June 4, 2003.
20. Message Maker. Developed by the National Institute of Standards and Technology (NIST) in conjunction with the HL7 Conformance Special Interest Group; http://www.nist.gov/messagemaker.
21. Snelick R, Gebase L. Dynamically Generating Conformance Tests for Messaging Systems. Sydney Henrard. In: Software Engineering Research and Practice (SERP06) conference proceedings, WORLDCOMP'06 June 26-29, 2006, Las Vegas, Nevada.
22. Open eHealth Foundation: http://www.openehealth.org/
23. Open Health Tools: http://www.openhealthtools.org/
24. Surescripts: company and network to enable and support e-prescribing http://surescripts.com
25. Trifolia Workbench HL7 Webedition. https://trifolia.lantanagroup.com/

Chapter 15
Testing and Certification Programs

15.1 Introduction

The final step in the cycle of implementation of standards is the certification process. Certification provides assurances to stakeholders that a HIT software product meets the requirements indicated in the specification Certification is a method that formally verifies conformance claims made by a vendor. Certification can be advantageous to the vendor, as it offers a certain degree of confidence to the purchasers. In some cases, use of certified HIT may be required in order for a health care organization or provider to participate in federal programs, such as qualifying to receive Meaningful Use incentive payments (in the US).

As discussed throughout this book, the development of reliable software products involves many steps and iterations of those steps. Figure 15.1 illustrates the key components in the life cycle of standards, implementation, and testing.

Standards usually are first developed as draft specifications. The development of implementations and testing tools inform the standard. An important outcome of

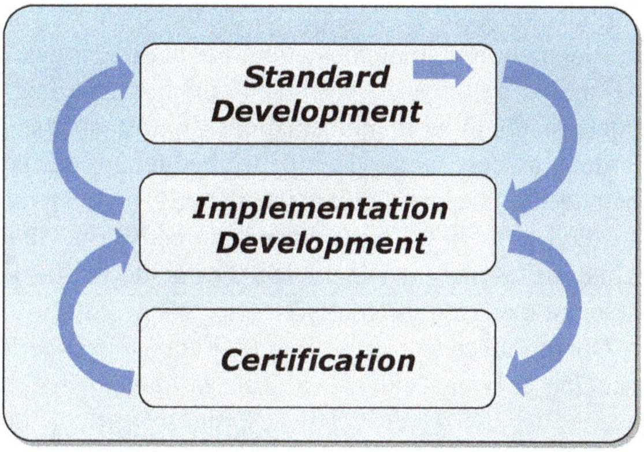

Fig. 15.1 Standards, implementation, and test life cycle overview

F. Oemig and R. Snelick, *Healthcare Interoperability Standards Compliance Handbook*, DOI 10.1007/978-3-319-44839-8_15

this step is to verify that requirements as expressed in those specifications are practical, implementable and testable. Before a final (normative) specification is published, this first verification cycle may go through multiple iterations. The development of conformance testing tools is a critical aspect of the implementation development step. Conformance testing at this point can be internal, or it can be an informal process using publicly available tools. Errors, ambiguities, and inconsistencies in the specification are reported. Certification is a formal process, and ideally it is conducted by a third party. Conformance testing and test tools are key components of certification. The certification process also informs issues in the standard, implementations, and test tools.

The Business Dictionary defines certification as a "Formal procedure by which an accredited or authorized person or agency assesses and verifies (and attests in writing by issuing a certificate) the attributes, characteristics, quality, qualification, goods or services, procedures or processes, or events or situation, in accordance with established requirements or standards" [1]. This definition is applicable for use in certification of the healthcare information technology. Note that in this chapter a distinction is made between Certification and Testing Programs. Certifications typically are rigid processes governed by accredited bodies; testing programs are more informal but perform similar functions. In some cases certification is based on a testing program.

In the remainder of this chapter, an overview is given of the role of certification and how it relates to standards development and conformance testing. A perspective on what certification testing means is given next. Finally, an overview of some of the most notable certification and testing programs is presented, including the US Health IT Certification and EHR Meaningful Use Programs and the IHE Testing Programs.

15.2 Certification Perspectives

Certification can be thought of as the final step in the life-cycle of standards development and implementation. Standards provide a set of requirements and are the means to an end. The intent of a standard is the eventual binding of the requirements to an implementation. Conformance is defined as the fulfilment of a product, process, or service of specified requirements [2]. Conformance testing is a method that seeks to determine directly or indirectly that the requirements in a standard have been implemented correctly. Standards, implementation, and conformance testing are interrelated. For a successful outcome, it is essential that all three are executed diligently.

Conformance testing is often (but not always) performed by testing laboratories, resulting in issuance of a certificate to implementations that pass all the tests. This process is called certification. Even if certification is not the goal, however,

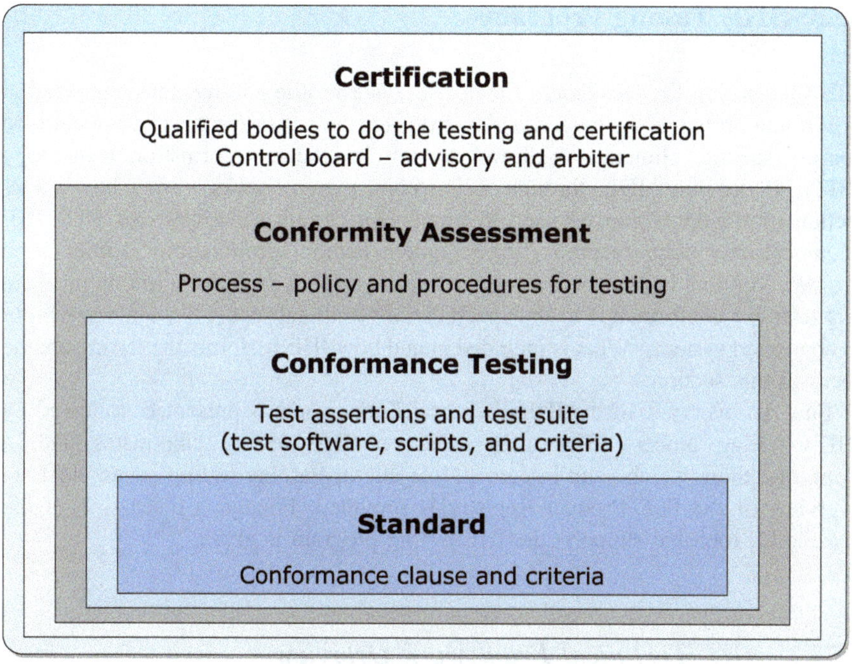

Fig. 15.2 Certification building blocks (adapted from [3])

conformance testing is still necessary, since it is the only way to ascertain if requirements in the standard have been implemented correctly. Additionally, conformance testing serves as a means of communication between buyers and sellers, allowing sellers to substantiate their claims and buyers to increase their confidence in a product.

The relationship among the standard, conformance testing, conformity assessment, and certification is similar to that of a set of inter-connected building blocks (see Fig. 15.2). None of the outer-layers of blocks can be performed unless the inner-layers of blocks have been completed. Thus, conformance testing can not be performed unless the standard (with its conformance clauses and clear, testable requirements) has been completed. Conformity assessment (processes and policies for testing) can not be implemented until the standard and the conformance testing test suite are in place. Finally, certification can only be accomplished when all of the three lower-level building blocks are in place, and one can stop anywhere along this spectrum. Many standards exist without conformance testing or certification. Some standards have associated conformance tests but no certification regimen, while some standards incorporate all the components up to and including certification.

15.3 IHE Testing Programs

IHE (Integrating the Healthcare Enterprises) is a profile enforcement organization (PEO) that promotes, leverages, and coordinates the use of established standards to address specific clinical workflows through healthcare information technology (HIT) [4]. In short, IHE, through their technical frameworks, shows how a collection of standards can be used to implement certain capabilities of HIT. IHE documents the requirements for these implementation specifications in Integration Profiles. Vendors implement the specifications and IHE provides a testing program that tests for conformance to the specifications and, subsequently, interoperability of connected systems. What is included in and how IHE performs the testing are the focus of this section.

First, an overview of the IHE Technical Frameworks is presented, followed by IHE's testing process. The main aspect of IHE testing culminates with a Connect-a-thon, which is an in-person, live interoperability testing event. Next, an overview of the IHE Product Registry is provided. Finally, a discussion of the Gazelle [5] tool that supports the IHE testing program is given.

15.3.1 IHE Technical Framework Overview

IHE develops technical frameworks that can be used by implementers to facilitate system integration. The technical frameworks define standards for common healthcare information technology use cases, such as managing patient identifiers. The technical frameworks leverage existing standards whenever possible and constrain/adapt them to meet the targeted use case. In the case of HL7 v2, this effort typically means leveraging the HL7 v2 standard and creating a set of conformance profiles. An example of this is in the Information Technology Infrastructure (ITI) Technical Framework (TF), in which a number of ADT (admit/discharge/transfer) messages and a query and response pair of messages are profiled for Patient Identification Cross-Referencing (PIX). The ITI TF for the PIX Integration Profile defines the associated actors, transactions, and functional requirements. For more information on IHE Technical Framework refer to Chap. 3.

15.3.2 IHE Testing Process

IHE testing is a multi-faceted and multi-phase process. Once the technical frameworks have been published, which is generally (but not necessarily) in August or September, implementers can begin reviewing and implementing. The typical testing cycle for the North American Connect-a-thon is depicted in Table 15.1. The

Table 15.1 North American connect-a-thon summary

Testing method	When	Testing type	Test environment
Pre-connect-a-thon	October to December	Conformance	Data instance testing Isolated-system testing
Virtual connect-a-thon	December to January	Conformance and interoperability	Peer-to-peer testing
Connect-a-thon	January	Conformance and interoperability	Peer-to-peer testing

European (and other) connect-a-thons have their own testing cycles. Each connect-a-thon tests a different set of integration profiles based on the capabilities and interests of the vendors for a particular realm.

IHE testing employs a number of incremental testing methods. First, vendors conduct conformance testing of their products. This task involves testing in isolation to determine if the system implements the requirements specified in the standard. These tests are called pre-connect-a-thon tests and correspond to the data instance testing and isolated system test environments. Interoperability testing (peer-to-peer testing) is conducted at an event called a connect-a-thon in which scores of vendors bring their products to a central site, and live-monitored tests are performed over a period of a week [6]. Such concentrated events are useful as vendors can interact with many other vendors in a short period of time; however, connect-a-thons occur relatively infrequently (once a year in the United States, Europe, and Asia-Oceania), and they are costly. An intermediate format in the form of an on-line virtual connect-a-thon, in which interoperability testing is always available, can supplement pre-connect-a-thon and connect-a-thon testing. This approach is a future direction, and a testing architecture to support it is being explored and developed by NIST and IHE. See the discussion of the Interoperability Test Bed (ITB) presented in Chap. 13 for an overview and a design proposal. The goal of the ITB is to conduct connect-a-thon-style testing virtually over the Internet, but there are technical challenges to overcome.

Regardless of the testing method, testing is performed at the integration profile[1] level not at the technical framework level. Vendors sign up for the integration profiles they wish to test; in essence, they are making a claim of conformance to one or more actors defined in the various integration profiles. The number of actors a given vendor tests is typically between 8 and 15 with an average of 12.[2] Testing

[1] In the IHE space, an integration profile is often simply referred to as a profile; but, to avoid confusion with the use of the term profiles in other contexts, e.g., message profile, we will continue to use the long name, integration profile.

[2] For the 2014 North American Connect-a-thon; Source: personal communication with Steve Moore, IHE.

will substantiate[3] or refute this claim. Since an integration profile often includes multiple actors, a particular vendor may claim conformance to only one (or a subset) of the actors in the integration profile. IHE has developed a test management tool (called Gazelle [5]), which, among other things, manages, records, and orchestrates tests and testing events. Its primary purpose is to conduct connect-a-thons, but it also is used to support pre-connect-a-thon and, more recently, virtual connect-a-thon activities. A more detailed overview of Gazelle and its capabilities is presented in a sub-section to follow.

15.3.2.1 Pre-connect-a-Thon

Pre-connect-a-thon testing is conformance testing and is typically performed with a validator (data instance testing) or a test system (isolated-system testing) with simulators. Data instance testing can employ context-free testing or context-based testing as described in Chap. 11. The goal of pre-connect-a-thon testing is to assess whether the vendor's implementation conforms to a certain degree to the requirements stated in the integration profile. Typically this assessment involves testing the creation of an artifact or a number of transactions and associated functional requirements. IHE, NIST, and the Mallinckrodt Institute of Radiology (MIR) are the main developers of testing tools that support pre-connect-a-thons. A list of pre-connect-a-thon tools can be found at [7].

15.3.2.2 Virtual Connect-a-Thon

A virtual connect-a-thon is a testing method that usually occurs between the pre-connect-a-thon and the connect-a-thon. Typical operation would involve a number of vendors connecting via the Internet and using a conference call or a chat service to coordinate testing. Often these events are organized by IHE program managers, target a small set of profiles, and are scheduled at a certain time. These events follow pre-connect-a-thon testing and focus on interoperability testing. In some cases, certain actors could be tested without pre-coordination. For example, a vendor may choose to provide access to a PIX Manager (server) via the Internet and publish necessary configuration information (e.g., IP address and port number). A vendor that wishes to test actors such as the PIX source and PIX consumer could do so without directly contacting the PIX Manager vendor. This approach gives the vendor some assurance of achieving interoperability before attending a

[3]As previously discussed, to a certain degree of confidence based on the quantity and quality of the test plan.

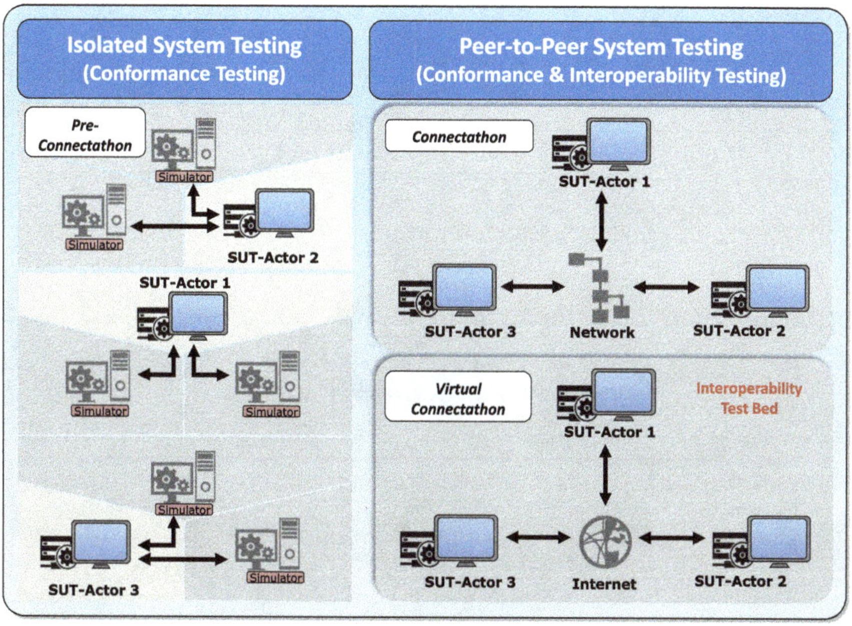

Fig. 15.3 IHE testing models

connect-a-thon. The testing is typically ad hoc, and conformance testing is not performed.

As mentioned before, the concept of a virtual connect-a-thon can be realized via the proposed ITB. The ITB affords a more controlled environment that allows for both conformance and interoperability testing. IHE Gazelle would serve as an ideal platform for the test bed since it manages vendors, configurations, and test cases.

15.3.2.3 Connect-a-Thon

Connect-a-thon testing consists of live-monitored tests performed over a period of a week and held at a particular geographic site [6]. The focus of connect-a-thon testing is interoperability. The basic setup is a large room in which vendors' systems are networked. Participants indicate what they want to test and then publish their availability. Once testing partners are coupled, their systems are configured in the Gazelle management tool, and they can proceed with testing. Once tests are completed, neutral monitors are employed to verify the tests. The typical number of tests verified at the North American Connect-a-thon is in the 3000–4000 range. Verification of tests includes a combination of automated tools and visual inspection. Typically, vendors are required to demonstrate successful integration with at least three different partners for a given test. IHE issues integration statements to

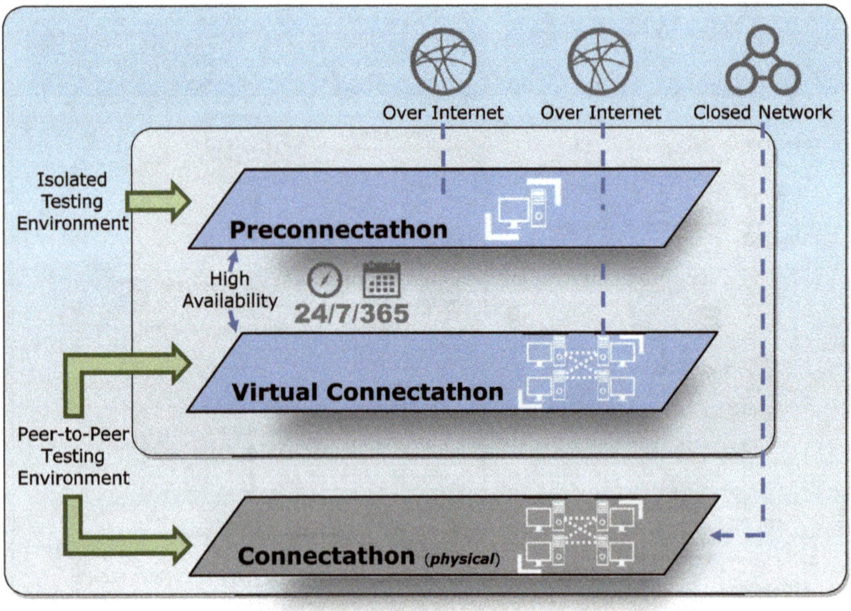

Fig. 15.4 IHE testing availability and approach

vendors for the software products and the IHE actors that successfully complete the testing. Connect-a-thon participation is a pre-requisite for the IHE showcase demonstration at the annual conferences of the Healthcare Information and Management Systems Society (HIMSS) or World of Health IT (WoHIT).

15.3.3 IHE Product Registry

Upon completion of testing, a list of Integration Statements is published in the IHE Product Registry [8]. Integration Statements, as defined by IHE, are documents published by vendors indicating their conformance claim for their products to specific integration profiles. Integration Statements include the vendor name, product name, product version, publication date, and additional information about the claim. The product registry on-line tool allows vendors to add and update their Integration Statements, and enables potential customers to browse and review them. This information can subsequently be used in requests for proposals. Table 15.2 provides an excerpt from an Integration Statement.

Table 15.2 IHE integration statement example (excerpt)

IHE Integration Statement			
Vendor	**Product Name**	**Version**	**Date**
XXX	YYY	3.2	03/03/15
This product implements all transactions required in the IHE Technical Framework to support the IHE Integration Profiles, Actors, and Options listed below:			

Integration Profile	Actor	Integration Profile Option
Healthcare Provider Directory	Provider Information Directory	None
Patient Demographics Query	Patient Demographics Supplier	None
Patient Demographics Query HL7 V3	Patient Demographics Supplier	None
Patient Identifier Cross-referencing for MPI	Patient Identity Cross-reference Manager	None
Patient Identifier Cross-referencing HL7 V3	Patient Identity Cross-reference Manager	None
Cross-Community Access	Initiating Gateway	None
Cross-Community Access	Initiating Gateway	Asynchronous Web Services Exchange
Cross-Community Access	Responding Gateway	None

15.3.4 Gazelle

Gazelle [5] is a multi-purpose tool that facilitates the operation of the IHE testing program. A central function of Gazelle is to manage connect-a-thons; i.e., Gazelle is the management tool that maintains all the integration profiles (actors and transactions), vendor declarations and configurations, test cases, orchestration of tests (including test views to vendors and monitors), and test results. In short, it automates much of the activities of the connect-a-thon. During the connect-a-thon, vendors use Gazelle to set up a test (i.e., match compatible actors). For example, Vendor A may be a PIX Source and is seeking to run a PIX Feed test with a PIX Manager. Gazelle facilitates making this match and setting up the test. Once the test instance has been established, it appears in each vendor's test list. The vendors then view the test case, proceed to run the test, document relevant results, and submit the results into Gazelle. The test instance then appears on the monitors' list (monitors who are trained to validate this type of test), alerting them that a test is ready to be validated. The monitor will then inspect the evidence in the test case and, depending on the type of test, may or may not request additional evidence by visual inspection of the vendors' products. Certain tests will never require visual inspection, while others always will; some may depend solely on the judgment of the monitor. Once the evaluation is completed, the monitor will submit their findings into Gazelle. Gazelle updates the vendor's test list status and internal histories. From this perspective, Gazelle is a test management tool; however, Gazelle offers additional capabilities to support conformance and interoperability testing, such as validators, simulators, and data generation tools. These aspects of Gazelle are addressed in Chap. 14.

Gazelle has proven to be a very effective and reliable tool for conducting connect-a-thons in which scores of vendors and hundreds of profile actors have to be managed and thousands of tests performed. Gazelle's operational aspects have to support a mix of automated and inspection tests. Gazelle has additional capabilities not described here and continues to expand its offering. For complete details see [5].

15.4 EHR Certification and Meaningful Use Programs

The US Congress has authorized creation and funding of federal programs to promote meaningful use of federally approved electronic health record (EHR) technologies aimed at achieving interoperability between information systems used in the health care setting. These programs, managed by the Centers for Medicare and Medicaid Services (CMS) and the Office of the National Coordinator for Health Information Technology (ONCHIT or ONC), began in 2009 and continue to the present day. This Section briefly explains the history and purpose of the federal EHR technology programs—in particular the ONC Health IT Certification Program—and provides insight into the reaction of the health care market. It also presents an overview of the ONC certification testing process, including the roles of the standards developers, the National Institute of Standards and Technology (NIST), the testing laboratories, and the certification bodies. These diverse groups work together to ensure that vendors' health IT products meet ONC's minimum functional and data exchange requirements.

15.4.1 Patient Safety and Federal EHR Technology Programs

According to the 2001 Institute of Medicine's (IOM) report [9], information technology (IT) has a critical role to play in health care delivery in the US. This report was a follow-up to the ground-breaking 1999 IOM report [10]. Anyone involved in providing health care is aware of the shocking statistics that were shared in that 1999 publication regarding the inexcusable number of deaths caused by preventable medical errors [11]. As of July, 2014, according to an article entitled

Deaths by medical mistakes hit records that was posted in the online journal *Healthcare IT News*, “Preventable medical errors persist as the No. 3 killer in the US—third only to heart disease and cancer—claiming the lives of some 400,000 people each year” [12]. In all of these reports and articles, proper use of health information technology (HIT) is listed as a key element for improving patient safety.

At the core of the HIT that is being praised in these writings is the electronic health record (EHR). The *Crossing the Quality Chasm* report of 2001 speaks of the 1991 IOM vision [13] for nationwide deployment of what were then called computer-based patient records (CPRs), and it also includes the IOM’s acknowledgment that progress had been slow as of 1991 toward achievement of this goal. The 2001 report recognized the continuing lack of significant progress toward the IOM goal 10 years later as it goes on to describe the potential benefits of using the EHR to reduce prescribing errors and to link all patient data across the continuum of care in order to provide quality health services and build a robust database for quality measurement [9].

Based on the overwhelming evidence of the need for deployment of the electronic record, President George W. Bush stated in his 2004 remarks to the American Association of Community Colleges Annual Convention that “Within ten years, every American must have a personal electronic medical record” [14]. It’s no wonder, then, that the EHR was the focus of the initial effort once federal funding was made available to assist and motivate adoption and specified meaningful utilization of HIT.

The facts about how routine use of EHRs in the practice of medicine—especially systems with clinical decision support capabilities—enables quality improvement as well as decreased cost of care were influential in convincing Congress to legislate the Health Information Technology for Economic and Clinical Health (HITECH) Act, a component of the American Recovery and Reinvestment Act (ARRA) of 2009. Among other provisions, the HITECH Act included funding for CMS incentive payments to Eligible Professionals (e.g., physicians) and Eligible Hospitals and Critical Access Hospitals that use HIT in accordance with specified requirements.

15.4.2 The Federal HIT Certification Program

Initially focusing on adoption of approved EHRs, approximately $18 billion in incentive payments were made available through the CMS HITECH-based EHR Meaningful Use (MU) Program. Those payments were to be disbursed by CMS to providers that attested to or demonstrated “meaningful use” (according to objectives and measures issued by CMS) of “certified” EHR technology (CEHRT). $2 billion of HITECH funds were allocated to the ONC with the mandate to create the necessary infrastructure to promote electronic exchange and use of health information in the US, along with numerous other related initiatives.

To support testing and certification of the EHR technologies/HIT, the ONC established a certification program, which included testing laboratories and certification bodies as well as EHR certification criteria that were published in the Federal Register. The ONC EHR certification criteria were related to the CMS EHR MU objectives and measures in that the ONC produced certification criteria that were intended to be used for testing EHR technologies' ability to support Eligible Professionals and Eligible Hospitals in demonstrating the CMS requirements.

Thus far, CMS has published Final Rule requirements for MU Stages 1, 2, and 3; and ONC has published Final Rules for four editions of EHR/HIT standards and certification criteria: 2011 Edition, 2014 Edition, 2014 Edition Release 2, and 2015 Edition. ONC CEHRT requirements are not a comprehensive list of all HIT features and functions that a physician's office or a hospital might want or need, nor do they include any usability standards that prescribe how HIT must be designed; rather, they represent the minimum capabilities HIT vendors must implement in their products in order to achieve ONC certification and to support users in meeting the CMS MU requirements. As such, the certification criteria are a subset of capabilities that a 21st-century HIT should support, and HIT developers are not prevented from including additional capabilities in their products that attain ONC certification.

The CMS Notice of Proposed Rulemaking (NPRM) for MU Stage 3 and the ONC NPRM for 2015 Edition HIT certification criteria were published in April of 2015. After a federally mandated Public Comment period, the CMS MU Stage 3 Final Rule and ONC 2015 Edition Final Rule were published in October of 2015.

As mentioned above, the ONC established a program to support testing and certification of EHR technology/HIT. The initial program (called the ONC Temporary Certification Program) was established according to the Temporary Certification Program Final Rule, which included creation of ONC-Authorized Testing and Certification Bodies (ONC-ATCBs) that provided both the testing and certification of EHR technologies. As stipulated in the HITECH Act, the National Institute of Standards and Technology (NIST) National Voluntary Laboratory Accreditation Program (NVLAP) tested ATCB applicants, and the testing laboratories that met the testing standards became ONC-ATCBs.

In order to institute a process that promoted integrity as well as robustness, the program authors always had in mind that the testing and certification activities would be performed by separate entities, or at least different divisions or personnel within a single entity. The ONC was given a very short timeline for establishing the certification program, however, and, in order to meet the deadline for starting initial certification testing, the Temporary Certification Program Final Rule allowed the identification of a group of ATCBs to perform both activities. This approach was faster than credentialing two separate sets of qualified entities, one set to do the testing and another set to do the certification, and also establishing the policies for their governance. Under this temporary Final Rule, the ATCB personnel who tested could also be the same personnel who certified the EHR technologies. This approach made the Certification Program vulnerable to criticism, since the personnel who performed the certification could be reviewing the testing results they themselves had documented about a given EHR technology.

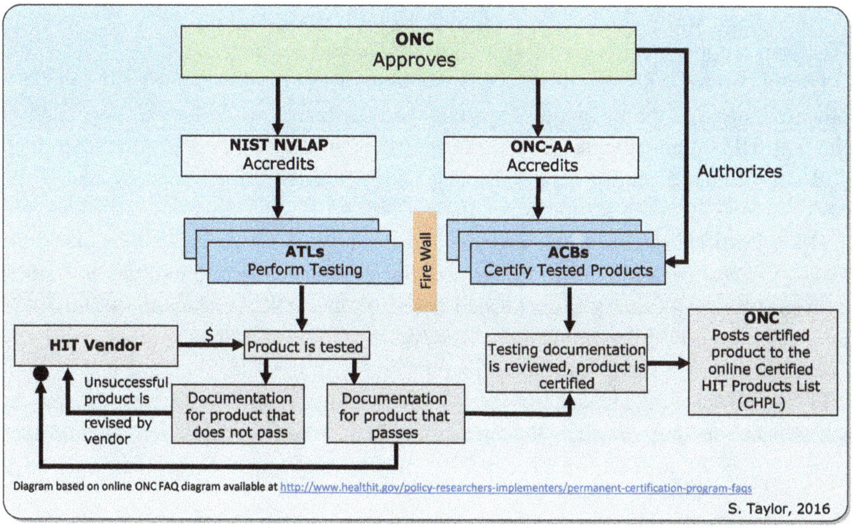

Fig. 15.5 ONC health IT certification program

When the permanent program (called the ONC Health IT Certification Program) was launched in accordance with the Permanent Certification Program Final Rule on October 4, 2012, the temporary program was sunset. Figure 15.5 illustrates key components of the ONC Health IT Certification Program, showing the testing and certification as separate and distinct activities—testing being the role of ONC-Accredited Testing Laboratories (ONC-ATLs) and certification being the role of ONC-Authorized Certification Bodies (ONC-ACBs).

As part of the establishment of the permanent program, the NIST NVLAP was named as the accreditor for the multiple ATLs. Testing laboratories applied to the NIST NVLAP and if they met the laboratory testing standards they became ONC-ATLs. In accordance with the permanent program Final Rule, ONC could approve *one* accreditor organization, called the ONC-Approved Accreditor (ONC-AA), to accredit and oversee the multiple certification bodies. ONC chose the American National Standards Institute (ANSI) for this role. Once the ONC-AA accredited them, each certification body had to obtain authorization from the ONC. A certification body is officially called an ONC-Authorized Certification Body (ONC-ACB) once it receives this authorization. The ACBs certify the health IT that pass the ATL testing under the ONC Health IT Certification Program.

As discussed previously, a given testing laboratory can qualify as both an ATL and as an ACB; but the lab must provide evidence to ONC that the testing and certification processes are kept completely separate, and that a "firewall" is maintained between the resources that perform the testing and the resources that award the certification.

When they are ready for their product to be tested, the HIT vendor selects an ATL from among the group of testing labs that have been accredited by ONC. If the ATL they choose is also an ONC-ACB, the vendor can have this one entity perform both activities for them, or they can choose a different ACB for the certification role. The HIT vendor pays the ATL to test their products. An ATL that also is an ACB can offer the vendor a package that includes pricing for both services. If the vendor selects a different entity for their ONC-ACB, the vendor would pay that ACB for certification services. Pricing and packaging are controlled by the individual ATLs and ACBs, and the exact dollar amount each one charges is proprietary information. Testing is performed based on the ONC certification criteria and ONC test method (test procedures, test data, and test tools—details about the development of the ONC test method are provided in the Sub-Section "The Role of NIST"), and each ATL usually develops their own proprietary test scripts to facilitate the testing process. Products that do not pass certification testing successfully may be re-tested, a process that may or may not require additional payment to the vendor's chosen ATL.

Results of the certification testing are carefully documented by the ATL, and, when the HIT module passes the testing, this documentation is submitted to the vendor's chosen ACB for review. If the testing results pass inspection by the ACB, then the product is certified and the necessary information about the product is submitted to the ONC, whereupon the ONC posts the information on the online ONC Certified HIT Products List (ONC-CHPL) accessible at http://oncchpl.force.com/ehrcert?q=chpl. Figure 15.6 provides an excerpt from one of the pages of the CHPL showing ONC 2014 Edition information about Epic ambulatory EHRs as an example.[4]

Each entry in the current version of the CHPL (as of early 2016) includes the vendor name, the original practice type of the product (i.e., ambulatory or inpatient), the product name, the product version, the CHPL Product Number,[5] and the product classification (i.e., Complete or Modular EHR).

By clicking on the name of the product that is listed in the Product column, one accesses a Web page containing supplemental detailed information about that particular product, as shown in Fig. 15.7. This view includes the name of the ATL that performed the testing, the ONC criteria to which the product is certified, the Clinical Quality Measures to which the product is certified, the CMS EHR Certification Identification Number[6] (listed on the CHPL as the "CHPL Certification ID"), and any additional software required for the product to achieve certification status.

---

[4]Inclusion of information about Epic is merely an arbitrary example and in no way implies an endorsement of this vendor or this vendor's products.

[5]Each certified Health IT Module on the CHPL has a "CHPL Product Number" assigned to it by the ONC-Authorized Certification Body (ONC-ACB) that certified the product.

[6]The CMS EHR Certification Identification Number is a number generated by the CHPL that represents a Health IT Module or combination of Health IT Modules, and that is used for reporting to CMS EHR Incentive Programs.

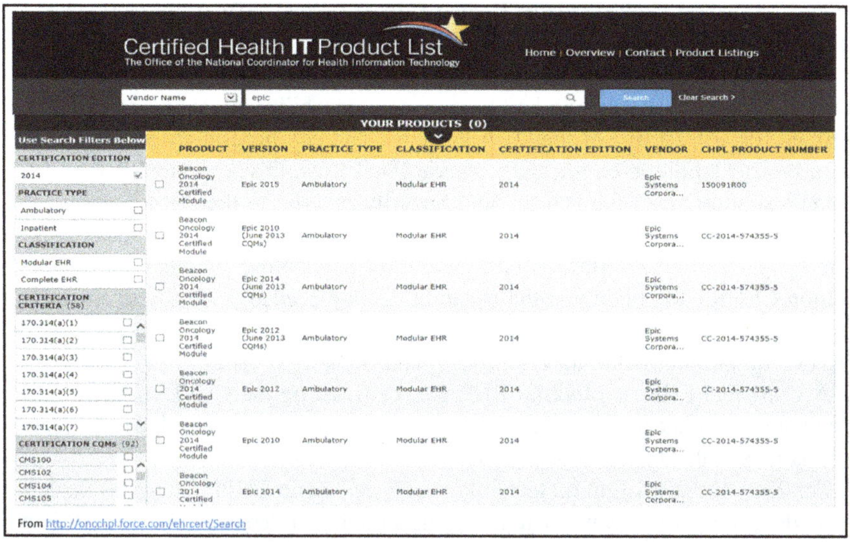

Fig. 15.6 ONC CHPL—vendor-specific view

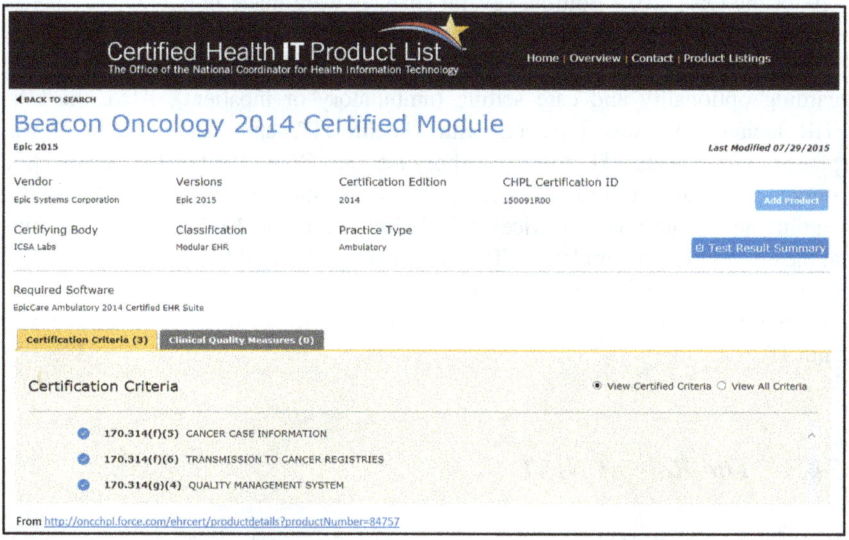

Fig. 15.7 ONC CHPL—detailed view

A 2014 Edition CEHRT can be certified and classified as a "Complete EHR" or as a "Modular EHR". The Complete EHR designation means that the EHR technology meets, at a minimum, all applicable Edition-specific ONC certification criteria published in the Federal Registry. In the ONC 2014 Edition Final Rule, EHR Module referred to any service or component, or combination of the two, that meets at least one ONC certification criterion published in the Federal Registry. In other words, an EHR Module had to provide a capability that could be tested and certified for at least one of the 2014 Edition ONC certification criteria.

In the 2011 Edition certification criteria Final Rule, ONC required that an EHR Module support all of the Privacy and Security criteria. In the 2014 Edition certification criteria, however, this requirement was eliminated in favor of making those criteria part of the "Base EHR definition", enabling purchasers of 2014 Edition CEHRT to obtain just the capabilities they needed from any given vendor so long as they ultimately had a combination of EHR technologies that satisfied the CEHRT definition, including the Privacy and Security criteria.

A Complete EHR or Modular EHR can be listed on the CHPL as having been tested for ambulatory use or inpatient use or both. The applicable certification criteria may differ for ambulatory EHRs versus inpatient EHRs.

For 2011 and 2014 Edition technologies, once a valid CHPL entry was made for a CEHRT, the entry was never removed. If an updated version of the CEHRT was posted, the entry for the older version(s) remained on the CHPL. Eligible Professionals and Eligible Hospitals use the CHPL to search for CEHRT that meet their needs.

As of the ONC 2015 Edition, several changes were made in how ONC labelled the certification criteria as well as what they called the technologies being certified. For example, the names of the certification criteria no longer included information regarding optionality and care setting (ambulatory or inpatient). Also, the term "EHR technology" was replaced with "health IT", and "EHR Module" was replaced with "health IT Module", because the ONC Health IT Certification Program as of 2015 Edition is open to the certification of all types of health IT, including healthcare-related devices. ONC disclosed in the 2015 Edition Final Rule that the designation "Complete EHR" will no longer be used for labelling a certified technology, which they indicated is in accordance with their decision to make the certification criteria agnostic regarding health care settings and open to all types of health IT.

15.4.3 The Role of NIST

NIST developed all of the test procedures, test data, and conformance test tools associated with the 2011 Edition ONC EHR certification criteria. NIST also developed most of the conformance test tools and their related test procedures for the Edition 2014 ONC certification criteria (and updated these items for 2014 Edition Release 2 where necessary), while working with subject matter experts (SMEs) from the Centers for Disease Control and Prevention (CDC), the Association of Public Health Laboratories (APHL), the International Society for

Disease Surveillance (ISDS), and other organizations to develop the associated test cases and test data.

For the 2015 Edition ONC certification criteria, NIST developed most of the conformance test tools and their related NIST Normative Test Process Documents, which provide the detailed testing actions. NIST worked with SMEs from organizations such as the CDC, APHL, ISDS, the National Council for Prescription Drug Programs (NCPDP), and the American Immunization Registry Association (AIRA) to develop Test Cases and Test Data for the test tools. The format and content of these test process documents are similar to the 2014 Edition ONC Test Procedure documents, but they exclude much of the background explanatory verbiage (such as quotes from the Preamble of the ONC Final Rule) in order to focus on the information that is most essential to developers and testers. Each test tool-specific document is accessible from the Documentation page of the 2015 Edition NIST HL7 v2 Immunization Test Suite, Syndromic Surveillance Test Suite, and Electronic Laboratory Reporting (ELR) Test Tool, and the 2015 Edition ePrescribing Test Tool.

The ONC developed two complementary documents for all of the 2015 Edition criteria: the *ONC 2015 Edition Test Procedure* documents and the *ONC 2015 Edition Certification Companion Guides* [see 15 for web-site]. The ONC Test Procedure document format is radically different and much shorter than the 2014 version. ONC stated on their Web site that the "2015 Edition Test Method has been constructed in an outcome-focused format with additional companion guide documents to aid stakeholder development of Health IT Modules".

Several of the ONC criteria designated data exchange standards, such as HL7 v2 implementation guides (IGs) and various vocabulary standards. NIST used the standard vocabularies and the conformance requirements listed in the IGs that are named in the ONC certification criteria in their development of the automated test tools used by the HIT vendors and ATLs for validation of test messages related to ONC certification testing.

ONC does not develop the data exchange standards that are named in the certification criteria, but ONC does support the development of these standards by communities of healthcare and HIT subject matter experts. One of the approaches ONC adopted for achieving its HIT interoperability mandate is known as the Standards and Interoperability (S&I) Framework, which provides a forum that empowers healthcare stakeholders from the public and private sectors to meet as work groups, discuss real-world healthcare interoperability challenges, and produce agreed-upon specifications to enable standardized healthcare data exchange.

NIST is an active participant in the S&I Framework Initiatives that are focused on HL7 v2 standards and provides input to the discussions to keep the associated work groups mindful of the necessity to produce "testable" specifications. As a member of these work groups, NIST also is able to seek feedback from HIT vendors and experts as "pilot testers" of draft versions of the NIST HL7 v2 test tools.

Figure 15.8 provides an overview of the EHR certification process (as of CMS MU Stage 2 and ONC 2014 Edition) where development and use of a NIST

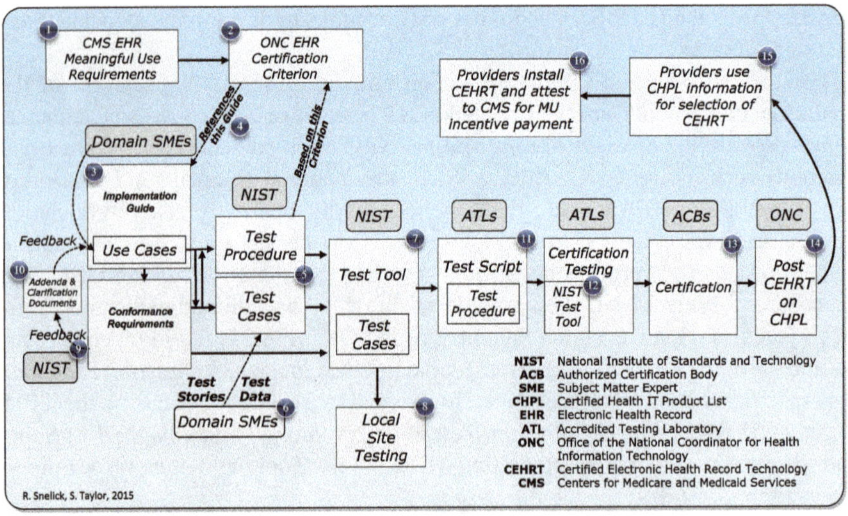

Fig. 15.8 Overview of the meaningful use and certification testing process

test tool was involved. The numbers in the diagram correspond to the numbered steps listed below the diagram that explain the process, including the relationship of the CMS EHR MU requirements to the ONC EHR certification criteria; the roles of various participants in the process; and the feedback loops that facilitate additional input to the standards authoring groups during the course of the NIST test tool development.

The following numbered list of steps corresponds to the numbers shown in Fig. 15.8 and provide an explanation for the process flow in the diagram:

1. CMS publishes a Final Rule listing EHR Meaningful Use (MU) Requirements for Eligible Professionals (EPs) and Eligible Hospitals (EHs)
2. ONC develops EHR certification criterion corresponding to CMS MU requirement
3. Domain subject matter experts (SMEs) develop an Implementation Guide for their discipline for specific Use Cases. NIST extracts and assesses the confor-mance requirements for tool development.
4. ONC criterion specifies the Implementation Guide
5. NIST develops the Test Procedure and Test Cases based on the ONC certification criterion and the Guide
6. Domain SMEs provide test stories and test data for the Test Cases
7. NIST develops the Test Tool for certification testing; the Test Tool includes the Test Cases (draft or beta versions of the NIST tools are published for public review, and comments sent to NIST are used to refine the tools and test data; once the official release of a NIST tool is published, NIST continues to collect feedback and to publish updated releases with related modifications)
8. The NIST Test Tool also can be used for local site testing/installations

9. The next version of the Guide written by domain SMEs includes feedback from NIST; and during development of the Test Tool, NIST provides feedback to the writers of the Guide regarding any need for clarification of the conformance requirements
10. Addenda and Clarification documents are written by domain SMEs as necessary
11. ATLs create their proprietary Test Scripts, which assimilate the NIST Test Procedure
12. ATLs use the NIST Test Tool for certification testing of EHR technologies, and submit results of successful EHR certification testing to an ACB
13. The ACB certifies the EHR technology based on results of the testing
14. ONC posts the CEHRT on the CHPL
15. Providers access the CHPL to view certified technologies and use the infor-ma-tion for selection of their CEHRT
16. Providers license or purchase CEHRT, install it, and then attest to CMS that they are using the CEHRT according to MU requirements in order to receive the incentive payments

The ONC HIT testing and certification process has been transparent, and all stakeholders were welcome to participate in the work groups that determine the data exchange requirements and standards.

15.4.4 Reaction in the Market to the Federal EHR Programs

The need for use of EHR technology in support of patient safety and control of the cost of healthcare in the US was recognized by HIT specialists in the late 1980s and reemphasized in the early 1990s. Motivating clinicians, especially physicians in their office practices, to adopt and use the available EHR technologies, however, proved to be difficult to achieve for all except a very small percentage of these users. At that time, a significant number of HIT mavens were telling each other that a government mandate and funding would have to be instigated before real progress could be made.

The CMS EHR MU incentive payments were legislated ultimately as part of a federal law focused on pulling the US out of a recession. The HITECH Act of 2009 that was part of that federal law has resulted in an increase in sales of EHRs and likely in additional HIT-related jobs, while also meeting the goal of prompting hospitals, and especially physician practices, to adopt EHR technologies at a far faster rate than during the previous decades. This Act brought the government mandate and funding that the pundits predicted would be needed. The targeted users of the EHR technologies, namely, the health delivery organizations and physician practices, understood from the beginning that HITECH and the CMS EHR Meaningful Use Programs would use persuasion initially (in the form of incentive

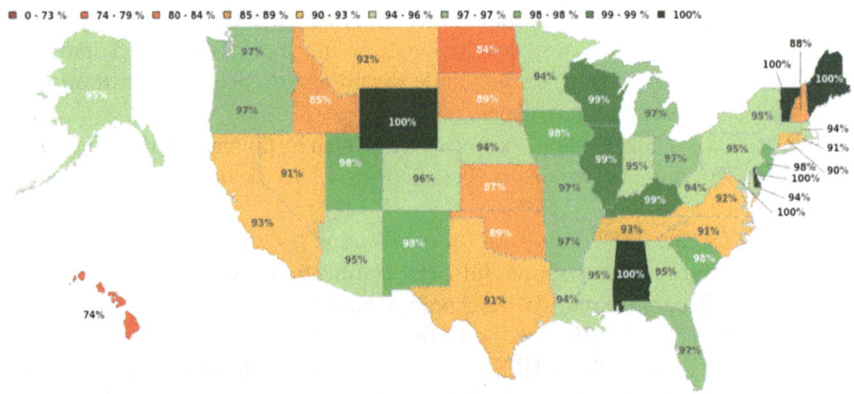

Fig. 15.9 Percentage of hospitals participating in the CMS EHR incentive programs (Health IT Dashboard 2014)

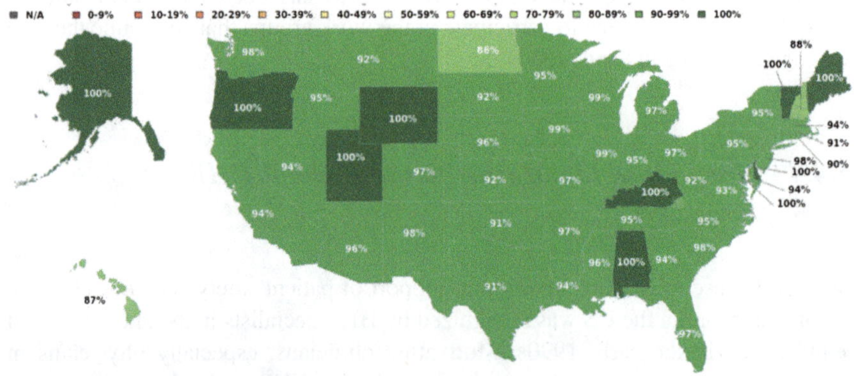

Fig. 15.10 Percentage of hospitals participating in the CMS EHR incentive programs (Health IT Dashboard 2015)

payments), but ultimately could use punitive methods (in the form of reductions in CMS payments for medical claims) against providers who do not demonstrate meaningful use of CEHRT.

According to the presentation given at the Healthcare Information Management Systems Society (HIMSS) conference in April of 2015 by Elisabeth Meyers and Elizabeth Holland of the CMS Center for Clinical Standards and Quality, nearly 305,000 Eligible Professionals and over 4000 Eligible Hospitals had successfully attested for EHR MU Stage 1 and Stage 2 [16]. Figure 15.9 shows by state the percentage of *Eligible Hospitals* that were participating in the CMS EHR Incentive Programs as of December 2014; and Fig. 15.10 shows an update of those data as of April 2015 [17].

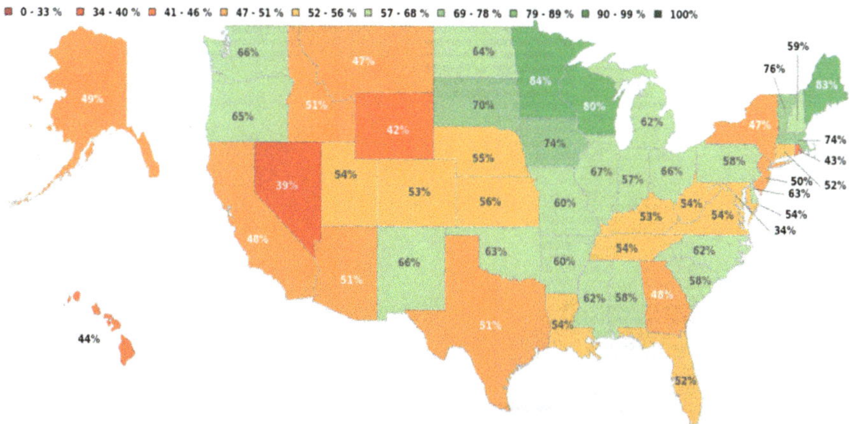

Fig. 15.11 Percentage of office-based professionals participating in the CMS EHR incentive programs (Health IT Dashboard 2014)

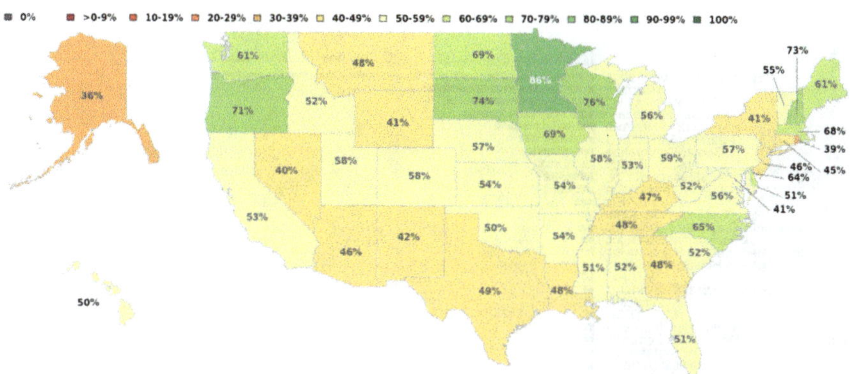

Fig. 15.12 Percentage of office-based professionals participating in the CMS EHR incentive programs (Health IT Dashboard 2015)

Figure 15.11 shows the percentage of office-based *Eligible Professionals* in each state who were participating in the Programs as of December 2014; and Fig. 15.12 shows the percentage of office-based Eligible Professionals in each state who were participating in the Programs as of April 2015 [17].

According to the statistics provided by the Health IT Dashboard, 95 % of eligible and critical access hospitals interoperability and 54 % of eligible office-based physicians had demonstrated meaningful use of certified HIT as of April 2015.

The EHR vendors have responded to the demand for CEHRT by providing certified products to Eligible Professionals and Eligible Hospitals. Figure 15.13 is a graph showing the leading EHR vendors that were providing their products to *hospitals* participating in the CMS EHR Incentive Programs as of March 2015; and

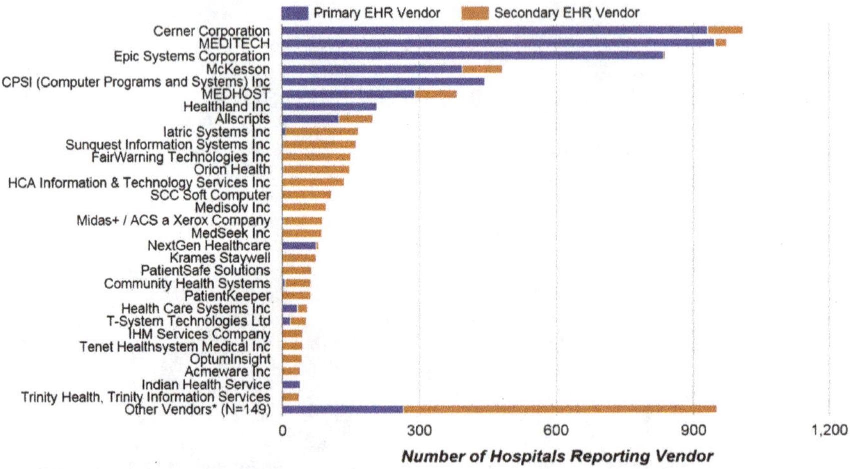

Fig. 15.13 EHR vendors reported by hospitals participating in the CMS EHR incentive programs (Health IT Dashboard 2015)

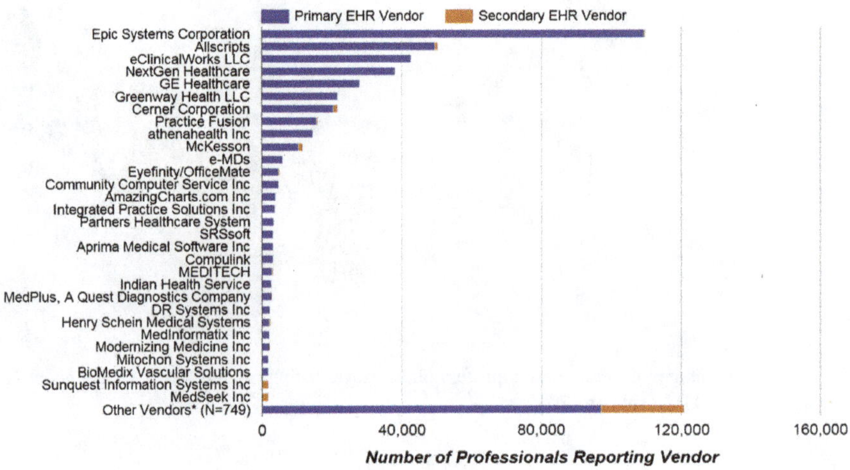

Fig. 15.14 EHR vendors reported by health care professionals participating in the CMS EHR incentive programs (Health IT Dashboard 2015)

Fig. 15.14 is a graph that shows the leading EHR vendors providing their products to *physician office practices* participating in the CMS EHR Incentive Programs as of March 2015 [17].

Figures 15.13 and 15.14 stratify the information about the EHRs into "Primary" and "Secondary" EHRs. Primary indicates that the EHR provides all or the majority of the capabilities needed by the user to meet CMS MU, and Secondary indicates that the EHR supplements the capabilities of the Primary EHR. This comparison provides insight into which vendors are providing ONC Certified EHR Modules and how these EHR Modules are being deployed.

The response of the market to the federal EHR programs thus far shows movement toward greater adoption and use by clinicians of EHR technologies that have been certified to support a specific level of capabilities (mostly those capabilities required for MU Stage 1) deemed to be necessary for achieving healthcare data exchange. As noted, however, in an online article, "The Meaningful Use program helped push providers to implement electronic health records systems that technically can exchange information, but it also fostered a "check the box" mentality that allows MU-stressed providers to settle for limited approaches for information exchange…" [18]. As this commenter is pointing out, data exchange is different from interoperability, which will be discussed in more detail in The Interoperability Factor sub-section. Even the acknowledged progress toward increased adoption of HIT has not been made without controversy related to several other issues.

While MU Stage 1 and 2011 Edition ONC certification were relatively easy to achieve, MU Stage 2 requirements and 2014 Edition certification criteria raised the bar quite a bit, causing push-back from users, in particular Eligible Professionals (physician office practices) as well as the EHR vendors. In addition to what was perceived by the market as an unrealistically short timeline for vendors to develop and deliver software with the additional EHR capabilities required for meeting 2014 Edition ONC certification–and for users to install and activate the certified versions of that software for MU Stage 2—CMS had initially scheduled the change-over from ICD-9 to ICD-10 for October, 2013. Even delaying that change until October, 2014, did not quiet the uproar over the heavy burden certification testing and EHR meaningful use placed on HIT vendors and users alike. Partially in response to this continued pushback, CMS announced another delay for implementation of ICD-10 until October 2015, as well as an extension of MU Stage 2 through 2017 and delay of MU Stage 3 until 2018.

The CMS EHR MU incentive payments, though better than no incentive payments at all, definitely do not cover the cost of licensing, installing, maintaining, and updating the CEHRT software, which can be quite expensive in terms of both time and money, especially from the perspective of a small physician practice. Much criticism of the usability of CEHRT has been voiced by the users; and, indeed, ONC certification criteria include *what* capabilities a CEHRT must support, but do not include specifications for *how* an EHR technology must be designed to support those capabilities.

The nursing profession has studied the CMS EHR MU Program and sought to guide the process by working with the groups established by the Federal Advisory Committee Act (FACA), whose policy-related deliberations affect nurses and nursing care. "While meaningful use criteria are not nursing specific, nurse leaders sitting on FACAs and measurement development teams are working to think about how to leverage MU to drive a patient-centered, quality and safety agenda that includes nursing input. There are many potential patient benefits to consider in

EHRs to encourage health IT adoption and use [19, 20]." The possibility that future ONC certification criteria could name a standard nursing vocabulary that is available in the public domain is vital to nurses. Nurses know coded patient care data documented in the EHR by nurses is essential for transforming information into a measurement of the depth of nursing's contribution to healthcare and patient outcomes.

The federal EHR programs initiated by the HITECH Act of 2009 have been met with a certain level of skepticism in the market as to the value the requirements are bringing to the delivery of healthcare in terms of patient safety and cost reduction. *With usability out-of-scope and interoperability remaining elusive, just pushing providers and provider organizations toward adoption and utilization of currently available certified HIT is considered insufficient.*

15.4.5 The Interoperability Factor

The US Congress expressed disappointment in the pace of advancing EHR interoperability under the federal programs, even stating that the draft ONC interoperability Roadmap that was published in January of 2015 [21] was not specific enough. This draft Roadmap, *Connecting Health and Care for the Nation: A Shared Nationwide Interoperability Roadmap*, outlined a proposal for key actions that both the private and public stakeholders needed to take in order to advance toward a more connected, interoperable health IT infrastructure in the US. During a Public Comment period, ONC "received over 250 comments which were used to shape the [Final] Roadmap… Additionally, the Roadmap was informed by the input from 25 federal partners, 90 individuals from 38 states from across the nation and the ONC Federal Advisory Committees (FACAs), whose membership includes 167 representatives from over 140 private and public organizations" [22]. The final version of this Roadmap [23] was published in early October, 2015. In this Roadmap, ONC defined interoperability as "the ability of a system to exchange electronic health information with and use electronic health information from other systems without special effort on the part of the user [23]." Included in the scope of this interoperability were all individuals, their families, and health care providers, all of whom are to be able to send, receive, find, and use electronic health information. The Roadmap anticipates that this information is accessible as appropriate, and that the access will be secure, timely, and reliable to support collaborative, informed decision-making.

Early reaction to the Roadmap from the healthcare community was mixed. The stakeholders want and need someone to take on the role of showing the way *and making it happen*. Soon after publication of the Roadmap, leadership of one physician organization stated, "We need more than a road map; we need action.", and then called for "increased accountability on the part of the [HIT] industry that creates these products and decreased accountability for physicians who have no choice but to use the 'inadequate' products [24]." An article published in January, 2016, expounds upon the way *true* interoperability needs to work, and laments the fact that "Interoperability is a moonshot challenge for the country…" [18].

15.4.6 Summary and Conclusions

The federal EHR programs that were initiated by Congress in 2009 as part of the HITECH Act have driven adoption of certified EHR technologies/HIT by the targeted users and have moved the nation closer to realizing the vision of an interoperable health IT infrastructure. The Centers for Medicare and Medicaid Services (CMS) and the Office of the National Coordinator for Health Information Technology (ONC), have established the EHR Meaningful Use (MU) Programs and Health IT Certification Program respectively. The EHR MU Programs have provided incentive payments to Eligible Professionals (e.g., physicians in office practices) and Eligible Hospitals for adoption of "certified" EHR technologies and demonstration of a specific level of "meaningful" use based on published CMS objectives and measures. The ONC Health IT Certification Program has established the requirements the HIT must meet in order to be deemed certified technology, and has instituted the testing infrastructure necessary for ensuring that vendors' HIT products meet the certification requirements.

Statistics as of April, 2015, show that a significant percentage of both Eligible Professionals and Eligible Hospitals across the US have received CMS incentive payments for either MU Stage 1 or Stage 2, which indicates adoption and meaningful use of HIT that is certified at least at a minimal level. Issues identified in this section—including the compressed timeline for development and deployment of certified technology; the expense of installing and maintaining it; additional federal mandates, such as changing to ICD-10, being placed on healthcare providers; and the reported lack of usability of the HIT according to clinical users—have impeded faster progress. While a considerable amount of work still needs to be accomplished and more progress needs to be made as of early 2016, the available statistics show that the CMS MU Programs and ONC Health IT Certification Program are driving the US toward more wide-spread use of HIT for providing patient care, for exchanging healthcare data, and for capturing data that are essential for measuring quality and cost of healthcare. Whether the actual impact of increased adoption and meaningful use of certified HIT on patient safety and healthcare costs is a positive one likely will be the focus of numerous research studies in the near future. Current lack of true interoperability between products marketed by disparate HIT vendors appears to be an inhibiting factor in achieving the ultimate benefits of effective and efficient use of HIT for patient care.

15.5 Other Programs

15.5.1 Surescripts

Surescripts [25] operates the largest electronic prescribing network in the US and offers various services and tools to support testing of electronic prescribing messages. Surescripts certifies EHR/e-Prescribing systems and pharmacy systems to use its network. Surescripts' conformance testing tools and certification are focused on message format and workflow in accordance to the Surescripts implementation guides, which are based on the NCPDP SCRIPT standard. The intent of Surescripts certification is to validate software that is used by prescribers, pharmacies and payers/PBMs for access to three core services: Prescription Benefit, Medication History, and Prescription Routing [25]. Surescripts also provides a Clinical Messaging service, allowing clinical information to be exchanged between healthcare clinics and physicians, and between pharmacies and physicians/practitioners.

While the majority of Surescripts transaction activity consists of NCPDP e-Prescribing messages, a portion of Surescripts volume is X12 eligibility messages, and it also supports exchange of certain HL7 standards (e.g., v2.x and CCDA), Direct messaging and prescription drug monitoring program (PDMP) reporting using the ASAP standard.

15.5.2 Certification in Australia

To complement the testing services described in Chap. 14, the Australian Healthcare Messaging Laboratory (AHML) also provides compliance and certification services. AHML certification of a given software product provides assurance to healthcare organizations using the product that their messages will conform to various standards and specifications.

The AHML certification process is illustrated in Fig. 15.15 (adapted from [26]). The customer (e.g., a Vendor) decides what they want tested and to what level. This testing can include additional requirements for message structure, content, and business rules that have been implemented locally. A certification officer works with the customer to setup and execute the tests, and assists in correcting any non-conformance messages. Certification includes the AHML testing processes described in Chap. 14. Customers submit a set of unaltered messages produced by the software products under test. A representative set of messages is validated, and results are reviewed and assessed. If any non-conformity is detected, modifications to the system under test can be made and the process is repeated. Upon successful completion AHML issues a certification certificate.

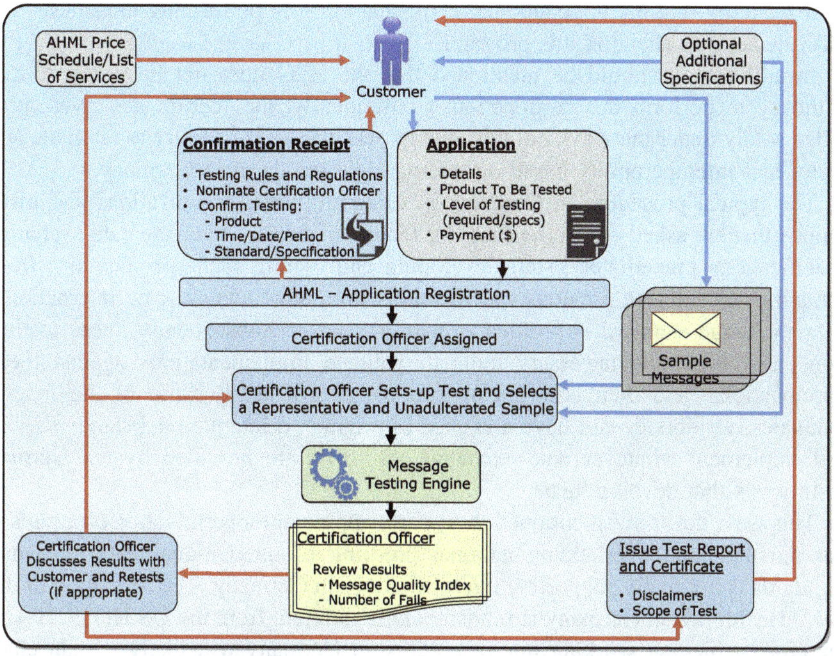

Fig. 15.15 AHML certification process [26]

The AHML certification services can be used to assess industry vendor products, government agencies' systems, and installed private and public healthcare organizations' systems. The AHML certification program is accredited by NATA, the National Association of Testing Authorities.

15.5.3 Certification in Germany

Between 2003 and 2006, HL7 Germany received a request to specify HL7 v2.5 standard message profiles for ADT on a national level. In response, the German project office of HL7 Germany worked on and successfully balloted a set of HL7 v2.5 message profiles. The originator of this request, the *Zentrum for Telematik GmbH* (ZTG), wanted to perform certification on a message level. Two vendors were found that passed this test successfully. However, due to a lack of resonance in the user community—no hospital and no provider practice used this as part of their tenders—and the huge amount of manual effort in performing those tests, the ZTG decided to abandon this program.

In addition, it should be mentioned that the ZTG does not have any formal authority to perform this certification. Consequently, the "certificates" were provided solely under the ZTG, but this attempt was the first one to try to facilitate and foster real interoperability based on international standards in Germany.

The typical procedure in Germany is straightforward: organizations and institutions that are asked—in some cases by federal mandate—to create data exchange specifications immediately, start developing and issuing such specifications from scratch or to enhance previous specifications. In almost all cases, no international data exchange standard is profiled to national needs. Subsequently, these institutions also build the necessary tools to validate implementations against these specifications, and then issue an appropriate certificate. Because of the federal mandates, vendors do not have a chance to migrate to international standards, but just implement whatever data exchange standards are provided by the German institutions that develop them.

This way, the above mentioned third-party approach for certification programs is not pursued, and overlapping national profiling of international data exchange standards is not really supporting interoperability in Germany. The formation of the new eHealth law in Germany is fundamentally different from the US HITECH Act, therefore achieving working interoperability in Germany will likely remain challenging for years to come.

15.6 Scope of Certification Testing

It is important to understand the scope, goal, and limitations of a certification and testing program. Awarding a certificate to information technology means "that with a reasonable amount of testing no errors could be detected". It does not mean that a software module is free of errors nor that it contains all expected capabilities. Certification of health IT is a critical step towards achieving interoperability for exchanging healthcare information, but it may not be the end-all. Purchasers need to understand what certification *buys* them. To elaborate on this point, a perspective on how the ONC certification program works, as it relates to meaningful use and implementation in practice, is given.

ONC certification testing related to meaningful use focuses on assessing the capabilities of the EHR product for a given set of requirements. It is not directed at site-specific installations. Purchasing a certified system provides a degree of certainty that the buyer is obtaining an EHR product[7] that meets the "national level"

[7]EHR Products are typically configurable to meet certified and non-certified uses.

capabilities established by the ONC as part of the EHR meaningful use program. End users of certified EHR products likely will need to configure their products according to their local requirements (which need to be in alignment with specifications in the regulation—as discussed previously, profiling can be employed to accomplish this).

It is also important to recognize that the ONC certification program targets the EHR technologies/HIT and not the systems that interact with them. For example, the transmission to immunization registries certification test assesses whether the EHR product can create HL7 v2 messages in accordance with the requirements given in the referenced standards. It does not, however, place any requirements on the receiving system, in this case the immunization information systems (IIS) used by the registries. Of course, in order to achieve interoperability the receiving systems must implement the corresponding requirements correctly and completely. The Meaningful Use Programs envision that these systems will, over time, acquire such capabilities due to market forces or because it is in their own best interest, as is the case for public health registries.

The named standards in the ONC certification criteria specify "national level" requirements. For the HL7 v2 messaging standards, these requirements are published in implementation guides and realized as constrainable conformance message profiles—meaning that a selected set of elements are fully specified while others are yet to be determined. This approach guarantees that certified EHR technologies have a certain level of common capabilities while providing flexibility for local customization. Local installations may need to complete trading-partner agreements. That is, they will build on the national level requirements to satisfy their local requirements for exchange of healthcare information. It is important that the trading-partner agreements don't relax or conflict with the national level requirements. Certified products will provide a minimum level of capabilities that won't necessarily coincide with local requirements (and often will not). Once local trading-partner agreements are put in place,[8] the EHR technology and partner systems will need to be implemented and configured accordingly. For example, a provider and their state immunization registry will coordinate exchange requirements. The referenced Meaningful Use interoperability standard provides the basis, but additional requirements may be necessary for this particular jurisdiction. In this case, the system receiving the HL7 v2 messages (i.e., immunization registry) must be able to import and understand the state-level information received from the certified EHR to achieve the desired interoperability. To ensure accuracy and integrity for this exchange of information, local site testing must be performed. At present, this aspect of testing is not part of the Meaningful Use Programs; however,

[8]Use of the profiling techniques described in Chap. 7 aids in the documentation and validation of these local requirements.

using a certified EHR provides a shorter pathway to achieving site-specific interoperability. Understanding the scope of the testing or certification program is important for purchasers and users of products that have been certified.

15.7 Summary

Certification is a formal process by which products, based on a vendor's claim, are assessed, validated for conformance, and verified. Upon successful completion, a certificate is issued to substantiate the claim. Various testing programs exist with different levels of rigor. Certification is the highest-level and has defined boundaries in its process; for example, there must be a firewall between the entities involved in the testing operation, the verification of results, and the issuance of a certificate. A number of testing and certification programs were presented, including IHE and the ONC Health IT Certification Program. It is important to understand the scope and limitations of any certification program.

References

1. Business Dictionary. http://www.businessdictionary.com/definition/certification.html
2. ISO Reference - ISO/IEC 17000 Conformity assessment - Vocabulary and general principles, first edition 2004-11-02.
3. Gebase L, Snelick R, Skall M. Conformance Testing and Interoperability: A Case Study in Healthcare Data Exchange. 2008 Software Engineering Research and Practice (SERP08), WORLDCOMP'08 July 14–17, 2008, Las Vegas, NV.
4. IHE, http://www.ihe.net/
5. eHealth Test Framework for Interoperability. http://gazelle.ihe.net/
6 IHE Connect-a-thon. http://www.ihe.net/connectathon/
7. http://wiki.ihe.net/index.php?title=IHE_Test_Tool_Information
8. IHE Product Registry. http://www.ihe.net/IHE_Product_Registry/
9. Institute of Medicine. Crossing the Quality Chasm: A New Health System for the 21st Century. Committee on Quality of Health Care in America. Washington, D.C.: National Academy Press, 2001. Chapter 7, Pages 164-180.
10. Institute of Medicine. To Err is Human: Building a Safer Health System. Eds: Linda T. Kohn, Janet M. Corrigan, and Molla S. Donaldson. Washington, D.C.: National Academy Press, 1999.
11. Institute of Medicine. To Err is Human: Building a Safer Health System. Eds: Linda T. Kohn, Janet M. Corrigan, and Molla S. Donaldson. Washington, D.C.: National Academy Press, 1999. Page 1.
12. Healthcare IT News. Deaths by medical mistakes hit records. Online. 2014. Available at http://www.healthcareitnews.com/news/deaths-by-medical-mistakes-hit-records
13. Institute of Medicine. The Computer-Based Patient Record: An Essential Technology for Health Care. *Eds:* Richard S. Dick and Elaine B. Steen. Washington, D.C.: National Academy Press, 1991.

14. The White House Archives: President Unveils Tech Initiatives for Energy, Health Care, Internet. Remarks by President George W. Bush at the American Association of Community Colleges Annual Convention, Minneapolis, Mn. 2004. Online. Available at http://georgewbush-whitehouse.archives.gov/news/releases/2004/04/20040426-6.html
15. ONC 2015 Edition Test Procedure documents and ONC 2015 Edition Certification Companion Guides. Available at https://www.healthit.gov/policy-researchers-implementers/2015-edition-test-method
16. Healthcare Information Management Systems Society (HIMSS). CMS Incentive Programs Overview. Elisabeth Meyers and Elizabeth Holland. Chicago, Illinois: HIMSS, 2015.
17. The Health IT Dashboard. Health IT QuickStats. Fast Facts about Health IT Adoption in Health Care. Online. http://dashboard.healthit.gov/quickstats/quickstats.php last accessed January 29th 2016.
18. Health Data Management. 2016. HIT Think—Emerging pressures on healthcare fuel need for true interoperability. Online. Available at http://www.healthdatamanagement.com/opinion/value-based-care-fuels-the-need-for-true-interoperability?
19. Office of the National Coordinator for Health Information Technology (ONC): Health IT standards committee: Recommendations to the national coordinator for health IT. 2012. Retrieved from www.healthit.gov/policy-researchers-implementers/health-it-standards-committee-recommendations-national-coordinator-h
20. Online Journal of Issues in Nursing (OJIN): An Overview of the National Quality Strategy: Where Do Nurses Fit?. Online. September 2013. Available at http://www.nursingworld.org/MainMenuCategories/ANAMarketplace/ANAPeriodicals/OJIN/TableofContents/Vol-18-2013/No3-Sept-2013/National-Quality-Strategy.html#ANA10a
21. HealthIT.gov. 2015. Connecting Health and Care for the Nation: A Shared Nationwide Interoperability Roadmap. Online. Available at https://www.healthit.gov/policy-researchers-implementers/interoperability. Draft Document: https://www.healthit.gov/sites/default/files/nationwide-interoperability-roadmap-draft-version-1.0.pdf
22. http://www.healthit.gov/buzz-blog/electronic-health-and-medical-records/interoperability-electronic-health-and-medical-records/connecting-health-care-nation-shared-nationwide-interoperability-roadmap-version-10/
23. HealthIT.gov: Connecting Health and Care for the Nation. A Shared Nationwide Interoperability Roadmap. Online. 2015. Available at https://www.healthit.gov/policy-researchers-implementers/interoperability, Final Document: https://www.healthit.gov/sites/default/files/hie-interoperability/nationwide-interoperability-roadmap-final-version-1.0.pdf
24. 2016 American Academy of Family Physicians. http://www.aafp.org/news/practice-professional-issues/20151012oncroadmap.html
25. Surescripts: Organization and network to enable and support e-prescribing. http://surescripts.com
26. Australian Healthcare Messaging Laboratory. http://www.ahml.com.au/, last accessed November 2015. (Offline since Feb. 2016)
27. Publication of the Integrating the Healthcare Enterprise (IHE) Technical Frameworks (TF). http://www.ihe.net/technical_frameworks

Appendix A
Additional Healthcare Data Exchange Standards

This chapter is provided to introduce additional healthcare data exchange standards beyond the standards presented in Chap. 4. The survey includes (among others) HL7 Version 3 (V3), HL7 CDA® (Clinical Document Architecture) as an instantiation of HL7 Version 3, ASTM (American Society for Testing and Materials), and DICOM (Digital Imaging and Communications in Medicine). To complete this survey, the German xDT family of standards for the ambulatory sector and the French standards Hprim Santé and PN13 are presented as well.

A.1 HL7 Version 3

HL7 V3 was introduced in 1995 with the goal of establishing a general model for healthcare that could be used globally. Work on this version continued for three years, during which time it became evident that the model would be difficult to define (if it could be defined at all), because the combined requirements of the different domains and different countries was preventing harmonization that would lead to ubiquitous acceptance [1].

Changing the strategy, an alternative approach lead to development of a meta-model called the Reference Information Model (RIM) [2]. The RIM can be thought of as a toolbox of elements that can be used for the construction of models for specific domains. (Examples of a domain are patient administration, billing, and pharmacy). The RIM consists of only four base classes and two additional classes for relationships (Fig. A.1). A detailed explanation of how to interpret the RIM can be found in the introduction provided with the HL7 V3 material or in the V3 Primer [3].

F. Oemig and R. Snelick, *Healthcare Interoperability Standards Compliance Handbook*, DOI 10.1007/978-3-319-44839-8

A.1.1 Reference Information Model (RIM)

Figure A.2 illustrates the entire *Reference Information Model* (RIM), including the Base classes, their specializations, and Relationship classes, in a print-optimized version.

In addition to these elements, the RIM contains special classes that are necessary for the generation of messages, management of queries and languages, and overall control. These classes are not represented in this figure.

As shown in Fig. A.1, there are six root classes consisting of four Base classes and two Relationship classes. The four Base classes include:

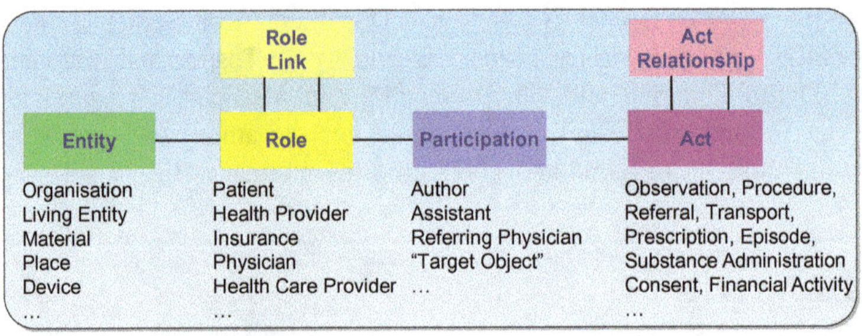

Fig. A.1 HL7 V3 RIM base classes

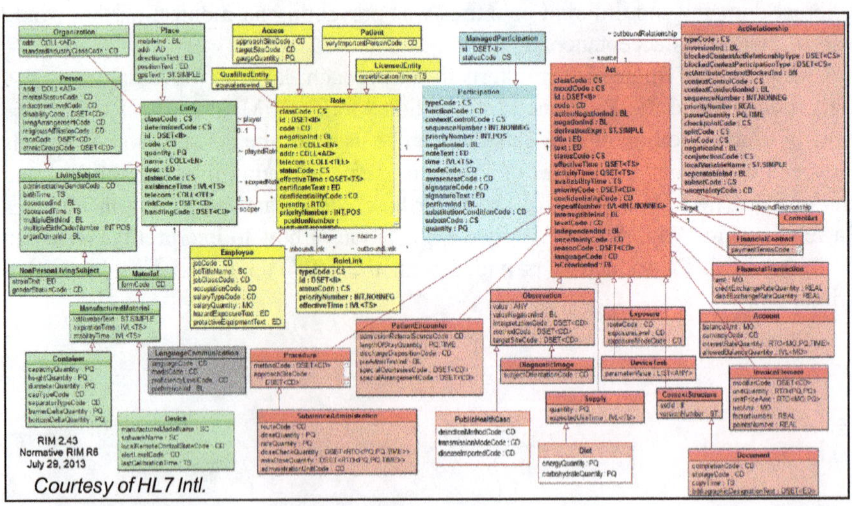

Fig. A.2 HL7 V3 RIM (reference information model)

- An *entity*—is the representation of physical, persistent objects. In addition to persons, materials and equipment, organizations and places also are an entity. An entity expresses a static thing.
- A *role*—expresses the ability that an entity has when being involved in activities. For example, a person may play the role of patient.
- A *participation*—describes the incorporation of an entity into a certain role in one act. For example, a person in the role of a physician participates in a surgery activity as the executive surgeon.
- An *act*—is the carrier for all information and expresses changes. For example, a *finding* is an observation and hence an *activity*.

Two Relationship classes are provided for the creation of linkages.

- A *role link*—is a direct relationship between various roles such as employer/employee (Fig. A.4). This class is used very rarely.
- An *act relationship*—combines various activities (Fig. A.5). For example, the activity of observing is the fulfillment of the activity order.

The six RIM classes can be combined in a myriad of ways to produce instantiations. For example, Fig. A.3 depicts a construct that represents "Person A" participating as a physician in the examination of a patient "Person B".

The two role classes related to the role link class, as shown in Fig. A.4, provide the direct linkage of roles and activities. In this example, Mr. Smith is employed by Miller Inc.

Similarly, two different activities, for example, the request and the corresponding result, are linked by an act relationship (Fig. A.5).

Another situation to consider pertains to the different relationships one role might have with two different to entities. Figure A.6 illustrates this concept indicated by the solid and the dashed lines. A role requires a certain context, and thus a person becomes ("plays") a patient in the context ("scope") of an organization (in this case a hospital).

As shown in the four examples (Figs. A.3, A.4, A.5 and A.6), the different options for creating relationships can be (arbitrarily) combined into more complex structures. Domain models are constructed from these classes (components of the toolbox) by linking them together, and the classes from the RIM are instantiated in such a domain model. The classes are given meaningful names to facilitate understanding of the domain models. For example, when the class "Person" from

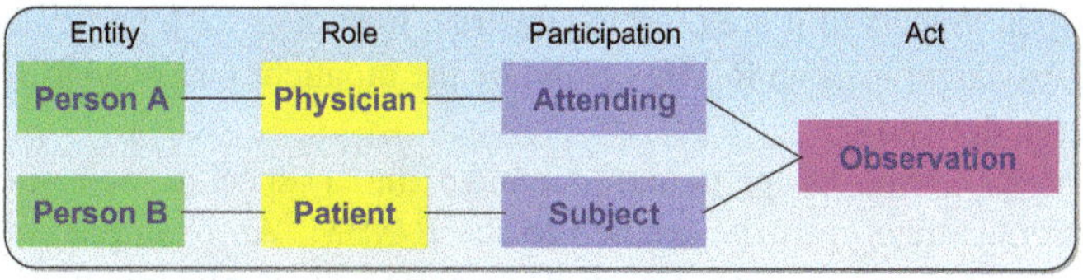

Fig. A.3 HL7 V3 Example 1 (simple activity)

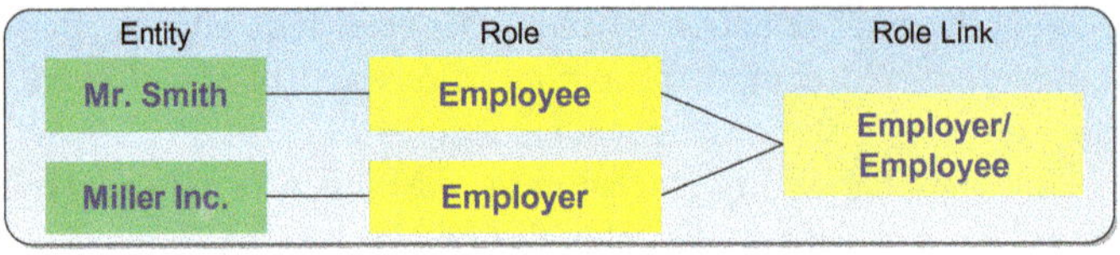

Fig. A.4 HL7 V3 Example 2 ("role link")

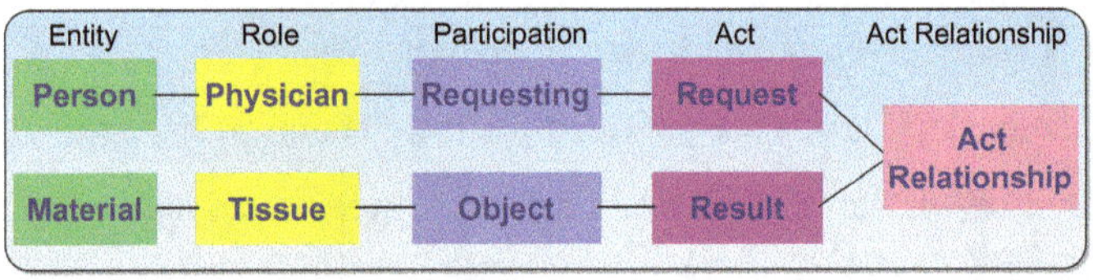

Fig. A.5 HL7 V3 Example 3 ("act relationship")

Fig. A.6 HL7 V3 Example 4 ("playing and scoping entity")

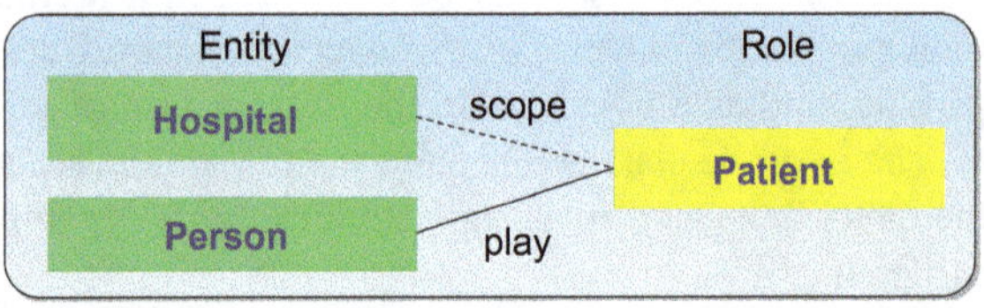

the entity hierarchy is used to represent the patient, the class is renamed "Patient" in the domain model.

To create such models, a customized Microsoft Visio™ module was employed originally to support the RIM and to validate classes (the necessary meta-information was stored in an Access database). This toolkit has been replaced by an application with more capabilities and features. The National Health Service (NHS) in the United Kingdom (UK) has provided a new program called Static Model Designer, which is based on Eclipse and, therefore, is free of any proprietary restrictions [4].

A *domain model* (D-MIM) is a conceptual (abstract) method used for illustrating the structure of the classes that are required for modeling a specific application domain such as administrative or billing. Figure A.7 shows an example of a domain model.

A domain model is further constrained to a *Refined Message Information Model* (R-MIM) when aspects of it are used to construct messages for a particular use case (scenario). An example of an R-MIM could be the inpatient visit scenario within the administrative domain.

In order to create a particular message in a specific scenario, further refinements/constraints must be applied to the R-MIM. An example could be the admission message in an inpatient visit scenario. This refinement leads to the *Hierarchical Message Definition* (HMD), which can be displayed either in a tabular

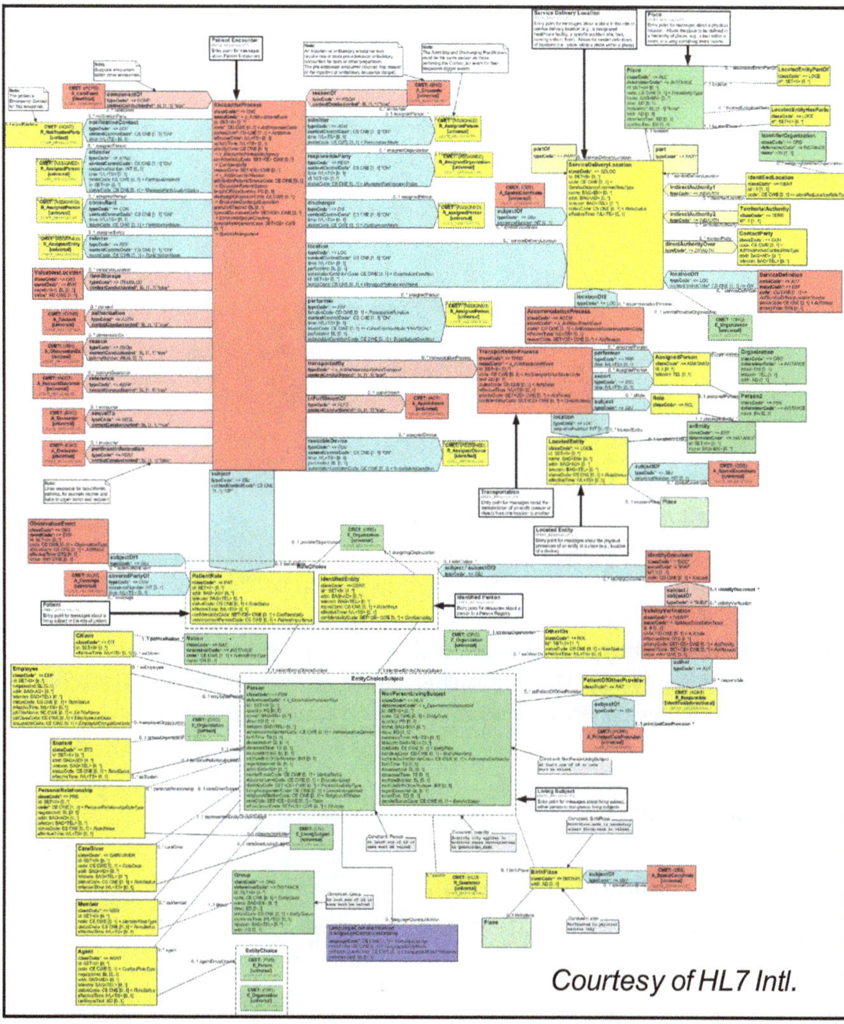

Fig. A.7 HL7® V3 example domain model

format or in an XML schema. Both the R-MIM and HMD form the basis for an implementation. The *Implementable Technology Specification* (ITS) then allows for and ensures the implementation of abstract models in a specific technology such as XML.

In addition to these abstract models that are based on the *Reference Information Model* (RIM) and that provide details for an implementation, two other areas of interest are important: the datatypes and the vocabulary (Fig. A.8).

The foundations for HL7 V3 are explained in more detail in the next subsections.

Fig. A.8 HL7 V3 implementation building blocks

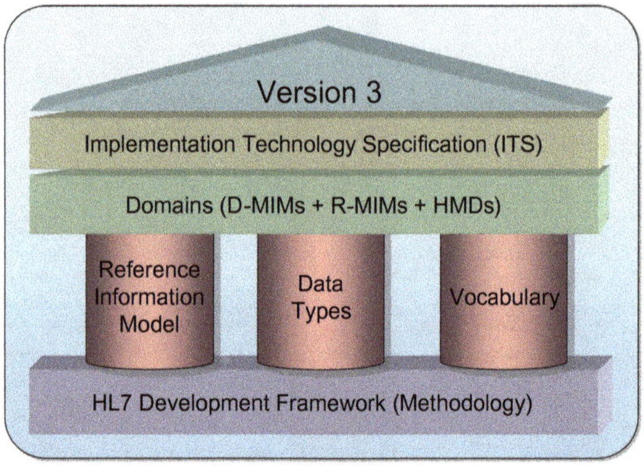

A.1.2 Structural Attributes

As mentioned previously, the RIM provides the domain modeling abstract classes, which can be used multiple times in the domain model. The process that enables multiple use of the classes is called *cloning*. Since the classes in the model are named individually, they must contain certain fixed information that is imperative for a correct interpretation. This information, such as *mood code* and *class code*, is provided as attributes called *structural attributes*, which are immutable.

A.1.2.1 Mood Code

The *mood code* (spelled *moodCode* in Fig. A.9) is an attribute that is assigned to abstract classes (entities and activities) to indicate their different functions. (A more technical term for this attribute would be "mode"). In the example shown in Fig. A.9, an observation ("OBS") in the "Request" Mood ("RQO", left act) is the order and an observation in the "Event" Mood ("EVN", right act) is the result.

The mood code is a static attribute, i.e., it cannot change once the class has been instantiated.

Using standard modeling techniques, one would normally create different classes—and, therefore, different class hierarchies—to represent different types of

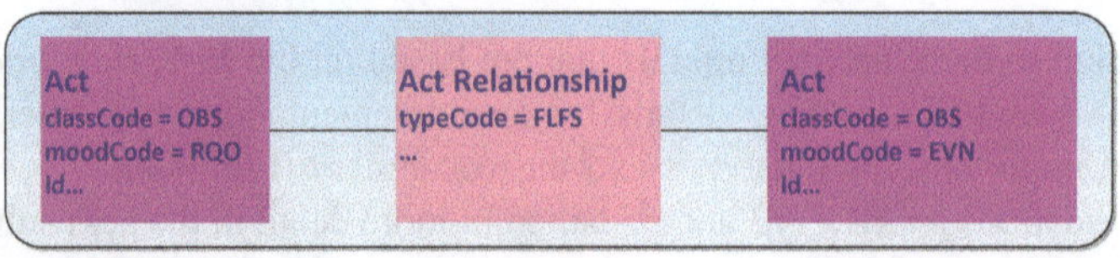

Fig. A.9 moodCode and classCode for HL7 V3 entities

Table A.1 HL7 V3 classCode hierarchy for acts (excerpt)

Level	Code	Description
0	ACT	Act
1	OBS	Observation
2	ALRT	Detected issue
2	BATTERY	Battery
…		
1	ActClassRecordOrganizer	Act class record organizer
2	COMPOSITION	Composition
3	DOC	Document
4	DOCCLIN	Clinical document
…		
2	CONTAINER	Record container

activities such as orders and observations. (This approach was used first (from 1995 to 1998) to develop a generic reference information model.) Creation of separate class hierarchies does not permit automated handling and processing of those classes. Consequently, the correct semantics of the classes must be set by the mood code attribute.

A.1.2.2 Class Code

In addition to the *moodCode*, another attribute, called the *classCode*, is used to designate the contents being conveyed through an instance of a class. Rather than creating a dedicated tree of classes in the class hierarchy, the same outcome can be achieved by using the appropriate classCode value.

Table A.1 provides an extract of the class hierarchy. The hierarchy is shown in the first column, with the numbers and lateral positions of the numbers relative to each other in that column indicating the level. The table shows that a detected issue

Table A.2 HL7 v2.x and V3 coding example for "administrative gender"

V2.x	V3	Explanation
M—Male	M—Male	
F—Female	F—Female	
A—Ambiguous		Not used with persons in V3
N—Not applicable		Not used with persons in V3
O—Other		Not used with persons in V3
U—Unknown	nullFlavor = "NI"-no information	"NI" and its descendants (specializations)
	UN-undifferentiated	

("ALRT") is a specialization of an observation ("OBS"), which is itself a specialization of the general activity ("ACT").

A.1.3 Null-Flavors

A notable difference between HL7 V3 and HL7 v2.x is the clear separation in V3 between "real" data and information about the absence of data. V3 generically supports the concept of a null-flavor, in which a non-data value is sent to indicate why the data are not available. This concept is built into V3 on an abstract level and is, therefore, available for all data types. Table 2.2 in Chap. 2 provides a list of null flavors.

As explained in Chap. 4, HL7 v2.x does not support null flavors. Null flavors are "simulated" in HL7 v2 in specific value sets (tables), and one of these simulated null flavor codes is selected based on the options available in the value set to which the message element is bound. Table A.2 provides examples that compare the v2.x approach to the V3 approach.

In V3, the implementation has numerous options for indicating the absence of data using the nullFlavor construct. As shown in the nullFlavor example in Table A.2, the different specializations of *no information* can be used as well.

In v2, the implementer has to choose from among the codes that are available in a specific table in order to indicate an absence of data in an element. In the Administrative Gender table example, *U* is for *Unknown*, whereas in other HL7 v2.x tables *UNK* or any other code could stand for *Unknown*.

A.1.4 Required and Mandatory Values

The explicit introduction of null flavors in the Development Framework of HL7 V3 (HDF) [5] led to an analysis about possible combinations of "valid (real) values", "valued information", and "no information". The term "required" in HL7 V3 means the information system must support the specific data element whether values are available for it or not. In contrast to HL7 v2.x, V3 does not imply a minimum cardinality of one, so the V3 term "required" is comparable to "required but may be empty" in v2.x. The introduction of the optionality indicator "mandatory" disallows the use of null values/flavors, so only valid values are conveyed. The V3 term "mandatory" is comparable to "required" in v2.x.

The use of valid values is closely associated with structural attribute where the use of a valid value means that absence of a value, even with a stated reason for its absence (e.g. "asked, but no response"), is not permitted. Table A.3 provides a list of constraints that have an impact on each other.

Table A.4 lists the allowed combinations of constraints derived from analyzing the possible values for each constraint and then combining them.

Table A.3 HL7 V3® constraint descriptions

Constraint	Description
Cardinality	This specifies the minimum and maximum number of occurrences (repeats) of the field/association. For example, 1…* implies the minimum number of occurrences (repeats) is 1 whereas the maximum number of occurrences (repeats) is unlimited
Mandatory	Valid values are M (mandatory) or Blank (not mandatory). M (mandatory) means that the field/association must be present in the message, otherwise the message is invalid and is non-conformant. For Mandatory fields, HL7 sets the minimum cardinality to 1 (a value must be present). Blank (not mandatory) means that the field/association does not need to be present in the message
Conformance	Valid values are R (required), NP (not permitted), and Blank (optional). R (required) means that the sending application must support this field/association. If the data are available, then the field/association is included in the message. If the minimum cardinality is 0 and the data are not available, the message is still conformant when the field/association is omitted. If the minimum cardinality is 1 and the data are not available, a NullFlavor is required (see below). NP (not permitted) means that the field/association is not included in the message schema and never included in a message instance. Blank (optional) means that the field/association may/may not be sent and support for this field/association is not required of sending applications. Conformance for this element is to be negotiated on a site-specific basis
Null-Flavor	For required fields/associations with a minimum cardinality of 1, a NullFlavor must be sent for fields/associations that are not available to a sending application. Sample NullFlavors are "no information", "unknown", "masked" (for privacy applications), "not asked" and "asked, but unknown" (patient was asked but did not know valid answer)

Table A.4 HL7 V3® cardinality requirements

Cardinality	Mandatory	Conformance	Null-flavor required?	Explanation of rules
0…, 1…			No	The field/association may or may not be present in a message. Conformance for this element is to be negotiated on a site-specific basis
0…, 1…		NP	Not allowed	The field/association is not present in the schema and cannot be included in a message instance
0…		R	No	Support for the field/association is required in a sending application. The field/association may or may not be present in a message

(continued)

Table A.4 (continued)

Cardinality	Mandatory	Conformance	Null-flavor required?	Explanation of rules
1...		R	Yes	Support for the field/association is required in a sending application. The field/association must be present in a message, but may not be valued. If the field/association is not valued, a NullFlavor must be specified
1...	M	R	Not allowed	Support for the field/association is required in a sending application. NullFlavor may not be specified. The field/association must be present and valued in a message

Use of default values is prohibited in HL7 V3. Some vendors manipulate the XML schemas, however, and use default values, which becomes very problematic since these values must be made available for evaluation in the message. Therefore, for each transmission the associated schema should be communicated as well, which increases the volume of transmitted data ("traffic") significantly.

A.1.5 State Transitions

Triggers for sending a message are an activity or a change in an internal state of an entity. The generic state transitions, which are implemented in the form of state machines, have been defined for this purpose. In the various scenarios, subsets of this generic definition of events are specified and communicated by messages.

The state transitions for activities (Fig. A.10) are different from those of entities (Fig. A.11). Entities as a representative of physical, persistent objects only support "active" or "inactive"—and a nullify to allow for virtually deleting those objects. Activities has a much richer state transition diagram to support complex workflows by interrupting the main statuses "new" and "active".

A.1.6 Application Roles

As explained in Chap. 1, messages are exchanged as the interaction between different actors. The trigger for the exchange of messages is either an event or a change in a state. In some cases, the exchange is not limited to a single message;

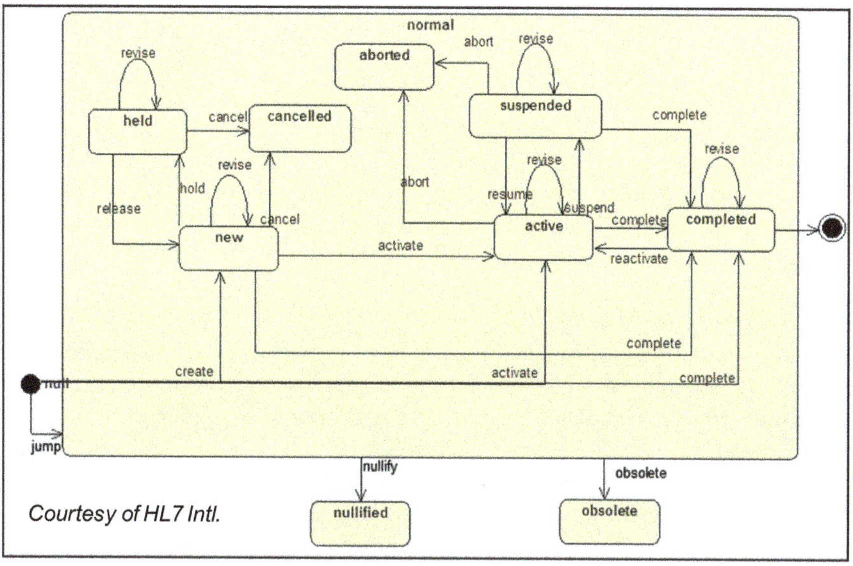

Fig. A.10 State machine for HL7® V3 acts

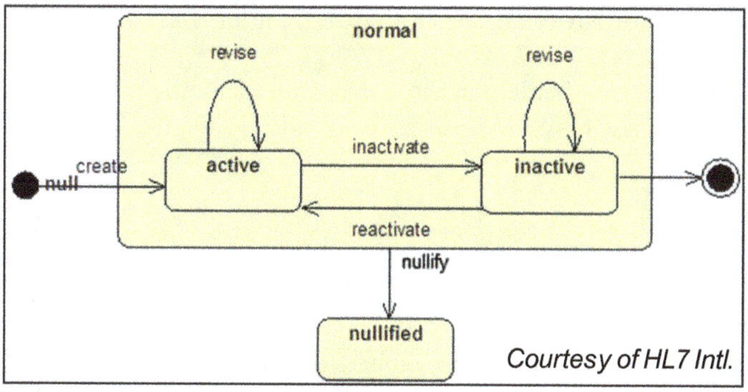

Fig. A.11 State machine for HL7® V3 entities

rather, several messages together comprise a specific scenario that can only be represented adequately in a system by considering all associated messages.

This capability is an enhancement over version 2.x, which does not have such a construct and cannot, therefore, represent multiple messages that have no relationship to each other.

It should be noted that an *application role* is a non-normative construct, i.e., there is no consistent understanding of its use. The basis for and conditions under which application roles are specified are not clear, nor is it clear what should be considered when implementing the static and dynamic behavior.

A.1.7 Data Types

Data are an essential prerequisite for an exchange of messages. These data often are presented as a single unit composed of several individual values that have a common connection, such as an address, which (in the US) consists of street number, street name, city, zip code, and state. (The state is not used in European countries.) Such a conglomeration of individual information is referred to as a datatype in programming languages. Quite often these languages specify operations that can be performed on these data types. The datatype *integer*, for example, uses the operations *predecessor* and *successor*.

The semantic properties of these data types are expressed by "invariant statements" that are valid at any time and for all possible values. In other areas of information science (computability and logic), such statements are regarded as fixed points.

V3 Data Types offer interesting built-in capabilities that are difficult to implement in general. These built-in capabilities are called Demotion and Promotion and are shown in Fig. A.12.

Demotion is the reduction of a data type to a simpler expression. A good example is the constraint of a set of identifiers ("SET <ID>") to a single identifier ("ID") where "ID" replaces the placeholder "T" for any data type.

The opposite direction is called *Promotion*, which allows a simple construct to be made into a more powerful one. In Fig. A.12, a timestamp (data type "TS") is enhanced to an interval ("IVL(TS)").

This feature places a burden on the implementer and, therefore, the underlying architecture of the software.

A.1.8 ITS

The data type specification is defined on an abstract level, independent of a given implementation. The same principle applies to domain models. For use in a practical scenario, a specific technology must be selected and mapping rules defined.

Currently for HL7 V3, only the *eXtensible Markup Language* (XML) [6] and Unified Modeling Language (UML) [7–9] are approved as technologies, and they are provided in the form of *Implementable Technology Specifications* (ITS).

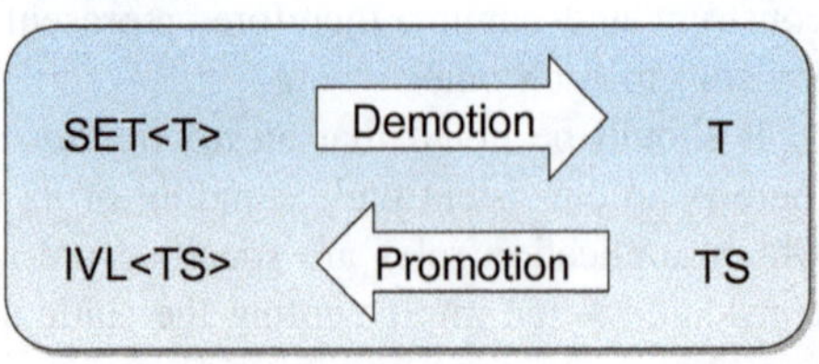

Fig. A.12 HL7 V3 promotion and demotion

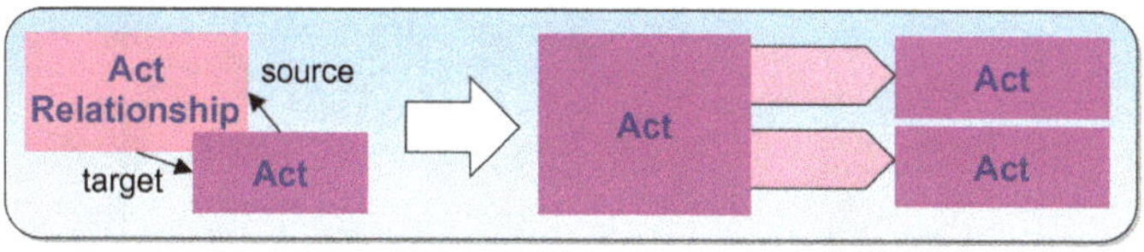

Fig. A.13 HL7 V3 recursive relationships

There are also other possible technologies that can be used for V3, including binary XML [10], JSON, and ASN.1 [11]. ER7, which is used by HL7 v2.x, could be, in principle, another option. ER7 requires a revision, however, because it currently does not allow for arbitrarily deeply nested structures with repetitions, thus making further delimiters necessary.

In March 2010, a proposal was submitted that recommended the definition of another XML ITS. To address backward compatibility, an ITS uses the names of the RIM classes directly as XML element names rather than names of classes from the domain model. This proposal has been rejected. Comparable to this approach, a second ITS called *green CDA* has been defined for CDA.

A.1.9 Recursive Relationships

HL7® V3 provides a powerful feature that appears to be simple but may cause a lot of interoperability problems: recursive relationships. The left-hand side of Fig. A.13 indicates how a recursive relationship is articulated in general. The right-hand side demonstrates a possible unrolling into concrete acts.

For implementers, this feature raises a challenge that is hard to meet, because it allows for multiple individual enrollments, especially when combined with specific semantics. The solution is creation of implementation guides that specify the resulting structures, including all details, so that an enrollment of recursive relationships need not be delegated to implementers themselves. On the other hand, providing the details in implementation guides decreases the chances that implementers will be aware that such a feature exists at all.

A.2 CDA

The HL7® *Clinical Document Architecture* (CDA) was originally developed to exchange any medical/clinical documents. CDA is based on HL7 Version 3 and, therefore, is created as a Domain Message Information Model (D-MIM) shown in Fig. A.14. Figure A.15 provides an overview of an extract from this detailed and complex model. (A very good introduction to this D-MIM is provided in *The CDA Book* [12, 13].)

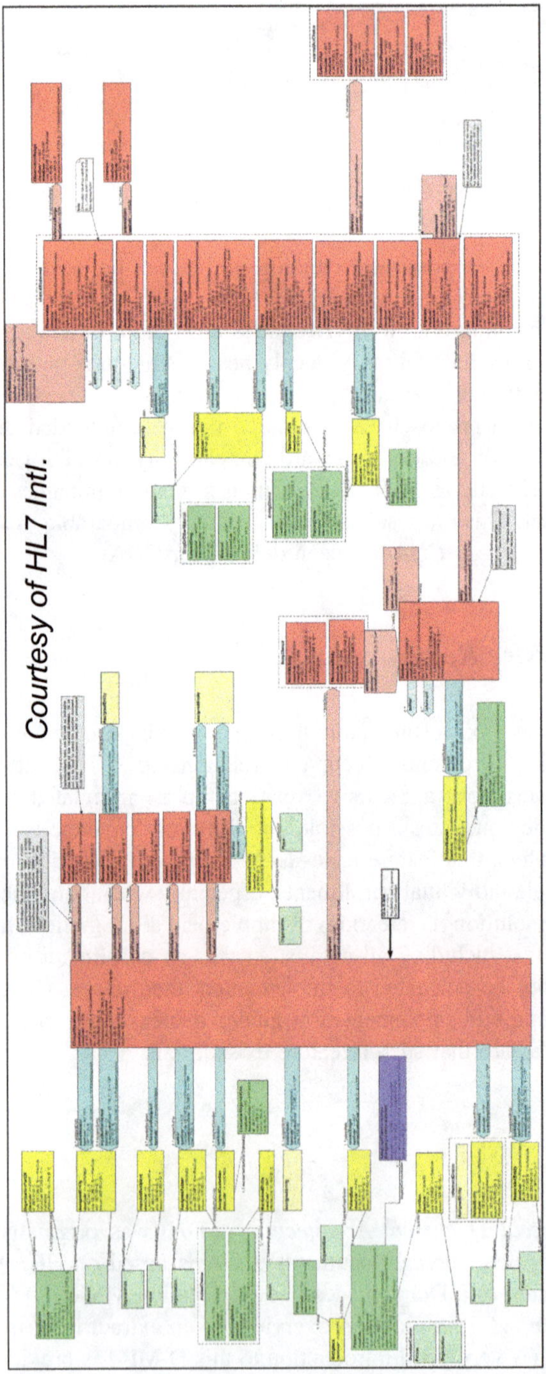

Fig. A.14 HL7® CDA domain message information model

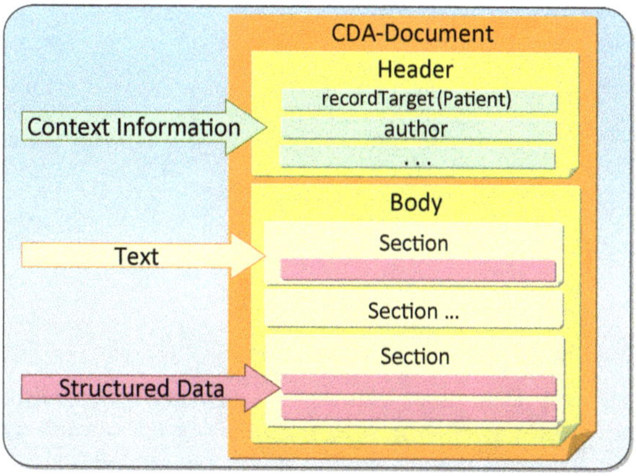

Fig. A.15 CDA general design

A CDA document mainly consists of two parts: the header with the metadata and the body providing the contents.

The header is used to provide identifying information about the document. Examples of this identifying information are the type of document (e.g. discharge letter or surgery protocol), the date of creation, participants involved in creating this document (e.g., author or data enterer), and, of course, a link to the patient themselves that is called *recordTarget*.

The body of a CDA document conveys the factual clinical information, which must be provided in a human-readable format—i.e., in a manner that a human consumer can read and understand it. The body normally is provided in textual form using natural language.

Figure A.15 shows the general design of a CDA document, including the relationship of the header section to the body section, as well as the use of text and structured data in the body section.

Figure A.16 shows an abbreviated example for a CDA document represented in XML. It is a valid XML document, but an invalid CDA instance because mandatory elements are missing. For simplicity, it only contains some meta-data, the patient (in record target), and a very short text in the main body.

An easy way to approach creation of a CDA is just to provide the necessary metadata and contents using the currently available document formats (PDF, DOC, JPG, etc.) and then encapsulate these elements into the body, as is illustrated in the left-hand side of Fig. A.17. In a second step, this content can be replaced by a set of sections containing text.

The strategy for accomplishing the migration from a contents perspective is shown in Fig. A.18. The green line demonstrates the quick initial integration of text, whether this integration is accomplished in an XML representation or just by encapsulating other file formats like PDF. In a second step, additional information can be added in structural form without compromising the previously negotiated textual data exchange. The red line in Fig. A.18 represents use of the second step.

```
<?xml version="1.0"?>
<ClinicalDocument >
      <id root="…"/>
      <code code="34133-9" codeSystem="2.16.840.1.113883.6.1"
            displayName="Summarization of episode note"/>
      <title>Good Health Clinic Continuity of Care Document</title>
      <effectiveTime value="20000407130000+0500"/>
      <confidentialityCode code="N"
            codeSystem="2.16.840.1.113883.5.25"/>
      <languageCode code="en-US"/>
      <recordTarget>
            <patientRole>
                  <id extension="12345" root="2.16.840.1.113883.19.5"/>
                  <patient>
                        <name>
                              <given>Henry</given>
                              <family>Levin</family>
                              <suffix>the 7th</suffix>
                        </name>
                        <administrativeGenderCode code="M"
                              codeSystem="2.16.840.1.113883.5.1"/>
                        <birthTime value="19320924"/>
                  </patient>
                  <providerOrganization>
                        <id root="2.16.840.1.113883.19.5"/>
                  </providerOrganization>
            </patientRole>
      </recordTarget>
      <component>
            <structuredBody>
                  <component>
                        <section>
                              <code code="48764-5"
                                    codeSystem="2.16.840.1.113883.6.1"/>
                              <title>Summary Purpose</title>
                              <text>Transfer of care</text>
                        </section>
                  </component>
                  ...
            </structuredBody>
      </component>
</ClinicalDocument>
```

Fig. A.16 Example CDA document

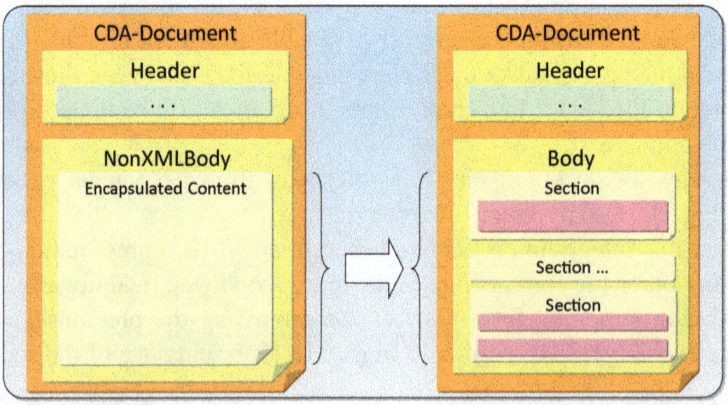

Fig. A.17 Content migration

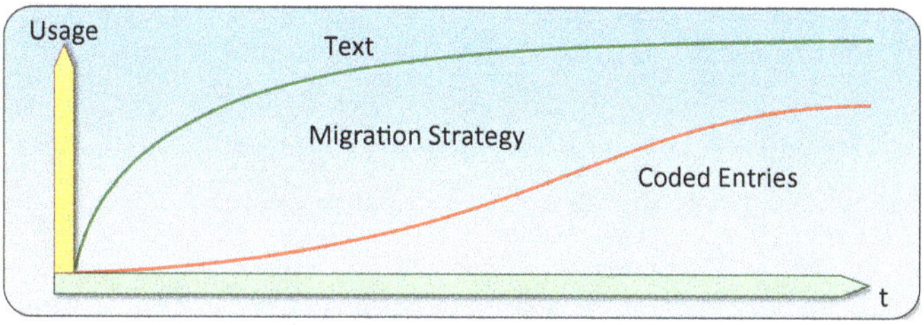

Fig. A.18 Migration strategy

A.2.1 Levels

An important concept in CDA documents is the notion of levels (Table A.5). CDA levels provide a mechanism for informing a consumer about how much information is available for machine processing.

When creating (or consuming) a CDA document, a minimum set of metadata must be provided; the text can be taken "as is" and encapsulated, facilitating a simple encoding that is used in almost all email clients. This process is demonstrated by the gray box in the lower left corner of Fig. A.19.

After the minimum set of metadata is provided for the document, the implementation can be expanded in different directions in parallel. On the one hand, further metadata may be added to the header to provide more details about the context of the document. This part of the continuing process is shown by the blue arrow in Fig. A.19. On the other hand, more details can be included in the document by adding different sections in the body, replacing the encapsulated document object. Adding more supported sections is another means of enhancing the use of CDA structures, as shown by the orange arrow in Fig. A.19. Along with implementing new sections, existing sections of the CDA document can be enhanced with structured data, as is shown by the red arrows in the diagram.

The different parts of a CDA document, which are represented by the different colors in Fig. A.19, can be augmented independently.

In Fig. A.20, the portions of a document representing the different CDA levels (described in detail in Table A.5) are marked by different colors.

As can be seen, levels 2 and 3 are somewhat orthogonal, as they are truly independent of each other. Processing of structured information provided in level 3

Table A.5 CDA levels

Level	Description
1	Text only: the document contains only free text that is neither structured nor clearly identifiable by its content
2	The different sections of the body are marked so that the contents become obvious, e.g., "this section contains a diagnosis"
3	The information is also provided in a structured form that allows for machine processing

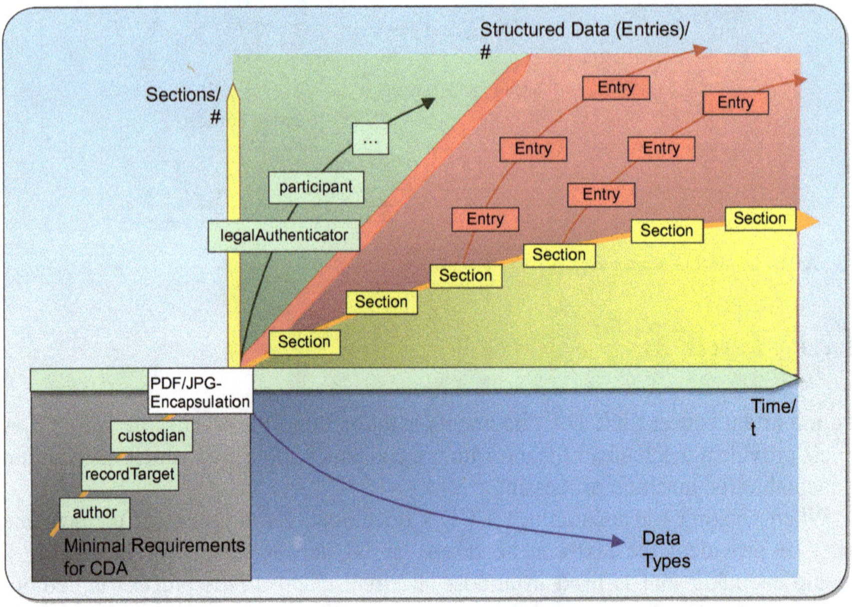

Fig. A.19 Integration states

```
        <component>
        <!—Anamnesis Component -->
        <section>
Level 2 <code code="10164-2"
        codeSystem="2.16.840.1.113883.6.1"
        codeSystemName="LOINC"/>
Level 1 <title>August 29, 2010: History of Past Illness
        <text>
        Chronical bronchitis for years, esp. with fresh cold air.
        Breathlessness with stress.
        </text>
Level 3 <entry>
        <observation>
        <code code="195967001"
        codeSystem="2.16.840.1.113883.6.96"
        codeSystemName="SNOMED CT"
        displayName="Asthma">
        </code>
        </observation>
        </entry>
        </section>
        </component>
```

Fig. A.20 Level 3 CDA Release 2 extract as example

Table A.6 "Enhanced" CDA levels

Level	Description
1a	Document contains a base 64 or hex encoded document in another format (in most cases it is PDF)
1b	Text only: the document contains only text and no clearly identifiable content
2a	Some sections follow a defined structure and provides information about the contents (either by class codes or a template identification)
2b	All sections follow a structure
3a	Some sections provide data in a structured form
3b	All sections contain structured information. (This may be hard to achieve because not all sections possibly allow for structured information)

is made easier, however, by including some information about the contents of that section in level 2.

Recent proposals advocate inclusion of a further subdivision, which could be a Level 0, containing only embedded objects, i.e., binary data that cannot be semantically processed. IHE ITI XDS-SD is an example of this approach.

Some specifications use a more detailed expansion of the levels within a CDA document, such as the levels listed in Table A.6.

Conversely, a level 4 could be added, which would indicate internal references (linking of the sections with each other). This enhancement approach is discussed in the 3rd release of the CDA specification.

A.2.2 Releases

The **first release** of the CDA specification occurred in 1999. At that time the goal was to define additional levels to enable the exchange of structured data. For Release 1 of the CDA standard, the authors attempted to allow a mechanism for conveying structured data in order to facilitate a smooth transition from communication of purely text-based information to communicating encoded information, but this mechanism never materialized. This planned enhancement in CDA Release 1 was then superseded by the development of a standard for CDA Release 2.

The **second release**, published in 2005, is now fully based on HL7 Version 3, and the data types were taken from HL7 V3 as well. This release also includes a collection of activities ("Act") in the CDA body that are known today as Clinical Statement Patterns today.

The **third release** is currently in development. All of the unimplemented requirements and additional ideas are being considered for this release, including the support of the HL7 V3 data types Release 2.

Another means to simplify creating and consuming CDA instances is the use of an alternative XML schema ("Green CDA").

A.2.3 Templates

Although the CDA Release 2 specification is provided in the form of an expansive model, it is composed of building blocks that allow creation of multi-faceted types of documents used for many purposes. These building blocks are called templates, and they apply to different levels (see Fig. A.21 and Table A.7 for details).

Figure A.21 shows where each kind of template is used.

Figure A.22 illustrates the stacking of the templates. The highest level template—the document-level template—specifies (among other details) which header-level templates and section-level templates are included. The section-level templates may

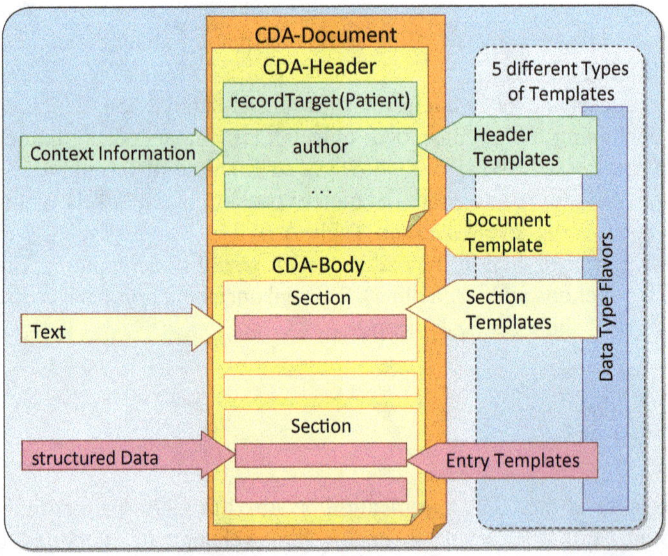

Fig. A.21 CDA template types

Table A.7 CDA templates

Template	Description	Location
Document	A document template specifies the type of document (e.g., discharge letter), necessary meta-data and the associated parts (header (light green in Fig. A.21) and body sections [light yellow in Fig. A.21]), which are represented by the green and yellow arrows in Fig. A.22	Header
Header	A header template is a building block to be used as meta-data in the header of the document. An example is the author of the document or the patient to whom this document is assigned	Header
Section	A section template describes a part of the main body of the document	Body
Entry	An entry-level template specifies structured information to be used with a section	Body (section)
Data Type	A specialization for a data type is normally called data type flavor and can be applied in all other templates. An example is the localization of names or addresses for a specific country	

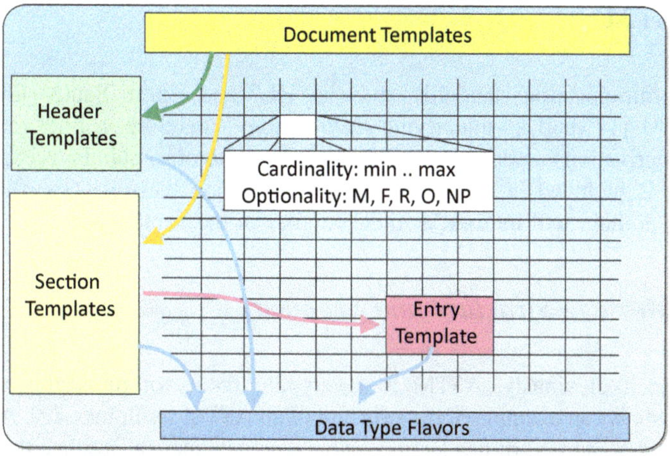

Fig. A.22 CDA template references

include entry-level templates. All templates make use of specific data flavors. Each usage has a specified cardinality and optionality.

A template can be defined as "open" or "closed". If the template is open, additional data structures and content can be inserted. If the template is closed, it is bound to the data structures and content defined by the template.

A.2.4 Implementation Guides

The entire Release 2 specification, together with the data types in Release 1, forms a very generic specification that can't be implemented completely by any application. Therefore, a document with additional guidance, an *implementation guide*, must be provided.

This guidance includes not only the IHE Content modules for section- and entry-levels published in the Patient Care Coordination (PCC) Technical Framework (TF), but also the well-known VHitG doctor's letter in Germany. Another good example of a document designed to provide additional guidance for use of the CDA Release 2 specification is the consolidated CDA Implementation Guide for the US realm known as C-CDA. This implementation guide is currently available as Release 2.0, and Release 2.1 is in development.

A.2.5 SDA—Structured Document Architecture

Another development is the *Structured Document Architecture* (SDA), which is more abstract than the CDA. The CDA is actually "only" a special version (constraint) of the SDA. Another example of a special version of the SDA would be *Structured Product Labeling* (SPL).

A.3 ASTM

Several communication standards—such as HL7 and Hprim Santé—are derived from ASTM [14] and its underlying methodology; therefore, a brief explanation about the derivations made from ASTM, in contrast to other standards explained in this book, is included in this section. Communication messages specified in the healthcare domain will be used as the examples in the explanation.

A.3.1 Message Structure and Segments

As mentioned previously, ASTM is a very old family of messaging standards. Table A.8 shows an example of the structure of an ASTM result message. All ASTM messages are composed of header and trailer segments that encapsulate the payload.

The braces ("{ }") denote repeating structures, which are expressed in a nesting format. Indentation is used to help with visualization.

Table A.9 uses the ASTM Patient Segment to expound on the information in Table A.8.

The ASTM segments are composed of a sequence of fields with attributes such as name, data type, optionality, repetitions, length, and a data element number.

A.3.2 Chapters

The structure of the ASTM chapters and the embedded specifications for segments are identical to these constructs in HL7 v2.x; therefore, we need not investigate that topic any more deeply and can just list a snippet of the ASTM documentation instead, which is shown in Table A.10.

Except for Chap. 1, which is the same as the introductory section in HL7 v2 specifications, ASTM documentation is more or less identical to HL7 v1 [15]

Table A.8 ASTM result message

Segments	Explanation
H	Header
{	
P	Patient
{	
O	Order
{ R }	Result
}	
}	
L	Trailer

Table A.9 ASTM segment P—Patient

Seq	Name	Type	Table	R/O	REP	LEN	ITEM#
1	Sequence number	SI		O	N		
…							
3	Lab assigned patient ID	ID		O	N	16	
…							
5	Patient name	PN		O	N		
…							
8	Sex	ID	1	O	N	1	
…							
14	Patient age	CQ		O	N		
…							
16	Patient height	CQ		O	N		
17	Patient weight	CQ		O	N		
…							

Table A.10 ASTM documentation overview

Chp.	Content	Segment	Description
1	ASTM result report	H	Header
		P	Patient
		L	Trailer
2	CNT—control/query	ADD	Addendum
		ERR	Error
		MSH	Message header
3	ADT—REG/ADT	PID	Patient identification
		NK1	Next of kin
		PV1	Patient visit
4	ORD—order entry	OBR	Observation request
		ORC	Common order
6	BLN—finance	DG1	Diagnosis
7	ANR—ancillary reporting	OBX	Observation
8	MFI—master files	MFI	Master file identification
		MFE	Master file entry

documentation. This similarity supports the assertion that ASTM is the standard from which the HL7 v2 family of standards was originally derived in 1987.

A.3.3 Conformance Methodology

ASTM has not specified a detailed conformance methodology. Because of ASTM's close relationship to the early versions of HL7 v2.x, however, the same methodology could be applied to both standards and would include the newest achievements of HL7 v2.8.

A.4 DICOM

DICOM is a communication standard for exchanging medical images [16].

A.4.1 Introduction and Overview

Originally, DICOM was designed to retrieve images from digital imaging devices such as the ones used for *computerized tomography* (CT), *magnetic resonance* (MR) *techniques*, and *positron emission tomography* (PET). DICOM quickly expanded to include storage of those images in *picture archives and communication systems* (PACS).

Data exchange for medical imaging is organized between a client and a server using DICOM commands—which are like function calls—on information objects (Fig. A.23).

DICOM also supports the different communication paradigms, as is explained in Chap. 2.

A.4.2 Information Model

DICOM provides a set of specifications for service classes, including:

- Storage Service Class
- Query/Retrieve Service Class
- Basic Worklist Management Service Class
- Print Management Service Class.

Each service class is an image object definition in combination with a group of services that can be invoked. Each image object definition makes use of attributes that are provided in the form of modules as shown in Fig. A.24.

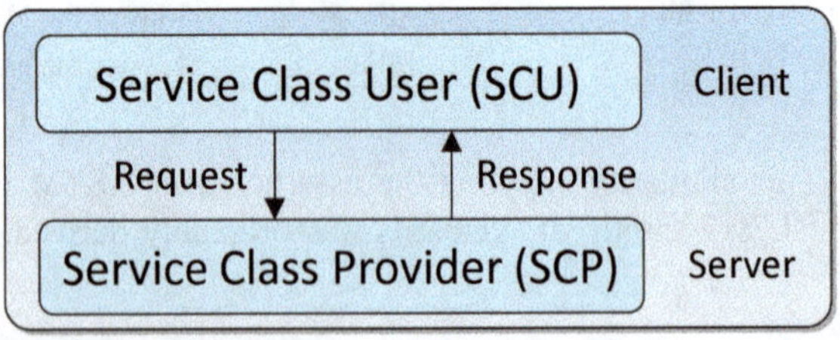

Fig. A.23 DICOM function calls

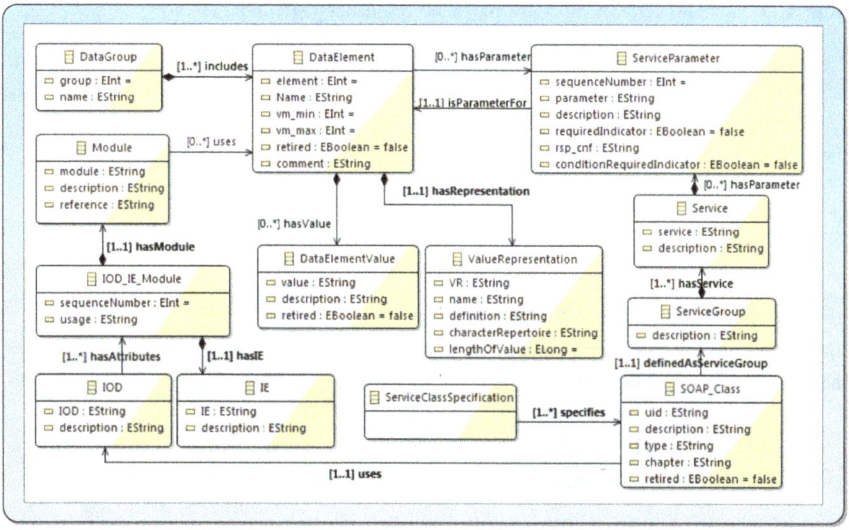

Fig. A.24 DICOM information model

A.4.3 *Information Object*

The different DICOM commands operate on information entities such CT scans, ultrasound images, or structured reports. Those entities are abstracted and called *information objects* as shown in Fig. A.24.

Figure A.25 shows an example of such an *information object* by using an entity relationship model that illustrates the information entities that comprise the object.

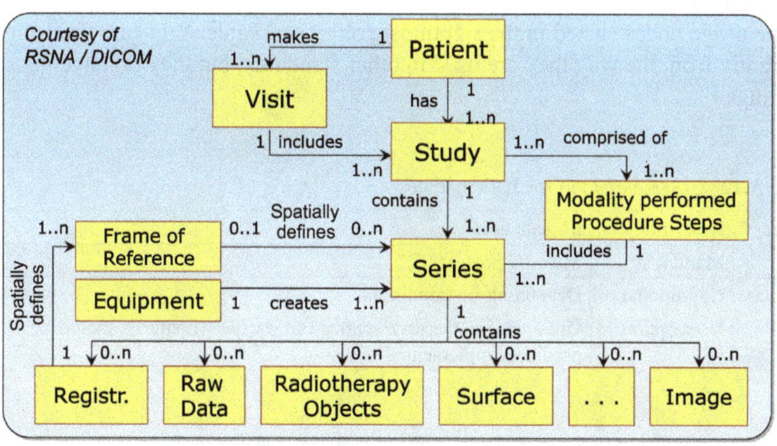

Fig. A.25 Example of a DICOM entity relationship model for information entities (IE)

Table A.11 DICOM IOD modules for magnetic resonance (MR) images

IE	Module	Reference	Usage
Patient	Patient	C.7.1.1	M
	Clinical trial subject	C.7.1.3	U
Study	General study	C.7.2.1	M
	Patient study	C.7.2.2	U
	Clinical trial study	C.7.2.3	U
Series	General series	C.7.3.1	M
	Clinical trial series	C.7.3.2	U
Frame of reference	Frame of reference	C.7.4.1	M
Equipment	General equipment	C.7.5.1	M
Image	General image	C.7.6.1	M
	Image plane	C.7.6.2	M
	Image pixel	C.7.6.3	M
	Contrast/bolus	C.7.6.4	C—required if contrast media was used in this image
	Device	C.7.6.12	U
	Specimen	C.7.6.22	U
	MR image	C.8.3.1	M
	Overlay plane	C.9.2	U
	VOI LUT	C.11.2	U
	SOP common	C.12.1	M

An *information entity* (IE), as indicated in Fig. A.25, is itself composed of components called *Information Object Definition* (IOD) modules. Each IE contains one or more IOD modules. Table A.11 shows an example set of these modules for magnetic resonance (MR) images. (The usage codes in Table A.11 are explained in Table A.12.)

The usage codes (listed in the rightmost column of Table A.11) are used slightly differently from the way they are used in other standards, but they do have the same meanings.

Table A.12 Usage definition for IOD modules

Usage	Description	Explanation
M	Mandatory	Must be present
C	Conditional	Depending on conditions
U	User option	Optional, i.e. the user/vendor can decide whether it should be provided/implemented

A.4.4 Data Element

A DICOM object (module) is composed of a sequence of bytes that is a concatenation of data elements, as is illustrated in Fig. A.26. The way DICOM data elements are defined is similar to ASN.1 [7], as the definition of a DICOM data element starts with an identifier.

VR, shown in Fig. A.26, is an acronym for *value representation* and denotes data types. VM, another acronym used with DICOM, stands for *value multiplicity* and represents the number of repetitions allowed (e.g., the cardinality of an element).

Each data element definition starts with a tag, which is a pair of positive (4-digit) integers. The first number in the pair denotes the group to which the element belongs. Table A.13 provides a small list of example DICOM data elements.

Within a given data set, the elements are sequenced by their tags in ascending order. The group number (the first integer in the pair of tag numbers) is used to keep closely related elements sequenced together.

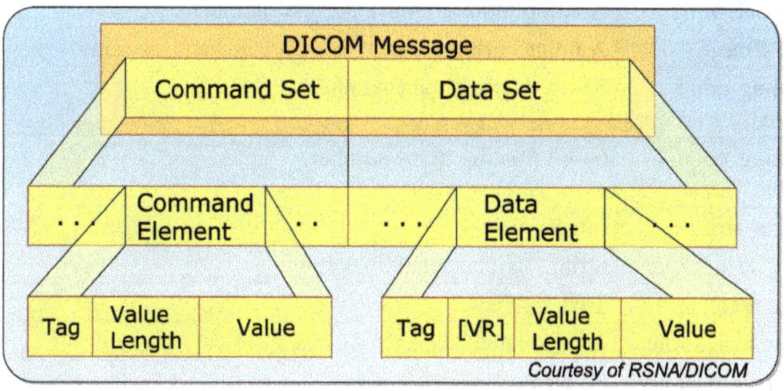

Fig. A.26 DICOM message structure

Table A.13 DICOM data elements (example)

Tag	Name	Keyword	VR	VM
(0008,0080)	Institution name	InstitutionName	LO	1
(0008,0081)	Institution address	InstitutionAddress	ST	1
(0008,0082)	Institution code sequence	InstitutionCodeSequence	SQ	1
(0008,0090)	Referring physician's name	ReferringPhysicianName	PN	1
(0008,0092)	Referring physician's address	ReferringPhysicianAddress	ST	1

A.4.5 Value Representation

The value representation (VR) specifies the data type and other constraints to which a data element must adhere. The VR can be combined with a regular expression, a set of assigned characters, and/or a specific length. Table A.14 provides a list of DICOM VRs along with a description and explanation for each one.

This list also shows that most of the VRs are purely technically oriented. The only two exceptions are the Application Entity (AE), which denotes a DICOM entity with some constraints on the string representation, and the Person Name

Table A.14 DICOM value representation

VR	Description	Explanation
AE	Application entity	A string to identify an application entity
AS	Age string	A 4-byte string to indicate a period of days, months, weeks or years
AT	Attribute tag	A pair of unsigned integers to declare a data element
CS	Code string	A short string to denote a code
DA	Date	A date
DS	Decimal string	A string representing a decimal number
DT	Date time	A point in time
FL	Floating point single	32-bit floating point number
FD	Floating point double	64-bit floating point number
IS	Integer string	Integer
LO	Long string	String, 64 characters maximum
LT	Long text	Text
OB	Other byte string	A negotiated sequence of bytes
OF	Other float string	32-bit floating point word
OW	Other word string	16-bit word
PN	Person name	Name of a person consisting of 5 components; the delimiter shall be fixed to "^" (caret) Note: This set of components is identical to the "old" XPN data type of HL7 v2.x, BUT the delimiter is fixed
SH	Short string	String, 16 characters maximum
SL	Signed long	Long integer
SQ	Sequence of items	A sequence of zero or more items
ST	Short text	String, 1 K maximum
TM	Time	A time
UI	Unique identifier	A character string denoting an UID (OID)
UL	Unsigned long	Unsigned long integer
UN	Unknown	A string of bytes with an unknown encoding
US	Unsigned short	Unsigned short integer
UT	Unlimited text	Text

(PN). Important to note is that the set of components associated with the Person Name VR is fixed at five, and the delimiter for PN has an additional constraint as well, because it is fixed to a caret ("^"). The HL7 v2 specification from which PN is derived allows some flexibility, so the encoding stack must be used correctly. If, as is done in most cases, a pure copy and paste is performed, an error will occur.

Some value representations are combined with additional constraints on the encoding, regular expressions (a set of characters, padding/leading/trailing spaces), and length (e.g., maximum and/or even number of bytes).

A.4.6 Conformance Methodology

With DICOM, the type[1] of data element determines whether this element is or is not required. In other words, the *DICOM type* is a representation of optionality, specifying whether a given element is mandatory or optional (Table A.15).

A.4.7 Proprietary Extensions

DICOM allows for the addition of proprietary data elements called *private elements*. These data elements must use the same value representations as the ones defined for the official public elements, and they must be assigned private data element tags that have odd numbers in a specific range.

Table A.15 DICOM® data element types

Type	Description	Explanation
1	Required	Data element shall be included and is mandatory, and this data element must be populated with valid information according to the value representation of length greater than zero
1C	Conditional	In principle, the same rules apply as with type 1, but only under certain conditions. Therefore, if the condition is true the rules for type 1 apply, and if not true the element is not allowed at all
2	Required if known	The standard declares this type of data element as mandatory, but with the exception that this data element can be empty if the value is not known, i.e., a value of zero length is allowed, but it must be present. In a subsequent paragraph is a statement saying that a data element of this type must be supported. In HL7 v2-speak this element would be called "required but may be empty"
2C	Conditional if known	This type of data element is comparable to type 2 using the same rules as explained with type 1C
3	Optional	A data element of this type may or may not be sent

[1]Please see DICOM Part 5: Data Structures and Encoding.

From this perspective, proprietary extensions are clearly marked and visible, and processing the appropriate information object is possible, in general; however, potential conflicts across different vendors may be found, because different vendors may use the same tag for different purposes.

A.5 XDT (Germany)

"xDT" is an abbreviation for a family of data transmission standards in the ambulatory sector. These standards mainly have been defined by the *Kassenärztliche Bundesvereinigung* (KBV), the *Zentralinstitut* (ZI) and the *Qualitätsring Medizinische Software* (QMS) [17, 18].

A.5.1 Introduction and Overview

The KBV defined a standard called *Abrechnungsdatentransfer* (ADT) for transferring billing data. The original intent for the development of Behandlungsdatentransfer (BDT), the first standard of the xDT-family outside the scope of billing purposes, was to define a standard format for data exchange between systems for *General Practitioners* (GPs) in case the HIT vendor declared bankruptcy. BDT (also known as patient related data transfer) was to allow for the export and subsequent re-import of all data about patients stored in GP offices. At the time BDT was developed, most of the clinical information was documented on paper, so an administrative data exchange, together with some medical data stored on index cards, was sufficient.

Later on, further specifications were developed for different kinds of use cases. Table A.16 provides an abridged overview of the xDT-family.

Features of BDT Versions 2.0 and 3.0 are presented in the following sections that describe the key aspects of the standard.

Table A.16 xDT family of standards

Standard	German description	English description/explanation
ADT	Abrechnungsdatentransfer	Billing data
BDT	Behandlungsdatentransfer	Administrative data/medical documentation
GDT	Gerätedatentransfer	Device data
LDT	Labordatentransfer	Laboratory data
KVDT	KV-Datentransfer	Billing data
…		

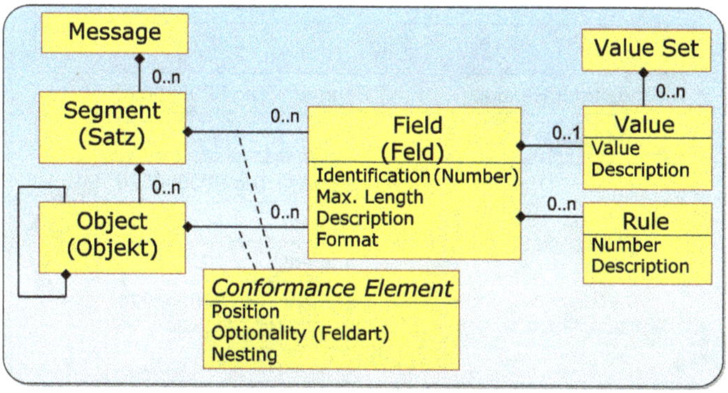

Fig. A.27 xDT information model

A.5.2 Information Model

The information model for xDT is very simple, as illustrated in Fig. A.27. Messages consist of segments ("Satz") that in turn may consist of objects ("Objekt"). An object is a relatively new concept that is designed to allow elements to be grouped together. Both segments and objects consist of fields ("Felder"). A field is a single object, such as a "family name of the patient" or the "zip code of the patients permanent address". Each field is identified by a four-digit number in combination with description, format (alphanumeric or numeric), and a maximum length. Furthermore, a field specification may be accompanied by a list of possible values (without any further identification) and a set of rules introducing constraints. The use of fields in segments and/or objects is controlled by the position (sequence), and, optionally, by a number indicating the nesting. Nesting is a mechanism to define dependencies of fields and to group them together.

A.5.3 Data Exchange

Data exchange and transport in xDT was originally based on files stored on disks. Nowadays, this method has been replaced by electronic file transport. In the German environment, D2D ("doctor to doctor communication") has been used in the past but is being replaced by KV-Connect from the KV Telematik GmbH, a subsidiary of the KBV.

The contents of each file is organized as illustrated by Fig. A.28. A set of messages is encapsulated by a file header and trailer.

The file header and trailer are represented by a single segment, whereas each message is composed of one or more consecutive segments.

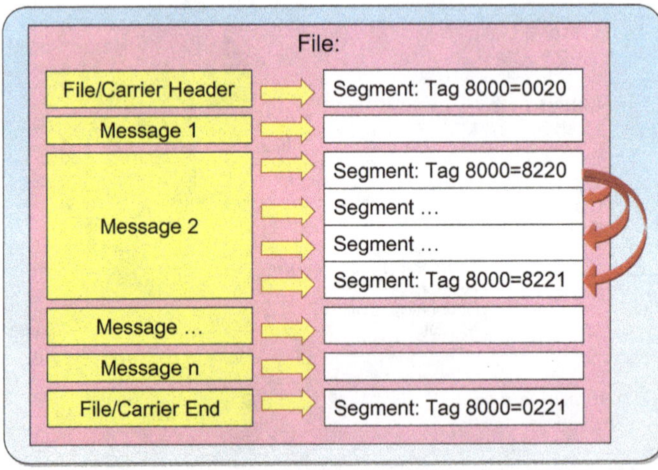

Fig. A.28 xDT File/transport

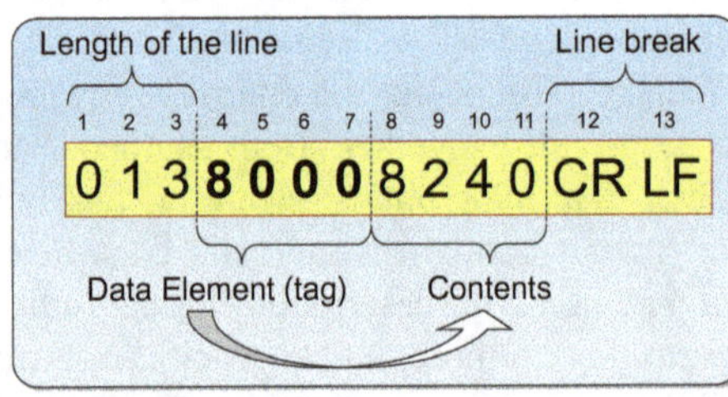

Fig. A.29 xDT encoding + parsing

A.5.4 Encoding and Parsing

The entire contents of the file, i.e., the messages containing the segments, are encoded in the form of lines, where each line represents a single data element. Figure A.29 provides an example of a single line with annotations about how to read it.

The first three characters of each line denote the length of the line (in decimal format) including the two bytes for Carriage Return (CR)/Line Feed (LF). Given the long history of this standard, the inclusion of the length should ensure proper encoding and integrity of the data.

The next four characters represent the identifier (tag) of the data element. This tag consists of four digits and clearly identifies the content (semantics), which is conveyed within the remaining characters. In Fig. A.29, the data element is identified by the tag "8000", which refers to and identifies the message type. The value for the message type in our example is "8240", which indicates that this is the header of the message.

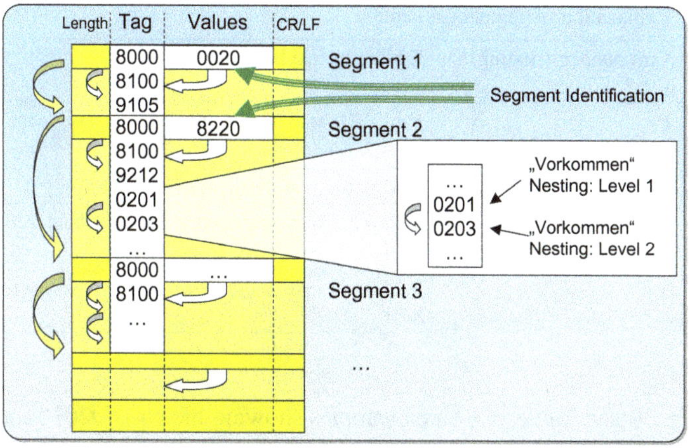

Fig. A.30 xDT encoding/decoding

The length of the content for the data element is calculated according to the following formula:

> The length of the data element equals the length of the line, minus 3 digits for the length itself, minus 4 digits for the data element tag, minus 2 digits for end of line (CR+LF).

The resulting structure, created by concatenating the different data elements into segments that are then concatenated into a message, is shown in Fig. A.30. An example of a message is demonstrated in Table A.31.

The *tag* attribute identifies the segment. As shown in Fig. A.30, the first segment (tag "8000") is identified as the *file header* (value "0020"). The second segment (2nd tag "8000") is the information about the *beginning of a message* (value "8220"). The third segment is the first segment with some contents (data), which is followed by more segments, until the next message begins or the transmission is concluded with a trailing file end segment (not shown in Fig. A.30).

The file header contains two items, which are marked by tag "8100" and "9105". The second segment indicates the beginning of a new lab order message (tag "8220"). The details for this message are included in subsequent segments.

A.5.5 Explanation of Segment Structure

Table A.17 provides an explanation of the segment structure, i.e., how the structure should be read. "FK" (Feldkennung) is the tag, and "*Vorkommen*" (nesting) indicates the repetition of the element relative to the previous element and a hierarchical structure. Indentation (higher value for nesting) is used to denote the dependence on the previous element.

Table A.17 Explanation of segment structure

FK (tag)	Vorkommen (nesting) 1 2 3 4	Erklärung (explanation)
8401	1	Feld 8401 may occur only once per segment
…		
0201	N	Feld 0201 may occur multiple times
0203	1	Feld 0203 may occur once for each field 0201
…		
8460	N	Feld 8460 may occur as often as necessary for field 8410

In Fig. A.30 and Table A.17 are examples showing the tags "0201" and "0203"; the second tag is nested depending on the first.

A.5.6 Overall Structure (Message Structure)

From a structural perspective, xDT defines a set of messages, which are organized in a layered system structure as "Kommunikation" ("communication"), "Datenpakete" (data packages/messages), "Sätze" (Segments) and "Felder" (fields). They are linked in a one-to-many relationship as demonstrated in Fig. A.31. From the perspective of an operating system, an xDT message is a file of the operating system.

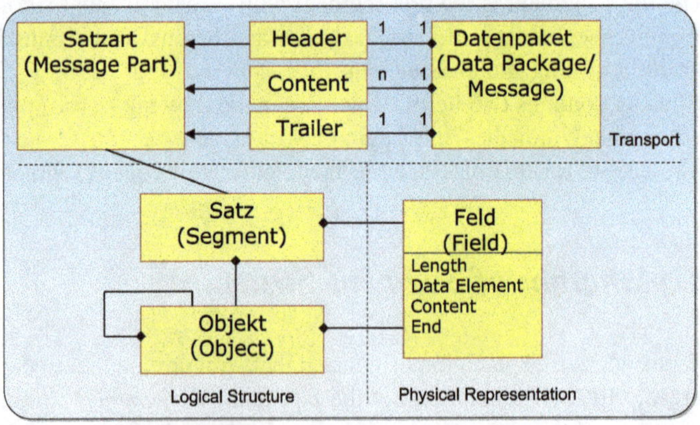

Fig. A.31 xDT overall structure

A.5.7 *"Datenpaket" (Data Package/Message)*

Table A.18 illustrates an example of a data package, which, as mentioned previously, is equivalent to a message in HL7 V2.x.

A.5.8 *"Satz" (Segment)*

Each segment ("Satz") is composed of a sequences of fields (data elements). Table A.19 provides an example of the Header Segment in xDT, which can be compared to an HL7 v2 segment.

Each segment definition is composed of the information listed in the "Columns" column of Table A.20: Segment Definition (Attributes). The information in the Example column does not appear in the original German specification but is provided for the readers' convenience.

It is worth noting that the *Vorkommen* (repetitions) column as used in Table A.19 also indicates the structure of the message: the numbers ("1 2 3 4") represent the nesting. Table A.21 provides an explanation for common patterns.

In order to understand how nesting (*Vorkommen*) works, Table A.19 has been copied and presented again below, but this time an HL7 v2.x equivalent representation is provided in the two rightmost columns in Table A.22.

Table A.18 Message for result reporting of laboratory to GPs

Segment	Description	Logical structure (HL7 v2.x AMS notation)
0020	Segment "0020" must occur on each transmission. It must be the first segment.	0020
8220	Segment "8220" must occur exactly once. It must be the second segment.	8220
8201 8203	These two segments can occur in arbitrary order and must follow segment "8220"	{< 8201 | 8203 >}
8221	This segment occurs exactly once and precedes segment "0021"	8221
0021	This segment occurs exactly once and is the last segment	0221

Table A.19 Satzart: P-Datenpaket-Header "8230" (header segment)

FK (tag)	Vorkommen (nesting) 1 2 3 4	Feldbezeichnung (German description)	Feldart (opt.)	Bedingung (condition)	Erläuterung (English explanation)
8000	1	Satzart	M		Message type
8100	1	Satzlänge	M		Total length of the message in bytes
9212	1	Version der Satzbeschreibung	M		version
0201	1	Betriebs- (BSNR) oder Nebenbetriebsstättennummer (NBSNR)	M		BSNR number
0203	1	(N)BSNR-Bezeichnung	M		BSNR description
0212	n	Lebenslange Arztnummer (LANR)	M		Replacement: 999999900
0211	1	Arztname	M		Physician name
0205	1	Strasse der (N)BSNR	M		Street BSNR
0215	1	PLZ der (N)BSNR	M		ZIP BSNR
0216	1	Ort der (N)BSNR	M		City BSNR
8300	1	Labor	m	Rule 425	Laboratory
8320	1	Laborname	m	Rule 425	Name of lab
8321	1	Strasse der Laboradresse	m	Rule 425	Street
8322	1	PLZ der Laboradresse	m	Rule 425	ZIP
8323	1	Ort der Laboradresse	m	Rule 425	Address of the lab
0101	1	KBV-Prüfnummer	M		KBV check digit
9106	1	verwendeter Zeichensatz	M		Used character set
8312	1	Kunden- (Arzt-Nummer)	M		Client (physician ID)
9103	1	Erstellungsdatum	M		Creation date
9472	n	allgemeine Informationen	K		General information
9300	1	Prüfsumme/Elektronische Signatur	K		Check digit
9301	1	Kryptoschlüssel	K		Cryptographic key

Table A.20 Segment definition (attributes)

Columns		Description	Example
Feldkennung	Tag	Data element number (tag)	8000
Vorkommen	Nesting	Number of repetitions	1
Feldinhalt	German description	Description	VKNR
Feldart	Optionality	Optionality (Muss = required/Kann = optional)	M
Bedingung	Condition	Conditions	Rule 425
Erläuterung	English explanation	Additional explanations	–

Table A.21 Nesting of fields

Vorkommen/Nesting	1 2 3 4	1 2 3 4	1 2 3 4

Example	1
	1
		1
		  1
			1
			  n

Explanation	Independent sequence: the second field is independent from the previous one	Depending sequence: the second field can only occur if the previous field is present	One-to-many relationship: the second field may occur multiple times given the previous one is present

Table A.22 xDT nesting of fields in HL7 v2 abstract message syntax

FK (tag)	Vorkommen (nesting) 1 2 3 4	Feldart (opt.)	Logical structure (HL7 v2.x AMS notation)	Rule/condition
8000	1	M	8000	
8100	1	M	8100	
9212	1	M	9212	
0201	1	M	0201	
0203	1	M	0203	
			{	
0212	n	M	0212	
0211	1	M	0211	
			}	
0205	1	M	0205	
0215	1	M	0215	
0216	1	M	0216	
8300	1	m	8300	C
8320	1	m	8320	C

(continued)

Table A.22 (continued)

FK (tag)	Vorkommen (nesting) 1 2 3 4	Feldart (opt.)	Logical structure (HL7 v2.x AMS notation)	Rule/condition
8321	1	m	8321	C
8322	1	m	8322	C
8323	1	m	8323	C
0101	1	M	0101	
9106	1	M	9106	
8312	1	M	312	
9103	1	M	9103	
9472	n	K	[{9472}]	
9300	1	K	[9300]	
9301	1	K	[9301]	

Table A.23 *Feldarten* (optionality)

Feldart	German description	English explanation
M (upper case)	Unbedingtes Mussfeld	Required
m (lower case)	Bedingtes Mussfeld	Conditionally required
K (upper case)	Kannfeld	Optional
k (lower case)	Bedingtes Kannfeld	Conditionally optional

A.5.8.1 "Feldarten" (Optionality)

Feldarten is optionality/usage. Table A.23 lists the possible options and their descriptions.

Upper and lower case representation distinguishes between the non-conditional and conditional. For example, *M* indicates *Required* and *m* indicates *Conditionally Required.* In hindsight, using upper and lower case as indicators was not a good choice, since specifications are vulnerable to unexpected automated text processing transformations that can alter the meaning. Therefore, newer versions of xDT standards only define "M" and "K".

A.5.9 *"Bedingung" (Condition/Rules)*

Rules are used to introduce additional constraints. Each field may be associated with one or more rules, which are organized by numbers. Table A.24 provides some examples.

Each rule falls into one of three categories, which have different purposes as explained in Table A.25.

Table A.24 "Rules" (conditions)

Regelnummer (rule number)	Kategorie (category)	Prüfung (rule including validation)	Erläuterung (explanation)
005	Format	HHMM	*Time* represented as four digits with: HH = hour and MM = minutes. The values shall be in the range of 0000–2359
…			
425	Context	Either field 8300 or one of fields 8320, 8321, 8322, and 8323 must be present	This rule specifies that some fields are mutually exclusive, but one must be present
…			

Table A.25 Rule categories

Category	Explanation	Example
Format	The representation of the data must follow certain guidelines	HHMM "Time" HH = hour, MM = minute, values: 0000–2359
Allowed content	In principle this is a set of possible values	"B", "K", "F"
Context	The value of a field must fulfill specific conditions	If content of field 4113 equals "6", then field 4106 shall be "02"

A.5.10 Feldtabelle (Data Element Table)

In addition to being listed in the segment tables (Table A.19), the standard lists each data element in a separate table along with further information, as shown in Table A.26.

Besides providing supplementary explanations, Table A.26 lists three important attributes for each data element: the maximum field length, the associated data types, and an optional set of associated rules, which are explained separately in several of the sub-sections below.

A.5.11 Feldtypen (Data Types)

xDT does not provide complex data types. Each data element is defined at a basic level by individual tags, as shown in Table A.27.

Table A.26 Field table

FK	Inhalt (description)	Feldlänge (Length)	Format	Regel (rule)	Erlaubte Inhalte und deren Bedeutung (explanation)
0080	ID der Fallakte oder Studie (record number)	≤60	alnum		Organisationsübergreifende ID, frei wählbar unter den Beteiligten (cross-enterprise identifier)
0101	KBV-Prüfnummer (KBV check digit)	16	alnum	F012 K050	KBV—interne Prüfnummer, die im Rahmen der Zertifizierung vergeben wird
0103	Name der Software (name of software)	≤60	alnum		Bsp.: Medistar (example)
0132	Version/Releasestand der software (version of software)	≤60	alnum		

Table A.27 xDT data types

Data Type	Explanation	Constraint
num	Numeric	For fixed field length the data shall be prepended by leading zeros, for variable field lengths no padding shall be done
alnum	Alphanumeric	Leading and trailing blanks are not allowed
date	numerische Datumsangabe im Format JJJJMMTT, wobei TT = 01–31, MM = 01–12, JJJJ = 0001–9999	
f	Decimal value (Beispiel: 15.1)	Decimal point is point

A.5.12 Vocabulary

As mentioned in Tables A.24 and A.25, the vocabulary (content) is managed by rules that provide a list of allowed values. In all cases, the values can either be listed or determined by a simple formula. In Table A.28 the values are listed in the column entitled *Prüfung* (verification). A more intuitive explanation is given the rightmost column; but, as is shown, there is no management, not as individual tables nor as code systems.

The information in the category (Kategorie) column only reflects where this rule is used, as explained in Table A.29.

The error status (*Fehlerstatus*) listed in Table A.28 is explained in Table A.30.

Table A.28 xDT allowed values

Regel-nummer (rule number)	Kategorie (category)	Fehlerstatus (error)	Prüfung (verification)	Erläuterung (explanation)
E001	QMS	F	1, 2	1 = Labor (laboratory) 2 = Einsender (submitter)
E002	KBV	F	1, 3, 5	1 = Mitglied (member) 3 = Familienversicherter (family) 5 = Rentner (pensioner)
E003	Basis	F	01–99	
E004	Basis	F	8220, 8221, 8230, 8231, 8205, 8215	
...				

Table A.29 xDT categories

Category	Explanation
QMS	used also outside statutory healthcare
KBV	only used within statutory healthcare
Basis	to be used in both use cases

Table A.30 xDT error status

Error status	Erklärung	Explanation
F	Fehler	Error
W	Warnung	Warning
I	Information/Hinweis	Information

A.5.13 Character Sets

xDT introduced a mechanism (i.e., a specific field) to denote which of the four character sets applies:

- 7-bit-Code
- IBM-Code (character table 437)
- ISO 8859-1
- ISO 8859-15

In all newer versions of the xDT standards, the ISO 8859-15 character set is mandatory, thus diminishing the problems with character sets.[2]

[2]This solution is not really sufficient, because most systems currently are migrating to UTF-8. The section about *character sets handling* in Chap. 5 explains why.

A.5.14 Example

Table A.31 provides an example definition of a laboratory test message instance. Note that the information in the four columns at the left of the table pertain to parts of the message instance, while the right column provides an explanation of the information.

This information shown in Table A.31 is transmitted via a file, hence, all lines are written into a file consecutively and separated by a line break.

The overall "visible" structure is shown in Fig. A.30.

Table A.31 BDT example for the definition of laboratory examination

Length	Field	(German) Content	End of field	Explanation
013	**8000**	8240	CR/LF	Segment: header
014	8100	00195	CR/LF	Total length of all field values for this segment
020	9212	SDEL1296.03	CR/LF	Version information
019	8320	Dr. Müller	CR/LF	Name of the laboratory
019	8231	Ottostr. 1	CR/LF	Street address of the laboratory
014	8322	50859	CR/LF	Zip code
013	8323	Köln	CR/LF	City
019	8324	02234/4094	CR/LF	Telephone number
020	8325	02234/71058	CR/LF	Fax number
010	9106	2	CR/LF	Character set
017	9103	09121996	CR/LF	Creation date
017	9104	20101996	CR/LF	Reference date
013	**8000**	8242	CR/LF	Segment: master data
014	8100	00201	CR/LF	Total length of all field values for this segment
014	8410	AMYLS	CR/LF	Test identification
025	8411	Amylase im Serum	CR/LF	Test description
011	8428	SE	CR/LF	Specimen identity
014	8430	Serum	CR/LF	Specimen description
010	8523	1	CR/LF	Necessary specimen amount
011	8521	ml	CR/LF	Unit
011	8471	kA	CR/LF	Clinically relevant information
010	8403	1	CR/LF	Fee schedule
015	5402	32.2.3	CR/LF	Chapter
014	5001	32072	CR/LF	Fee
010	8403	2	CR/LF	Fee schedule

(continued)

Table A.31 (continued)

Length	Field	(German) Content	End of field	Explanation
015	5402	32.2.3	CR/LF	Chapter
014	5001	32072	CR/LF	Fee
013	**8000**	8242	CR/LF	Segment: 8242
…	…	…	…	

A.5.15 Conformance Methodology

There is no explicit definition of a conformance methodology for xDT; however, given that the usage of the elements is similar to other communication standards, one can expect the set of challenges to be similar as well. The unidirectional transmission of information, mostly used in public health or insurance reimbursement scenarios, does not cause any severe problems, since the definitions of the exchange format and the fields contained in that specification are oriented towards the receiver requirements. This statement is substantiated by the fact that the xDT specification was developed by an organization responsible for processing the GP's billing claims. Under these circumstances, the receiver is likely to be capable of supporting all specified fields whether they are optional or not, and the optionality definition is more of a concern for the sending application.

The standard defines the fields to be used, together with an indication of whether each field is required or optional. There is no concept of deprecated or withdrawn elements, therefore backward compatibility is neither implied in the specification nor discussed explicitly. The different xDT releases allow fields to be moved around in the structure without needing to take compatibility issues into account.

In contrast to other SDOs, KBV has defined a testing scenario ("certification") that every healthcare information technology vendor must pass, and QMS also is preparing such certification procedures that will be voluntary.

Finally, one has to keep in mind that data exchange among GPs is not very well established due to competition between the vendors of GP systems as well as the GPs themselves; therefore, the interoperability problems are inevitable due to the lack of communication among trading partners.

A.6 Hprim Santé (France)

Another communication standard for exchanging data among health(care) facilities is Hprim Santé, which is used in France. The abbreviation Hprim Santé comes from *Harmonie et Promotion de l'Information Médicale*. It is a derivation of ASTM E12-38 and was defined in 1990. The maintenance of this standard stopped in 2004. One of the weaknesses of this deprecated specification is that it does not support important capabilities, such as Assigning Authorities for identifiers or code system OIDs. It is still in use today for data exchange between clinics and labs, but it is being superseded by HL7 v2.x messages embedded in IHE profiles (PAM, LTW) for intra-hospital messaging.

The primary purpose of Hprim Santé is the exchange of patient related administrative data (admissions, discharges and transfers), orders, result reports, invoices and financial data.

A.6.1 Introduction and Overview

From their common ancestor ASTM E1238, the content of Hprim Santé is very similar to the content in HL7 version 2.x, with some essential differences. Figure A.32 shows an example of an Hprim Santé administrative (ADM) message that is the equivalent of an HL7 ADT message.

It is quite easy to understand the content and purpose of this message if one knows the definition of HL7 v2.x, even though some essential differences can be detected.

A.6.2 Segments

Similar to HL7 v2.x, the Hprim standard uses segments ; but, due to the limited scope of this standard, only a few segments are used. Table A.32 lists those segments.

The asterisk in the second column indicates that this segment is an extension to the original ASTM E1238 standard and has been defined by the Hprim association.

Table A.33 shows an example of the message header segment (H) as it could appear in Hprim Santé.

See Table A.34 for the definitions of the Properties codes.

A segment is composed of a list of fields, also known as elements. In contrast to HL7 v2.x, the fields do not have an identifier, just a short description. The properties and data type aspects of these fields will be explained later. The length indicates the maximum allowable length for the field.

The Value column in Table A.23 lists either the allowed values for populating the field in the segment or the table that contains the allowed values. The referenced table is defined separately in the Hprim Santé specification. “Table HPRIM 1” listed in the Value column for the “Message Type (context)” field in Table A.37 is an example of one of these tables, and it is explained in the “Vocabulary” subsection below.

```
H|^~\&|||76001^SIH||ADM|||IPAT||P|A2.2|200502071617|

P|7924|000000228064||002280640036|BOUTAUD^MARIE^^^^|DELAHAYES
|19230804|F||100 RUE GEORGES LAFAURIE^^LE HAVRE^^76600^F||02 35
54 02 75||||||||||20050207161535|OP|^^CA25^CA25|

P|7925|000000377092||003770920009|BELLENGER^PAULETTE^^^^|HERO
UARD|19300924|F||FRONT DE MER 37 QUAI DE LA
VIC^^FECAMP^^76400^F||02 35 29 12
22||||||||||20050207161631|OP|^^CA21^CA21|

P|7926|000000199066||001990660009|DALIFARD^IRENE^^^^|BORGES|19
550828|F||621 HAMEAU DE LA BRIERE^^GRAIMBOUVILLE^^76430^F||02
35 13 68 75||||||||||20050207161639|OP|^^CA21^CA21|

P|7927|000000414927||004149270006|COMONT^BERTHE^^^^|COMONT|1
9310517|F||46 RUE DE ZURICH^^LE HAVRE^^76600^F||02 35 24 17
78||||||||||20050207160000|OP|^^MG21^MG21|

P|7928|000000219512||002195120042|BUCCHIOTTY^MARIE
YVETTE^^^^||19130823|F||93 RUE VIVIANI^^LE HAVRE^^76600^F||02 35
51 28 04||||||||||20050207161554|OP|^^MG21^MG21|

P|7929|000000351611||003516110009|ROBILLARD^JENNIFER^^^^||19850
530|F||162 RUE DE LA VALLEE^^LE HAVRE^^76600^F||02 35 24 04
32||||||||||20041221172000|OP|^^GO40^GO40|

P|7930|000000210494||002104940033|SCHAFFNER^RAYMOND^^^^|SCHA
FFNER|19270928|M||27 RUE CLAUDE DEBUSSY^^LE
HAVRE^^76620^F||02 35 46 66
89||||||||||20050207160500|MP|^Dechocage 2^UR23^UR23|

P|7931|000000441956||004419560001|ENZ^LEONE^^^^|BREDEL|1922010
9|F||63 RUE DU GENERAL SARRAIL^^LE HAVRE^^76600^F||02 35 19 90
06||||||||||20041213153942|OP|^^GA11^GA11|

L|1||||
```

Fig. A.32 Example Hprim Santé ADM message

A.6.2.1 Properties

The *Properties* attribute of an Hprim Santé field has dual purposes. One purpose is to indicate whether the element must appear in the message or not (often referred to as Optionality or Usage in other standards). The other purpose is to provide a qualifier for the element indicating whether the element can contain delimiters. More than one property can apply to an element, but these properties can't be in conflict with each other (see Table A.37 Hprim Santé Message Header Segment as an example).

The codes for the properties are defined as shown in Table A.34.

Table A.32 Hprim Santé Segments

Segment	Hprim extension	English description	French description
H		Message header	Identifie le message, l'émetteur et le récepteur
P		Patient	Identifie le patient
OBR		Observation request	Contient les informations relatives à une demande d'analyses ou d'acte de radiologie
OBX		Observation result	Contient les informations relatives aux résultats d'un test ou acte appliqué à un patient
FAC	*	Invoice header	Contient "l'en-tête" de la facture d'une demande d'analyses
ACT	*	Invoice line item	Contient une "ligne" de facture
REG	*	Payment details	Contient les elements de règlement
C		Comment for the previous segment	Commentaire se rapportant au segment precedent
L		End of message	Marque la fin du message
A		Appendix (extension of the previous segment in a message)	Addendum prolongeant le segment precedent
AP	*	Insurance (primary)	Contient les informations relatives à la couverture "primaire" du patient (caisse primaire d'assurance maladie)
AC	*	Insurance (secondary)	Contient les informations relatives aux couvertures complémentaires du patient
ERR	*	Error	Contient un message d'erreurs relatif au contenu des segments et champs reçus

A.6.3 Message Types

The Hprim Santé standard aggregates messages into message type groups that are not very sophisticated. Identification of the discrete purpose of a given message in the group is not possible; for example, as shown in Table A.35, an administrative message, whether it is for an admission or a discharge, is referenced by the message type "ADM".

A.6.4 Message Structure

Looking at the message structure specification in the Hprim Santé standard, it is very hard to identify a correct structure with regard to optionality. Tables A.36 and A.37 provide two examples for appropriate message instances.

Table A.33 Hprim Santé message header segment: H

#	Description	Properties	Length	Data type	Value
1	Segment type	O	1	ST	H
2	Delimiter	O	5	ST	
3	Identification of message (filename)	F	12	ST	
4	Password	F	12	ST	
5	Identification of sender	O	40	SPEC	
6	Address of sender	F	100	AD	
7	Message type (context)	O	7	CM	Table HPRIM 1
8	Phone number of sender	F R	40	TN	
9	Transmission properties	F	40	ST	
10	Identification of receiver	O	40	SPEC	
11	Comment	F	80	ST	
12	Processing mode	F	1	ID	P, T or D
13	Version and type	O	10	SPEC	Table HPRIM 2
14	Date/time of message	O	26	TS	

Table A.34 Hprim Santé segment properties

Code	English description	Original French description
O	Required	obligatoire
F	Facultative (optional)	facultatif
E	To be provided by filler	renseigné par l'exécutant
R	Repeatable field	répétiteur autorisé
C	Recorded (to be returned as is if it has been informed by the transmitter)	consigné (à retourner à l'identique s'il a été renseigné par l'émetteur)
INTERDIT	Prohibited (This code is not listed officially in the table, but it is used)	Interdit

Table A.35 Hprim Santé Table 1 (message type)

Code	English description	Original French description
ORM	Order	transfert de demandes d'analyses = prescription
ORA	Order with administrative data	
ORU	Results	transfert de résultats d'analyses
ADM	Admission	transfert de données d'admission
FAC	Invoice	transfert de données de facturation
REG	Payment	transfert de données de règlement
ERR	Error	transfert de messages d'erreur

Table A.36 Hprim Santé ADM message structure (Example 1)

Level → Optional	1	2	3	4		Logical Structure (HL7 v2.x notation[3])
	H					H
		P1				{
*			AP1			P
*				AC1		[{
*				AC2		AP
		P2				[{ AC }]
*			AP1			}]
*				AC1		}
	L					L

[a]This column represents what is shown in the first five columns and does not have a row-to-row equivalence

Table A.37 Hprim Santé ADM message structure (Example 2)

Level → Optional	1	2	3	4	5	6	7		Logical Structure (HL7 v2.x notation)
	H								H
		P1							{
*			AP1						P
*				AC1					[{
*				AC2					AP
					FAC1				[{AC}]
*						REG1			}]
							ACT1		FAC
							ACT2		[{
		P2							REG
*			AP1						[{ACT}]
*				AC1					}]
					FAC1				
							ACT1		}
	L								L

In Table A.36, the columns with headers "1" to "4", and in Table A.37, the columns with headers "1" to "7" contain named segments and represent the nesting hierarchy of the segments. The indenting of the content on the rows under the different columns is used to indicate how the segments are nested within a message. The numbers appended to the characters of the named segments indicate one or more instances of the given segment in the message.

The Hprim Santé standard has not defined an appropriate abstract message syntax, so it is difficult to create a correct representation of it. The two example message instances above would need to be analyzed further in order to extract a proper abstract message syntax that supports the understanding of the message structure. The resulting structure would be listed as a translation of an Hprim Santé ADM message structure to an HL7 AMS notation, as shown in the "Logical Structure" columns of Tables A.36 and A.37.

A.6.4.1 Comparison to HL7 V2.X

The message definition and representation in Hprim Santé has one advantage and several disadvantages compared to HL7 v2.x.

Advantage:

- Hprim Santé eliminates a structural disadvantage of the HL7 v2.x ER7 encoding by keeping the old ASTM E1238 segment denoting the end of the message (L segment, see Table A.32).

Disadvantages:

- Hprim Santé has used the same segment identifiers as those used by ASTM, including their weakness of not having the same fixed length of 3 characters.
- Since Hprim Santé is an old deprecated standard (developed in 1990) that was defined when the size of the message was important because of memory constraints, the encoding allows for extending a segment. The segment "A" (see Table A.32) has been defined to allow insertion of a line break if the overall length of a single (encoded) line becomes too long. The maximum allowable length of a single line is 220 characters.
- The notation for an overall message structure is difficult to read and can hardly be understood.
- Messages that contain information for more than one patient are allowed. Because messages are normally processed in total, encountering and dealing with errors on application level does cause problems, so this fact is classified as a disadvantage. Splitting the data into separate messages should not cause any problems.

Table A.38 Hprim Santé data types

DT	English description	French description	# of components
AD	Address	Adresse	6
CD	Coded element	Identifiant codé	6
CM	Composite datatype	Identifiants composites	
ID	Identifier	Identificateur	
NM	Numeric	Valeur numérique	
PN	Person name	Nom, prénom et qualité	6
CNA	Person identifier	Identifiant d'individu	3
ST	String	Chaîne de caractère	
TN	Telephone number	Numéro de téléphone	
TS	Timestamp	Date et heure	
TX	Text	Texte long	

Table A.39 Hprim Santé Table "Statut de l'admission" (segment P-25)

Code	English description	French description
OP	Discharge	Sortie
IP	Admission	Entrée
IO	Outpatient admission	Entrée—Sortie (externes ou ambulatoires)
ER	Emergency	Entrée urgence
MP	Movement or update	Mouvement interne ou modification
PA	Preadmission	Pré-admission

A.6.5 Data Types

The Hprim Santé standard defines a limited number of data types for the most common types of data elements (see Table A.38).

A.6.6 Vocabulary

Hprim Santé makes use of vocabulary that is defined inline, i.e., without a specific markup. The allowed values (codes = "valeurs") are listed in the field description of the segment table and explained in the detailed field descriptions. A good example of this approach is the admission status of a patient, as listed in Table A.39.

A.6.7 *Encoding*

In principle, Hprim Santé is using a similar encoding strategy as HL7 version 2, because this strategy is derived from the same parent (base) specification. The encoding is based on flexible delimiters transmitted with the message header.

In contrast to HL7 v2.x, the Hprim Santé encoding rules limit the size of a single line to 220 characters; therefore, a segment must be spread across multiple lines if the content of the segment exceeds the predefined limit. In this case an "A segment" (i.e., a continuation segment) is used to convey that the segment's content continues in this line in the message. This process can be repeated, resulting in multiple consecutive "A segments". The "A segment" is not a special segment, and it can be used everywhere.

A.6.8 *Conformance Methodology*

The conformance methodology for Hprim Santé is not defined explicitly; however, since this standard is similar to HL7 v2.x, the same conformance methodology could be applied (though application of a methodology for Hprim Santé is no longer relevant since it is deprecated).

A.7 PN13 (France)

PN13 is an XML-based communication standard in the pharmaceutical domain and is used for exchanging prescriptions, pharmaceutical consultations, data related to dispensing of medications, and reports about administration of medications. This standard is dedicated to hospital medication workflows [19].

The PN13 standard was defined in France in 1998, as a request from the ministry of health. (PN13 was the name of that request). It has had some influence on the design of CEN "ENV 13607" [20]. Though consistent with 13607, PN13 has not been the basis for 13607. 13607 covers prescriptions in the community pharmacy while PN13 is dedicated to prescribing, dispensing and administration of medicine in hospital only. PN13 is still in use in French hospitals today.

PN13 was the 13th French PreNorm initiated by the Health Ministry. PN13 has been published as a document of the Health ministry "Bulletin Officiel" in July 2002. The Phast-SIPh community is in charge of PN13 implementation, which is an XML implementation. The current release of this implementable standard is called Siph2v3, and is made available only to members of the Phast-SIPh community (editors of EMR and editors of hospital pharmacy software).

Table A.40 PN13 message types

Defined message type (French)	English explanation
Prescription de medicaments	Prescription of drugs
Compte-rendu d'analyse pharmaceutique	Pharmaceutical analysis report or pharmaceutical advice
Dispensation nominative	Nominative dispensation with individual doses
Dispensation reglobalisée	Multi-patient dispensation
Distribution des médicaments	Distribution of drugs for local stock refill
Compte-rendu d'administration des médicaments	Report of drug administration to the patient

A.7.1 Introduction and Overview

This standard has defined certain actors to help in specifying the interactions:

- le prescripteur—prescriber (creates the prescription)
- le pharmacien—pharmacist (validates the prescription, provides a pharmaceutical advice on it, and dispenses the medications)
- le préparateur—pharmaceutical assistant (involved in the dispense process)
- l'administrateur—the care provider who administers the medication to the patient and reports on this activity
- le gestionnaire des approvisionnements—supply manager
- l'automate—robot.

A.7.2 Message Types

PN13 has defined a set of message types, such as the ones listed in Table A.40.

The message types are composed of data elements defined as UML classes and implemented as XML element "complex types".

A.7.3 Data Elements

PN13 has defined the data elements shown in Table A.41 (the ones that are used for prescriptions are marked with an "X" in the rightmost column of the table).

The elements are organized hierarchically within a prescription message (Fig. A.33).

The segments are composed of fields. Table A.42 lists the fields, and their associated attributes, that are used for patient demographic data.

Table A.41 PN13 segments

French element	English explanation	Level	Prescription
Patient	Patient	1	X
Séjour	Visit/encounter	1	X
Prescription	Prescription	1	X
Compte-rendu d'analyse	Pharmaceutical advice	1	
Elément de Livraison	Delivery detail	1	
Bon de Livraison	Delivery report	2	
Compte-rendu d'administration	Administration report	2	
Elément d'administration	Administration details	2	
Renseignement complémentaire	Additional notes (clinical information relevant for the prescription)	2	X
Element de prescription	Prescription item	2	X
Composant adminstré	Item/component administered	3	
Composant prescrit	Prescribed item/component	3	X
Elément de posologie	Dose	3	X
Elément liés	Associate element	3	X

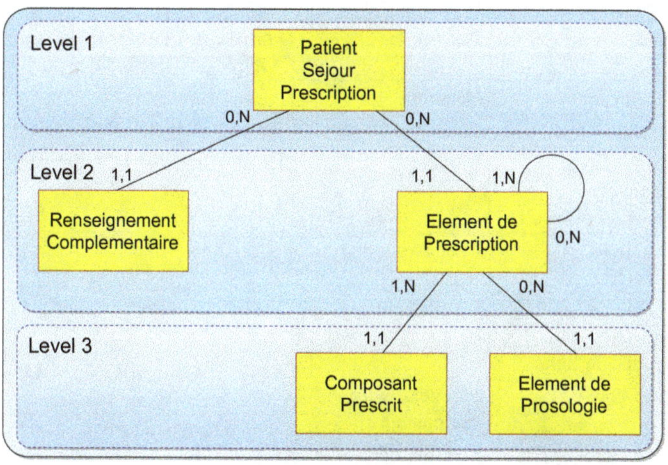

Fig. A.33 PN13 message type for a prescription

A.7.4 Data Type

PN13 uses a very limited set of data types, which are shown in Table A.43.

Table A.42 PN13 segment (patient)

Object: patient		Obligatoire	Unique	
Attribute (French)	(English)	Présence (optionality)	Exigibilité	Type
IPP	ID	O	Exigible	AN
Nom usuel	Usual name	F	Exigible	AN
Nom de naissance	Birth name	F	Exigible	AN
Prénoms	Given name	F	Exigible	AN
Date de naissance	Date of birth	F	Exigible	DH
Sexe	Gender	F	Exigible	Codé

Table A.43 PN13 data types

Type	French description	English explanation	
AN	Alphanumérique	Alphanumeric	
B	Booléen	Boolean	"0" = No, "1" = yes
C	Codé	Coded element	1–16 characters It has four attributes which allow strong semantic conformance checking. Quantities are managed as a unit code (type C) plus a number (type N)
CS	C ou S	C or S	
D	Date	Date	Format: AAAAMMJJ or AAAAMMJJHHMMSS
DH	Date-heure	Date/time	
H	Horaire	Time	Format, HH, HHMM or HHMMSS
N	Nombre avec séparateur décimal optionnel	Number	Decimal number with optionally a decimal point
S	Chaîne de caractères	Character string	
S32	Chaîne de caractères sans retour à la ligne	Character string on a single line	Max 32 characters
T	texte libre	Free text, which can contain multiple lines	

As a consequence of having so few data types, higher level data types for information like addresses or a person's names must be achieved using a set of fields, which in turn is vulnerable to inconsistent definitions. Table A.42 contains an example in which three components are used to represent a person's name.

The current version of PN13 defines the following structured types:

- IDP "Identification de Personne"—Person Identifier
- CMT "Commentaire"—Comment

Table A.44 PN13 presence (optionality and cardinality)

Code	French description	English explanation
E	Exigible	Mandatory
F	Facultatif	Optional
O	Obligatoire	Required
R	Répétitif	Repeating
U	Unique	Single occurrence

A.7.5 Optionality and Cardinality

Certain codes used for presence can be combined for the same element since they provide different concepts, as shown in Table A.44.

PN13 has no explicit concept of repetitions. Repeating elements are simply marked as "repeating" without any further constraints.

A.7.6 Representation

PN13 is encoded using XML as its encoding language. Figure A.34 shows a snippet from an XML schema definition.

A.7.7 Conformance Methodology

PN13 has no explicit conformance methodology. According to the specification, a conformance methodology can be established, although no conformance methodology for PN13 is known to exist.

Conformance to PN13 implies the use of a full set of code systems, which are provided by Phast. The Phast-SIPh implementation guide (460 pages) contains detailed explanations for most current use cases.

A.8 Summary

This chapter presented an overview of additional healthcare data exchange standards. Together with the standards presented in Chap. 4, the reader is given insight into the diverse set of available standards.

```
<xs:complexType name="Messages">
  <xs:choice maxOccurs="unbounded">
    <xs:element ref="M_Prescription_médicaments"/>
    <xs:element ref="M_Compte_rendu_analyse_pharm"/>
    <xs:element ref="M_Dispensation_nominative"/>
    <xs:element ref="M_Dispensation_reglobalisée"/>
    <xs:element ref="M_Distribution_médicaments"/>
    <xs:element ref="M_Compte_rendu_administration"/>
    <xs:element ref="M_Autre"/>
  </xs:choice>
  <xs:attribute name="Phast-libellé" type="xs:string"
                fixed="Messages PN13"/>
  <xs:attribute name="Phast-version" type="xs:string"
                default="SIPhIIv2alpha4.02"/>
  <xs:attribute name="Phast-application" type="xs:string"/>
</xs:complexType>
<xs:element name="Messages" type="Messages"/>
<xs:complexType name="M_Prescription_médicaments">
  <xs:sequence>
    <xs:element ref="Patient"/>
    <xs:element ref="Séjour"/>
    <xs:element ref="Prescription"/>
  </xs:sequence>
  <xs:attribute name="Phast-libellé" type="xs:string"
                fixed="Prescription de médicaments"/>
</xs:complexType>
<xs:element name="M_Prescription_médicaments"
            type="M_Prescription_médicaments"/>
```

Fig. A.34 PN13 XML encoding (XSD snippet)

References

1. Health Level Seven International, www.hl7.org
2. HL7 Version 3 Reference Information Model http://www.hl7.org
3. Hinchley A: Understanding Version 3 - A Primer on the HL7 Version 3. Communication Standard, Alexander Moench Publishing, ISBN: 3-933819-0
4. National Health Service, http://en.wikipedia.org, http://en.wikipedia.org/wiki/National_Health_Service_(England)
5. HL7 Development Framework, http://wiki.hl7.org/index.php?title=HL7_Development_Framework, *last accessed December 28, 2015.*
6. Extensible Markup Language, http://www.w3c.org
7. Unified Modeling Language, ISO/IEC 19501:2005, http://www.uml.org
8. Booch G, Rumbaugh J, Jacobson I. Das UML-Benutzerhandbuch: Aktuell zur Version 2.0. Addison-Wesley, 2006. ISBN 978-3827325709.
9. Booch G, Rumbaugh J, Jacobson I. The Unified Modeling Language User Guide. Addison-Wesley, 2007, ISBN 0321267974.
10. Binary XML, http://www.w3.org/XML/Binary
11. ASN1. Standard. http://www.itu.int/ITU-T/studygroups/com17/languages/
12. Boone K. The CDA Book. Springer, 2011, ISBN 978-0857293350.
13. Clinical Document Architecture, Normative Edition. May 2005, http://www.hl7.org
14. American Society for Testing and Materials. http://www.astm.org
15. An Application Protocol for Electronic Data Interchange in Healthcare Environment, HL7 Inc., Sept.1987, scanned version, http://www.hl7.org/documentcenter/private/standards/v2xIG/HL7v1_specification_19870928.pdf
16. DICOM: Digital Images and Communication in Medicine. Version 3. http://www.rsna.org/Technology/DICOM/index.cfm
17. Mainz R: BDT 3.0 für Einsteiger. Books on Demand. ISBN 978-3-7386-0752-9, http://www.bod.de/buch/reinhold-mainz/bdt-3-0-fuer-einsteiger/9783738607529.html, last accessed July 13th, 2015.
18. Qualitätsring Medizinische Software. http://www.qms.de
19. Boux O: Interopérabilité & circuit du médicament, Le standard PN13 – SIPh2 v3. Manuel de référence, Seconde édition. Copyright © 2014 Phast, 460 pages.
20. DIN V ENV 13607. Health informatics - Messages for the exchange of information on medicine prescriptions. English version ENV 13607:2000.

Appendix B
Trademark Information

All figures and tables marked with "Courtesy of" contain copyrighted material the owner of which is named. All rights are reserved by the indicated owner and the material is used with explicit permission.

HL7®, HL7 CDA® and FHIR® and are registered trademarks of Health Level Seven International, Inc. and are used with permission. HL7® Version 2.x, HL7 Version 3.0, HL7® CTS2 is copyrighted material owned by HL7® International and are used with permission. Use of these trademarks and material does not represent endorsement of HL7® International of this text.

DICOM® is the registered trademark of the National Electrical Manufacturers Association for its standards publications relating to digital communication of medical information. © Copyright 2015 by the National Electrical Manufacturers Association. All rights including translation into other languages, reserved under the Universal Copyright Convention, the Berne Convention for the Protection of Literacy and Artistic Works, and the International and Pan American Copyright Conventions.

IHE International grants to each Member Organization, and to any other user of these 1315 documents, an irrevocable, worldwide, perpetual, royalty-free, non-transferable, nonexclusive, non-sublicensable license under its Copyrights in any IHE Profiles and Technical Framework documents, as well as any additional copyrighted materials that will be owned by IHE International and will be made available for use by Member Organizations, to reproduce and distribute (in any and all print, electronic or other means of reproduction, storage or 1320 transmission) such IHE Technical Documents (http://ihe.net/uploadedFiles/Content/About_IHE/Governance/IHE-International-Principles-of-Governance.pdf).

Reproduced by permission of DIN Deutsches Institut für Normung e.V. The definitive version for the implementation of this standard is the edition bearing the most recent date of issue, obtainable from Beuth Verlag GmbH, Burggrafenstraße 6, 10787 Berlin, Germany.

Copyright © OASIS® 1993–2016. All Rights Reserved. OASIS trademark, IPR and other policies apply. Reproduced with permission.

F. Oemig and R. Snelick, *Healthcare Interoperability Standards Compliance Handbook*, DOI 10.1007/978-3-319-44839-8

IETF Trust hereby grants to each person who wishes to exercise such rights, to the greatest extent that it is permitted to do so, a non-exclusive, royalty-free, worldwide right and license under all copyrights and rights of authors to copy, publish, display and distribute unmodified portions of IETF Contributions and IETF Documents and translations thereof, provided that:

- each such portion is clearly attributed to IETF and identifies the RFC or other IETF Document or IETF Contribution from which it is taken,
- all IETF legends, legal notices and indications of authorship contained in the original IETF RFC must also be included where any substantial portion of the text of an IETF RFC, and in any event where more than one-fifth of such text, is reproduced in a single document or series of related documents. (http://trustee.ietf.org/license-info/IETF-TLP-5.htm, Section 3.c.iii)

From United Nations Directories for Electronic Data Interchange for Administration, Commerce and Transport, by TBG10 Healthcare, © (copyright 2010) United Nations. Reprinted with the permission of the United Nations.

Hprim Santé recommendation is the intellectual property of association Interop'Santé made available to its members PN13. SiPh2 version 3 is protected by copyright Phast, and made available to the members of the SIPh community.

The xDT family is a family of standards for system neutral data exchange among applications in German physician offices. More information is available on the website of QMS—Qualitätsring Medizinische Software, http://www.qms-standards.de/.

Use of these trademarks and referenced materials does not represent endorsement by these organizations for the text provided with this book.

The information in this book was compiled with great care. However, mistakes cannot be completely ruled out. Authors assume no legal responsibility or liability of possible errors, incorrect data or the resulting consequences thereof.

All product names are used without guarantee of their unrestricted applicability and are possibly registered trademarks.

Certain commercial products or materials are identified in this book in order to explain a concept or to provide realistic examples adequately. Such identification is not intended to imply recommendation or endorsement by the National Institute of Standards and Technology, nor is it intended to imply that the products or materials identified are necessarily the best available for the purpose.

Index

F. Oemig and R. Snelick, *Healthcare Interoperability Standards Compliance Handbook*, DOI 10.1007/978-3-319-44839-8

Printed in the USA
CPSIA information can be obtained
at www.ICGtesting.com
CBHW081344070624
9724CB00003B/191

9 783319 448374